BRONSON WOMEN

AND THE

SCHOOL OF NURSING

BRONSON WOMEN AND THE SCHOOL OF NURSING

Journeys Through One Hundred Years

by

Jacqueline L. Wylie, RN, MSN, MA

and

Anna M. Stryd, RN, MA

Alumni Association of
Bronson Methodist Hospital School of Nursing
2005

ISBN 0-9763413-0-1

Wylie, Jacqueline L., 1940–
Bronson Women and the School of Nursing: Journeys through one hundred years, by Jacqueline L. Wylie and Anna M. Stryd. Edited by Hazel Starcher. Kalamazoo, Mich.: Alumni Association of Bronson Methodist Hospital School of Nursing, 2005.
xviii, 774 p. Includes photographs, appendices and index.
1. Bronson Methodist Hospital School of Nursing. 2. Kalamazoo County—Nursing schools—Bronson Methodist Hospital School of Nursing 3. Nursing schools—History I. Title II. Stryd, Anna M., 1941–

RT80.M52 .W983 362.W983

Printed by Fidlar Doubleday, Inc.
Kalamazoo, Michigan

Dedicated to

All Bronson School of Nursing Graduates

and Other Nurses who practiced

at Bronson Methodist Hospital,

committing their lives to the care of others and to the advancement of the nursing profession.

TABLE OF CONTENTS

PREFACE

I never intended to write a 100-year story about Bronson Methodist Hospital and the loyal nurse graduates who chose to practice nursing there. I kept thinking, there must be a writer out there who wants to write this story! So I kept looking while listening, collecting stories and continuing the search for an author. Eventually, it was I who sat at the word processor overwhelmed by the formidable task because no one whom I had asked volunteered to write the story after all.

Bronson stories that I heard told over 45 years often came to my mind, especially during the 1980s when I felt the school was destined for closure. I thought about all of the untold stories that will never be revealed: stories imprinted in graduate memories, ours to keep, some to share, and others never to be heard; stories left in files, buried in old news clippings, left in the hearts and minds of deceased alumni and others who worked at Bronson, never to be opened, never to be told—a loss of a rich, 20th-century nursing story.

Recording Bronson stories occurred to me in the 1980s, after I became the director of the school. Hospital-based programs were closing their doors at a rapid rate, and springing up in their place were numerous community college and a few university programs. Nursing education was quickly moving into higher education and out of the work-study, apprentice model that had provided inexpensive labor for charity-based hospitals and had offered young women a career choice at the turn of the century. I wanted Bronson to transform into a university baccalaureate program, but not without acknowledging the local 100-year legacy of nurses who cared for patients and community and, at the same time, cared for the profession they loved. I felt nurses needed to move into academia and build new relationships, in addition to the clinical practice roles.

Mary Lou Stewart whetted my appetite for documenting Bronson history. She was hired to archive Bronson documents for their preservation. I listened to her stories, one in particular—the taped interview with Amy Bailey Seward, 1914 Bronson graduate. Geneva Williams was the second archivist hired at Bronson who supported this work.

I watched the chronology grow from 1900 and learned names of nurses who were the first hospital superintendents, directors of nursing, nurse educators and graduates. Linda K. Strodtman, PhD, RN, was a Michigan nurse historian who became known to me through organizational networking, and I communicated with her about how to proceed with the project. She offered suggestions and a reference on oral history. After reading excerpts, she believed that I could at least start by collecting stories. In 1989, Marge Kars, the Bronson librarian, accompanied me to interview Cornelia Veenhuis Cody, 1921 graduate, at her family home on Vine Street, whose story was rich with details of the past, and I was fascinated to learn about her early nursing experiences. The interview was typed verbatim by the School of Nursing Administrative Assistant, Mary Beth Sanders, and stored for inclusion in the soon to-be-written Bronson story. The process of interviewing, taping and verbatim recording was tedious and too time consuming for a young director and the school staff. I wanted to establish an alumni ad hoc committee, making the Bronson book project into a three- to five-year group task with a lead writer arising in the process. The project did not come together, and five years passed too quickly.

During the summers of 1996 and 1997, I had the help of Wanda Boekhout, Kelley Hempsall and Joyce Branch in scouring the Bronson archives. We found more stories about Bronson nurses and the hospital in *Kalamazoo Gazette* articles which had been clipped, dated and saved; Bronson in-house publications, including all School of Nursing records and Board of Trustee minutes; and Bronson pictures. The Sisters of St. Joseph Archives at Nazareth, and the State of Michigan Archives in Lansing, and other saved documents from various sources were also searched. Boxes of information were piling up at my home, and still there was no one to write the story.

How else could stories be found and recorded? The next tactic was the 1997 request for stories from Bronson graduates published in the monthly alumni newsletter, *The Bulletin,* sent to all active members. I asked alumni to write or tape their stories for inclusion in a Bronson history. Soon I would find someone to put the whole story together. Questions came to mind along with who would write it: How could it be funded? Would the book have an audience? When would I know that enough material had been collected?

Stories flowed in weekly, during 1997 and 1998, that were emotionally moving about significant events that had transformed naïve, immature girls into caring, professional nurses. It was a privilege to read them and to be given approval to include them in the soon-to-be written story. Some of the quotations used herein have been edited to assure clarity and consistency throughout this publication. These changes have in no way altered the intent of the writer or speaker.

Nurse colleagues and friends, Barb Groh and Judy Hoelscher, encouraged me to begin writing. Just do it. Barb sent me a Chinese proverb, "The palest ink is better than the best memory," which tapped some internal courage and provided support along with ideas for framing the story. I began writing, still always looking for a motivated author. Beth Johnson, a free-lance editor who had worked at Bronson helped at first by reviewing some of the beginning work in 1997. Annie Stearns, a young Bronson graduate with a graduate degree in writing, listened and offered suggestions. Kelley Hempsall helped bring historical context to the decades and introduced me to the Sisters of St. Joseph who had recorded the Borgess nursing and hospital history.

Two years after early retirement from Bronson, I committed myself to begin writing the story in 1997. I rashly projected a 1998 completion date, a novice writer without a clue. The Alumni Association agreed to publish the book. The hospital gave $15,000, one of the few times that the alumni received a gift, given their role of giving, not getting. Robert Doud suggested I put together a captioned picture-book souvenir for the commemorative event being planned to coincide with the May 1998 last school graduation. Too much time had been invested to hear his sound advice for a novice writer. The stories had to be honored and preserved.

Linda Ickes, past School of Nursing office manager, helped transfer manuscript from my home computer when it was updated so that none of the work, however rough, would be lost. Diane Wittig Peters, a friend, helped enter numerous written stories submitted earlier by alumni.

The new millennium came. Progress was slow. Friend and retired Western Michigan University colleague, Hazel Starcher edited drafts to facilitate progress. Diane Worden expressed interest in indexing the final product, sight unseen, and concluded that the book would not be completed until perhaps the next millennium without steady editorial support. By encouraging monthly progress, she might actually get the opportunity to create the index one day! She became our faithful, friendly editor. Anna Stryd then offered to select pictures to reinforce the story. It was an incredible task that included sorting pictures from alumni and the hospital's files, with help from its photographer, Larry Wolf, and reviewing of news clippings and pictures sent by alumni as well as those in WMU's Archives (where Bronson material was sent when the school disbanded) and in the Kalamazoo Valley Museum. Next Anna put together all of the appendices and helped with revisions after initial editing.

In an ongoing process of weekly support, Anna Stryd became coauthor. Her major contributions to the book made it a stronger, more accurate story. Her persistent drive to complete the project kept me on target. Diane and Anna decided to restrict my open-ended attempt to continue the story *ad infinitum* despite accumulated alumni stories that were gathered during 1999–2004. I couldn't seem to find a cut-off point. Over and over I hear them say, "Stop, Jackie, stop. One hundred years is enough!"

Storytelling is now up to you, the graduates with a long tradition of compassionate service and cutting-edge nursing education. Complete your untold story. Enrich the world of caring with nursing stories. As long as Bronson graduates practice and retire, more stories will be remembered, told and hopefully recorded. Maybe a more refined, second Bronson story will document the next 100 years. I'm looking for that writer now. You who have given your love, stories, suggestions, and encouragement know about the need to continue the story. You are in my heart, and I thank you for your contributions with every cell in my body.

Acknowledgments

Besides all the people already mentioned, crucial contributors included friends and colleagues:

- Rosemarie Nedeau-Cayo responded graciously to every request for specific School of Nursing data. Dick and Betty Vander Molen '51, answered many, many questions and provided memories in written stories. Hazel Latondress cordially told me about challenging years at Bronson.
- Sr. Kathleen Walsh invited me into the Sisters of St. Joseph's historical archives to kindly tell the story of Borgess Hospital's beginning in 1889 and how Bronson came into being 11 years later.
- Julie VanderNoot, Volunteer Services, offered information about the women and men who supported Bronson care—how the women's auxiliary services morphed into the present-day model of hospital volunteerism.

- Jo Ulrich '73, described the new hospital's design, and Nancee Hofmeister '82, elaborated on Bronson's move to attain magnet hospital status and its resources in the magnet hospital movement. Mary Ann Eldred, Senior Vice President of Patient Care Services (1998-2003), during phone interviews and e-mail, added nursing's input about new hospital design. Jackie Wahl described her work in the new hospital design and on researching the environmental impact on nurses' workdays after the move.
- Chief Nurse Executives Roberta Utrecht and Katie Harrelson, during the last 15 years, provided information in interviews, recent e-mails and phone communications on transitional times in nursing, hospital-nursing management, current Bronson nursing philosophy, and goals and desired outcomes.
- Susan Ulshafer, Senior Vice President of Human Resources, told about her role in managing the school closure and magnet hospital designation.
- Frank Sardone, Chief Executive Officer, shared his commitment to the development of a strong, professional practice nursing team as part of the overall hospital organizational structure, supported by Susan Ulshafer, Vice President, Human Resources.
- Robert Doud, Vice President, Public Relations, and Marge Kars helped share the Bronson story in the community. Susan Watts, Director of Corporate Communications, is appreciated for her assistance in marketing this book.
- Kurt Haenicke, College of Health and Human Services, listened and answered questions.
- Bronson graduates who directly contributed to the story are noted by asterisks in Appendix D, List of Graduates.

Permissions granted for copying, quotes or pictures came from Bronson Methodist Hospital; The Fetzer Institute, Kalamazoo, Michigan, in the person of Amy Ferguson; *Kalamazoo Gazette*; The Florence Nightingale Museum, London, England, and the contemporary Florence Nightingale scholars, Deva-Marie Beck, Barbara Dossey, and Louise Selanders; Western Michigan University Archives, especially Susan Husband, Curator of the Regional History Collection, and Carrie Cummings, Supervisor, Records and Registration at Western Michigan University; The Kalamazoo Public Library; the Kalamazoo Valley Museum; and the University of Pennsylvania Press.

Not only does it take a village to raise a child, fellow Bronson graduates learned that it takes the effort of a hospital community to write a 100–year story about the School of Nursing and its beloved Bronson Methodist Hospital.

Jackie Wylie '62
July 2004

During the 1980s when Jackie began talking about finding someone to document the history of our alma mater, I thought it would be an interesting, but time-consuming project. I knew Jackie had the incentive and knowledge to write the story, but that she needed encouragement and support for this huge undertaking.

I was a resident of Truesdale Hall for three years and an active participant in student government, which helped to create my interest in the School of Nursing, and helped mold me into the person I am today. With this background and loyalty to Bronson Methodist Hospital, I felt this would be a project of interest to me personally, as well as others from the school and in local communities. During the initial story-gathering period I was involved with a business venture and without time to assist.

In the summer of 2003, I offered help to find pictures. Little did I know what I was getting into! Pictures led to gathering other graphic materials needed for the appendices, which led to more and more. People graciously shared their time and resources. Larry Wolf, Bronson Methodist Hospital photographer, helped us to search the photo archives for prints and was helpful finding additional pictures when requested; Darrah Barnes and Rebecca Pierce quickly responded to my request for permission to reprint pictures from the *Kalamazoo Gazette;* Thomas Dietz and Paula Metzner accommodated my request to look through boxes and more boxes, for information to strengthen the story. Alumnae provided pictures, and the alumni files held other documents used in this book.

I have learned so much while working on the book, from the initial stages to its completion. Jackie and Diane Worden are great teachers and it was a pleasure working with them. At times we were disappointed because we were unable to include more stories as they came to light. Diane's tenacity kept Jackie and me aware of the need to produce a printed volume that was light enough to be lifted, and we thank her once again. It is my hope that this story will honor all Bronson nurses—a monument to their caring and healing service!

Anna Stryd '61
February 2005

Section I.

APPRENTICES

CHAPTER 1

CAREGIVERS AND HOSPITALS IN KALAMAZOO, 1889–1920

A quote of H.B. Osborne, MD, supported the Bronson Methodist Hospital School of Nursing story. He wrote that the hospital would not have happened ". . . were it not for the women who have fostered the work so nobly. It only proves what a man is he owes to woman."[1] Hospital beginnings were recorded in stories told in the Bronson Hospital and Sisters of Saint Joseph archives and the *Kalamazoo Gazette*. Bronson and Borgess Medical Center have different beginning stories and influences. Together they progressed into a dominant technological, allopathic medical model.[2] Feminine influences were less obvious in public versions of the story.

General hospitals opened in response to a growing group of residents moving to the city to work in the paper mills—away from family care (mother, aunt, daughter) and, when available, one attending family physician who often practiced medicine in an office attached to his/her home and in the homes of patients. Three general hospitals opened at the turn of the 19th century: Borgess Hospital, the first, in 1889; second, Queen City Private Hospital in 1896 with closure in 1900; and the Kalamazoo Hospital (later to be renamed Bronson Hospital) in 1900. The Kalamazoo Asylum, specifically designed to treat the indigent and mentally ill, preceded the three. It opened in 1859, and successively became the Kalamazoo State Hospital, the

Kalamazoo Regional Psychiatric Hospital and the Kalamazoo Psychiatric Hospital. All had nursing schools, except Queen City.

BORGESS HOSPITAL

Borgess Hospital opened in 1889,[3] and was well established with plans to enlarge by 1900 when the Kalamazoo Hospital came into being.

Originally, the first hospital was ". . . a Christmas gift from the Bishop Borgess of Detroit to Father O'Brien, who devoted it to the good of suffering humanity, in establishing a model general hospital on a small scale, filling a want, the lack of which would be a shame to a city of importance of Kalamazoo."[4] This gift converted the home of Reverend Moses Hill into a 20-bed hospital, located on the corner of Portage and Lovell Streets, where the first expansion in 1901 added 30 beds. By 1910 Borgess had a total capacity of 100 beds.

The new hospital was staffed by 11 well-educated women who came from Watertown, New York, at the request of Father O'Brien. They were nuns from the order of the Sisters of Saint Joseph. Sister Mary Raphael, the biological sister of Father O'Brien, was a homeopathic physician educated at the University of Michigan, and so the hospital took on the appearance of a homeopathic practice.[5]

There is evidence in early *Kalamazoo Gazette* articles that the local physicians found fault with the Borgess system overall—the environment was too homey—not medically aseptic. The rooms had carpets and draperies. The nuns wore flowing robes, possible contaminants in an age that had embraced the germ theory and surgical asepsis. A description of the environment included ". . . private rooms with home comforts where patients can be treated as privately as in their own home. Special baths, massage, wine, extraordinary diet and constant attendance of a nurse."[6] a healing house—forward thinking in many ways—creating a healing environment, and in conflict with aseptic practices according to the allopathic physicians.

The nuns and Florence Nightingale seemed to hold healing principles in common. Nightingale's *Notes on Nursing* agree with many homeopathic principles and practices, including medical asepsis within a healing environment:

> In watching disease, both in private houses and in public hospitals, the thing which strikes the experienced observer most forcibly is this, that the symptoms or the sufferings generally considered to be inevitable and incident to the disease are very often not symptoms of the disease at all, but of something quite different—of the want of fresh air, or of light, or of warmth, or of quiet, or of cleanliness, or of punctuality and care in the administration of diet, of each or of all of these.
>
> [Nursing] has been limited to signify little more than the administration of medicines and the applications of poultices. It ought to signify the proper use of fresh air, light, warmth, cleanliness, quiet, and the proper selection and administration of diet—all the least expense of vital power to the patient.[7]

Many of the people who used Borgess Hospital's services were poor and could not pay for their hospital or medical care. The Sisters did not receive money from their diocese or church.[8] They were a self-supporting order, expected to collect fees and donations to cover their living expenses as well as the costs for operating a hospital. Borgess was surviving, rather than thriving, according to its own accounts and the 1892 newspaper story in which the city pondered the question, should the city own the hospital? The city of Kalamazoo did provide limited financial support to the new hospital.[9]

Father O'Brien, as spokesperson for the Sisters of St. Joseph,[10] and understanding their financial difficulty, offered the hospital for sale to Kalamazoo. But the city sang the nuns' praises, not wanting to be involved in the hospital business. The city provided less than adequate funding to assist with charity care. There seemed to be no way to offset citizen inability to pay for the care.

Since Borgess Hospital had never been self-sustaining, the city and the taxpayers had no reason to complain. They should have been thankful for the economical methods of caring for those who have been unfortunate and have been inmates of the institution at the expense of the city, explained the *Gazette*. The city did not exceed $8300 a year for the care of people at the institution. As long as the rates and arrangements continued, the city was better off having the hospital owned by its owners than own and operate it.[11]

The only way to sustain a hospital venture was to accept donations, provide charity care, and limit labor costs. In other words, the nuns basically worked for their board and room. The money from the city, private donations, and the nuns' solicitation of funds, as well as austere management, was used to build several social services in Kalamazoo and the surrounding area. The Sisters of St. Joseph were the first charity hospital administrators, nurses, social workers, caregivers for the "feeble minded" and parochial school teachers in Kalamazoo County.[12]

THE FIRST SCHOOL OF NURSING IN KALAMAZOO

The St. Camillus School of Nursing originated in 1895 with Sister Mary Raphael O'Brien, MD, conducting lectures and clinical instruction in the ways of homeopathic medicine. Nuns were the first students. The need for nurses grew quickly in the booming paper-producing town. Seven years later, because of a shortage of nuns, the Sisters invited applications from women of all denominations to create an adequate student nurse supply of bedside caregivers. Nursing students were needed to continue operations within their budget and meet the supply demand.

SISTERS OF ST. JOSEPH SOON TO FORM NON-SECTARIAN TRAINING CLASS FOR NURSES

> The new Borgess hospital building was opened Monday (March 11, 1902) and some of the new patients were placed in this portion of the building. In the evening the building presented a beautiful

> sight for the lighting arrangements are very effective. The night-lights in the hall are a dark red and very soft in color tone and quite appropriate when a mild light is needed.
>
> It is the intention of the Sisters of St. Joseph to form a training class for nurses in the near future and while none of the plans have been formulated as yet, it is certain that members of any creed will be allowed to join and study.[13]

The nuns continually gave a verbal message of their nonsectarian practices. They stated that "the business of the sisters is to care for the sick and not to meddle with religious opinions of patients. They have no fight with any one. No religious discussion will be tolerated on the premises."[14]

The school that was established followed the modus operandi of the times: an apprenticeship model. Under this plan, hospitals provided training, and room and board to would-be nurses, with services 24 hours per day, seven days per week.

ONE "TRUE" WAY TO TREAT ILLNESS AND DISEASE—ALLOPATHIC MEDICINE

Major concerns of the allopathic physicians involved the practice of homeopathic medicine at Borgess Hospital and the right of their physician colleague, Sister Mary Raphael, to admit and care for patients who did not already have an attending physician. Her acceptance of patients would be expected of a charitable religious order,[15] but doctors perceived that she was taking potential business away from them.

By 1896, the nuns felt that they were forced to ask for the dismissal of the Borgess Medical Staff, which included the physicians who later organized the Kalamazoo Hospital. Dr. Oliver LaCrone, for one, looked on homeopathy as being medically and scientifically irrational. His retirement speech from the Kalamazoo Academy of Medicine was a scathing criticism of healthcare practices at Borgess

Hospital. His speech left no recourse except to request the dismissal of Dr. LaCrone and his allopathic-practicing colleagues from Borgess.[16]

The nuns' reply was recorded in the local newspaper.[17] They asked for the resignations of all staff physicians (apparently a closed, exclusive group), and immediately invited all of them back in an inclusive hospital staff model that "will hereafter be open to all honorable physicians of either school." The reference to either school refers to physicians practicing in either an allopathic or homeopathic model.[18]

Three days later the *Kalamazoo Gazette* carried an editorial, "The Staff Replies."[19] Father O'Brien was the spokesperson for the nuns, and the physicians blamed him for the problem. The divergence now appeared to be both medical and denominational.

> That Father O'Brien should use his influence to destroy the original staff of Borgess Hospital and in its place so shuffle the cards of circumstances as to confer position and power upon his own sister might be excusable, but to accuse the staff as a body of actions which have had a detrimental influence upon his church and his hospital, is a statement which is untrue and anything coming as untrue from an ecclesiastical dignitary may rightfully be branded as infamous.
>
> In referring to that institution as his hospital, we simply mean that as far as the staff knows, Father O'Brien is the power behind the throne.[20]

Dr. H.B. Osborne chose not to return. Some of his colleagues followed his example.

Queen City Private Hospital Exists for a Short Time

Dr. Orton H. Clark opened the private hospital in a house at 203 South Street, in 1896,[21] perhaps as the first dissenter from Borgess. He closed it four years later on September 7, 1900, unable to simultaneously manage both the hospital and his private practice. No documentation was found regarding nursing care or the management practices at this hospital. The 1900 closure of the Queens City Hospital forced the physicians who were unhappy with the Borgess Hospital philosophy to initiate their new hospital venture.[22] Medical care of the 20th century was beginning to turn into a business.

In 1897, Dr. Osborne's nephew, Rush McNair, MD, rented a small house at 419 John Street (later 138 E. Lovell) with the intention of creating another hospital. He then convinced his patient, Henry Brees, to donate the land adjacent to the house to build a modern hospital.

Bronson Hospital's Forerunner Incorporated as Kalamazoo Hospital Association

On December 4, 1900, Bronson Hospital's predecessor was created as the Kalamazoo Hospital Association. Newspaper headlines touted the event: "New Hospital Assured, Will Open its Doors to Public in About a Month, Capital of $30,000, Institution Will Be Located on the Corner of John and Cedar Streets."[23]

Local physicians acquired more land, bordering on Lovell and John Street, next to the land donated by Mr. Brees. The *Gazette* further reported that the Kalamazoo Hospital Association had been formed by Doctors Cornelius Van Zwaluwenberg, O.A. LaCrone, E. H. Van Deusen,[24] H.B. Osborne, Rush McNair, and J.W. Bosman. The capital investment was $30,000.[25]

> Many of the physicians and citizens have long fostered the idea of a nonsectarian hospital and the plan is now practically materialized. It will be remembered that the late Henry Brees left in trust a lot at the corner of John and Cedar Streets for hospital purposes. This has been enlarged by purchase of adjacent land. . . .
>
> A hospital association has been formed and incorporation papers have been forwarded to Lansing. . . .

> The dwelling house at 419 John Street is now being fitted up for hospital purposes which will provide limited quarters for the winter until the new building can be erected. . . .
>
> The management of the hospital will unite with all charitable individuals and organizations in providing relief in the way of hospital treatment to those worthy of such benevolence.[26, 27]

The "house at 419 John Street (on the property now owned by the six physicians) was fitted for hospital purposes which will provide limited quarters for the winter until the new building can be erected."[28] The opening of the new hospital in the old Fish home would not be celebrated to save the fanfare for the dedication of the "real" hospital, once built:

NEW HOSPITAL TO OPEN SOON

> We have perfected the organization and have supplied the temporary institution with all the modern improvements which the hospital department can command. The hospital will open in a few days, but there will be no formal opening. The organization has already gotten all kinds of gifts and offers from friends who have proffered their assistance. We have received several applications from patients out of town, who ask for admission as soon as the hospital is opened. The hospital will be known as the Kalamazoo Hospital and has its temporary quarters at 419 John Street (the old Fish home). The local fraternity, the majority of whom will comprise the visiting and house staff, have engaged the present quarters as a nucleus of what, they say, will be one of the best modernly equipped hospitals in the country, to be erected during the present year [said Dr. Rush McNair].
>
> Miss Jessie Yancey, a graduate nurse of considerable experience in Chicago hospitals, who comes highly recommended by the faculty of the Northwestern Medical School, has been engaged as the head nurse of the new institution.[29]

COULD KALAMAZOO AFFORD OR DID IT NEED ONE MORE HOSPITAL?

The ability of the city to support two hospitals did not seem to be a question at the time the Kalamazoo Hospital was being developed. However, according to city officials as reported by the *Gazette*, it was not particularly needed. Borgess Hospital was rated as highly satisfactory in care provided by the Sisters of St. Joseph.[30] The public was satisfied, and the Borgess community responded to growing demands.

A "Nonsectarian" Hospital Takes Shape

"The hospitals of the city have been crowded the last few years and the general growth of the city and the prevalence of the hospital idea renders another hospital a necessity."[31]

The "hospital idea" had arrived in Kalamazoo, requiring plans for new buildings and staff. Affordable staff began with the nuns and later, poor and uneducated women from the community. Schools of nursing became the foundation and financial base for available, inexpensive, female labor: nursing students. Another door opened to women seeking independence.

When the hospital opened in the Fish home, nursing assistants were needed. They came in the form of nursing students. A hospital could not operate twenty-four hours a day without people who had a reason to "train" long hours for little pay. Reward would come in commitment to duty—that is, to care for others until they were again able to care for themselves. This approach was a legitimate extension of women's work from the home into the community when most all work for women (nurses, teachers, librarians, housekeepers, sales clerks, *etc.*) received low pay.[32]

Meanwhile, the new Kalamazoo Hospital took longer to plan and build than originally planned. Fundraising was not an easy task. Some community members did not think that a new nonsectarian hospital, owned by physicians, would be in the best interests of its patients. Could physicians own the hospital and not have a conflict of interest? This same concern is heard today about physician-owned stock in illness care technology and medical services.

To overcome this barrier, the Kalamazoo Hospital Association reorganized on March 28, 1902, under a new board of directors on which only retired physicians could serve. Dr. E.H. Van Deusen and Dr. W.E. Upjohn met the new criterion and could be depended upon to support an allopathic model of practice. In addition, ladies auxiliary groups formed to rally the community behind the nonsectarian hospital cause. The physicians' wives set out to complete the task started by their husbands.

Charity care was certainly a major part of hospital care, as well as the beginning of illness care as a business entity, especially with the support of a thriving pharmaceutical company in Kalamazoo whose leaders provided their fair share of charity (donations to the hospital), but which also benefited their business with the sale of drugs. No doubt, the Upjohn family of physicians played a major role in setting the stage for medical care in this region. The pharmaceutical business was beginning to boom, and the Upjohn Company was part of it. Pharmaceutical production fit into the allopathic framework, focusing on cure and management of disease with extensive use of drugs.

The Role of Women

At the turn of the century, Kalamazoo nuns represented expert nurses, nonsectarian women were willing to train as nurses, and a group of affluent women were ready to take on a cause.

How did affluent women support the "hospital idea?" The Women's Auxiliary of the Kalamazoo Hospital Association included members who were physicians' wives and who envisioned a plan engaging the community to fund a new hospital building, its maintenance, and its charity care. The women's group, led by Mrs. O.A. LaCrone, president,[33] initiated the task. Kalamazoo women made a promise to the community to build and equip a modern hospital with free beds for adults and children and with a full-fledged school of nursing.

Physicians' offices were often attached to their homes. No doubt the women in the family played the role of physician assistant. They understood the illness business well. Not only were they the original physician assistants, they were 24-hour caregivers, seven days a week when family fell ill. As late as the 1930s, many operations and assistance at births were performed in the patient's home with the help of nurses and family members.

Thus, physicians' wives took on the role of hospital fundraisers while their husbands had a place to practice and people without a family physician had a place to go for medical care. This change in the development of health care would cost Americans more than imagined. The focus would be on illness and disease, with little attention to and consciousness of women's family role in maintaining wellness and preventing disease.

Another hospital gave physicians more space to practice and prosper outside of their office and home domain. How charitable was the movement? What were the intentions of prominent community members? Benevolence as well as a desire to practice medicine without the perceived control of a religious group of women were likely two major factors. The developing Upjohn Company with numerous physician family members was also influential in the development of the nonsectarian hospital. The lack of reference to women physicians in documents reviewed while writing this book is notable.[34]

By 1903, the Kalamazoo Hospital was staffed by a head nurse, four assistant nurses, a cook and an orderly. The title "nurse" was not protected by license. Most likely, Miss Yancey gave the four assistants on-the-job training. Eventually they were recognized for their work-study with certificates of completion, although the school was not officially registered by the Michigan Board of Nursing until 1904. The graduates were Minnie Johnston, Rena Koster, Mary Legge, and Elizabeth (Bessie)

Pyle.[35] They were considered to be the first graduates of what would later become the Bronson School of Nursing.[36]

The *Gazette* also supported the "hospital idea" with requests for donations tied to the recovery of patients. Nine patients were mentioned in the May 22, 1903, *Kalamazoo Gazette* article as well as in a report on donations, three of whom were a: "15-year-old boy . . . who is ill with appendicitis and was taken to the hospital a week ago," a man who, "underwent an operation last week for empyema . . ." [and] a woman, "who had been in the hospital since April 21 and will soon be sufficiently recovered from her illness to return to her home in Otsego." The article continues:

> The institution is often remembered with very acceptable donations, such as old linen for bandages and like articles. Fruits and flowers, gifts very acceptable to the patients, are also generously donated from time to time and bring cheer and patience to those who are suffering with pain. Such gifts show that the outside world is not wholly without sympathy and that those who are ill are not forgotten.[37]

For the next five years (1902-1907) the women continued to play a major role in creating positive public sentiment and gaining financial support for the institution. By number, they held majority power on the hospital board of directors of ten women and five men. How did this happen? One of the early fundraising ploys was to sell stock in the new hospital. No earnings would be gained, but the stockholders would have voting rights in the management of the new hospital. The Women's Auxiliary, in providing financial support, had a substantial amount of this stock and gained majority board privileges for a brief five-year period in the one-hundred-year history of the hospital. Dr. E.H. Van Deusen became board president the first year, with Dr. W.E. Upjohn taking the helm in 1903 when Dr. Van Deusen became ill and resigned.

In late 1903, hiring an architect prompted the women to step up their fundraising efforts. A loan of $10,000 was secured to build the hospital, which included an elevator!

In the meantime (1902), Borgess Hospital opened its new building at Portage and Lovell streets. It was four stories, had an elevator, and was just around the corner from the Kalamazoo Hospital, still located in the little Fish family home on John Street. This modern Borgess expansion did not deter the Women's Auxiliary. Fundraising efforts continued, led by the Kalamazoo Hospital Association Board of Directors and its Women's Auxiliary. According to Mary Lou Stewart,[38] every fundraising idea one could envision was used. The women sold personal belongings and conducted a variety of yearly benefit programs around social and entertainment themes[39] such as benefit dances and minstrel shows.

Two popular fundraising events were auto days and trolley days, organized by the women and supported by the *Kalamazoo Gazette*, as evidenced by numerous articles encouraging participation. Cars were a novelty. For a donation, most people were thrilled for the opportunity to secure a ride to local events. On trolley days, the women ran the trolleys for the city and collected the money for the building fund. Community picnics were planned that featured baseball games between lawyers and physicians. On one spectacular day, the women raised $825! However hard the women worked to secure hospital dollars, they were unable to raise the $18,000 pledged.

Nevertheless, the cornerstone was laid on May 22, 1904, in the building at Lovell and John. A *Kalamazoo Gazette* report on the following day, recognized the accomplishments of the women:

> Honorable J.W. Osborn, mayor of the city, was master of ceremonies and he presided most acceptably. His introductory remarks were appropriate and in them he gave praise to the women

> of Kalamazoo, who had worked so hard for the success of this enterprise.

Rev. E.J. Blekkink offered prayer.

> The story of the four years' effort to raise the money to make possible the erection of this structure is interesting and at the same time a valuable lesson in earnest and conscientious effort on the part of the women of Kalamazoo to advance the interest of the community. There has been no let up on the part of these enthusiastic and courageous women who have met and overcome many obstacles on their march to ultimate success in their vast undertaking.[40]

The report continues with details on fundraising, "Probably the youngest contributor to the fund was little Virginia Connable who earned $1.17 by the sale of lemonade."[41] Dr. H. B. Osborne was the principal speaker at this event:

> This is one of the happiest days of my life, for it means an important step forward in the realization of a fond hope. Twenty-four years ago I came to Kalamazoo, when this place was a village. We needed a hospital then and under the leadership of Dr. Hitchcock, an effort was made to build one, but for various reasons it proved unsuccessful. In fact, all our effort seemed to show how not to have a hospital. Kalamazoo then became a city and the need for a hospital still existed. It is doubtful if the city would have one underway now, were it not for the women who have fostered the work so nobly. It only proves that what a man is he owes to woman.[42]

It is interesting to note that the new Borgess hospital, just around the corner, was not mentioned.

A second, modern, state-of-the-art hospital on the corner of Lovell and John streets had become a reality. Gray fieldstone walls formed the base of the 50-patient, three-story, brick building, which boasted an elevator "for convenience."[43]

The *Kalamazoo Gazette* reports on June 4, 1904, "It has been decided to close the present Kalamazoo Hospital. The board of directors took this action owing to the work on the new building." Was cost a factor in closing? Resources were limited. It would cost $50,000 to complete the new hospital with an outstanding debt amounting to $16,000.[44]

What happened to Miss Jessie Yancey when the temporary hospital quarters closed in 1904? A newspaper report implicates an earlier departure and return.

> Miss Jessie Yancey, formerly in charge of the Kalamazoo Hospital, but of late connected with the Visiting Nurses' Association of Chicago, arrived in Kalamazoo Tuesday morning. She will enter upon her duties here today under direction of the Women's Civic Improvement League (WCIL) of this city.[45]
>
> [She was quoted,] " I hope the people here will regard me as their friend and will call upon me in every kind of need and I will help them in every way which lies in my power. I want the people to feel that I am here for their good. I hope too, that the physicians will regard me as their friend and call upon me to aid them whenever they are in need of help."[46]

It is worth noting that Miss Yancey was hired by the WCIL, not by a hospital or a physician. Her statement gives one the impression of an independent nursing-practice model that was well developed at the beginning of the 20th century. A follow-up story a few months later described her practice caring for the poor.[47] The physicians expressed their thanks to the nurse for taking the patients unable to pay for services. Nursing and medical services were interdependent, although nurses seemed to lose or give up their autonomous role as their affiliation with hospitals and physicians grew.

Visiting nurses began their work in Kalamazoo on February 24, 1904, with Miss Frances Bottling as director.[48] It is not clear whether they too were part of the WCIL.

Nurses were leaders in community health efforts as evidenced by the work of public health and visiting nurses' associations (VNA). An example is the VNA of Chicago, controlled by a board of women. Reference is made to their president's, Miss Harriet Fulmer, attendance, at the Woman's Congress in Berlin, Germany. [49]

New Kalamazoo Hospital near Ready to Open

The "new" aseptic hospital model fit within the practice standards written by Florence Nightingale a half century earlier. Hygiene, asepsis, clean air, water, and attention to the physical surroundings were part of the therapeutic milieu that she advised.

The interior, as described in a *Kalamazoo Gazette* article, gave the impression of order, discipline, and asepsis: a truly modern hospital! It was built for and by the physicians to do their work in accordance with the prevailing science of the times. The support of influential Kalamazoo women and men made it happen. The walls were white. Furnishings were sparse, and no draperies or carpets were used to eliminate a place for unwanted microscopic-size visitors to grow. Medical asepsis was a necessary practice.

> Hall floors of marble mosaic . . . in the rooms cement floors admit thorough washing without injury to the building. There are no corners in which dust may collect . . . the building is as nearly aseptic as improved methods of architecture permit. The operating rooms are on the top floor. No dust can reach them from the street; skylights provide excellent light. On one side of the hall are the surgeons' apartments, on the other the nurses' washrooms. When the surgeon comes from the street, he enters a washroom where he leaves his outer clothing . . . washes his hands and face and dons his surgical gown. At the end of the hall are other wash bowls with running water where he continues his ablutions. After he has entered the operating room further sterilizing apparatus makes it possible for him to put his hand into practically aseptic condition. [50]

Philosophy Supports the Perceived Need for a Second Hospital

The Sisters of St. Joseph seemed to have their own style of power. Would the story have been different if the Sisters had participated in direct negotiations with the Kalamazoo Academy of Medicine? Was it an embarrassment to the physicians that the Sisters were able to fund the first modern hospital just a few blocks from the location of the Kalamazoo Hospital? Could a new hospital at the beginning of the 20th century have it all? Could the allopathic physicians accept interdisciplinary practices with homeopathic physicians and nurses? Could different schools of medicine and nursing exist side by side?

Inclusivity, diversity, and tolerance were obviously not buzzwords of the day. No, the only thing that could happen, happened. Acceptance of diversity was not a pattern for American social institutions. Strengths in cultural pluralism and inclusive practice still elude us one hundred years later.

In the past twenty years (1980s-2000s) Bronson Methodist Hospital has accepted doctors of osteopathy on the medical staff.[51]

The Kalamazoo Hospital's commitment to the poor and aged was not different from that of the Sisters of St. Joseph. Charity care had been provided at the Borgess Hospital since it opened in 1889. Both hospitals struggled to find the resources needed for numerous patients who could not pay.[52] As early as 1892, the Sisters of St. Joseph had offered the sale of the hospital to the city of Kalamazoo in order to reduce their fundraising struggle and increase caring services.

The shift in the care of the sick from a feminine to a masculine model becomes quite evident in 1900 hospital structures. They were spartan in appearance, lacking in aesthetics. Hospitals were meant to be healing places. An aseptic environment was essential to prevent the spread of communicable diseases, but abandoning a healing home-like environment can be questioned.

Another major deterrent to having one hospital was the perceived religious differences between Christian denominations, Catholic and Protestant. Fear of the unknown and egocentric behavior continues to be a discomfort that leads to exclusive practices in all social arenas. Clearly, for the Protestant physicians, the local Catholic hospital organization with its homeopathic model was unsettling. Recognizing differences seemed to be easier than fitting the pieces of the great health care puzzle together. Caring similarities abound although they were ignored. Differences were perceived as threat-producing insecurity and lack of control.

Gender inequity was a third major barrier to the establishment of one, strong, healing organization. The Sisters of St. Joseph could not negotiate directly with the physicians to resolve their differences. The message had to be carried through Father O'Brien. The allopathic medical staff eventually won, with Borgess following suit with federal funding for development of allopathic schools of medicine at the expense of other health care philosophies and models of practice. Other health caregivers were essentially relegated to second-class positions, the power residing with allopathic physicians. Outwardly, nurses, like "good" submissive women, simply fit into this allopathic system and followed their call to caring.

Philosophical differences were major barriers to harmonious collaborative efforts. The name of the game was not partnership or acceptance of diverse practitioners. It was competition for recognition and credibility.

A FULL-FLEDGED SCHOOL OF NURSING

The Bronson School of Nursing opened within this environment of differences. From the very beginning, it was known as a first-class school. From 1904 to 1909 students were sent to New York's Women's and Children's Infirmary for additional training and, by 1910, affiliations were established with Michael Reese Hospital in Chicago. Amy Bailey, 1914 graduate, recalled that the extra training at Michael Reese was in the care of children. She and one other student took the train to South Haven and then boarded a boat to Chicago. She did not recall practicing at the Kalamazoo Insane Asylum which started its own school of nursing in the early nineteen hundreds and boasted the presence of Linda Richards, America's first trained nurse in 1904.[53]

Minnie Goodnow, was the superintendent of Bronson Hospital from 1909 to 1911. She served with three units in France during World War I and wrote a book *War Nurse in France. War Nursing,*[54] about her experiences. She successfully authored several books on nursing including several editions of *Outlines of Nursing History,*[55,56] *Nursing History in Brief,*[57] *First Year Nursing,*[58] and *Technic of Nursing.*[59] The hospital was very fortunate to have such a qualified administrator in its organizational years and one who attained international status during her nursing career.

Early graduate, Ruth Hinds '21 recalls, "I taught [at Bronson] for a year after I graduated. I worked at the hospital with one other nurse. We changed off with three months of night duty and three months of obstetrics. Then I got married and you could not work at the hospital if you were married. So, I did a little private duty, . . . we needed the money. I never liked to do private duty. I never liked to sit with one person and hold their hand. It was not my way of doing nursing."[60] Ruth was related to the Reverend Dr. William Puffer, the first Methodist minister to become superintendent of the hospital. Most likely her ability to secure a scarce hospital position was related to the family connection to Dr. Puffer.

THE HOSPITAL'S AILING FINANCIAL SYSTEM, 1910-1920

The new hospital struggled, unable to keep up with bills and non-collectable debts from patients who had no money. The women's auxiliaries worked hard to keep up with the need but were unable to do so. People with resources still preferred private care by physicians and nurses in their home, not with strange caregivers in public institutions.

Information varies about the solvency of the hospital. Mr. Boyles (or Broyles)[61] was appointed manager in 1916. He was asked to resign when trouble became evident in 1918. The debt had grown to $40,000. Borgess offered to buy the hospital for $40,000, not an option for those who had labored so intensely to build a separate entity.

Bad debts continued to be a daily reality and most likely supplies were hard to obtain without cash. A recommendation was made to turn the hospital over to the Michigan Methodist Conference and, in late 1919, the Conference agreed to assume leadership and control of the hospital. It appears that Dr. William Puffer, himself a Methodist minister, used long debates and arguments to convince other Methodists of the merit of this proposal. What of those who lived hundreds of miles from Kalamazoo and, most likely, would never benefit? Why would they want to take on this burden? How would their parishioners gain?

A Michigan White Cross brochure provided an answer with the following words of Jesus Christ, "I am among you as he that serveth," and this opening statement,

> One of the best uses of money in the world for people, who want their money to accomplish all possible good, is to help the work of Christian Hospitals, which exist to relieve human suffering in a Christian atmosphere, using the best methods known to modern medicine and nursing science.
>
> The Methodist Episcopal Church has 77 Hospitals in 28 states and the District of Columbia. They have 9,374 beds. Last year [1930] these 77 hospitals gave care to 281,778 persons, . . . with part pay and part free care. . . .
>
> Hospitals give doctors the best place in which to do their work. . . . Hospitals provide modern equipment and expert nursing care. Hospital service is expensive. Many sick and injured persons have little money. . . . There is not one of all the Hospitals in Methodism, now doing such a vast amount of good, that could continue to exist without the support from churches. This church has done very important work for our nation in Evangelism and

> Education, but all its organized philanthropic work has been built up since 1881.[62]

Contributions of Women Continue

In 1920, the hospital's name officially changed to Bronson Methodist Hospital (BMH). Dr. Puffer became the first Methodist minister superintendent. His reports refer to the philanthropic ladies and their role in continuing in volunteer endeavors such as the Women's Auxiliary, What-So-Ever Free Bed Associations, Crib-side Society, *etc.* Once their services were provided, however, the women were to experience less direct input into management decision making.

Organization of White Cross guilds within the state Methodist system expanded the volunteer work of women across the entire state. This kind of effort kept costs in control until the public later would bear the burden, as insurance became the major third-party payer.

School of Nursing Changes

In July 1985, Mary Lou Stewart, BMH Archivist, engaged two early graduates in conversation with each other about the school. They were Ruth Hinds, 1921 graduate and Amy Bailey from 1914. Ruth's student tenure crossed the years when Bronson moved from its nonsectarian status into a 40-year relationship with the Methodist Church. Ruth recalled the improvement in hospital resources with the church's intervention and consistent donations.

Nursing education began to be more formalized. Most of the classes continued to be taught by doctors when Ruth started the nursing program in 1918. A nurse, however, started teaching nursing arts in a classroom and practice format and arranged for doctors' lectures. When asked by the archivist, "Was the hospital desperately poor?" Ruth said, "No. We had enough to work with—maybe not enough to decorate [the patient's rooms to create an aesthetic environment]. We made up sterile packs for operations and would need to wait for supplies to turn around from laundry. It didn't matter if the turn around took 10 or 15 hours. There were no short cuts, even though supplies were limited. We had almost no infections!"

CHAPTER 1 NOTES

---

[1] *Kalamazoo Morning Gazette,* 1904 May 23, "Corner stone exercises: large crowd gathered at Kalamazoo Hospital."

[2] Turn of the century physicians were trained in different philosophical models of practice, *i.e.,* allopathic, homeopathic, naturopathic and osteopathic.

[3] *Kalamazoo Gazette,* 1889 August 3, reported that the, "hospital will not be open to receive patients before the middle of October."

[4] *Kalamazoo Gazette,* 1892 July 7, "Borgess Hospital."

[5] Oral interview with Sister Kathleen Walsh, Nazareth Archives, Nazareth, Mich., with Jackie Wylie, 1997 August 23.

[6] Sisters of St. Joseph Historical Archives, Nazareth, Mich.

[7] Nightingale, F. *Notes on Nursing.* New York: D.Appleton, 1894. p.8.

[8] Oral interview with Sister Kathleen Walsh, *op.cit.*

[9] *Kalamazoo Gazette,* 1892 February 6, "The Borgess Hospital, what is to become of it? Three offers received."

[10] The Sisters of St. Joseph did not participate in public meetings, thereby limiting their ability to negotiate directly with city officials, or attend formal meetings of the Kalamazoo Academy of Medicine.

[11] *Kalamazoo Gazette,* 1892 February 6, *op.cit.*

[12] Nazareth Archives and Historical Collection, Nazareth, Mich.

[13] *Kalamazoo Gazette,* 1902 March 11, "New hospital open to the public, several patients taken in at Borgess Monday, Sisters of St. Joseph soon to form non-sectarian training class for nurses."

[14] *Kalamazoo Gazette,* 1896 March 27, "They all complied, Borgess staff resigns, Dean O'Brien's views of the controversy which led to the trouble and final severance of the relations between the staff and himself—the hospital and the physicians."

[15] Oral Interview with Sister Kathleen Walsh, Sisters of St. Joseph Historical Archives, Nazareth Mich., 1997 August 23, with Jackie Wylie.

[16] *Kalamazoo Gazette,* 1896 March 27, *op.cit.*

---

[17] *Ibid.*

[18] According to Webster's New World Dictionary, 3rd edition, allopathy is the, "treatment of disease by remedies that produce effects from or opposite to those produced by the disease: loosely applied to the general practice of medicine today, but in strict usage opposed to homeopathy." Homeopathy is defined as a system of medical treatment based on the theory that certain diseases can be cured by giving very small doses of drugs which in a healthy person would produce symptoms like those of the disease: opposed to allopathy.

[19] *Kalamazoo Gazette*, 1896 March 29, "The staff replies, their views of the hospital controversy, respect the sisters, and lay blame on their advisor—they make some strong statements and sign their names."

[20] *Ibid.*

[21] *Polk City Directory,* 1899.

[22] *Kalamazoo Gazette*, 1900 October 13, "Project for a new hospital, one said to be under way by local physicians, to be established at corner John and Cedar streets—doctors not talking."

[23] *Kalamazoo Gazette*, 1900 December 4.

[24] E. H. Van Deusen, MD, was a pioneer in medical mental health care and was past superintendent of the Kalamazoo Insane Asylum. In 1893, he gave the Kalamazoo Public Library to the community.

[25] Michigan White Cross, *Annual Report 1930 June–1931 July.* Dr. E. Ames and Dr. J. H. La Huis joined later.

[26] *Kalamazoo Morning Gazette,* 1900 November 14, "New hospital is assured."

[27] *Kalamazoo Gazette,* 1976 July 7, "Acceptance was slow but Bronson grew to major hospital." "Brees, an early Kalamazoo land developer, . . . conveyed a piece of land . . . for construction of a hospital. That conveyance, on Dec. 24, 1896, included 75 feet of frontage on John Street and 100 feet of frontage on Cedar Street. On Dec. 19 of that year, there also had been a deed recorded conveying an aging, moderate-sized house and a 40-foot lot on John Street from Mary C. Miller to the six doctors for $2,395.59. Land was deeded on Sept. 23, 1902 for two lots on either side of the Miller lot, increasing the John Street frontage . . . to 193 feet." Those two lots were gifts from Mr. and Mrs. Herbert H. Everard.

[28] *Kalamazoo Morning Gazette*, 1900 November 11.

[29] *Kalamazoo Gazette,* 1901 January 20, "New hospital to open soon, is supplied with all modern improvements, Dr. E. H. Van Deusen is president, experienced nurse and cook have been engaged."

[30] *Kalamazoo Gazette*, 1892 February 6 and 1882 July 7.

---

[31] *Kalamazoo Gazette*, 1900 November 14.

[32] D'Antonio, Patricia, *Reflections*, 1997 3rd /4th Quarter. "Nineteenth century nursing: science and the value of duty, will and power."

[33] *Kalamazoo Gazette,* 1902 October 10, "New hospital now assured, building committee has been appointed, will proceed at once."

[34] Not all of the physicians in the area were men, as evidenced by Kalamazoo Academy of Medicine Records and Sister Mary Raphael, a practicing homeopathic physician at Borgess Hospital. The Kalamazoo Academy of Medicine has record of women who were medical doctors; however, they did not appear to be part of the early hospital movement, if records reviewed accurately portray their involvement.

[35] Bronson Hospital School of Nursing records.

[36] *Kalamazoo Gazette,* 1903 May 22, "Kalamazoo Hospital conducted by five nurses, a cook and an orderly, nine patients now in the institution, all on the way to recovery—many visitors call with acceptable donations."

[37] *Ibid.*

[38] Oral interview with Amy Bailey Seward, by Mary Lou Stewart.

[39] *Kalamazoo Gazette,* 1904 June 7, "Auto day for hospital aid, will you have a ride on circus day, will cost small sum, and you can go to the circus looking like ready money—auto parties promise to be numerous—for Kalamazoo Hospital."

[40] *Kalamazoo Gazette,* 1904 May 23, "Corner stone exercises, large crowd gathers at Kalamazoo Hospital, interesting program, an important step forward in erection of this structure for good of greater Kalamazoo—strong box with documents laid away."

[41] *Kalamazoo Morning Gazette,* 1904 May 23, *op.cit.*

[42] *Kalamazoo Gazette,* 1904 May 23.

[43] *Kalamazoo Gazette,* 1903 December 5, "Change in plans for the hospital."

[44] Taped history, Mary Lou Stewart, Bronson Archives, "Forty significant hospital events."

[45] Obviously, collaboration occurred with physicians because the WCIL quarters was set up in the house first remodeled for the Kalamazoo Hospital.

[46] *Kalamazoo Gazette*, 1904 June 15, "Miss Yancey begins work, new visiting nurse has had much experience, returns to old home."

[47] *Kalamazoo Gazette*, 1904 September 20, "Miss Yancey and her work, visiting nurse gives aid in many homes, calls on sick poor, her services and counsel appreciated by lead physicians—makes an average of ten visits daily—under league's direction."

[48] VNA Archives

[49] *Kalamazoo Gazette*, 1904 September 20, *op.cit.*

[50] *Kalamazoo Gazette*, 1905 April 19, "Hospital is nearly ready."

[51] Bronson Methodist Hospital has given practice privileges to osteopathic physicians, nurse practitioners and nurse midwives in recent years. Integrative medicine, holistic or complementary alternative medicine may be the beginning of transdisciplinary, inclusive practice.

[52] *Kalamazoo Gazette,* 1892 February 6, *op.cit.*

[53] Richards, Linda. *Reminiscences of America's First Trained Nurse.* Reprint. Philadelphia: J.B. Lippincott, 1948.

[54] Goodnow, Minnie. *War Nurse in France. War Nursing*. Phildelphia: W.B. Saunders, 1917.

[55] Goodnow, Minnie. *Outlines of Nursing History,* 4th ed. Philadelphia: W.B. Saunders, 1929.

[56] Goodnow, Minnie, *Outlines of Nursing History,* 6th ed. Philadelphia: W.B. Saunders, 1938.

[57] Goodnow, Minnie, *Nursing History in Brief.* Philadelphia: W.B. Saunders, 1943.

[58] *Bronson Bulletin, 7(2):* 1949 Spring; 3.

[59] *Ibid.*

[60] Taped interview with Ruth Hinds Phelps by Mary Lou Stewart, 1985 July 3.

[61] Spelling of name was not confirmed.

[62] Michigan White Cross, *Annual Report 1930 July–1931 June.* p.5.

CHAPTER 2

RECOLLECTIONS FROM EARLY GRADUATES, 1913–1929

MINA WEBER MACGRAYNE '13

Alumni Association minutes throughout the 1920s attest to Mina Weber's loyalty and commitment to the young, growing group of Bronson graduates. Her story provides evidence of her leadership qualities that positioned her for influential roles within the association and Bronson Methodist Hospital School of Nursing affairs for the following four decades.

Mina Weber's name is in a handwritten list, titled "Charter Members," on the back of Dr. Ralph Balch's office stationery. Weber worked for Dr. Balch after graduation. Most likely she wrote the list of graduates from classes from 1909 to 1917 or provided the piece of paper on which they were written, and very likely Weber assumed a leadership role in the Alumni Association. Minutes of the association's meetings were recorded since January, 1923,[1] but no record was found to document officers or business conducted prior to 1923. Alumni associations represented the local branches of state nurses' associations and the national American Nurses Association.

Enrolled at the School of Nursing in 1910, when she was nineteen years old, an admission requirement, and two years after her May 1908 graduation from Centreville High School, Weber[2] was president of her senior class whose speech upon graduation was entitled, "A Crown to be Won." What could she have meant? We can guess from stories told about her that her topic related to giving service to one's community: a crown would be won by those committed to serve others. As uncommon as it was for young women to graduate from high school in 1908, Weber served as class president.[3] Weber was not afraid to be recognized. She knew how to negotiate in ways not offensive to others who believed woman's place was in the home. Her demeanor was most often reflective and practical in public and at home, characteristics typical of nurses from hospital-based programs. She never touted her leadership skills in giving service to Bronson, the School of Nursing, the community and the Alumni Association.

An early school picture provided by her daughter during a 1998 interview demonstrated evidence of Weber's role as a team player on a girl's basketball team. Not many young women at the turn of the century would risk such sporting behavior. She started her community involvement early, not only as a class speaker, but also as one who enjoyed team relationships, strengths often found in directors of nursing, a role she would later assume.

Why did she choose Bronson and why did she wait until 1910 to enroll? She was seventeen when she graduated from high school. It may have been that her family thought that she was too young to leave home or family responsibilities may have required her presence. Though Bronson was not officially affiliated with the Methodist Church until 1920, graduate stories prior to this date validate a Methodist presence with continuous donations of linens and food.[4] Weber's family belonged to a Methodist Church. Possibly she heard about the program through her church affiliation. Kalamazoo may have provided the closest program to home and also the comfort of a protestant religious connection, a place for Weber to "win her crown."

Becoming a registered nurse by passing a licensing exam authorized by the Michigan State Board of Nursing came into being in 1917. The new law required that graduates be 21 years of age to take the exam.

Professionalism Personified

Miss Weber was a picture of professionalism and beauty in her nursing school uniform. She exemplified the young graduate nurse of her day—a sister of Florence Nightingale to be sure. Her quick ability to learn principles of nursing and hospital techniques and to give effective, efficient nursing service made her a favorite of nursing superintendent Edith Cowie Partridge and the Bronson physicians. Weber was hired by Dr. Ralph Balch, when she graduated in 1913, to assist in surgery at Bronson, in patient's homes, and in his office.

Later, she practiced nursing for a period of time (dates are not documented) on the East Coast where, it is believed, she was involved with the use of radiation in medical care.[5]

Weber must have had an adventurous side, as well as an incredibly strong sense of duty. Her next professional choice may have related to Dr. Balch's decision to become a military surgeon in World War I. She joined the Armed Services as a Red Cross Nurse and took the oath of office on February 15, 1918. She saw the ravages of the war directly in the field treatment of injured soldiers, spending a year on the front lines in France. The story she told her daughter about a nursing care experience on Armistice Day involved assisting with a surgical procedure for a colonel who had a self-inflicted gunshot wound (one of the many war ravages rarely discussed then or now). As she worked desperately with her teammates to save his life, they received word that the Armistice agreement had been signed, a significant emotional event in her life, always remembered.

Weber also described a holiday with a group of nurses on an old Mediterranean ship that was not exactly a cruise liner. According to her story it left something to be desired with its infestations and unclean condition. The holiday (perhaps a gift to the Red Cross nurses) probably took place immediately after her time in France and did not meet her standard. She sent a postcard to her father to document the event, but the postmark date is illegible.[6]

She returned to the United States on March 27, 1919, entering at the port of Newport News, Virginia, and she was relieved of her active war duty on April 17, 1919.[7] It is possible that she returned to work for Dr. Balch, although dates are not documented, but she became director of nursing of the hospital and School of Nursing in 1922. She is identified in pictures with the entire hospital staff of thirty-nine, posed in front of the hospital. Even as director she continued an active role in the Alumni Association according to meeting minutes throughout the 1920s. Her election to president, recorded in the January 2, 1923, minutes, came from a total of seven votes cast: Miss Weber, five and Miss Lemmer two.[8]

Motherhood and Continued Service

Weber remained as director until her 1925 marriage to Daly Macgrayne, the secretary-treasurer at Brody Chevrolet in Kalamazoo. It was common for nurses to resign their positions when they married, but she continued to be active in the Alumni Association. Affluent women then could not have it all—nurse and homemaker were incompatible full-time roles. September 29, 1925, minutes recognize her name change to Macgrayne. Her daughter Janet[9] was born in 1926, and twin sons, Paul and Daly came four years later.

Why she chose nursing may be evident in some of the character traits and relationship attributes she bestowed on her children. When her daughter, Janet '48, recognized a "bossy" trait of her own she was quick to see the behavior as an inheritance from Weber who was a present, loving, and serious no-nonsense mother who provided a healthy home for her family.

Daily attention to nutritious meals, a known fact for wellness, was just one way that she promoted family health. Weber abided by dietetic rules she had learned in nursing school and from her dear friend, Alice Worman, a dietician at Kalamazoo State Hospital. There was hot cereal for breakfast, nutritious lunches packed for school (no Twinkies!), and always one big hot meal a day which, according to Alice, was a must for a healthy body. It mattered not how hot the weather or the kitchen, a hot meal was prepared!

A lifelong friendship developed through her professional relationship with surgeon, Dr. Ralph Balch and his wife, who became Uncle Ralph and Aunt Otha to the Macgrayne children. The Macgrayne home on Bronson Boulevard was built on property adjacent to the Balch's. Many family vacations were shared. It was as if the Balch's took on parent–grandparent roles.

Weber's daughter recalled her mother's temporary return to Bronson to serve as the interim director of nurses; however, the appointment to this position and exactly when it occurred are not clear. Janet believes that it might have been in 1935, 1937 or 1940 because a maid was hired to assist the family. It appears that her return was a brief episode until a permanent director could be hired.

Mina Weber served on the Nursing Education Committee of the Board of Trustees for several years in the 1940s[10] and assisted in the planning of the 50th anniversary celebration of the Bronson School of Nursing in 1954 as part of her alumna involvement. In later years she belonged to a Methodist Church, a church women's circle, and a local garden club, along with the Nursing Education Committee at Bronson. She became ill with diabetes mellitus later in life, and was an invalid preceding her death in 1978 when she was 87 years old.

AMY L. BAILEY SEWARD '14

Amy Bailey was born August 7, 1894, to a farming family in Fulton, Wakeshma Township, Michigan, the daughter of Mary Jane (Withey) and Charles

Bailey.[11] She was the youngest, the eighth child,[12] with four brothers and three sisters. Most likely her older siblings were at home and able to care for family and farm.

Nursing was not Bailey's childhood career choice. She wanted to be a teacher and perhaps knew of the Western Normal School for teachers in Kalamazoo. Most likely the family did not have the resources to send her to college.

For a young, poor woman, an apprenticeship or work-study program with a monthly stipend was the only career option outside of the home. It was not uncommon for daughters of farmers to leave rural areas and seek work in growing cities. When an opportunity to attend nursing school came along she took it. She applied to the Bronson School of Nursing upon graduation from high school in Athens, Michigan, on June 7, 1911, and was accepted for the fall of 1911.[13] Bailey graduated from Bronson in 1914. "We earned our diplomas. We did it the hard way."[14]

Hospital-based schools of nursing provided a way to get family consent to leave home and receive board and room, plus training for respectable work. Romanticized stories drew poor women to this choice.[15] Many hands were needed in the new hospital as it struggled to make ends meet. It wasn't easy to find young women to do this work. Recruitment efforts were obvious in early readings about the hospital.

Most patients coming to the hospitals for care were the working poor from Kalamazoo paper mills. They could not pay for the services rendered 24 hours a day, seven days a week. Charitable care was provided when payment wasn't possible. Past bills were often not collected. The working poor did not have disposable income beyond needs for food, shelter and clothing.

Arriving for Training

Seventeen-year old Bailey, upon arrival, saw a new, state-of-the-art hospital on the corner of Lovell and John Street with gray fieldstone walls that formed the base of the 50–patient, three-story, brick building. It boasted an elevator "for convenience,"[16] and its interior gave the impression of order, discipline and asepsis.

The hospital met Bailey's expectations and offered promise of a life more exciting than the farm had to offer. Pictures of her in uniform, along with her many stories, present a woman who seized the day by taking opportunity when she saw it. Bailey's training was rigorous. The lifestyle fit her no-nonsense, determined personality.

> I entered the hospital as a student nurse following my graduation from Athens High School. Our uniforms were gray and white striped with high starched collars, long sleeves, and stiffly starched white aprons and bibs. Probationers earned the right to wear nurses caps the first year, the second year narrow black velvet bands were placed on the caps, and in the third year wide black velvet bands were added. After graduation an all-white uniform was worn and the original Bronson Hospital blue and gold pin. I have always treasured my memories of in-training days at the hospital and my blue and gold pin.[17]

Her education included hours of on-the-job training seven days (or nights) per week with a few hours off for church. Classes were taught by the nursing superintendent and, when their schedules allowed, by physicians when, or if, students were available off duty at times that matched physicians' availabilities. Patient services, however, came before student classroom learning. Students were the direct-care staff under the supervision of a nurse superintendent. Experiential learning preceded academic knowledge within the context of the hospital environment.

By all accounts, Bailey was a strong-willed woman with a demeanor that fit the expectations of the environment. She knew her place and did not outwardly push the hospital norms, which could call for dismissal at a moment's notice. Bailey found ways to manage the strict environment and to move "around" the rules. Fire escapes provided "unnoticed" exit and reentry with a little help from a colluding friend.[18]

Escape from the rigid rules provided a few hours of fun. Students were not always ready to give up the pleasures of youth. They managed the duality of being individual free spirits and still conformed to a controlling environment. Later they gained the powers that led to becoming the controlling, sometimes oppressive, ones themselves.[19] Secrets for survival were passed on from student to student and class to class, unwritten but a major part of Bronson's hidden nursing curriculum. Outwardly, nursing followed the dominant medical model. Inwardly, nursing care took precedence. We lived in a counterculture. Nursing care was well integrated into the nurses' management of medical care for which nurses were responsible 24 hours a day, seven days a week.

Upon graduation most of the Bronson students were not hired by the hospital. They registered as private-duty nurses and, if they had physician allies and a "good" reputation, they worked for families who could pay for their services at home or as inpatients at the hospital and with beginning visiting nursing services. When Bailey graduated, she became a special-duty nurse caring for one patient at a time, often at the request of a physician.[20]

Private-duty practice required a major commitment to the patient and her or his family, staying for the duration of the illness at the hospital and later at home. Bronson food came from the kitchen on a dumb waiter, and the nurses took the trays to their patients. As Bailey recalled, she served a lot of baked custard and apples. She was on duty with her hospitalized patient all day and night, except for two hours when a staff nurse provided relief. She slept in the room on a folding cot provided by the orderly. The patient would call out to her during the night when her assistance was needed.

Bailey knew the value of presence, nutrition, aesthetics and asepsis, using them to bring healing to her patients. "I brought my own dishes to put on their tray. They had pink roses on them. I tried to make the tray as beautiful as possible." Her caring side was noticed and remembered by Ruth Hinds '21, in a taped conversation. Hinds described Bailey and her famous dishes. "Once I was sick when I was a nursing student, and Amy took care of me. I will never forget her china. It was white with little pink rose buds. You got well just eating food on her china. It was such a treat."[21]

Bailey's strong will matched the nature of the nonsectarian, community hospital. She loved the institution, and in the late 1930s fulfilled her teaching dream as a teacher of nurse aides. If she had any regrets about her career choice, they were not obvious to the people who knew her and recorded her story.

Once a private duty case took Bailey as far as Cody, Wyoming. Her niece tells the story about Bailey's love for horses and her acquisition of a pony from an Indian chief in return for nursing care provided to his family.

Becoming a Recognized Professional

Bailey passed the Michigan State Board of Nursing examination to become a professional registered nurse on January 15, 1918, four years after graduation. State licensure had become mandatory to call oneself a professional nurse. She said the exam was hard for those who had graduated years before, quite understandable given the amount of attention paid to on-the-job experiential learning and the little paid to preparing for examination. Competency was demonstrated in work and daily patient outcomes.

What kinds of resources were available to the nurses and physicians in the provision of care? When Bronson Methodist Hospital Archivist, Mary Lou Stewart, discussed the topic with Bailey and Hinds, incongruencies were evident. Dr. Boys had once indicated that the hospital was so poor the nurses had only one towel each that they kept under their apron. Rumor was that linens were so scarce that sheets were taken off the nursing students' beds for patients. He also said that they could not afford commercially prepared catgut for surgical sutures. Bailey said, "No! That's absurd! He's wrong. Standards were high. Everything was very clean." Both Bailey and Hinds agreed everything was immaculate. Asepsis was one of the most important aspects of care and cure. Perceptions evidently varied with the position of the observer, or hardships could have been forgotten in place of a romantic, idealized healing place.

Bailey reiterated, "Everything was new and fresh." Maybe so in 1911 in her first memories; maybe not so by 1918 or 1919 when the hospital was failing to pay its bills and not managing to find resources to maintain it. All accounts describe the new hospital as unable to pay bills and collect its debts from patients who had no money. The women's auxiliaries worked hard to keep up with the need but were unable to do so. People with resources still preferred private care by physicians and nurses in the comfort of their homes, not with strange caregivers in public institutions where exposure to disease was likely to be eminent.

A Claim to Fame

Eleanor Roosevelt's thank you note to Bailey was a special remembrance of the part she played in the national movement to train nurse aides as auxiliary staff for delegating care to nurses aides to relieve the nursing shortage during World War II. The note is protected in the Bronson alumni historical files.[22] Bailey administered the first Bronson nurse aide training program including celebratory events such as luncheons to reward the women who passed the nurse aide course.

Nurse aide training continued after WWII as a strategy for cost containment in hospitals. It continues to this day, with titles such as patient care assistants or technologists. Nursing homes often use the nurse aide title.

One Last Professional Nursing Care Experience, 1990

The last years of Bailey's life were spent home bound, managing her own nursing care from a hospital bed positioned in the middle of her dining room, facing the living room and front door. She had hired visiting nurses and meals-on-wheels as two of the main services to sustain her independent lifestyle even when she became bedridden.

When she was dying, nurses from the Visiting Nurses Association cared for her at home, assisting her as she directed her own care. She chose not to be transferred to an institution, without worry of dying alone and placing a high value on independence and self-control.

The VNA nurses, however, did care, and did not want her to die alone. They expected that she would die within the week and called for help. They asked the Alumni Association of the Bronson Methodist Hospital School of Nursing to help care for her around the clock. The VNA representative told Jackie Wylie that they wanted to follow Bailey's wishes despite her lack of money. Wylie said "yes" to support her care decision, wanting to meet this woman, after having heard her strong voice on tape as she reminisced about early nursing student days.[23] Other alumni also rose to the call. They contributed money to the VNA and time when they could be present at Bailey's bedside.

> I picked up the key to Bailey's house from the VNA office in the late afternoon and, according to the instructions, drove to her small bungalow on Woodward Street, parked, and entered through the front door. Once inside, I could see her hospital bed in the middle of the dining room. She was alone and bedridden, as I had expected. My mind wandered back to the visiting nurses' courage, strength and trust in supporting Bailey's precarious position. I familiarized myself with her general appearance and physical surroundings. She appeared to be sleeping, a big woman without apparent physical wasting, her purse tucked under her pillow. She had a urinary catheter, but no other obvious tubes, and she looked well cared for.

> After I introduced myself and explained that I would be with her for the evening and night, what did we do for each other that evening? We exchanged a bit of history, a bit of care and my presence. When I offered her water to hydrate dry mucous membranes, Bailey didn't seem able or willing to suck through a straw. I found a teaspoon in a kitchen drawer and gave her water, which she accepted and swallowed without difficulty. She communicated only with body language and appeared to rally with the small amounts of hydration. I repositioned her with a pillow to get her off her back. Her skin was intact—no pressure sores. She and her previous caregivers had not let this common complication of a bed-bound body from occurring. She received no medications.

Bailey was surrounded by her story at the end and was playing it out in her way. I noticed some of the documents on her wall—Bronson diploma, September 23, 1914, and State of Michigan Registration as a registered nurse, January 15, 1918. Maybe nursing wasn't her first love but it was her last. She died at home on March 7, 1990.

Nursing became Bailey's greatest love and a lifelong practice for her personally and professionally. Nursing and Bronson Hospital appeared to be synonymous for her. She remained loyal to the school of nursing even beyond her dying day. Funeral instructions, written in her hand, stated that she was to be buried in her Bronson cape of royal blue, wearing her gold graduate pin, shaped like a Maltese cross. The blue enamel center was inscribed, 1914, the date of graduation. Her initials, ALB, were on the back. She was buried wrapped in her cape as she had planned, a faithful member of the Bronson Hospital sisterhood.[24, 25]

CORNELIA VEENHUIS CODY '21

Cornelia Veenhuis[26] grew up in Kalamazoo. Her family's home was located at 821 West Vine Street, and they moved into it in 1919. Seventy years later Wylie interviewed her there on February 28, 1989. The furnishings appeared to be of early nineteen-hundred vintage. She told her story, including that of her 1921 graduation, with pride and she stopped often to laugh.

Her father was a brick mason. Veenhuis was proud of the quality of his work—solid and lasting. With this heritage she made an early commitment to find a way for self-sufficiency by making the best of existing resources. Nursing school was one of them.

She started working at 15 in the hardware department of Woolworth's on Burdick Street. Her older sister worked in the candy department. The five dollars a week she earned wasn't going to get her very far. She didn't want to be poor, and there had to be more to life than clerking.

"My mother was sick a lot, . . . with nine children and all." Once when the doctor came, he said, "You'd make a good nurse. Why don't you go into training?" I asked, "What do I have to do?" He said that I should get in touch with someone who knew more about it than he did and that he would write a letter of reference." As she walked to work, Veenhuis crossed paths with Mary T., a Red Cross field worker, and asked her what she needed to do to go into training? Veenhuis learned what she needed to know in order to apply.

"I continued to work at Woolworth's, and I also took care of Mrs. U. who wanted me to stay [and work for her]. She knew I wanted nurses' training. So, she told me, "Go talk with Mrs. Wildermuth[27] and let me know." Then Mrs. U. made all the arrangements for me. No tuition was paid but we had to have money for eight uniforms, caps, bibs, aprons and new shoes along with one good dress-up dress that I made with the help of my sister. It was a dark blue silk or taffeta. It hung in the closet and I never used it except on special occasions which were very few, such as a tea put on by the Methodist ladies at capping."

One of her sisters, Josephine, also interviewed for nurses' training at Bronson. The interviewer was Dr. Boys. Why did he say no to Josephine and yes to Veenhuis? What was Josephine's problem? She was too pretty (and "flirty," according to her sister). Dr. Boys told her: you won't last two months and you'll be married. She was not admitted. Neither did another sister whom Veenhuis felt had not been a strong student in high school, yet the doctor, trying to be kind, did not tell her she was weak in academic skills. Veenhuis recalled taking a test as another part of the application process.

An Opportunity Beckons!

Lucky Veenhuis! Here was her chance, and she would not fail. She started school in October of 1918. When asked to describe her first year of school, she said, "We did a lot of scrubbing," and laughed. "We didn't have much help. We had a woman who scrubbed the floors, but we had to wash everything else with soap and water for the three to four patients assigned. We were responsible for their rooms and utensils."

Also, as a "probie,"[28] the students took care of the doctors. They had to see that the doctors had soap and towels to wash up in the service room when they came to the floors. "Probies did the dirty work." After three months, probationary status was removed or the student was dismissed. Veenhuis was given her nurse's cap and greater duties: responsibility for the personal care of patients such as bed baths and back massage, which were part of the daily routine.

"There was a shortage of linen. If you didn't get your patient's linen early, none was left. When we ran out, we called the Methodist church ladies. They would bring us towels, washcloths, sheets and pillowcases. They also provided canned goods and fruit, such as bananas and oranges, for patients and staff.

"The third-year nursing students helped doctors with surgical procedures. They'd tell us what to do. The doctors also had graduate nurse assistants. Blanche Hermann[29] was one. We'd help the doctors, including preparation of sterile linens. We had to have instrument trays ready. While a probie helped him wash before a procedure, more seasoned students set up the sterile trays, first by boiling the instruments, taking them out with forceps, arranging surgical trays, and assisting the physician and assistant.

"One day we weren't very busy. Mrs. Wildermuth sent me to the storeroom to give it a good scrubbing. I think she was testing me. We all got a turn. I didn't want to go home and do nothing."

Another time, "We were assigned to wash the operating room walls when they needed it, and Dr. Puffer[30] happened to come by. He did not approve of the students up on ladders washing walls and so he called Mr. Kindleberger[31] who then planned for a group of men to scrub the walls."

A Student's Day (1918 through 1921)

"The day started with Chapel at 6:30 A.M. Somebody had donated an organ. Everyone was half asleep. We sang out of old Methodist hymnals. That meant an awful lot to me. We took care of patients from 7:00–10:00 A.M. and 10:30 A.M.–1:00 P.M., with lunch, and 2:00–4:00 P.M. was time off though we rarely got the two- to four- o'clock time. We had classes from 1:00–2:00 P.M. every day the first year, and the rest of the day we worked on the halls, a 7:00 A.M.–7:00 P.M. [shift.]"

Mrs. Wildermuth, and one other nurse taught nursing classes, and several doctors taught about their specialties. From doctors Boys, Balch and Fulkerson students learned aseptic technique, dressing changes, "so many things . . . ." Veenhuis lived in the nurses' home next to the hospital. Bedrooms were shared and there was one bath for all. "If you wanted a bath you needed to light the Humphrey heater for hot water. I went to bed at 9:00, never later than 10:00." Nursing supervisors also lived at the nurses' home where they could monitor student and hospital activity 24 hours a day.

The hospital bought another house across the street to accommodate more needed students as patient numbers increased. Senior students moved to the newly purchased home. It was nice, with double rooms and more sinks.

Veenhuis remembered that three girls dropped out. One girl couldn't find her high school diploma after the school burned and that seemed to be an irresolvable issue. A couple of girls, who did not like nurses' training, left.

If a student became ill, she got excellent care at the hospital and then was sent home to recover. "One of the years there was terrible flu but we all had flu shots. I did get ill in April and was in the hospital for two weeks and then home for two weeks. I had to make up the time after my class graduated in October. I really felt badly about the absence but I was mostly left on my own after I returned and ended up getting my first private duty job."

What did students do for fun and relaxation? Veenhuis recalled one activity—students going to movies that lasted later than 10:00 P.M., the curfew. She dared not risk breaking this rule. "I had worked too hard to get this far." They swam at the YWCA, a function that seemed to have been organized by the Methodist Church ladies. Attendance was encouraged at the Methodist Church. The last row in the church was reserved for students who were admitted in uniform so that they could easily return to work.

Veenhuis recalled coming back in June for a graduation ceremony with all of the graduates in lovely organdy, pastel dresses for a reception and everyone wearing uniforms at graduation at the first Methodist Church, on the corner of Rose and Cedar streets, before it burned down.

First Graduate Nurse Assignments

Veenhuis' first assignment was negotiated while making up her "ill" time after graduation. She was hired to care for Mrs. K., two weeks in Bronson Methodist Hospital and two weeks at home after childbirth. She was paid $7.00 a day! What a difference from the $5.00 a week she had earned at Woolworth's.

For three years she continued private duty practice at Bronson Methodist Hospital and in patients' homes, recalling a case in Schoolcraft assisting Dr. Boys and

Mrs. Wildermuth. No longer the director of nursing, Mrs. Wildermuth worked for Dr. Boys as a nurse anesthetist. The patient had acute appendicitis and, subsequently, an appendectomy on the kitchen table in his home.[32] Veenhuis stayed for 10 days to care for the patient during his crucial recovery. To facilitate wound drainage, the head of the bed was elevated on concrete blocks. Keep it draining! No antibiotics meant that the body's immune system had to rid itself of virulent pathogens. The process was helped by keeping the wound open so that purulent drainage would not accumulate and healing would occur from inside to out. Dressings had to be changed three to four times a day, and the doctor came by every day to check the patient's progress. Veenhuis' patient was ". . . a big, strong man, a good patient, no trouble . . . ," who survived the insult of a ruptured appendix and abdominal surgery at home before the days of antibiotics. "I was thankful Dr. Boys had taught me about sterile dressings."

> ***Ruth Hinds Phelps '21***
>
> Ruth as president, addressed her senior class at graduation, excerpts from which follow:
>
> We have had our share of work and fun—we have shed many tears during our "probie" days—we have laughed at our own mistakes.
>
> The time has not seemed long since we entered training—afraid almost to breathe for fear that might not be the proper thing to do—anxious to please but not knowing how—and learning rapidly that many are the trials of a probationer.
>
> Probably our happiest memory is of the day we received our caps, after the three longest months. Milestones along the way were our narrow and wide black bands, received at the end of our first and second years.
>
> Looking backward we are sure we have chosen rightly and, could these three years repeat themselves, we would find ourselves again as we are tonight—the graduating class of 1921.

Another early case was located on Gull Lake Island for the family who owned Saniwax Paper Company. Mr. I. had a ruptured appendix and subsequent appendectomy at Bronson. He was hospitalized for three weeks under Veenhuis' care before she accompanied him home. She stayed with him day and night because he needed so much care. "I was up and down a lot. I didn't mind. I was young" (inferring that she had the stamina to be present such long hours). She slept on a screened cot in the corner of the patient's room. I went downstairs to dress and undress. Days were enjoyable as the patient's wife would play the piano and entertain them. Veenhuis was paid $10.00 per day! After seven days, a relief night nurse was hired to assist until Mr. I. needed less attention. Later the family moved the patient to his Kalamazoo home on West Main where Veenhuis continued to provide care for three months, draining the wound and enhancing family morale!

Once she was called to a case in Vicksburg, taking the train and, arriving early in the evening, expecting a family member to pick her up. No one came. The custodian let her into the depot and said that she could stay all night if she didn't let anyone in, to which she agreed. Veenhuis welcomed the morning train and returned home. After that experience her family agreed that, if people wanted her in the evening, they should come for you at the house. About 10 years later, at a class reunion, her classmates admitted their prank. They had made the call and set her up for this disappointment. Why? She thought perhaps it was jealousy related to her connections with people, such as the U. family who had been nice to her. Wylie believed they were envious of her ability to see opportunities and take advantage of them. Veenhuis had learned a skill many nurses lacked, to be assertive and directly market her nursing skills.

Listening to early stories, it is important to note that nurses competed for available private-pay assignments. Almost no one was hired by the hospital after graduation with care provided by a nursing supervisor and students. Veenhuis's private duty practice seemed to be bolstered by her professional relationships with local physicians. She belonged to the Alumni Association of Bronson Methodist Hospital School of Nursing and the Michigan Nurses Association, a common practice. The nurse registry in Kalamazoo was connected to the Alumni Association giving physicians and families a way to directly contract with nurses. Private duty nursing, according to many of the Bronson nurses' stories, had a lot of "down-time." The pay was good, but there were too many days off for a stable, secure position for a single woman. Other barriers to work were the relatively few families who could afford private duty nurses and absence of an open referral system.

Continuing to live at home, whenever the telephone rang she expected her dad to say, "You'd better answer it. It's probably for you but don't go out into the country."

"In three years I'd had it." Twenty-four-hour-per-day duty took its toll. She didn't want to work full time forever, and once more the thought returned from her Woolworth days, "I don't want to do this forever." By 1924 Veenhuis learned of an opportunity to go to the University of Michigan.

Return to School: More Education, More Opportunities, 1924–1930

Again, Veenhuis spoke with Nurse Mary T. who told her about a meeting in Battle Creek where a professor, Barbara Bartlett, was to lecture about the need for public health nurses as well as scholarship money that was available for relevant courses. Veenhuis attended the lecture. As a result she enrolled at the University of Michigan. She was in class in Ann Arbor from September through February where she studied public health theory. After completing fieldwork in Detroit she received a B.S. degree from the University of Michigan. About Detroit, she described riding the streetcars in her white uniform and other passengers helping her find her way to her destination.

In City Hall one day she spied a hiring notice: Public Health Nurse Wanted in Monroe, Michigan. The pay was $1,100 a year! She was hired and stayed for five years. Her responsibilities included the establishment of a dental program for children, as well as daily health promotion/disease prevention activities that included checks for head lice on all children. Rich or poor, every head was examined. Well-to-do mothers were insulted by the head lice checks. Veenhuis pointed out that lice do not discriminate by social class. When cases were found, she taught mothers how to irradicate pediculosis with a chemical and fine combs, as well as how to prevent the ailment. "We had very little pediculosis, but it took constant surveillance to avert infestations."

She visited schools once a week. Schools furnished bathing facilities, including towels, washcloths and scrub brushes. Rubber caps were provided for girls with long hair. Children were able to shower twice weekly in the basement of the Lincoln School (probably a voluntary program for children whose families chose to participate). They would bring clean clothes with them. The showers provided an opportunity to play and so were popular with the children. Veenhuis supervised their hygiene activities and was responsible for disinfection of supplies and the environment. She boiled the little scrub brushes.

She bought a car the second year in Monroe. Her salary had increased to $1,500 and, with a car, she could get around faster plus do home calls.

Veenhuis was "just wandering around" at a Michigan Nurses Association meeting in Lansing when she noticed another job posting: Public Health Nurses Wanted. The position was with the Children's Fund of Michigan. She recalled that a senator established the fund with $10 million he withdrew from General Motors and Ford stocks. The fund's purpose was to bring healthcare, provided by a nurse, to every county north of the Bay City line.

Big Bay Camp in Marquette offered an all-summer program for children. "One of my jobs was to identify and take children there. My mother and two sisters helped me to transport the children to the camp destination. Once the children got over their homesickness, they loved it."

She accepted a job in Reed City as her next position. "We established committees in every county to provide support from each community. The people were lovely. All of the railroad people had cars. They transported children to clinics for us. We had the best of everything!" Visiting physicians assessed the children for dental and medical problems. They came from Grand Rapids, St. Ignace, and

Newberry, just to name a few. Veenhuis arranged for the monthly visits by setting up makeshift clinics in rural schoolhouses. The teachers would supply a table and sheets on her request. Veenhuis boiled two dozen syringes and needles at a time over a little sterno burner to sterilize them for small pox, diphtheria and influenza vaccinations. The doctors would draw up ten units of vaccine at a time and would change needles with each child. No electric was available in these rural areas. When the money ran out 12 years later, in 1942, Veenhuis left the position.

Extended Career Opportunities

With a summer off, she was on her way to New York Hospital Maternity Center for training in Obstetrics. "I wanted to know more about Obstetrics and I thought I needed a little change. That's when the fair was on, and I really enjoyed it."

Upon her return, she worked in St. Ignace until family illness required her to change direction—back to Kalamazoo. Her father had diabetes and her mother was not well. Her mother, father and one set of grandparents were living in the family's Vine Street home, so she moved in again to be present for them.

Veenhuis worked for the Kalamazoo City Health Department for a short time and then as an emergency nurse for a Navy tank-building company in town at the North Plant on Pitcher Street. Three years later the company relocated to Riverside, California. She loved California, had been there once on vacation, and would have moved with the company, but felt she could not leave her ailing family.

"All the time I was working I took courses at Western [Michigan College.] I studied a little Spanish now and then, which I enjoyed. The professor said nobody was going out the door until they could speak Spanish. I earned my degree in biology and nursing and graduated in 1949. I was granted credit for my previous nurses' training."[33]

While she was at Western, another avenue of work presented itself in the form of the Metropolitan Life Insurance Company (MLIC) as a part-time relief nurse.

Veenhuis recalled having lunch at the Van Avery Drug Store on the north side of town where "the agents were good about referring moms and new babies for nursing care. MLIC offered $500 life insurance policies to families for $0.10 per week. A visiting nurse came with the policy.

As a side note, at an earlier time nurses had sold insurance policies and also provided healthcare, what a great way to provide insurance and health promotion for a broad population. However, the nurses perceived this approach as a conflict of interest and chose to back out of the agreement with Metropolitan Life. It was unfortunate for patients and nurses that a suitable compromise to their dilemma could not be found so the program was dropped. MLIC was wonderful and even paid mileage according to Veenhuis.

Audibly sighing, she recalled her 1950 marriage to Mr. Cody, a man she met at the Ingersoll Steel Company while working in industrial nursing. His untimely death, four years later, left her widowed but not without her wit or ability to work. He may have had leukemia but would not seek the care he needed at the Veterans Center in Fort Custer, Battle Creek. Before her marriage, his mother had told her that he had some health problems. During our interview, it was as if the married part of her life was quite insignificant, and her grief was either well hidden or had been forgotten years ago.

After her husband's death, Veenhuis went back to Western Michigan College. She believed that nurses should continue their education because of the constant change in practice, and her advice was, "Take a foreign language!" She found her ability to speak Spanish helpful to her career and making friends. An outsider, she could quickly become an "insider" by her ability to speak the language. "If I said something in Spanish, they opened the gate for me."

She returned to private duty, caring for a Kalamazoo woman, Mrs. G., off and on, for six years. She was paid well but, toward the end, the 24-hour duty became too much to manage at this time in her life.

Close to retirement she worked as a Girl Scout Camp nurse for two summers. "Then I decided I had had enough and would enjoy life instead." She retired at 64 years of age with social security. Retirement didn't last long. Her sister was ill with Parkinson's disease and diabetes. Veenstra moved her from a nursing home in Holland, Michigan, to the family's Vine Street home. "I cared for her in this room [the room in which the interview was conducted] for nine years until she died."

Veenhuis seized the day over and over throughout her life and nursing career. I never heard her utter a word of disappointment other than the moment when she discovered that her classmates had played a trick on her early in her career. That too seemed to have been forgiven with no hard feelings. She lived her life as a devoted nurse and family member and also took care of herself. Always on the lookout for opportunities, she found academic and work experiences—moving on when the challenge was gone and interest had waned. She was a strong, hard-working woman, not a saint or martyr. I wonder who cared for her in her last years? I suspect that she died with her boots on. I hope so.

MARGARET KITZMILLER LA MAR '27

At the time, a nursing superintendent's power rested in her ability to interpret and implement medical culture needs and wishes. Students were the conduit. Kitzmiller shares excerpts (which have been edited herein) of her 1920s nursing school story in a letter written September 13, 1997. Her story is upbeat, and says how much she enjoyed nurses training. The medical-driven culture comes to mind throughout her story.

"I was in the class of 1927 and loved every minute of it. I roomed with Harriet Troxell Stetler in West Home during our last two years. We had one bathroom with a tub and, if you wanted a bath, you shared it with two to five girls.

"Mina Weber was the superintendent of nurses for my first year and a half. Ann Draher followed her. Half way through my second year, I almost quit the program because Mrs. Draher continually made changes in the curriculum and student routine. I hung in there because nursing was my life. I couldn't remember when I didn't want to be a nurse, and I had never been in a hospital until I went to nurses' training.

"Once, in my second year, the student nurses were assigned by Mrs. Draher to scrub the floors. When the doctors found out, they had a fit. Ten hours was enough they said. Still, we cleaned the patient rooms when they left, and I mean, cleaned!

"I loved night duty but had a terrible time sleeping. Once I took three sleeping pills and could barely waken at 7:00 P.M. for night duty. I was on the OB floor with three new women in labor by 10:00 P.M. I never took pills again. We had two hours off during the night if we weren't too busy. Our cook was Blanche, and she favored the night crews!

"I signed up with mortuary for early morning autopsies. I would take notes for the pathologist. I learned more anatomy that way! I helped in this way when I was on night duty and before I went to bed. Sometimes, after working all night, I had to attend Dr. Hubbell's lectures at one to two o'clock in the afternoon. Most of the lectures, however, were at eight o'clock to nine o'clock, after night duty.

"I loved surgery and I worshiped Dr. Charles Boys. We called him "Charley my boy!" I loved surgery. One of the first times I scrubbed for him he jabbed me with his elbow and said, "Come on, come on, what's the matter with you?" I was devastated and got tears—had to blow my nose several times, but hung in there. Mrs. Wildermuth who administered anesthesia for his patients, remarked about how awful he was that day. After the surgery was over, I was in the service room blowing again. Dr. Boys came out, put his hand on my shoulder, and said, "Going to bawl about it?" I said, "No, I'm not, I'm too damn mad!" After that encounter, I could do no wrong. He often asked for me to scrub.

"One day Dr. Boys scheduled a woman for a hysterectomy and repair at the South Haven Hospital. He asked Mrs. Draher if I could go with him to scrub and look after his instruments. She let me go! I was in seventh heaven, walking on air! Mrs. Wildermuth did not go that day.

"After graduation, I did private duty for a short time. Then Dr. Boys called and asked if I'd like a surgical job in Battle Creek, working for a Dr. Stone. I said, "Of course I would." This practice included going to the hospital, helping with surgery in the morning and assisting in the physician's office in the afternoon.[34] I applied, was hired, and went to work two weeks later.

"After nine months in Battle Creek, my ex-roommate, Harriet Troxell, visited from California where she had moved and married. She told me about a 30-bed hospital in South San Francisco. Her husband went to see the doctor there and asked if they needed a surgical nurse. I got the job after he told the doctor about me. I traveled to California on the train with Harriet and went to work three days after arriving. Work was a ten-hour day, the same as Michigan. I worked in surgery and as head nurse throughout the war and for the next 22 years.

"In retrospect, I think I would have been a good doctor. Nursing was next best. I hung in there because it was my life."

JENNIE BAST BELL '28

Entering Bronson's nursing school was a way for Jennie Bast to get an education. At the time she had never been in a hospital! In September of 1925 she came prepared with blue and white chambray dresses, and black shoes and stockings. She remembers every morning, at 6:30 A.M. standing at breakfast and singing:

Be present at our table Lord
Be here and everywhere adored
These mercies bless and grant that we
May feast in Paradise with thee.

At first, Bast was homesick and asked her parents to come take her home. They came, bringing a lunch which she couldn't eat because she was so sick. Her father encouraged her to come home with them, but her much wiser mother said, "Stay two more weeks—if you still want to come home we will come back." After her parents left, never again was she so homesick.

About her schooling, she relates that her chores were numerous, and the students were more or less maids. They did everything except mop floors, including: changing flowers, washing bed pans, rubber sheets, and bed sheets; making up vacant rooms, and then going to class when the staff doctors had time to teach.

It was Christmas season at Detroit's Herman Kiefer Hospital in 1927 and Bast recalls these "Laughable Memories":

> We six girls were about at the close of our Contagious Disease training. We were all feeling sorry for ourselves because we would be away from home over the holidays. It was decided that we would pool our food parcels from home and have a real bash on Christmas Eve.
>
> So it was we gathered in Abbott's and Bast's room for the spread. We were ready to enjoy the goodies—the beds were put together and everything looked delicious. What happened next remains an indelible memory. Someone bumped the beds! What a catastrophe we faced!!
>
> Shall we pick our precious goodies off the floor and risk contracting all these horrible diseases we were nursing? Resounding in our ears was the admonishment: NEVER, NEVER, eat anything that drops on the floor! We even had seen visible evidence of all the germs that were under our soles!
>
> What was our decision? It was unanimous that we risk exposure to all those germs. The food was enjoyed and a happy hour shared that none of us would ever forget.
>
> ***Merry Christmas to the Survivors!***

ANNE REIFF RAISCH '29

This 1929 graduate spoke of her student experience in third person and provided a window into a student's life, from beginning training to graduation. Her story describing the ordinary days of nursing students included numerous significant emotional events, showing her emotional state as a "sister of confusion." For her, the educational highlight was that friends made in training were cherished for a lifetime. Wylie sensed why their shared experience unified the nursing students for the rest of their lives.

Reiff remembered being eight years old and sitting through the long night with her father, by her mother's hospital door. On a hard bench in the darkened corridor, she watched through sleep-dimmed eyes as the nurses, in their softly rustling, starched uniforms, drifted waif-like in and out of her mother's room, always closing the door firmly. They spoke in hurried, staccato whispers and carried covered basins, and trays or armloads of neatly folded linens. It was eerie, a little frightening, but intriguing, too. Her mind focused on what the nurses were doing to her mother behind that closed door. She decided to find out one day, even if she had to become a nurse. There was no idealistic motive, just curiosity that brought a naïve country girl to Bronson in September of 1926. Three months after graduating from high school at age 17, Bronson Methodist Hospital admitted an unsophisticated farm girl, Anne Reiff, into its Nurses' Training Program. A wide-eyed, eager, but frightened novice stepped into the world.

First Came Probation

On arrival Reiff was assigned to a room in an old Victorian house which had been converted into a dormitory upstairs and classrooms on the first floor. In the large upstairs front bedroom, she met two roommates who seemed relaxed, enthusiastic, and friendly. Four other probies occupied the back two bedrooms. Alarm clocks were set for 6 o'clock. Chapel was a daily ritual. It preceded breakfast with prayers and Bible readings. Breakfast was served at 6:30, and the first duty shift was at 7 A.M.

The probationers presented themselves in their blue and white striped uniforms trimmed with detachable, stiffly starched, white collars and cuffs, plus a gathered white apron which matched the hem length of the dress. Black oxfords with black cotton stockings completed the uniforms. While the staff hurried off to the floors on that first day, probies were given a tour of the facility and classes began. The instructor was a patient, compassionate and kind nurse. We were further indoctrinated in patient care by daily contacts with nurses and physicians whose kindness and compassion did not always extend to students.

The days were filled with learning rules, duties and theory. Everyone addressed each other as “Miss.” First names were a no-no. Students were to stand whenever an attending physician or other VIP came within speaking distance. Duty hours were from 7 A.M. until 7 P.M. with class time off. If the workload permitted, the supervisor scheduled a three-hour break for each nurse, which was usually possible if no classes were scheduled. Two half days off, one during the week and another on Sunday, were given to all students.

When class ended, other tasks were assigned, such as fixing flowers, putting away linen, passing or collecting dinner trays, and then there was always the service room with its stacks of bedpans and enamelware to be scrubbed and sterilized. If work was slack, 4”x4” gauze sponges were waiting to be folded, “Be sure the loose ends are tucked inside.”

The newcomers became “sisters in confusion.” They studied together and practiced bed-making and applying splints using each other as patients, in lieu of a mannequin, Mrs. Chase. They commiserated with each other over myriad things not understood and, through the trying months, became friends for a lifetime.

During Reiff’s probation, the hospital had acquired a handsome Victorian house, the Dewing House, adjacent to its property. One colorful, warm, autumn day, the probies, with their heads swathed in diapers and wearing discarded patients' gowns, cleaned the basement of the house. It was filled with shelves of ancient canned fruit and the usual accumulation of debris, not touched for generations. The leader of this policing detail was no less than the superintendent of nurses. Some probies grumbled about the indignity of the task but for most it was a welcome change from the routine. The old mansion hosted a hilarious Halloween party that year, when all the slimy, chain-rattling, practical jokes, known by generations of nurses, were trotted out by the upper classmen to frighten the wits out of the probies.

Boyfriends visited on weekends, the visits limited by a 10 o'clock curfew. The dorm doors were locked at that hour, and woe unto any wayward young woman who climbed down the fire escape to go for a joy ride. Scuttlebutt had it that two seniors, attempting an escape, ended in the police station following an automobile mishap. They were suspended, but received their diplomas in late August, months after their classmates graduated.

After duty hours came study time, with a few exceptions such as making fudge on the Bunsen burner in the makeshift lab behind the classroom. Many attended the movie matinee at the theater down the street on their half-days off, paid for out of the five-dollar stipend they received each month. Gossip, girl talk, and singing, accompanied on a ukulele, also made for fun and relaxation after a stressful day.

After the six months' probationary period, the candidates were judged on their scholastic and practical abilities. The lucky ones were given a starched school cap and a white bib. This capping ritual was held in the parlor of one of the dorms. The ceremony was complete with punch, cookies and congratulations.

Patient Care Begins

As full-fledged students the freshmen advanced to more complicated procedures on the floor. The routine, daily care of the patients included bed care, enemas, temperatures, blood pressures, *etc.* Until a new class arrived, service room chores, with their everlasting bedpan detail, always awaited.

By the middle of the second year fundamentals of patient care had been mastered, and textbooks, with unfamiliar names like materia medica, anatomy, principles of nursing, pathology, dietetics, and pediatrics were part of the vocabulary. Obstetrics occupied most of the second floor, and it was next on the list of services to be learned. To a student who had been raised on a farm, witnessing the birth of calves and puppies, obstetrics was not entirely a mystery. Reiff, however, was not prepared for her first experience as an observer in the delivery room. After a difficult labor the patient was delivered of hydrocephalic twin babies. They were mercifully left on the table where they died peacefully, without interference.

Eventually, a senior student was assigned to night duty as the obstetrics charge-nurse, while several other students cared for the mothers and their babies. It was a busy time, with both labor and delivery rooms needing attention. One day, at evening report, one student did not answer roll call and no one knew where she was. When the graduate in charge of the hospital that night came on the floor, however, she said very matter-of-factly that the missing student had given birth to a full-term baby that afternoon and had been transferred to another facility.

Reiff was stunned. In her first term as a charge nurse, her first real responsibility, she had been unaware that one of her staff was carrying a full-term baby under her gathered apron. There was some comfort in the knowledge that no one else knew either.

In the obstetrical labor room, the continual need of rectal examinations to determine the dilatation of the cervix in the final stages of labor was a problem. This was a crucial responsibility. Without resident physicians it was necessary to call the attending doctor at precisely the right time; if too early the culprit who made the error was open to severe censure by both the nurse supervisor and the doctor and an additional ribbing by the other nurses. Fortunately, the obstetrical supervisor, Miss

Marie Wantz, was a compassionate person. At night she made the final decision for an indecisive student.

As for nursery duty, one baby would surely be a joy, but 20 or so could be frustrating. Sometimes a loud mouth boy, often at least nine pounds, sounded as though he belonged in Pediatrics when he woke up a peaceful nursery at 3:00 A.M. Understandably, a busy nurse might shove the delinquent into the hall or even the linen closet for a time.

Diapers were not disposable; they were thoroughly cleaned before being deposited in the diaper pail. Bottles and nipples were sterilized, and the formula came from the diet kitchen.

Because it was part of the well-rounded nurse's experience, all were required to "special" a patient for a 24-hour shift. One second-year student was assigned to an adult tonsillectomy patient and seeing that her post-op care—ice-collar, emesis basin, *etc.*, was provided properly. When it was time to "put the patient to bed," the student carefully filled the ice-collar, and attended to the back-rub and any other TLC that came to mind. It was spring so an extra blanket was folded on the foot of the patient's bed and another on the nurse's cot. The window was opened a bit, as requested, before the nurse retired to her cot along the opposite wall. Even though the student tried to sleep lightly, she wasn't awakened until she heard the morning noises in the hall. Horrified lest her patient had hemorrhaged or choked to death during the night, she was relieved to see that her charge was sleeping quietly. She was chagrined, however, when she realized that the patient had closed the window and neatly spread the blankets on both bed and cot. When the patient was dismissed that afternoon, she gave her embarrassed "special" nurse a silver compact and a box of candy. All patients were not that understanding.

There were perks when on diet kitchen duty, but the dietician's eyes appeared to be in the back of her head when goodies for a study-hour snack found their way into a uniform pocket. Kitchen duty wasn't exciting work, but you couldn't kill anybody either. Many of the classes were taught by doctors who specialized in particular fields.

Learning Advanced Nursing Practices

To further prepare for any eventuality, students spent three months at the Herman Keifer Communicable Disease Hospital in Detroit, known as the pest house. Again, the prospective nurses were reminded of the rigid discipline required in identifying "clean and contaminated" areas when dealing with quarantined patients. As a student nurse, to contract a communicable disease was a disgrace to the training school, and a blot on its record. Classmates, too, were inclined to be reproachful, even though the sinner was sick as a dog. Unfortunately, when one of the girls ended up with a strep throat, she also faced the wrath of the superintendent of nurses when she returned home potentially to infect other members of her family. Medical aseptic practices literally meant the difference between health, morbidity and mortality. Infectious diseases accounted for most morbidity and mortality. Prevention of disease contraction was expected—not to get the disease or to pass it on.

By the third year, sterile procedures, such as performing catheterizations, giving hypodermics, preparing sterile trays for intravenous, and spinals, *etc.*, were routine, and surgery duty was assigned. Students were not allowed to give IVs.

The OR was special. Maybe it was because the suite was on the top floor. Most girls approached those big, white, swinging, double doors with apprehension and awe. All had been warned from day one that, in surgery, there was no room for error. Discipline and strict compliance with every rule were imperative. Even with the background acquired on the floors, in the OR there was much more to remember. The surgeons were big, brisk, and generally intimidating; to the unsophisticated student, they seemed from another planet, remote and unapproachable.

The trainee newcomer to surgery served as the prep nurse. An orderly did the male preps.[35] The evening preceding surgery the trainee collected specimens and did the urinalyses. Whatever skin preparation was needed, shaving and applying antiseptic, was also her job. She was a "gofer" during the day, honed hypo needles, and washed syringes to be sterilized. Instruments were washed and put in the cabinets. Instruments were boiled in small sterilizers and carried, hot and dripping, by the circulating nurse to the scrub nurse. The rubber gloves were washed, tested for holes and sterilized. Sponges, not the disposable kind, were usually woven and were called "lap pads." Big metal drums, packed with the carefully folded linens with which to drape the patients and tables during surgery, were autoclaved. Floors were washed, along with furniture if needed. Discipline for some rules infraction or for breaking sterile technique had the culprit washing down the O.R. walls.

The operating room supervisor, Miss Dena Wolters, was a superb teacher. She put the fear of contamination so firmly in students' minds that they never forgot it. Ever! Surgical asepsis was an awesome responsibility.[36] It seemed a miracle to become a scrub nurse, pass instruments to the surgeon, and not suffer his wrath when a clamp instead of a suture was passed into his outstretched hand. Satisfaction came in knowing that after months of hard work and frustration, the effort had been worthwhile. Your work could really matter.

Many procedures practiced 50 years ago are archaic today (Reiff related her story February 2, 1989). For instance, pneumonia patients and the nurses who took care of them once were subjected to icy rooms. Open windows provided oxygen, while layers of blankets and hot water bottles kept the patient from freezing to death. Along with mustard plasters, turpentine stupes were commonly used for abdominal problems. After 15 minutes, when thick flannels were twisted in the stupe wringer and put in place, both the nurse's hands and the patient's belly were red from the counterirritant.

The primary thrust of nurses' training was for the patient's well-being and comfort. Instructors admonished their students over and over again to, "Turn at the door after attending the patient and ask, 'Are you comfortable?' 'May I get you anything else?'" It saved a bell sometimes, and ensured a warm, friendly atmosphere.

It was a hard school for Reiff and her classmates. They learned a great deal: discipline, a respect for the patient—even the cantankerous ones—and a feeling of contributing substantially to the health field. Best of all, the friends made in training were cherished for a lifetime.

CHAPTER 2 NOTES

---

[1] Bronson Methodist Hospital School of Nursing Alumni Association's minutes are held in the alumni archives.

[2] Born September 10, 1891, daughter of Emma and Joseph Weber, raised on a farm in St. Joseph County, MI. Mina was the third child of four, Leo, Carol, Mina and Lulu.

[3] Oral interview with Janet Camery, by Jackie Wylie, 1998 August 8.

[4] Oral interview with Cornelia Veenhuis Cody, by Jackie Wylie, 1989 February 28.

[5] Kalamazoo pioneer roentgenologist, Dr. Augustus W. Crane, was world-renowned in the early 1900s for his clinical applications of the roentgen ray in diagnostic procedures. His practice would have made it necessary for local nurses to learn about nursing care related to radiologic procedures.

[6] Oral interview and perusal of personal family documents with Janet Camery, by Jackie Wylie, 1998 August 8.

[7] Mina Weber Macgrayne included dated notes of important events in her personal journal.

[8] Jean Lemmer Vander Molen is the stepmother of Richard Vander Molen who is the only honorary Bronson graduate.

[9] Janet Macgrayne Camery was Mina Weber's daughter.

[10] Mrs. D. C. Macgrayne's name appears as a member of the School of Nursing Committee in an annual report submitted to the Michigan Board of Registration of Nurses and Trained Attendants for the year ending April 30, 1944.

[11] *Kalamazoo Gazette,* 1990 March 8, Amy Bailey Seward obituary.

[12] Oral interview with Amy Bailey Seward, by Mary Lou Stewart, 1985 July 3.

[13] Age for admission apparently was lowered to 17 years or an exception to the general rule was made for Bailey.

---

[14] Oral interview with Amy Bailey Seward, *op.cit.*

[15] Reverby, S. M. *Ordered to care: the dilemma of American nursing, 1850–1945*, n.p., 1987. pp.77–84.

[16] *Kalamazoo Gazette*, 1903 December 5, "Change in plans for the hospital/"

[17] *Catalyst,* 18(4): 1979 April; 9. "Amy Bailey Seward."

[18] Oral interview with Janet Swain, by Jackie Wylie, 1997 July 30.

[19] Freire, P. *Pedagogy of the oppressed,* 20th ed. Continuum Publishing, 1997.

[20] Oral interview with Amy Bailey Seward, *op.cit.*

[21] Oral history with Ruth Hinds Phelps, taken by Jackie Wylie, 1989.

[22] Eleanor Roosevelt's thank you note was donated to the Alumni Association by Janet Swain, Amy Bailey Seward's great niece. It is housed with the Alumni Association files at the Western Michigan University Archives.

[23] Oral interview with Amy Bailey Seward, *op.cit.*

[24] Funeral Instructions for Mrs. A. L. Seward (Amy Bailey Seward), n.d.

[25] Men in nursing were scarce in the nonsectarian world and so the term, sisterhood, applies. Records show that one man, Earl Cowlbeck, graduated in 1908 followed by William Huber in 1913. Another man does not graduate until Paul Johnson in 1975. According to a *Kalamazoo Gazette* account, Mr. Cowlbeck served in the U.S. Army Medical Corps. He quit nursing after marrying and fathering three children, since one could not support a family on nurses' wages.

[26] Oral interview with Cornelia Veenhuis Cody, by Marge Kars and Jackie Wylie, 1989 February 28.

[27] Mrs. Edna Wildermuth was the superintendent of nurses at Bronson Hospital from 1917–1920.

[28] The "probie" designation was given to nursing students during the first months of their education and training. They were on probation and were very conscious that dismissal would occur if they did not meet all rules, regulations and course requirements.

[29] Blanche Hermann Winslow was a 1919 Bronson graduate.

[30] Dr. Puffer became the hospital superintendent in 1920, the first Methodist minister to lead at Bronson when the Michigan Methodist Episcopal Church took over hospital management.

[31] Mr. Kindleberger was an executive of the Kalamazoo Vegetable Parchment paper mill.

[32] Kitchen operations were not uncommon. People often preferred care in familiar surroundings and did not choose to be in the hospital with strangers or, could not afford to pay. (I heard about numerous home operation stories as I listened and read numerous graduate stories about family illness experiences.)

---

[33] Western Michigan University, formerly Western Michigan College, offered a BS degree with a major in nursing to RNs who had completed Bronson Methodist Hospital School of Nursing plus completed two more years of study at the College. The program existed in the 1940s and early 1950s before being disbanded.

[34] RNs working for physicians in their offices and as their private scrub nurses was a common model still being practiced in the 1960s at Bronson.

[35] A surgical prep consisted of cleansing and shaving body hair from the operative site and surrounding area.

[36] Remember, this was a day without antibiotics. If patients developed the complication of a wound infection, recovery depended as much on their innate immune systems as on incision and drainage of the infected wound. The risk of death increased significantly.

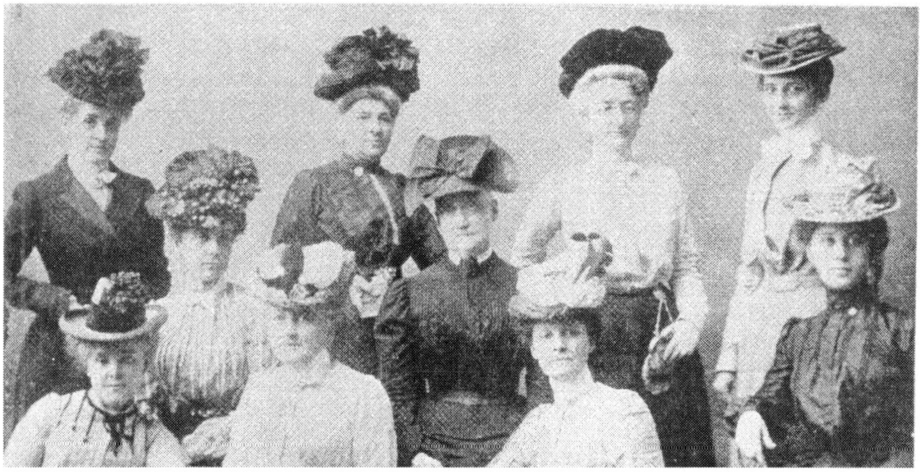

1. (above) The Trolley Day volunteer ladies raised local money for the downtown Bronson Hospital. (left to right, top) Mrs. A.K.Edwards, Mrs. Samuel Rosenbaum, Mrs. Ira Ransom, Miss Elizabeth Holtenhouse; (middle) Mrs. F.F.Rowe, Mrs. J.M.Edwards; (bottom) Mrs. Mary Cobb, Mrs. Shellmire, Mrs. Charles Peck, Mrs. Perley Abbey.

2. (below) Bronson Hospital in 1904, when the School of Nursing was founded. The 46-bed institution had seven nurses. Four, including Rena Koster Bosker, had had two years training, and the other three were students.

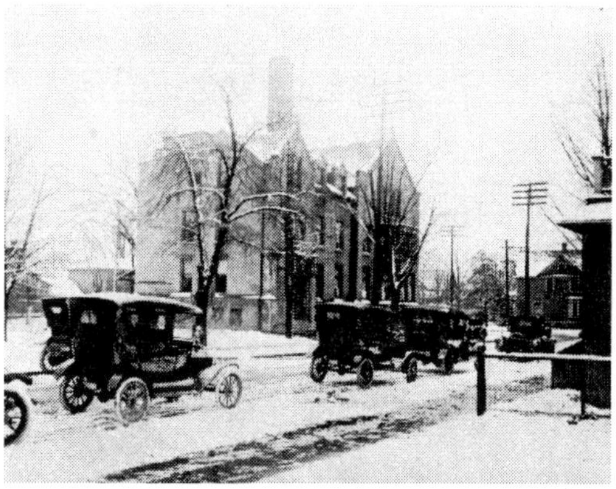

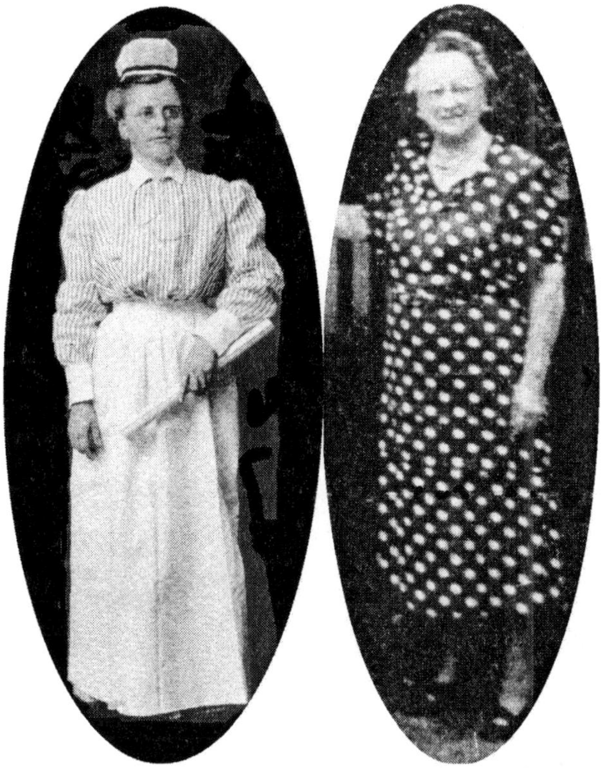

3. (left) Rena Koster, first graduate of Bronson Hospital 1903, and Rena Koster Bosker 1954. Students graduated from the hospital before the official establishment of the School of Nursing in 1904.

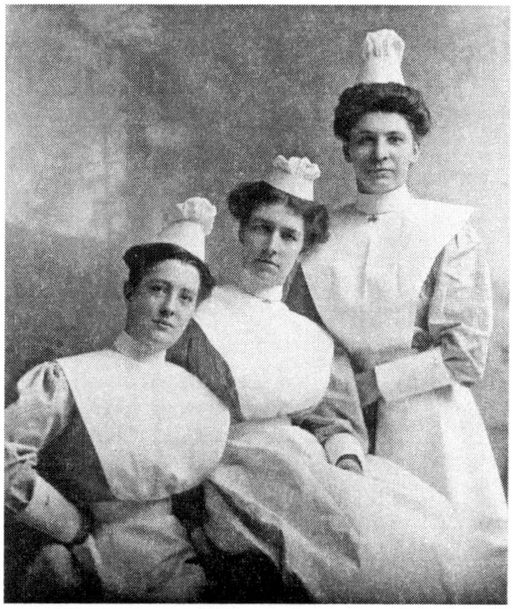

4. (above) Graduating class 1909, left to right: Theresa Norberg, Mae Fye, Nellie Brody. Notice how the caps are folded and worn.

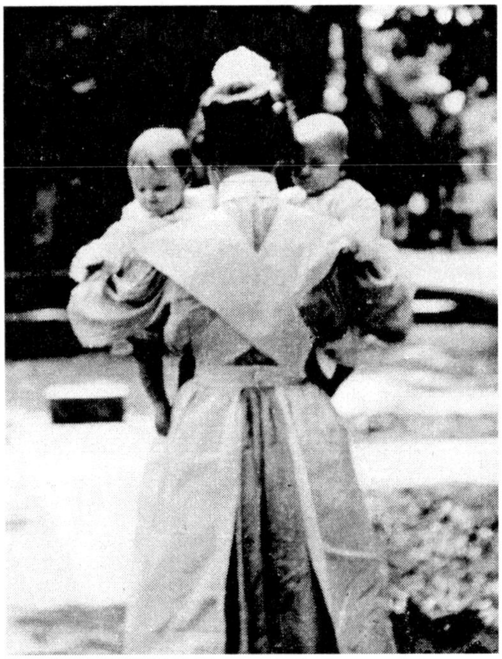

5. Frances Flower holding unidentified twins. Frances, who graduated in 1911, is wearing her student uniform.

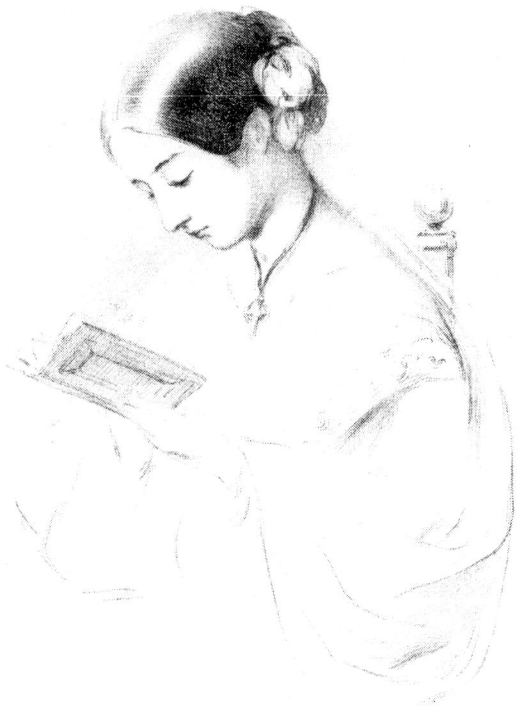

6. Florence Nightingale, drawing by Hilary Bonham-Carter.

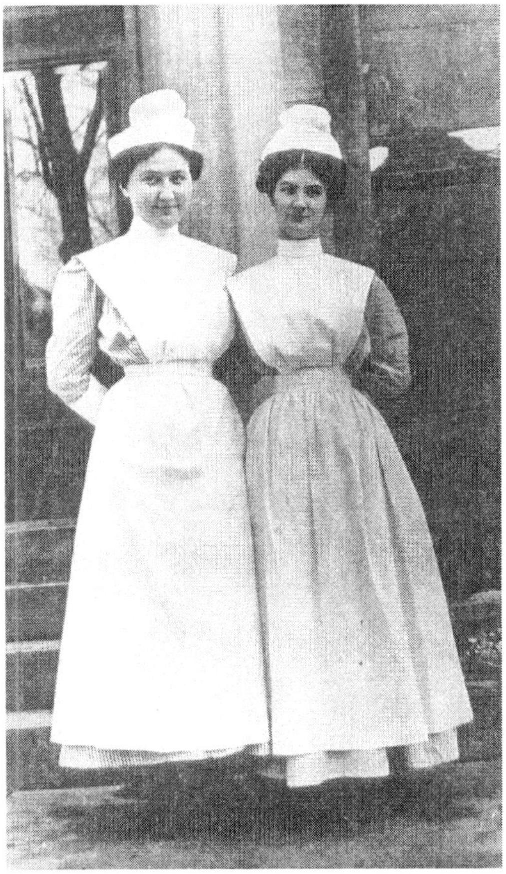

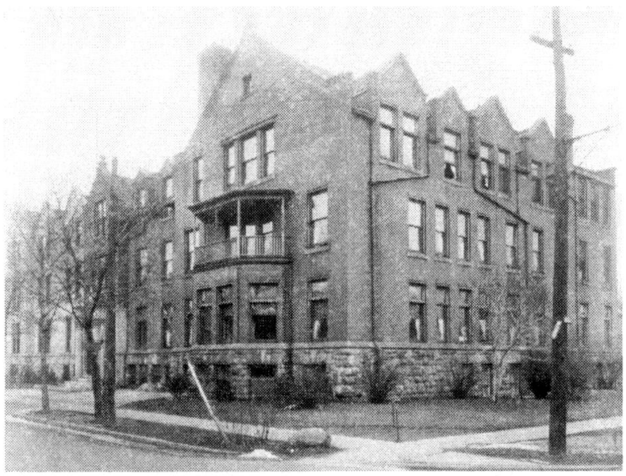

7. (above) Bronson Methodist Hospital, circa early 1900s. Entrance door is also door into what more recently was known as Wesley Hall.

8. (left) Students Mina Weber and Lulu Teller standing in front of the hospital, circa 1911–1913. Mina Weber graduated in 1913.

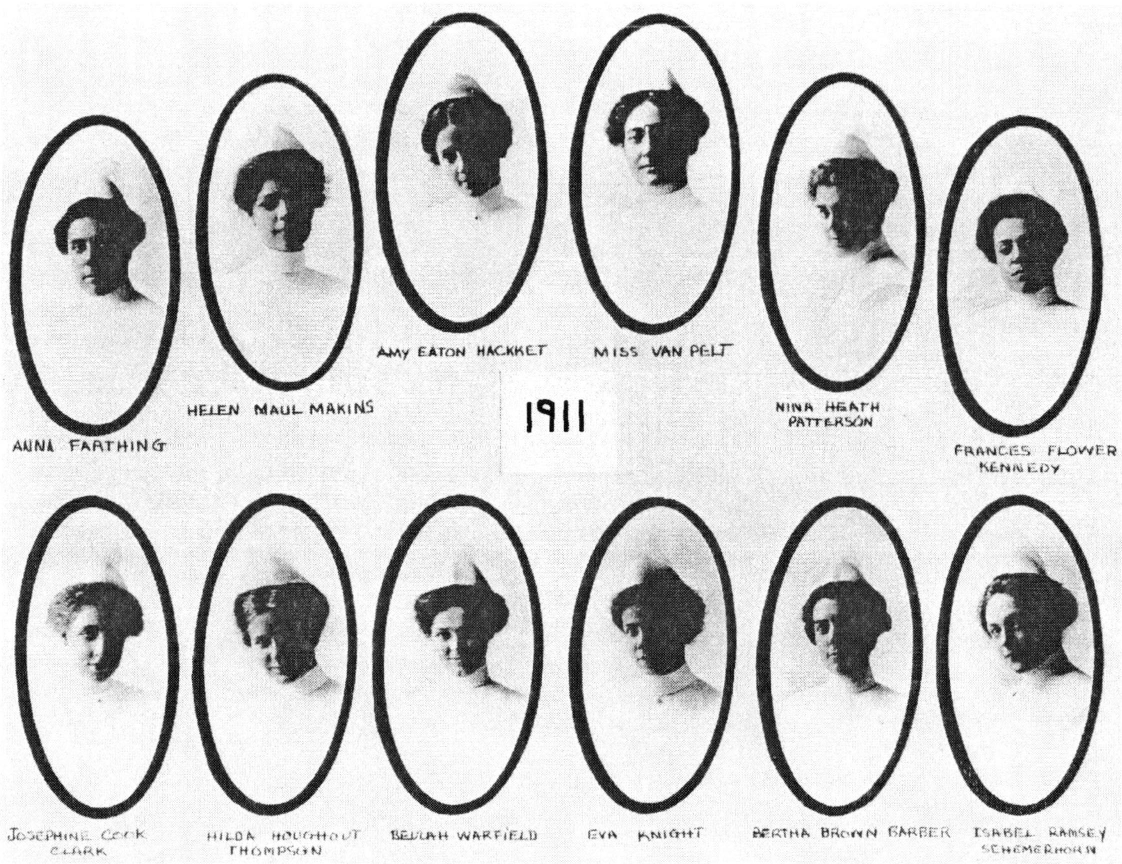

9. Miss Van Pelt was Director of Nursing for School of Nursing graduates in 1911.

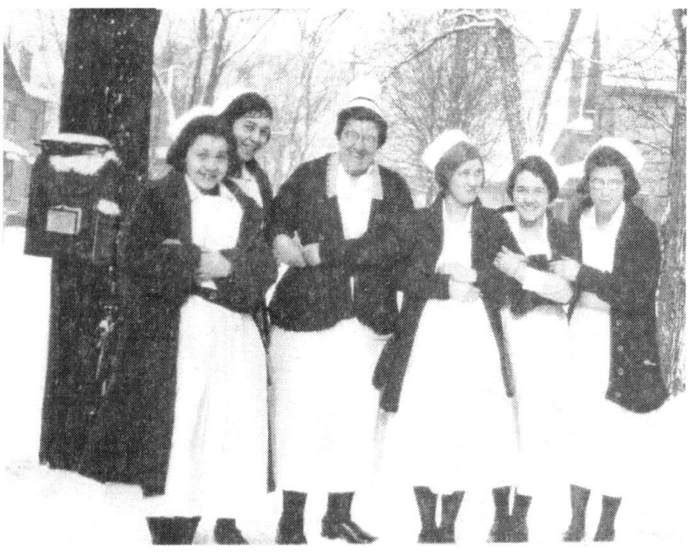

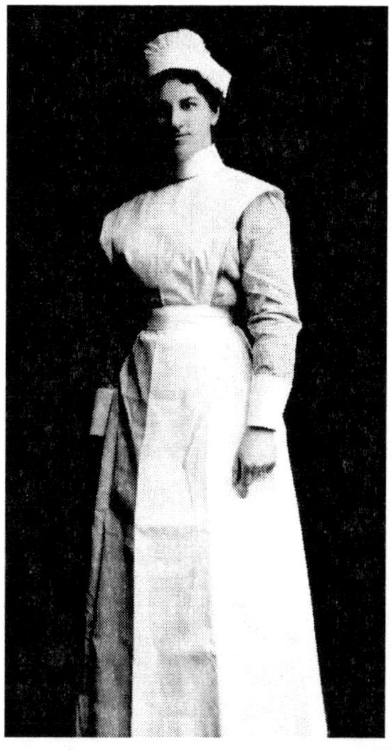

10. (above) Student nurses wore black stockings and shoes before they wore capes, 1918.

11. (right) Anna Heethuis wore a student uniform in 1914.

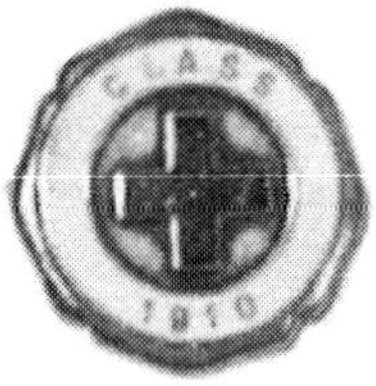
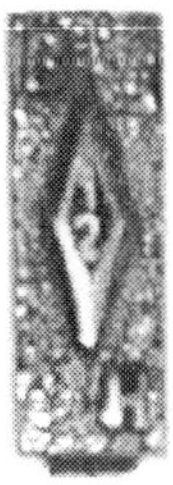
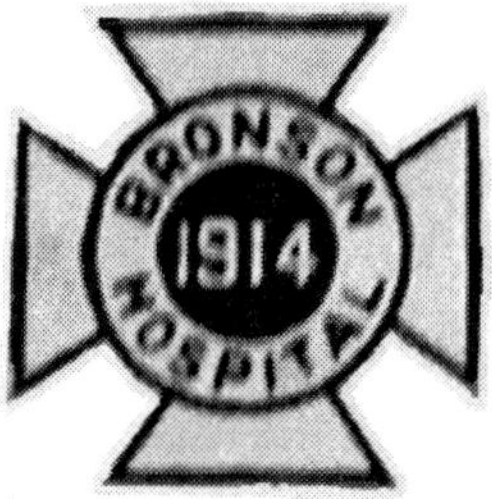

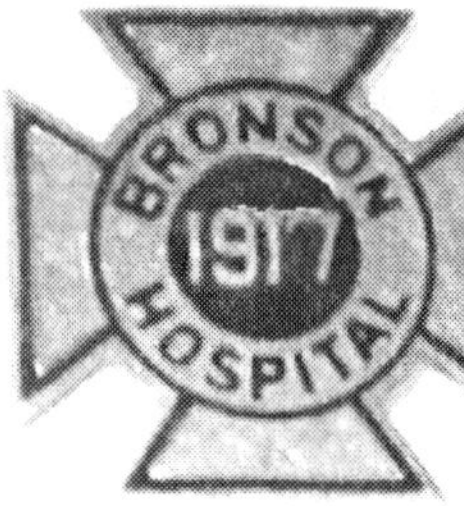

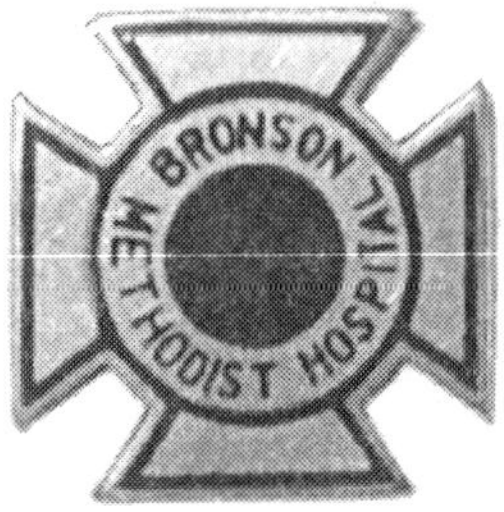

12. Class and graduation pins, 1910 – 1928

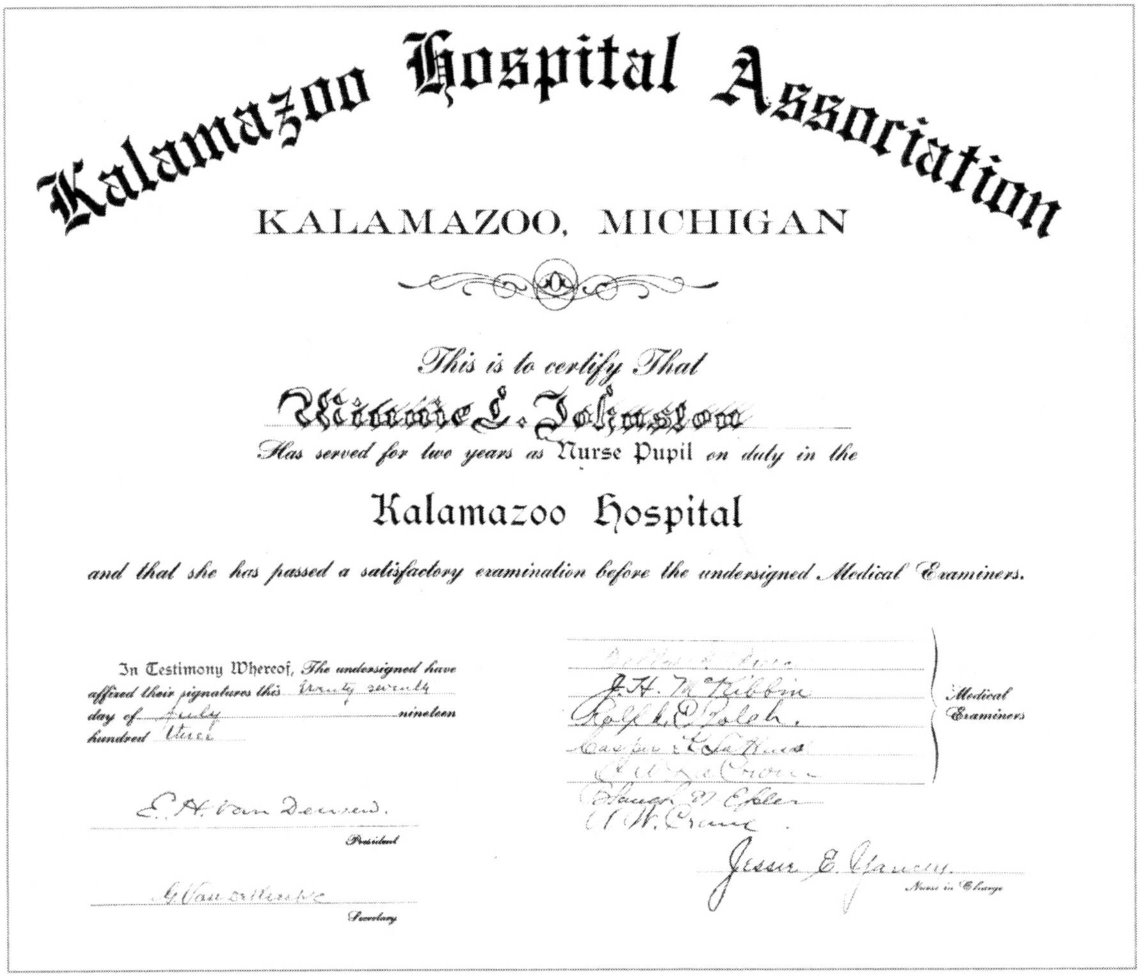

Kalamazoo Hospital Association

KALAMAZOO, MICHIGAN

This is to certify That

Minnie L. Johnston

Has served for two years as Nurse Pupil *on duty in the*

Kalamazoo Hospital

and that she has passed a satisfactory examination before the undersigned Medical Examiners.

In Testimony Whereof, *The undersigned have affixed their signatures this* twenty seventh *day of* July *nineteen hundred* three

E. H. Van Deusen.
President

Secretary

J. H. McKibbin
A. W. Crane
Medical Examiners

Nurse in Charge

13. Minnie Johnston was in the first graduating class before the school of nursing was officially established. Her graduation certificate certified that she had served for two years as a "nurse pupil" and satisfactorily passed her examination before seven medical examiners, 1903.

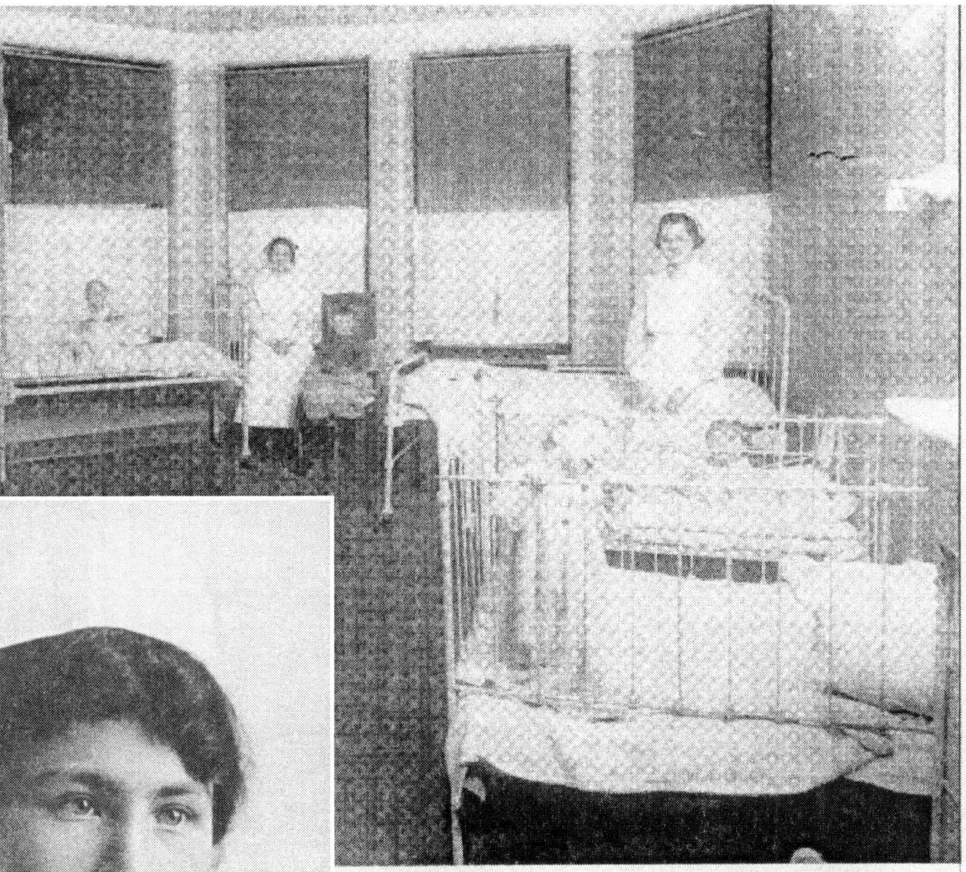

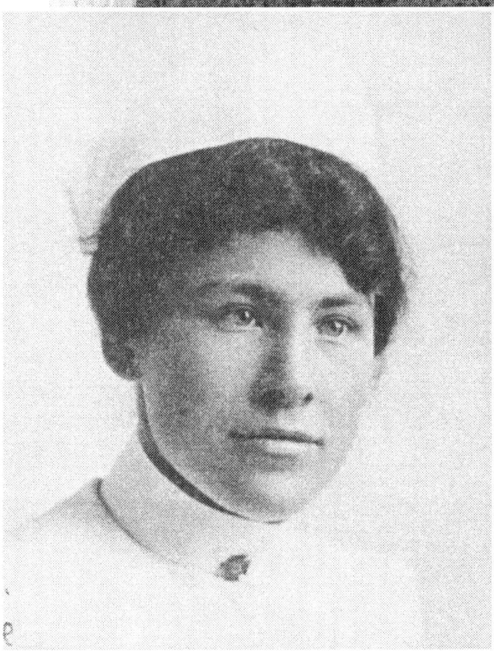

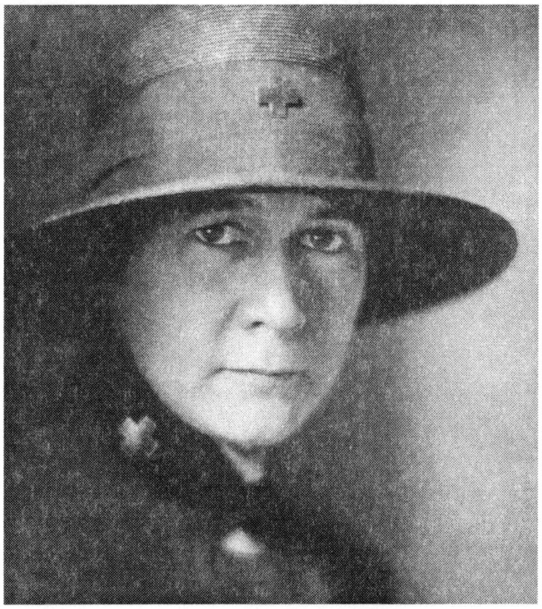

14. (clockwise from above) Lois Zerwis, Class of 1915;

15. Pediatric unit, circa early 1900s. There was no equipment in the rooms, just cribs and a wheelchair;

16. Mina Weber, 1913 Bronson School of Nursing graduate, served in France during World War I as a Red Cross nurse.

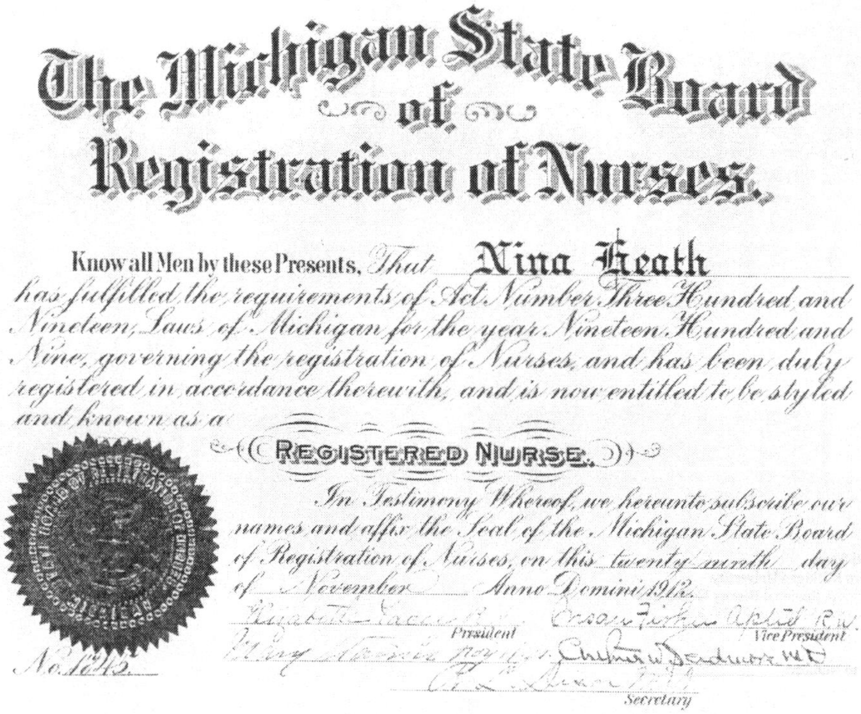

The Michigan State Board of Registration of Nurses.

Know all Men by these Presents, That Nina Heath has fulfilled the requirements of Act Number Three Hundred and Nineteen, Laws of Michigan for the year Nineteen Hundred and Nine, governing the registration of Nurses, and has been duly registered in accordance therewith, and is now entitled to be styled and known as a

REGISTERED NURSE.

In Testimony Whereof, we hereunto subscribe our names and affix the Seal of the Michigan State Board of Registration of Nurses, on this twenty ninth day of November Anno Domini 1912.

President

Vice President

Secretary

No. 1245

17. Michigan State Board of Nurses Registration for Nina Heath dated November 29, 1912.

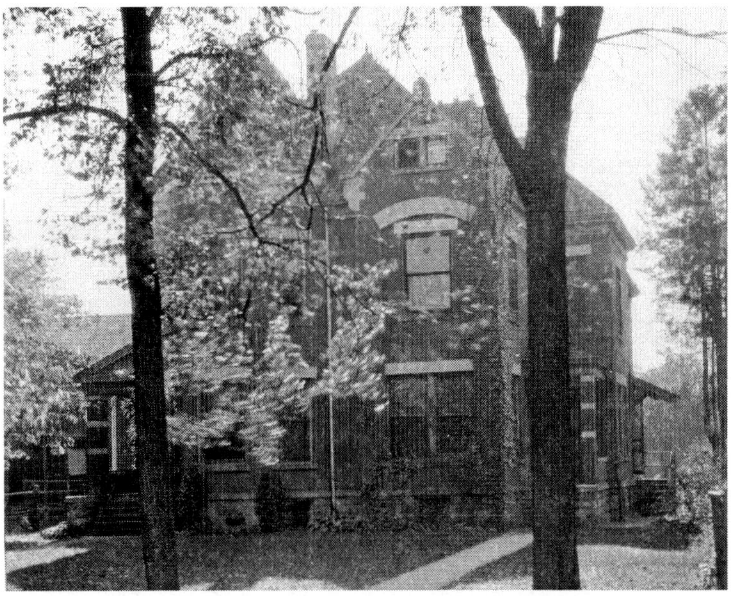

18. Osborne Home, purchased with accompanying land September 8, 1921, for $20,000, was formerly the home of a greatly honored physician for whom it was named. Twenty-six student nurses and the superintendent of nurses lived here.

19. Dr. William Puffer, the first Methodist minister who served as Superintendent of Bronson Methodist Hospital, 1920–34.

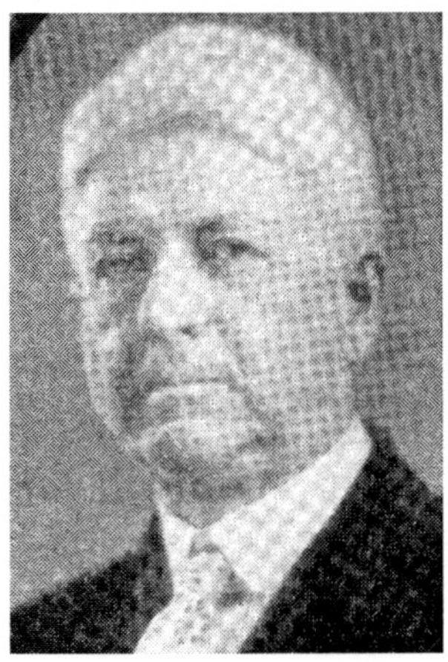

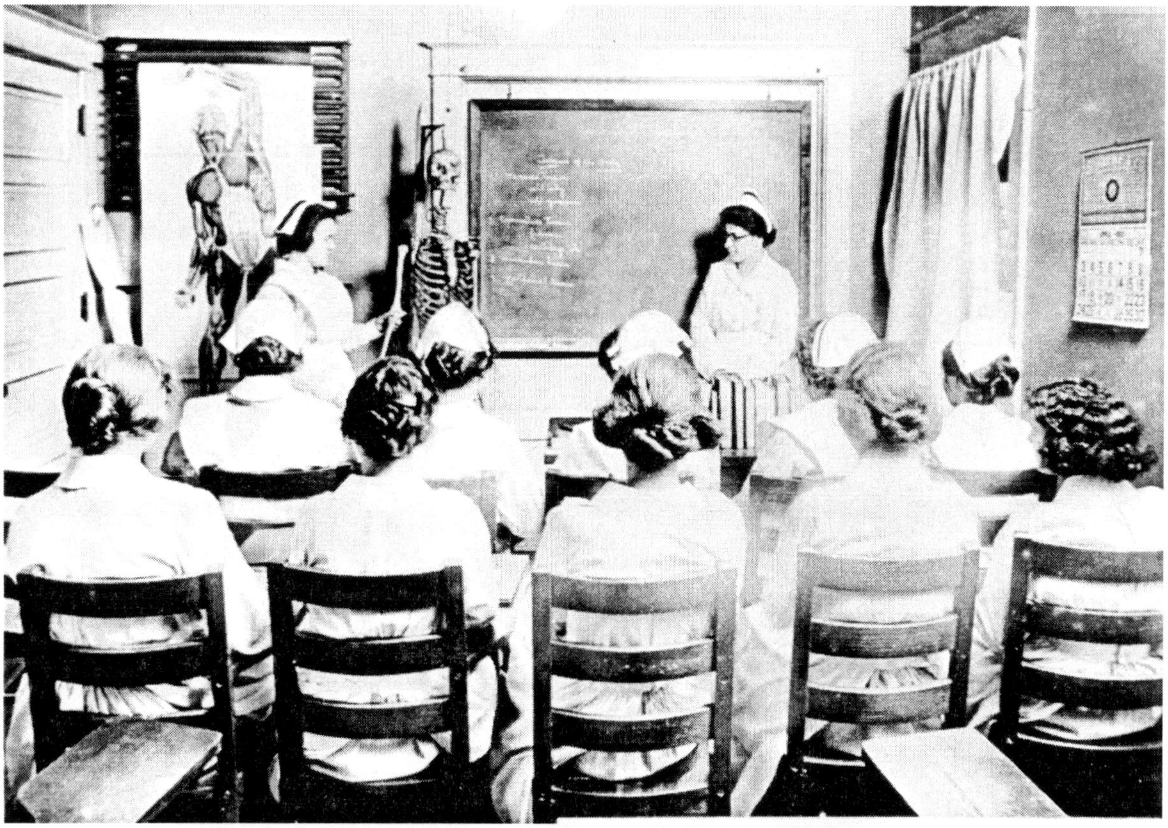

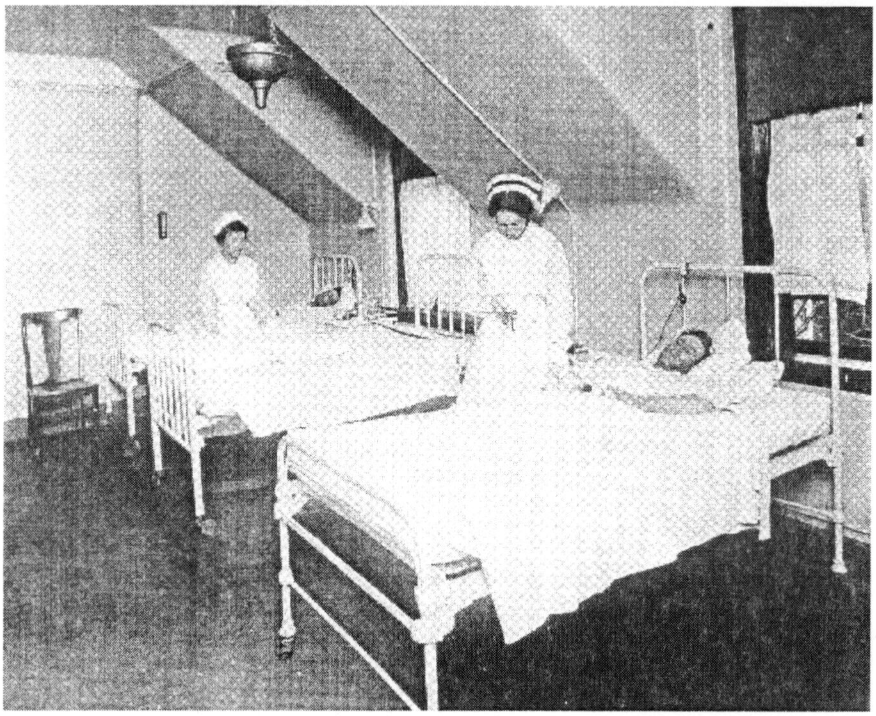

20. (above) In 1921 a contemporary noted that classroom "work is of high order, with an able faculty."

21. (left) Bronson ward, circa 1920.

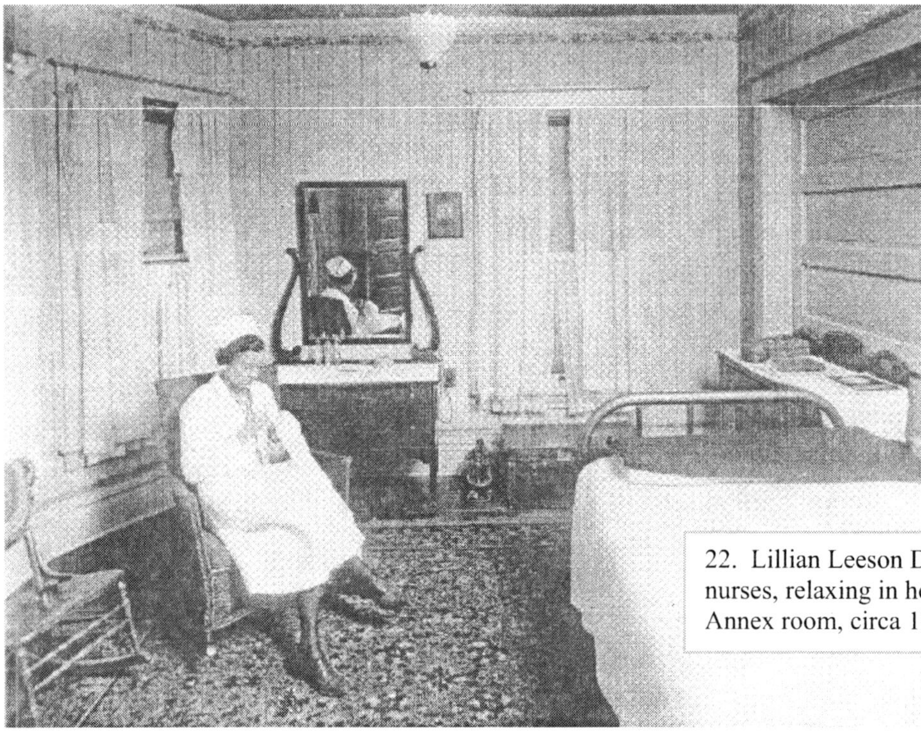

22. Lillian Leeson Daviell, director of nurses, relaxing in her room, a typical Annex room, circa 1922.

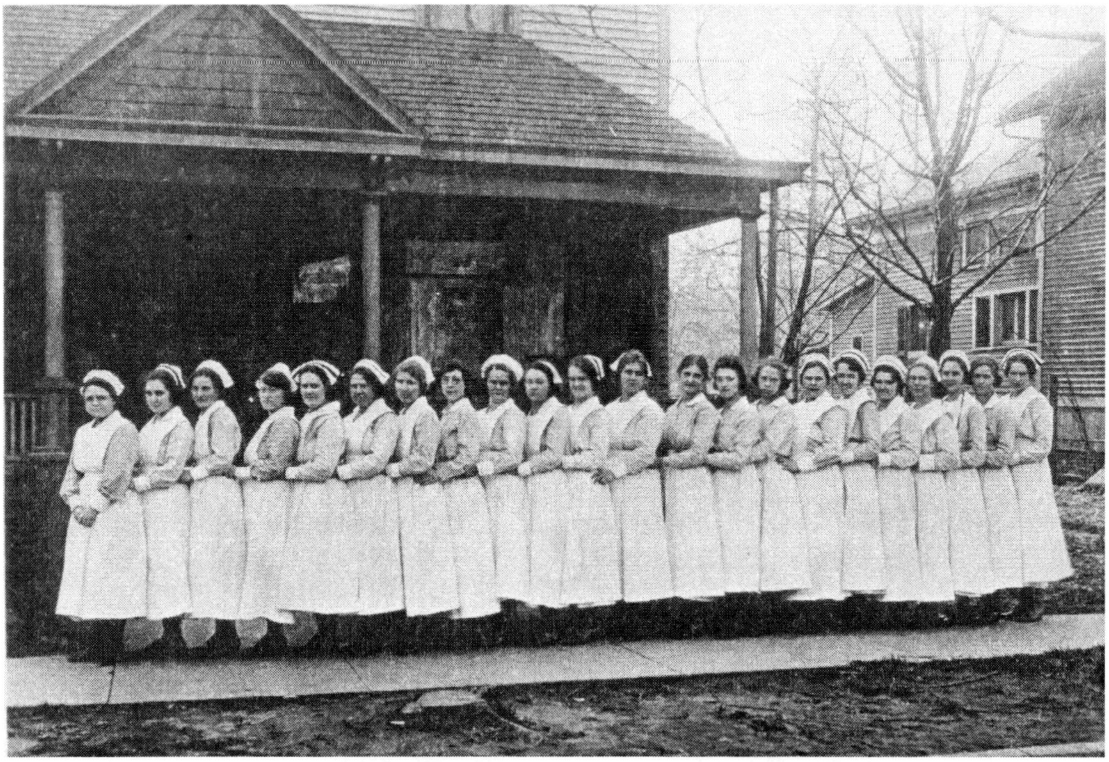

23. Entire student body in front of Old West Home, Classes 1922, 1923 and 1924.

24. (right) Herman Kiefer Hospital was added as the Communicable Disease Affiliation in 1924. (left to right) L.O.E.Menq, Jennie Bast, Bertha Robertson, and Ruth Homer at the hospital, about 1927–28.

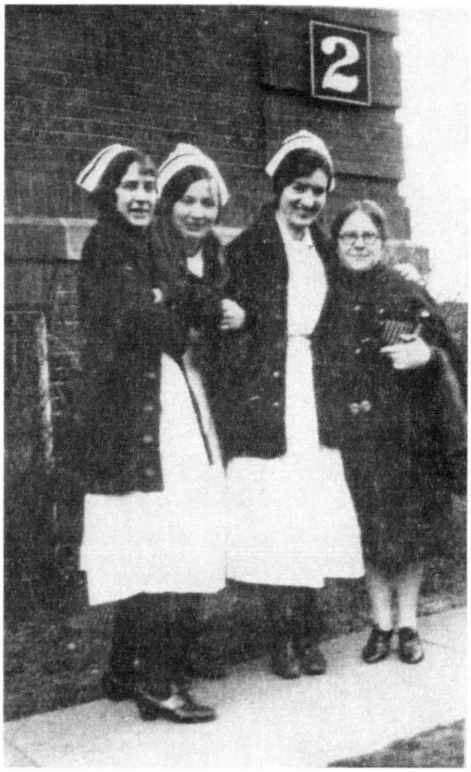

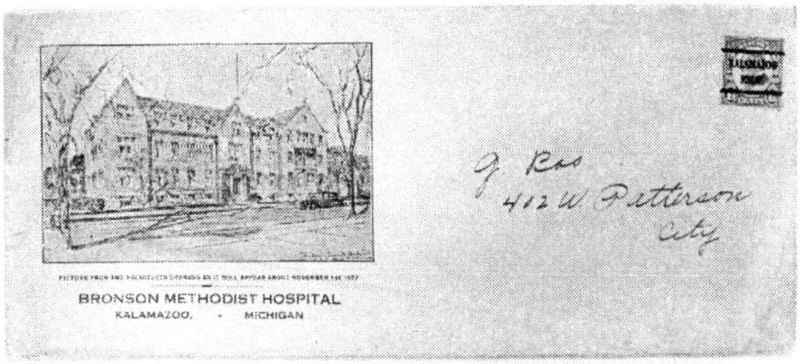

25. Subscriber solicitation envelope for new hospital.

26. (below) Bronson female ward, circa early 1920s. Beulah Pike, who graduated in 1923, is on left.

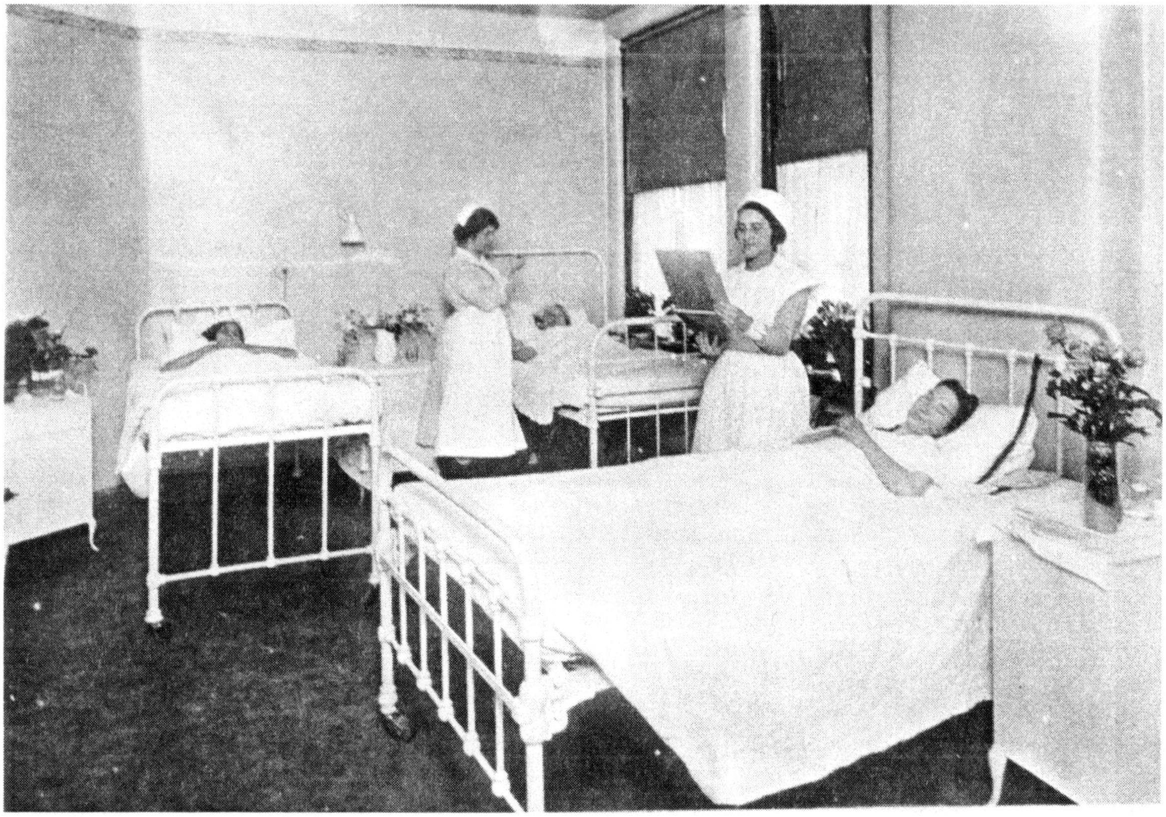

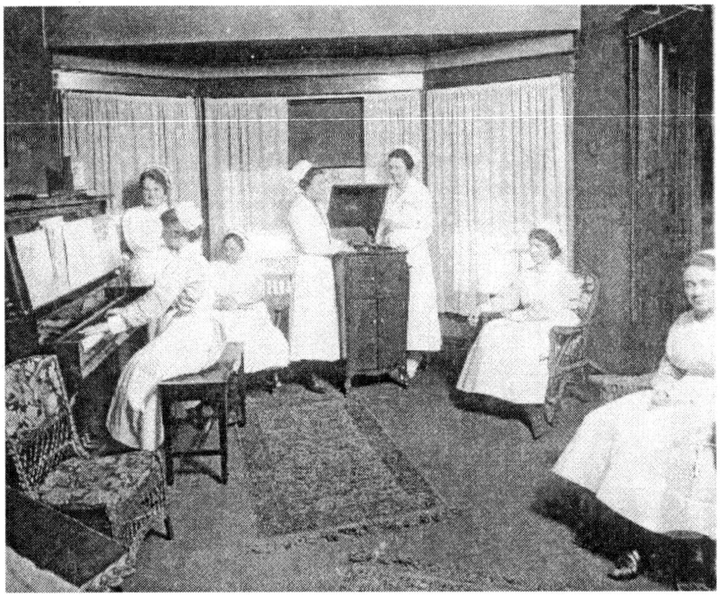

27. (above) The parlor in West Home, circa 1924. Lillian Leeson Daviell and Blanche Hermann Winslow at victrola and nursing students taking time away from hospital duty.

28. Class of 1928 as probies, 1925. Ann Draher on right was superintendent of nurses.

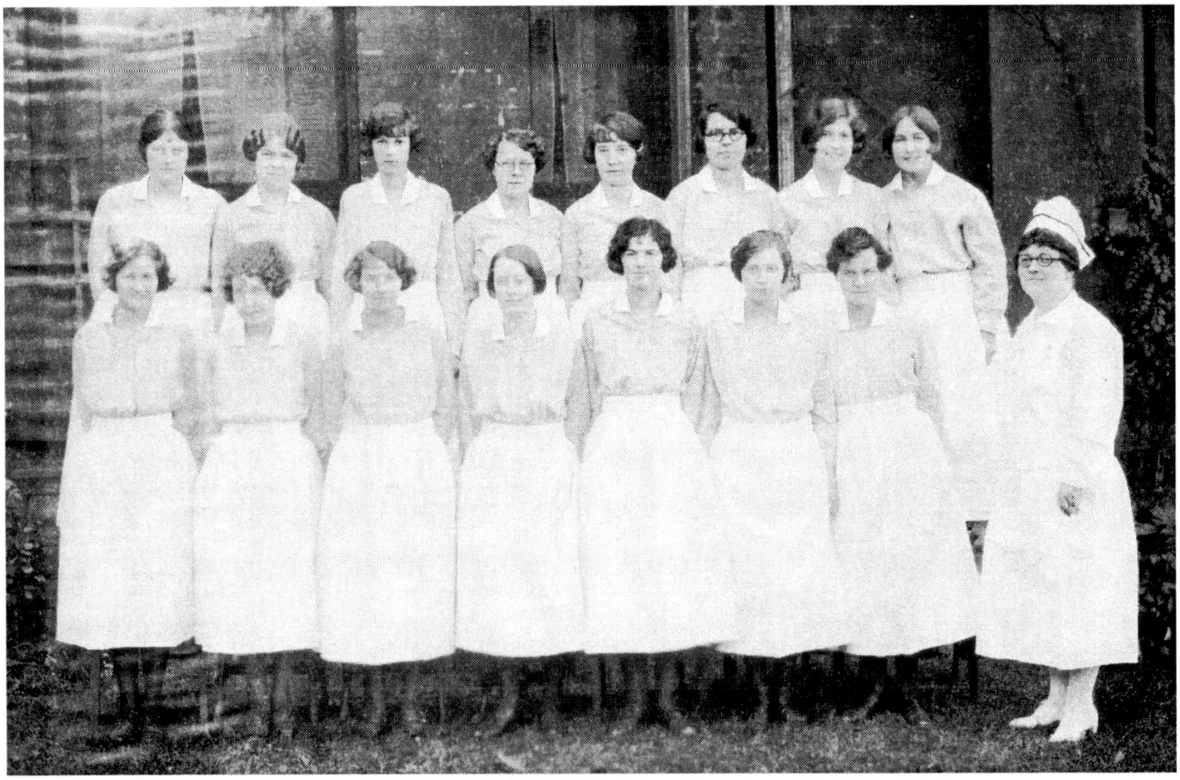

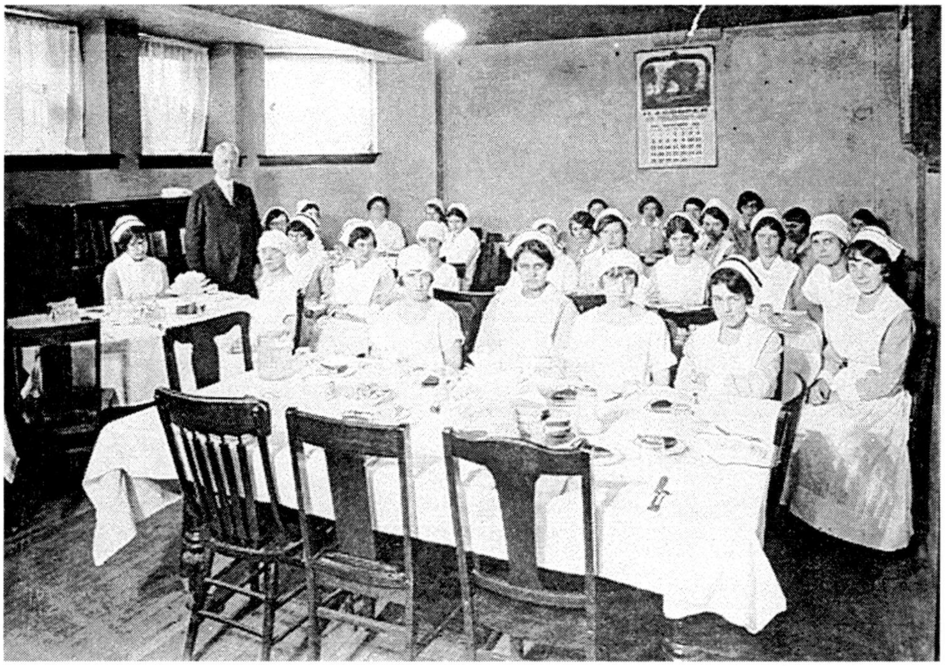

29. Banquet for the graduating class of 1925, with Dr. Puffer standing.

30. Operating room—three nurses assisting with surgery, 1924.

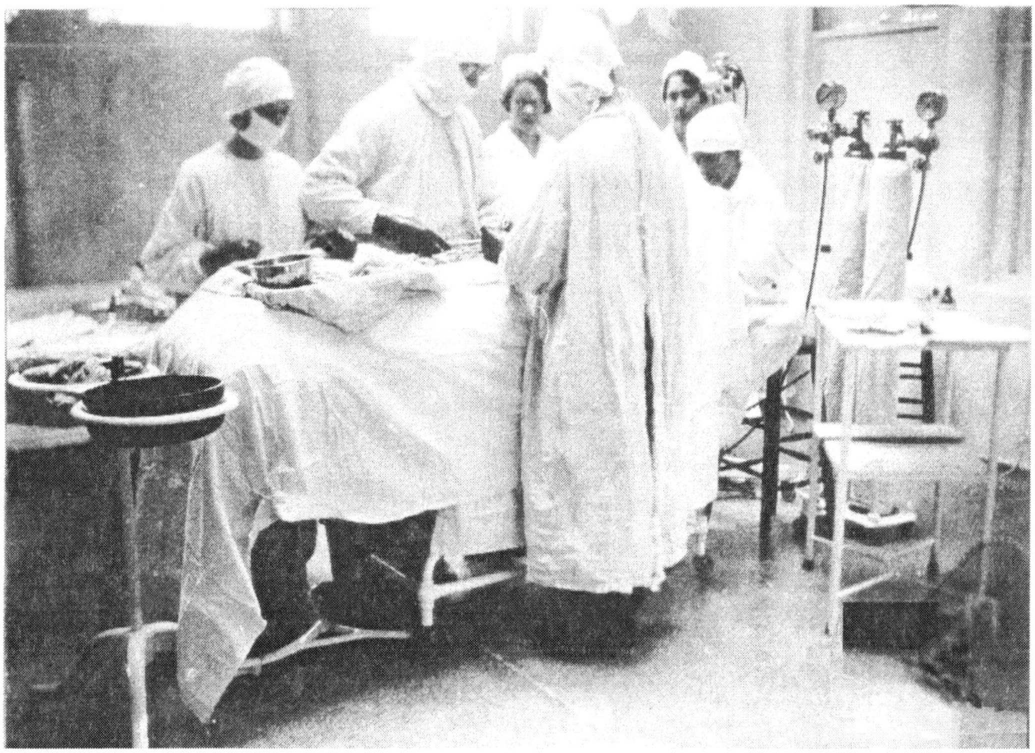

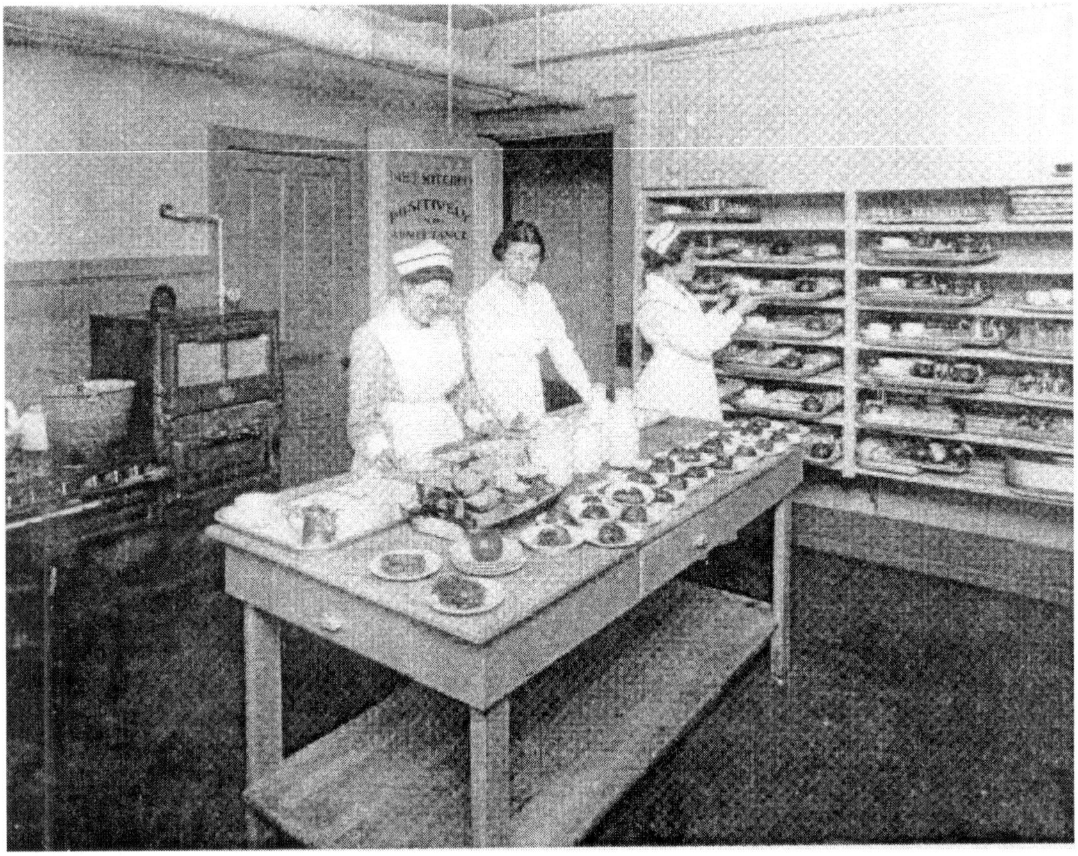

31. Eva Kingsley on left and Bertha Ory on right preparing food trays under the watchful eye of dietician Helen Madden, ca early 1920s.

32. Entire nursing staff and faculty, Classes 1926, 1927, 1928, 1929. Students were used as staff nurses and the supervisors were considered faculty.

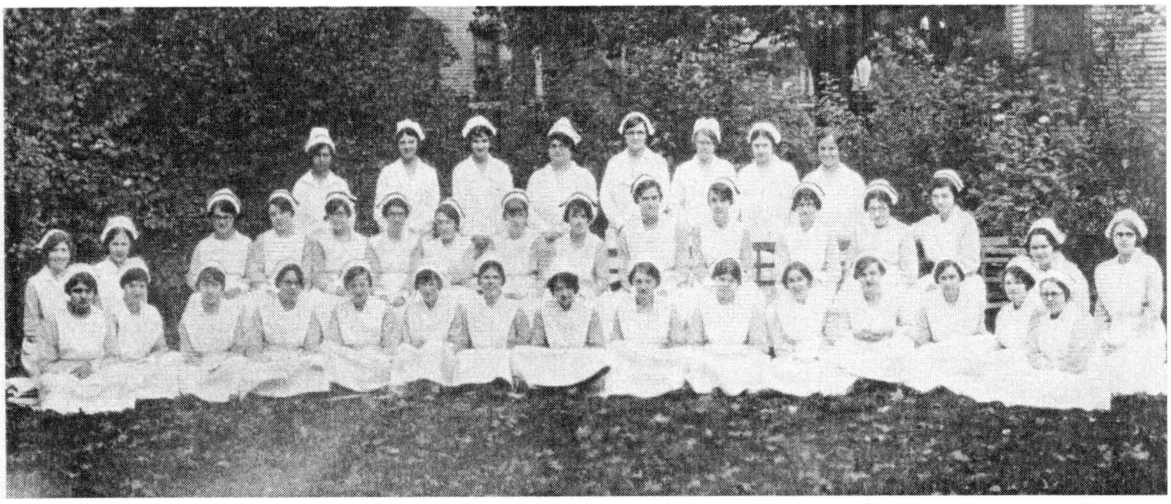

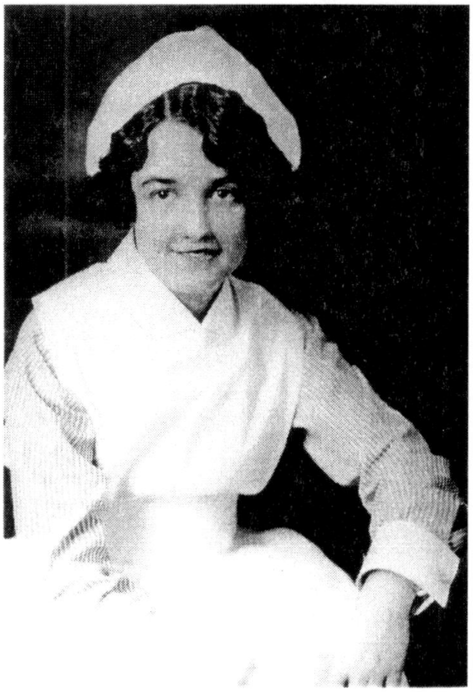

33. Anne Reiff Raisch, Class of 1929, who learned "discipline, a respect for the patient and a feeling of being able to contribute something worthwhile in the health field."

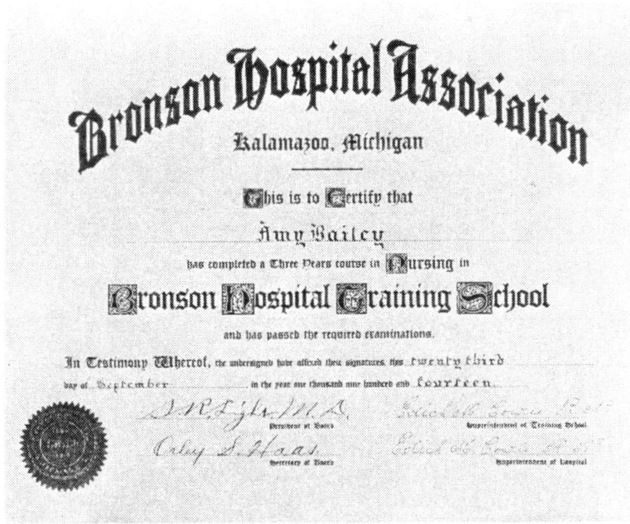

Bronson Hospital Association
Kalamazoo, Michigan

This is to Certify that
Amy Bailey
has completed a Three Years course in Nursing in
Bronson Hospital Training School
and has passed the required examinations.

In Testimony Whereof, the undersigned have affixed their signatures this twenty third day of September in the year one thousand nine hundred and fourteen.

President of Board — Superintendent of Training School
Secretary of Board — Superintendent of Hospital

34. As seen on the wall of Amy's home by Jackie Wylie during Amy's last days, Amy Bailey Seward's certificate for successful completion of three years of nurses' training at Bronson Hospital Training School, 1914.

35. Nurses assisting with an operation, 1926. Note the lack of masks, the open door, and others learning by observation.

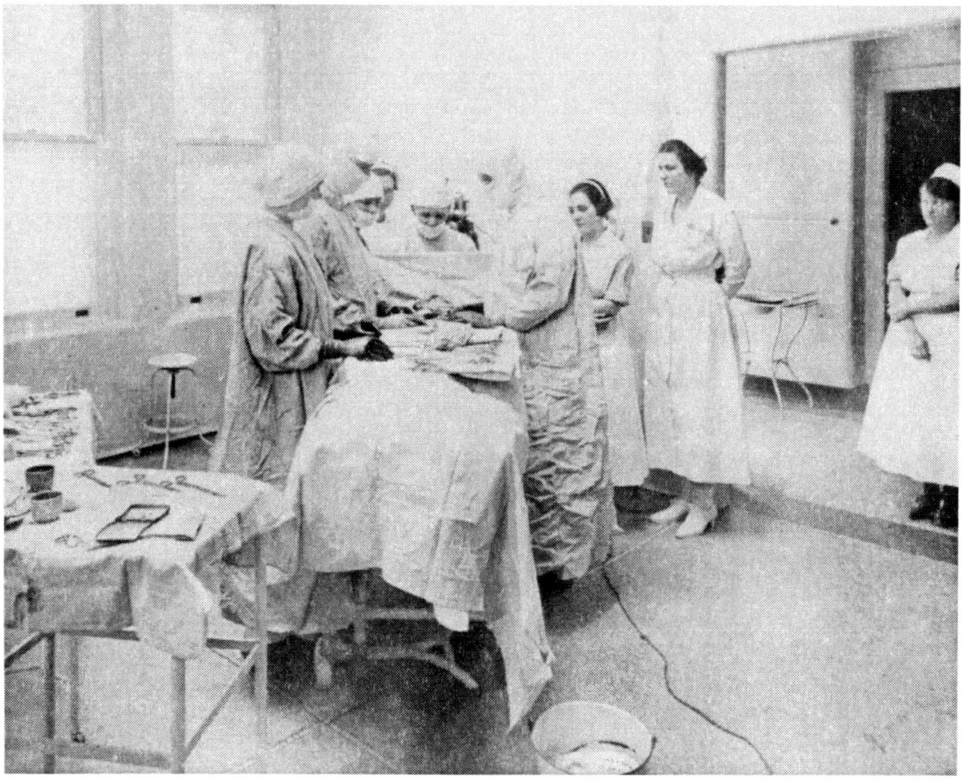

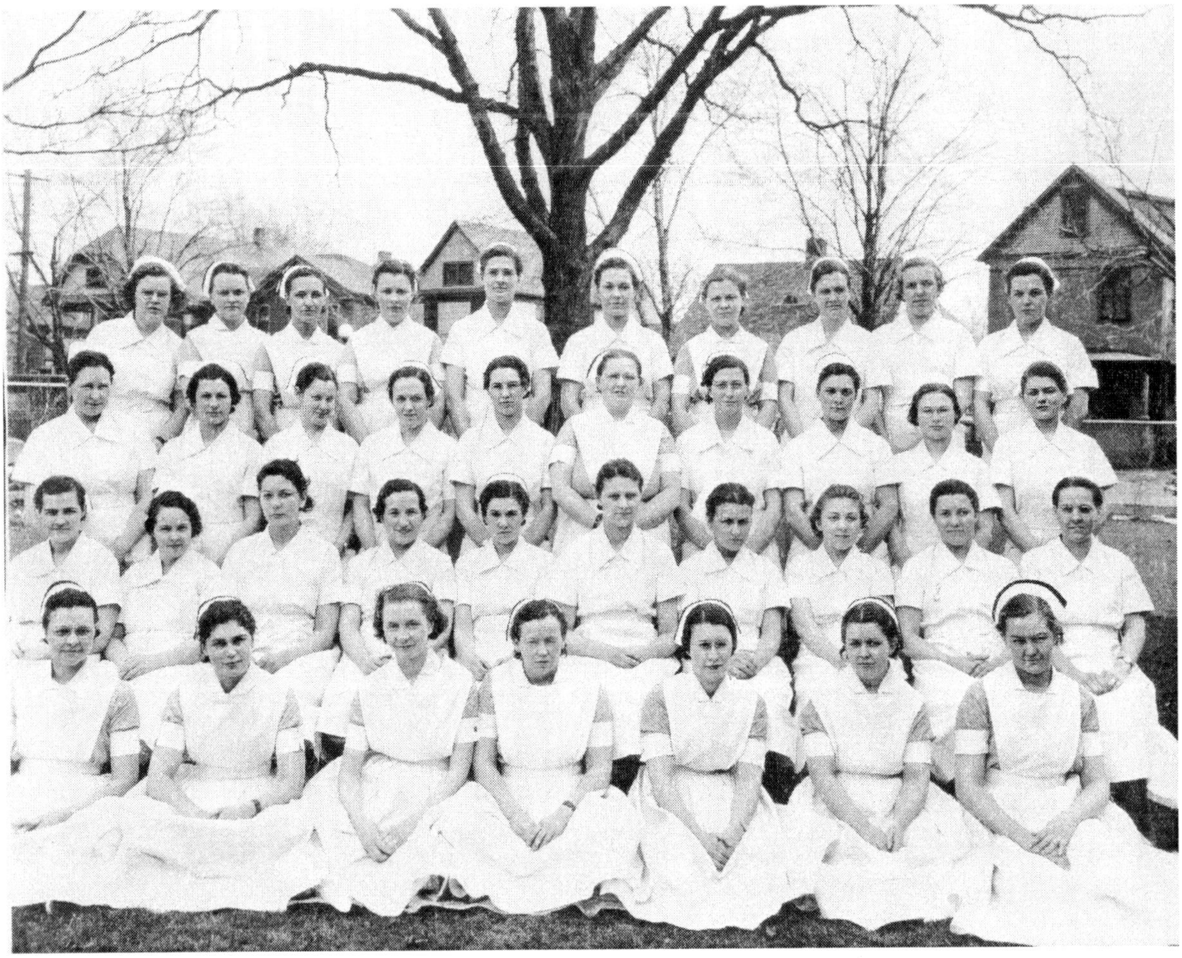

36. Student Body, 1936. Back row: Helen Latimer, Mary Simmons, Elaine Stover, Margaret Martin, Mary Geschwendt, Anne Althaus, Viola Frohrep, Mildred Walker, Dorothy Smith, Hazel Schulke. Third row: Jennie Ingle, Anna May, Gladys Thornburg, Frances Wyers, Arvilla Wilson, Lucretia Rose, Elizabeth Frutig, Ruth Gall, Margaret McNeal, Mary Cunningham. Second Row: Theodora Martin, Betty Seymoure, Jena Newell, Kathryn Pohly, Marian Watts, Mary VanderWeele, Dollie Paull, Arlene Denaway, Geraldine Crane, Thelma Kinney. First row: Doris Walton, Alta Conklin, Lorraine Raymont, Nola Vandenberg, Estina Sherrod, Charlotte Maloy, Dorothy Nelson. Notice Cedar Home in back at far left.

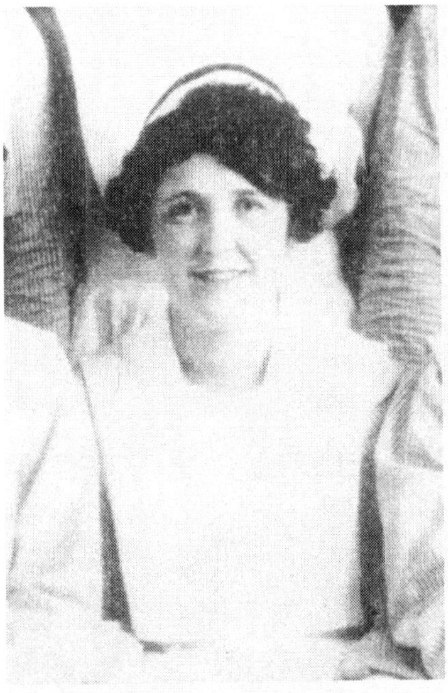

37. Margaret Hanna, 1925 graduate. Margaret married Franklin Varney, an Upjohn Company executive. She remembered the hospital as a beneficiary in her will and some of these funds supported the atrium in the *New* Bronson Methodist Hospital, opened in 2000.

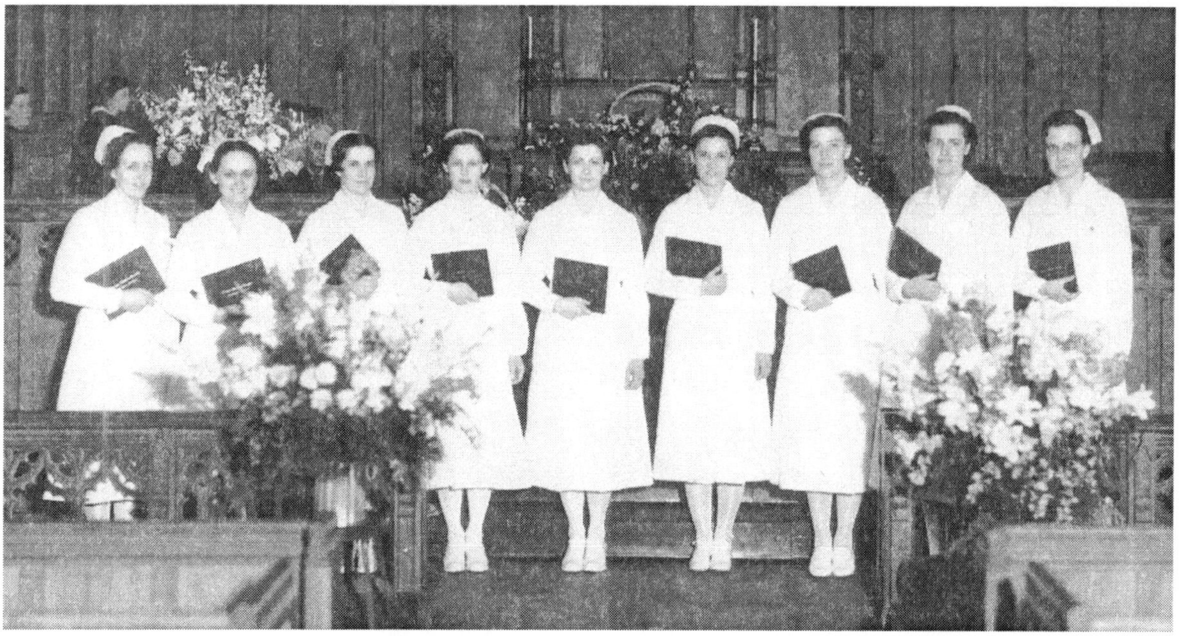

38. (above) Graduation class at the First Methodist Church, 1938. Left to right: Frances Wyers, Velma Smith, Marian Watts, Gladys Thornburg, Anna May, Ruth Gall, Elizabeth Frutig, Theodora Martin, Mildred Walker.

39. Nursing faculty (the entire nursing staff other than students), October 1924. Front row: Mina Weber, Superintendent of Nurses. Second row: Mary Mohney, night supervisor and Sena Holke, operating supervisor. Top row: Helen Madden, dietician, Lucy Evans, obstetrics supervisor, Myrtle Showerman, educational director.

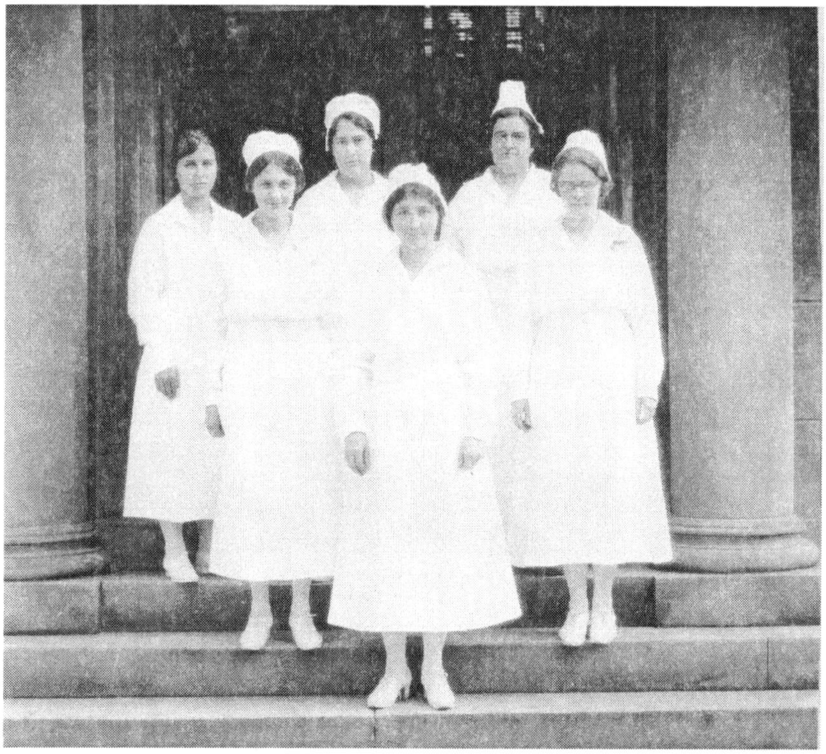

40. Freshman student Margaret Ruth Martin by fire escape at Osborne Home, 1935. Notice black shoes and stockings.

41. Schoolhouse, later known as the Annex.

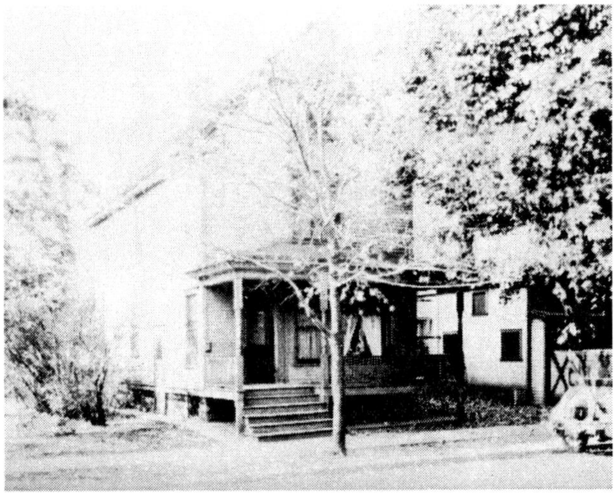

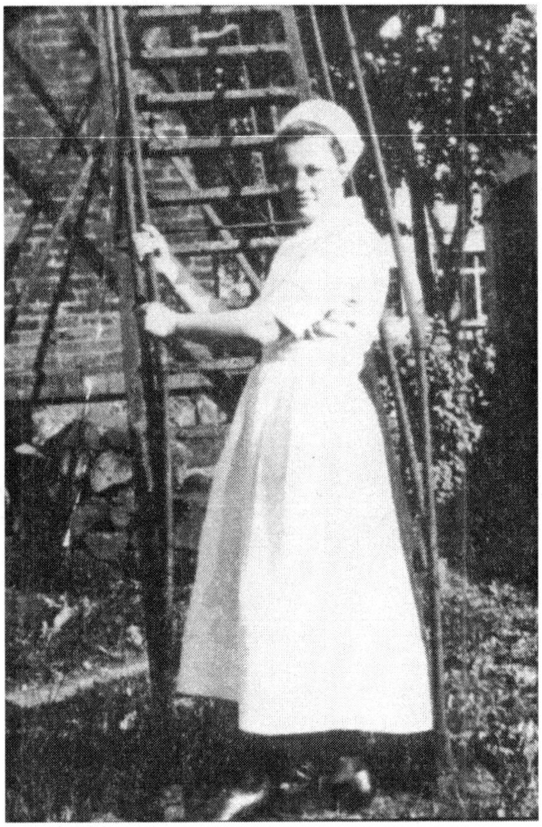

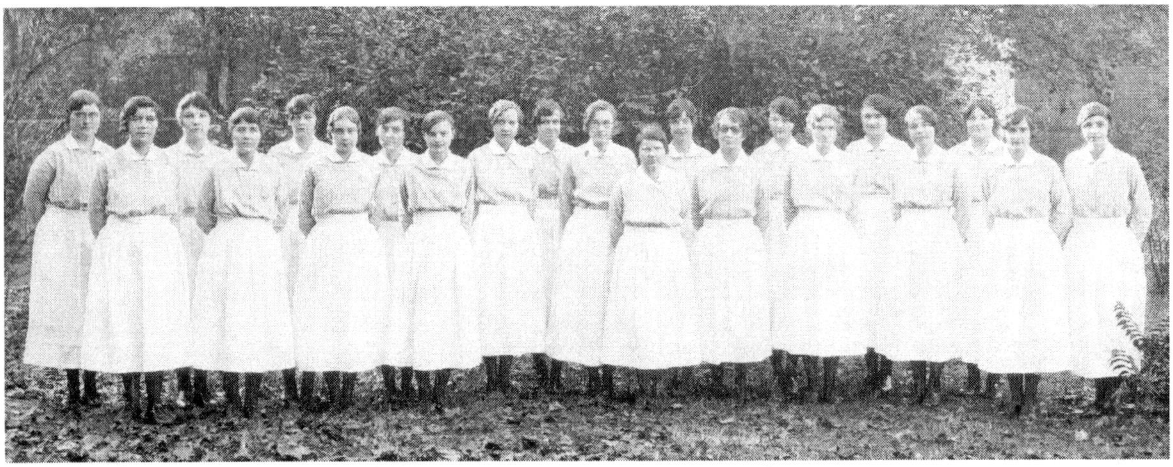

42. Freshman in 1929 graduated in the Class of 1932. Left to right: Edna Baker, Ruth Putney, Ena Kraft, Esther Tucker, Wanda Leach, Unidentified, Virginia Minogue, Ruth Hudgins, Unidentified, Velva McLeod, Dorothy Armstrong, Mary McCormick, Charlotte Wallis, Frances Britton, Unidentified, Hope Harding, Beatrice Wilcox, Marie Dainer, Unidentified, Wilma Rowe, Alethea Crawford.

CHAPTER 3

WE WERE CALLED—
CHOOSING NURSING, CHOOSING A SCHOOL

FLORENCE NIGHTINGALE

"As Florence Nightingale's lantern pierced the darkness of the 19th century hospital care and lit the way to modern nursing methods, so do hours of careful study lead to a nursing career . . . ." [1] As a reminder, Nightingale's picture carrying a lantern, which illuminated the woman in her dark-colored dress, white apron, and head covering, hung in the Bronson library. Hours of tedious study were required to become a registered nurse.

Nightingale's Early Life and Education

Born in Florence, Italy, in 1820, she was named after her birthplace. Her birth occurred during the second year of her well-to-do parents' extended three-year honeymoon and one year after her sister Parthenope's birth in Greece. Her parents, William Edward Nightingale (WEN) and Frances (Fanny) Smith Nightingale, were Unitarian, which accounted for the way Nightingale conducted her life as well as her philosophical approach to nursing and public health. She and her sister were raised in the affluent Anglican Church, however, because of their mother's desire that her daughters have the English advantage and the best marriage prospects.[2]

Because the family was part of the upper ruling class and the Nightingales had the proper social connections to assure a bright future for their two daughters, bringing her daughters into society was a major life work for Nightingale's mother. Though her plan worked for Parthenope, it did not for Florence who had her own deeply religious ideas of what she could become if she stepped out of the nineteenth-century limitations placed on affluent women. She entertained no ideas of becoming either the spinster daughter living at home or a wife, positions bound to family, home management, and what she considered boring social events. Nightingale had chances to marry and, in one case, was courted for several years before finally refusing her suitor's hand.

Her father was a gentleman, well educated at Edinburgh and Cambridge, with family money to support his family's lifestyle. He owned two mansions, Lea Hurst in Derbyshire, near Sherwood Forest and a distance from London, and Embley Park near the village of Wellow. The latter was close to Salisbury with its easier access to London and high society, which her mother favored.

WEN, as he was called, educated his daughters at home. Nightingale was his star pupil, learning history, philosophy, Latin, classical Greek, German, Italian, and French. She wanted to understand more about mathematics, apparently not her father's strong suit. When he did not comply with her wishes, she found herself a tutor who enhanced her natural ability as a statistician and analyst. She collected and used data about British social conditions and military hospital system to convince influential politicians (often friends of the family) of the need for social justice and social welfare reform. WEN allowed the strong-willed Nightingale to have her way, while trying to appease his wife and Parnethope who desperately wanted Florence to conform to social norms for upper-class English women.

Nightingale's education included lifelong correspondence with nationally and internationally known government and religious officials. People respected her genius and sought her for consultation on national matters, but she agonized over the family discord created by her unpopular break from traditional upper-class life. Her decisions became a constant source of distress for herself and her family until she reached the age of 30 when her relationship with God ameliorated the stress.[3]

Why Nightingale Chose Nursing

Nightingale wanted to be a nurse when she was six years old, and God's talk with her at 17 mandated nursing as her life work. Nursing was her divine calling, which she could not compromise.[4] Her story of "being called" is similar to the stories told repeatedly by numerous Bronson graduates.

Doing charitable work was what made her happy. Taking care of the sick in the village and within her extended family was work condoned for upper-class women.

She used the advantage of European travel (an appropriate activity for rich young women with chaperones) to visit systems of charity and nursing not found in England or the Anglican Church. Nightingale spent time in a Roman Catholic convent and at Kaiserwerth, a German Protestant deaconess nursing school, where women were trained as nurses. Her findings built on her own intuition about ways of caring for the sick.

Nightingale's calling, along with her genius, spirituality, passion, and curiosity, became a winning combination for building a public health movement and effecting nursing reform in the nineteenth century.

A Mystic

First, she fit the definition of a mystic, ". . .one who professes to undergo mystical experiences and so to comprehend intuitively truths beyond human understanding."[5] She informed herself through her observations, spiritual and earthly experiences, and knowledge of statistical analysis, along with her incredible ability to network and learn from the science and religions of her time. Ahead of her time, she ". . . sought to unify science and religion in a way that would bring order, meaning and purpose to human life."[6]

Second, her passion was to bring heaven-like qualities to Earth for the betterment of all humankind around the globe. She believed that all humans evolved in consciousness and in " . . . the mind's capacity to arrive at ultimate Truth."[7] She did not limit herself to parochial thinking, an influence of her extended Unitarian family. Though Nightingale criticized the Anglican Church regularly, and often thought about changing religions, she stayed in its confines, probably very aware of the political influence she could have being associated with the most affluent church, whose members—her family's friends—were well connected to Parliament.

For her, statistics linked daily life to concepts of unity and to universal laws that she believed came from God.[8] Nightingale was certain that God's laws were not attached to any one religion but provided a framework on which all religions were built, ". . . any religion will do which you yourself think a good thing."[9] She did not believe in miracles. Inner work was necessary to find God within one's self and to be in touch with and use God-given skills!

> Where shall I find God? In myself. That is the true Mystical Doctrine. But then I myself must be in a state for Him to come and dwell in me. This is the whole aim of the Mystical Life; and all Mystical Rules in all times and countries have been laid down for putting the soul in such a state.[10]

And so, when 17 years old, sitting on a stone bench under Cedar of Lebanon trees at her family's Embley Park estate, God first spoke to Nightingale. Nursing was to be her calling. Her education combined art, science, and religion into a unified framework on which she built nursing theory and practice. She believed that people could be raised to higher levels of consciousness and, in doing so, bring tolerance and heaven-like qualities to Earth. Furthermore, she believed that people could create heaven or hell on Earth. Her work focused on the betterment of all humankind—the impoverished, the ill, and the women who were considered to be second-class citizens, even in the ruling class. In a sense, she was a mystical scientist with an unheralded vision and dream for a healthier world. She combined the observable and knowable with a spiritual connection. Science alone could not change human behavior or society.

Given the proper circumstances, people and society could live in unity and harmony. Well-being could be achieved by integration of will and spirit within God's universal laws. According to Nightingale, these laws were not to be equated with Moses' laws or other prophetic teachings. They were laws, if understood, which would lead toward heaven on Earth, a perfect society. Her God was loving and benevolent, and would never condemn people for not understanding his laws. "Man's suffering is rather the result of his ignorance of the consequences of his actions."[11]

A Reformer

God spoke to her again when she was 30 years old, when Nightingale broke away from her family. At this time her passion to help others converted from building a base of theory and data into a plan of action. Believing that human behavior was the result of nurture, she set about to provide that nurture throughout England by establishing a nursing school that would teach caring and give women a respectable profession.

Mainly self-educated, Nightingale did receive three months of training in 1851 at the Institute of Kaiserwerth, founded by Pastor Theodor Fliedner.[12] Her stay at Kaiserwerth was cut short by the death of her Grandmother Shore, which required time and attention to her grieving family in the fall of 1852.

Puzzled by the limited education available to nursing pupils, she felt she had gained as much knowledge from previously listening to her own intuition, and through conscious observation, experience, and documentation while caring for the village sick and her own family. These activities gave her life meaning, while she was still within the confines and constraints of her family home.

After meeting family obligations, and before seeking a position as nursing superintendent, she visited the Sisters of Charity, Paris, France. The nuns' lifestyle and training in the care of the sick and poor worked within an efficient structure[13] making them desirable role models for Nightingale. With 33 years of synthesizing and combining academics, religion, and life experiences she was ready to assume a position of authority that would enable her to change the existing, unhealthy English medical system.

A modernist and progressive activist, Nightingale opposed class distinctions and women's status in English society. She hid from public view and consciously did not participate in the women's suffrage movement. Instead she laid the groundwork for women to gain lawful rights as citizens with rights equal to those of men. Her plan was to create a legitimate profession for women. She hoped to establish English nursing programs similar to the training programs she had observed and studied at Kaiserwerth in Germany and with the Sisters of Charity in Paris.

Nightingale became well known for her philanthropic ideas and charitable work in caring for the sick. She convinced her liberal father to allow her the freedom to pursue her passion. Lady Charlotte Canning, a friend of Nightingale, recommended her, at the age of 33, to the Ladies Committee as the superintendent of the Institution for the Care of Sick Gentle-women in Distressed Circumstances. Located at Number One, Harley Street, in London, it was a small hospital with 30 beds for physically and emotionally debilitated governesses—women who most often were paid so little and worked so hard as to present a case for slave labor. Only destitute, previously affluent, women could apply for a governess position.[14] Women without connections to a father, husband or brothers were outcasts, and women's work was limited so that any job, even if seven days a week, 24 hours per day, would provide them with a roof and food. Poorer women faired worse. They were often homeless and on the streets. They were the ones who turned to hospital drudgery for food and a bed when prostitution was no longer an option.

The institution was in a poorly managed process of renovation. Nightingale orchestrated some architectural changes, including the inclusion of a dumbwaiter so that equipment and food could be moved from floor to floor. Her architectural genius came from her intuition and watching her father build Embley Park Estate.

She hired the best nurses, aides, housekeepers and cook whom she could find. If they were not trainable or had a bad attitude, she dismissed them quickly since labor sources were readily available. By the end of one year, the facility was running efficiently with three good nurses and support staff, and Nightingale was ready to move on.[15]

Her father gave her an allowance of 500 pounds a year (not an uncommon action with sons) for her own apartment in London where she could work toward reforming nursing, public health, hospitals and the British army's management of soldiers' health. Often she used her own money to pay for hospital services or equipment when other funding did not materialize.

Reform and the English Military

Nightingale's work to reform the archaic English military medical system emerged during the Crimean War when wounded soldiers were left to die in deplorable conditions. She made the best of all her social connections. Sir Sidney Herbert, husband of her friend, Elizabeth Herbert, recommended that she go to Scutari, where the military hospital for wounded soldiers offered nothing but death for the majority. Nightingale accepted the appointment and became the first woman chief in command at an English military hospital. She took her own housekeeper,

Mrs. Clarke, and several trained nurses, mostly nuns. They were the first women to care for the many English war-wounded.

When Nightingale arrived in Scutari, 3,000 wounded soldiers had been evacuated to the hospital and lay dying, mostly from infected wounds. She and her staff cleaned everything in sight, including soldiers' bodies, their clothes, linens and bandages, equipment, and rooms. They offered nutritious food and fresh air. Nightingale became known as the "lady with the lamp" as she made rounds during the night, a comforting sight for the soldiers and a nursing tradition for which she is most famous. Making constant rounds on patients ensured their care and best conditions for healing.[16]

By December 1854, 5,000 wounded men were under Nightingale's care.[17] She herself often worked a 20-hour day,[18] and the outcomes were amazing. The death rate dropped from an astounding 44 percent to 2.2 percent! The drop was attributed to introducing medical asepsis, and better nutrition and instituting a fresh-air, clean, and healing environment. Nightingale's philosophy applied to practice was successful! Nurses could indirectly heal the sick and wounded by promoting a healthy environment so that the body could heal itself.[19]

Nightingale never backed away from contagious patients. At Scutari, in May of 1855, she fell ill with Crimean fever and fatigue, requiring rest and nursing care for several weeks. She would not tolerate even the thought of returning to England until the war was over.[20] Her favorite Aunt Mai came to help her manage as superintendent while she was ill.[21] The soldiers got better and sang her praise in letters to their families. In later years, she would continue to supervise health-care reform from her own bedside, never fully recovering from the debilitating disease she had acquired. Some believed she used illness as an excuse for not leaving her home and for having ample time for writing.

She became known as a heroine, and her work was even noticed by Queen Victoria.[22] Because of her reclusive nature, however, the public never had a chance to meet her. She refused any engagement meant to honor her stellar work.

Nightingale's medical military reform did not end with Scutari. Upon her return to England her influence was even greater in Parliament. She continued to suffer from a debilitating condition, most likely brucellosis, but with family, domestic and clerical help, she pursued her public health statistical work for several years, documenting her research findings (data collected and analyzed from her direct observations and examination of medical records). Nightingale established standards of nursing care with ethical underpinnings similar to those in nursing education and services seen today.

National Nightingale Fund and the Nursing Training School

Out of Scutari came the National Nightingale Fund, instituted by Sir Sidney Herbert in Parliament, to recognize her valor and to fund nurses' training programs in England. Nightingale had earned the resources to make her dream become reality![23] Local governmental units through all of England donated seven thousand pounds. Her mother was extremely proud and happy for her daughter's fame, while Nightingale praised God for bringing the resources to build a school of nursing.

As an invalid, Nightingale never directly managed the Nightingale School of Nursing but led the movement to organize the first nurses' training program at St. Thomas Hospital in London from her bedside. Admired by Nightingale, Sarah Elizabeth Wardroper, hospital matron, took on the dual role as the first matron of the Nightingale School of Nursing. Wardroper, not a nurse, was the only available woman Nightingale trusted to lead the school. Funding for the school was separate from the hospital's resources, a way to protect it. The opening of the training school, even with considerable support from Parliament, met opposition from physicians who did not believe nursing care could be improved with education—nurses were nothing more than servants trained to care for the sick and dying.[24] Their uniforms and dust caps testified to the lowly role.

The school opened on June 24, 1860, with 11 probationers who signed a four-year contract and, in return, received their training, board and room, plus a stipend.[25] Applicants were judged to be of good character and intelligent. The program was not without voluntary terminations and dismissals of students viewed as unfit for the training.

From 1872 to 1900, behind the scene, Nightingale wrote annual addresses to be read aloud to probationers, reminders of the need for high character, decent morals, good nursing practice and spiritual[26] unity. She also influenced the administration with regard to funding for the Nightingale School.

The Nightingale School of Nursing was one of Nightingale's dreams and her most-remembered accomplishment, although it was somewhat tangential to her incredible feats in improving healthcare for the poorest of the English population and sanitation standards in India and, in particular, decreasing the mortality of English soldiers during the Crimean War, as well as overall improving the British military medical system.

Nightingale's private funds from her family enabled her to secure equipment and services on occasions when other funding sources fell short or were not available. For most nurses who came out of poor working-class conditions and followed her, financing nursing services was not an option.

She authored numerous manuscripts and books. Her famous 1860 *Notes on Nursing: What It Is, And What It Is Not*, was widely disseminated in the United States, with 15,000 copies published in 1859, a year before the London nursing school was opened. The document outlined all of the philosophical underpinnings of unity principles and described ways to place the patient in the best possible condition to heal by the use of interventions such as, ". . . color, light, music, pets, relaxation, nutrition, and exercise. . . ."[27]

Nightingale's work did not go unnoticed by her American friend, Elizabeth Blackwell, the first woman physician in the U.S., and Dorothea Linde Dix, Superintendent of the first Union army nurses. Dix offered advice to the North American military medical system, which mimicked the English system prior to Nightingale's involvement—deadly for all who sought care.[28]

Impact on Nursing Education in America

Bronson Hospital's early school most likely looked like the two-year Nightingale Training School for Nurses.[29] The Nightingale School had no religious affiliation and was financially independent of the hospital,[30] and although most American schools were modeled after it, they were dependent on their hospital affiliation and often church donations. Bronson did not have a religious affiliation until the Methodist church rescued the financially ailing organization in 1920, but the school was never autonomous from the hospital.

The caring concepts that distinguished the Bronson School of Nursing connect to the writings of Nightingale, who was always progressive, utilizing new findings and discoveries in caring science. The training was rigorous, and slowly hospital schools either dissolved or moved into institutions of higher learning and away from hospitals, with the understanding that nursing science and practice required a college educational base similar to all professions. The movement started at the beginning of the twentieth century as numbers of hospital nursing schools swelled, then declined in the last 30 years of the century, and was mostly completed by 2000. Nursing students were no longer probationers at hospitals but received traditional, college education with theory, laboratory and clinical practice part of community colleges and universities. Advancement of education to graduate and doctoral levels began early in the 1900s but advanced degreed nurses fell short of numbers needed for healthcare managers, educators and researchers.

Last Years

The year 1887 was Nightingale's self-proclaimed Jubilee Year—50 years since her divine calling to nursing. To recognize the event and to the advantage of nursing, Queen Victoria asked that donations be made to the Queen Victoria Jubilee Institute for Nurses and given to home nursing care for the poor.[31] Philosophically, Nightingale had begun to see that public health and home nursing care were advantageous compared to hospital care. These beliefs also migrated to the United States, although most nurses continued to find employment in hospitals.

Burial in a Small Church Cemetery

True to her private nature, Nightingale would not hear of being buried with kings and queens in Westminster Abbey. She was buried a few miles from Embley Park in a cemetery adjacent to St. Margaret's of Antioch Church. Names of her mother, father, sister and herself are on each side of one headstone that has the full names of the other three, but only her initials, F.N. After her incredibly productive invalid years, she was the last of her family to die, living to 90 years of age.

Her life ended in 1910, during the early years of the "modern" Bronson Hospital and School of Nursing when many women, like Nightingale "called" to nursing, found a way to leave home by a path other than marriage, and enter a life that they considered of their own making, not different from the decision of women who chose to become nuns. Nursing was a professional discipline that lighted the way to a path of service beyond the home.

CHOOSING BRONSON

Hospital-based nursing program recruitment of women was driven by the need for an available, inexpensive labor force. Bronson recruited mostly from working-class families, the daughters of white craftsmen, paper-mill workers, farmers, and

Methodists. Societal expectations of the "good daughter" had expanded to cover the growing need of caregiving for strangers.[32]

Nursing, therefore, offered the choice to move away from one's family since residency near the hospital was a requirement. Consider the women who chose not to marry or who had limited suitors.[33] Entering a convent or leading a celibate life became an option whereas nursing offered a secular alternative.

Romanticized ideals about healing and alleviation of suffering are common altruistic themes in Bronson graduates' stories. Others admitted to wondering, "Why did I make this choice?" Some of the graduates gave practical reasons. College was not an option for poor women. Nursing seemed better than working as a servant/housekeeper or a paper-mill or garment-factory laborer. Nursing school provided an opportunity to leave home and to receive specialized training. Many, similar to Nightingale, believed that God had called them to the nursing profession.

Nursing school offered a work-study model, plus room and board, with a small, monthly stipend provided in the earliest years. Sometimes it was more work than study and, depending on the informant, the pursuit was either a great learning experience or just plain drudgery. The graduates who shared their stories mostly provide positive recollections. The stories of those who would have preferred a different career or who quit school are not included in this volume but would tell another story about women's career choices if they were.

> "My aunt was a nurse. I never wanted to do anything else.
> ***Margaret Gould Carter '47***

> The message is clear, "I came from a poor family. I always wanted to help others, and really enjoyed medical science but could not afford college. Bronson had an excellent reputation and a small tuition fee that I could afford."
> ***Virginia Brouse '56***

Occasionally, up to the 1950s, graduates mention career options other than nursing. Graduates of the 1960s begin to include more frequent accounts of previous college experience and nursing as a second career choice. For others, nursing was a lifetime script.

First thoughts of nursing career possibilities were implanted by relatives, nurses and teachers who were influential in a girl's life. "You would make a good nurse someday," was a phrase repeated by many Bronson graduates. Family illnesses or being a young patient oneself provided the chance to experience nursing care. In the first half of the century, private-duty, home-care nurses served as role models and often became heroines for young observers who hung around the bedside. Dorothy Armstrong, 1932 graduate, on the other hand, stated, "When I was fifteen my mother received poor care during an illness so I resolved to learn nursing. Having heard of wild parties in hospitals, my parents wanted me to attend a church hospital like Bronson." Most stories reveal the heroine theme.

Family

> My motivation to become a nurse was a remark made by my mother (a so-called practical nurse) who had rheumatic fever when I was 10 years old. I helped wait on her while she was confined to bed, and she said, "Helen, you would make a good nurse!" From then on, I thought of nothing else. I did not think nursing school would be possible because we didn't have any money. I knew of Bronson through church and the women's society. I was encouraged to forward my application and was accepted, then needed the money, 110 dollars. A family friend loaned it to me. Many years later she was one of my patients in a home-nursing program.
>
> I was called on the carpet for dating a college student who was working in the hospital kitchen. Dr. Puffer explained to me that that behavior was a "no-no." I expected to be sent home but wasn't. I have always been thankful that I completed nurse's training in 1937, especially since later I was a single parent for 20 years. With the help of family and working as a RN, I was able to make it!
>
> ***Helen Hjortholm Molyneux '37***

When I began my high school junior year in Yale, Michigan, in 1932, my older sister, Helen, began her first year of training at Bronson. I had given no thought to the nursing profession. As I neared graduation in 1934, I started to consider career options. My mother and father would return from visits with Helen with glowing accounts of how well my sister liked Bronson and how well she was doing. The reports were largely responsible for my growing interest and curiosity. It was mutually agreed that I would follow my sister's footsteps and I entered training in the fall of 1934.

Margaret Ruth Martin Correll '37

My motivation to go into nurses training began at home. My mother was a Bronson graduate of 1918. She chose Bronson Hospital based on the recommendation of Dr. L. V. Rogers of Galesburg. She worked in the home of the Roger's family. I spend a lot of time looking at my mother's photo album and the old striped uniform, the white starched apron and bib along with the voile cap. Eventually, we became the first mother[34] and daughter who graduated from BMH.

Marilyn E. Newton '45

My father called me his 'little nurse.' I was always caring for and helping my siblings.

Winifred Mein Terpstra '44

I grew up wanting to be a nurse. My mother, Mina Weber Macgrayne, graduated from Bronson in 1913.

Janet Macgrayne Camery '48

My favorite great aunt, Marie Wantz, worked at BMH so, I guess, this was the primary motivation to attend Bronson.

Edythe Merrill Rivers '66

I chose nursing after a nurse helped my sister who was very ill with scarlet fever. I was 10 years old. I chose Bronson because it was a "good" Methodist hospital. I was Methodist.

Ione Bailey Ambrose '49

My motivation was to break free from the isolation of my first career choice in the medical research laboratory and to learn to interact and help others in difficult circumstances.

Amanda Speedy '93

I always dreamed of being a nurse. My aunt was a nurse's aide at the Ann Arbor University Hospital, working in pediatrics, and I loved hearing her talk about the children she cared for. My mother was my driving force, pushing me to go on to higher education, a chance she never had. We were Methodists, and I remember how pleased our minister was with my school selection.

Janice McClellan Duryea '53

All of my life I wanted to be a nurse. I loved being a baby sitter and caring for family members. I was an avid reader and, for a while in high school, changed directions toward college to become a physician. I lasted two years and fell in love. My husband was in the Navy then, so I had time to finish nurse's training at Bronson.

Suzanne Barrett Van Dyken '53

My mother was a diploma-prepared registered nurse and, from the time I was five, I was determined to be just like her. I never seriously considered another school. Living in Battle Creek, Bronson seemed ideal geographically and academically. I was convinced that the diploma route would give me the necessary clinical experience.

Susan Ammon Robinson '81

Nursing is something that I always wanted to do. I'm sure my mom was the biggest influence. I remember her coming home from work and talking about the people she cared for, and this sounded pretty exciting to me as a small girl. She also went to Bronson for her education, which is why I chose to go there even though I grew up on the east side of the state. I'm not sure that she's aware of the impact that choice made on my life.

Patti Harner '83

As far back as I can remember I wanted to be a nurse. A big influence was my grandmother who had severe rheumatoid arthritis. The affliction progressed to the point where she could barely walk, and the doctor advised her to remain in bed. She was bed-bound for 13 years. Just touching the foot of the bed would cause her to cry out in pain. After the death of my grandfather, my mother and aunt cared for her in their homes, with a live-in woman to assist. I remember Marian Vandenberg Vanderweele '31, a registered nurse, giving suggestions to my mother. She had a wealth of information and her simple suggestions made care easier. I felt that this was the vocation for me.

Florence Clementz Manning '49

Healthcare Professionals Impact on Choice

I was eight years old when I had a ruptured appendix and peritonitis. It was the last day of school in Legget Grade School in Akron, Ohio, and I insisted, against my mother's wishes, on attending to receive my report card. I had a very difficult walk home and that night, with a lump in my right side, I went by ambulance to Children's Hospital in Akron. The nurses and doctors were such kind and lovely people, the best I had ever met. So I decided to become a nurse, taking all the classes in high school that were required for a nursing career.

Mary Schanzlin Lietzke '34

I was inspired by a private duty nurse who worked a 20-hour shift taking care of my mother in our home. I chose Bronson because I heard about the hospital from the Methodist church I attended. I was homesick the first months because I was 500 miles away and couldn't go home for a year.

My greatest joys in nursing were my classmates, who were like sisters, and taking care of patients. My fear was making a mistake and being sent home.

Ruby Kemp Kanaar '36

When I was 12 or 13 years old, my mother became ill and had to be hospitalized in Sault Saint Marie, Ontario. I became intrigued with the nurses and their expertise. At the same time I became acquainted with a newcomer in town. She was from Kalamazoo, Michigan, of all places. We got to be close friends, but she returned to Kalamazoo after a year. We vowed to be friends forever. I graduated from high school too young to be accepted into a nursing school in Canada. My friend gathered all of the information she could find about the two hospital nursing programs in Kalamazoo, and sent it to me. I applied. Lo and behold, I was accepted and on my way immediately.

Late in the 1930s, Canada was at war. I had another choice to make. I could return to Canada and be drafted into the service immediately. I was not a citizen of the United States, but I was allowed to stay and finish [nurse's] training; however, if I were to go back, if only to visit, I would not be allowed to leave Canada. You know my decision, which I have never regretted.

My greatest joys in nursing school were twofold. It was always gratifying to give care to someone and then see him or her discharged in good health. I volunteered with the Red Cross for several years, working bloodmobiles and teaching volunteer aides who were indispensable during the war years. My second joy was meeting my husband-to-be, with whom I have shared 52 years.

Jewel Curry Pikkaart '41

In junior high I knew I wanted to go into physical therapy or nursing. By high school I knew that it would be nursing. I lived in Grand Rapids so I applied to Blodgett Hospital School of Nursing. The summer before my senior year, I attended the Methodist Church camp at Lake Louise, where I met the camp nurse, Jane Mayfield. You could tell she loved her profession and was proud of her school, BMH. She asked me to apply. I was accepted at both Blodgett and Bronson, and chose Bronson. I have never regretted it. I was very homesick but knew it was where the Lord wanted me to be.

Betty Gosling Vander Molen '51

I attended a summer church camp at Lake Louise when I was in the sixth grade. The camp nurse was from BMH. I was so impressed that I decided I would be a nurse and go to Bronson.[35] I never wavered in my decision. I had a scholarship offer from Harper-Grace Hospital in Detroit but did not give it a second thought.

Jane Sny Hartman '67

I'm one of those people who always knew what I wanted to be: I was going to be a nurse. The crisp, starched, white uniform and cap of the nurse at my doctor's office, and the old radio program, Dr. Christian and his nurse, June, played by Rosemary DeCamp, reinforced my desire. I was always a compassionate person and had a strong desire to help others deal with illness and pain.

Marilyn Newcombe Bryant '54

My grandparents lived on the east side of Kalamazoo. I can recall seeing student nurses from Borgess Hospital shopping in a drug store on more than one occasion. They were dressed in white uniforms and navy blue capes. As a seven-year old, I was impressed. I knew in junior high school that I wanted to be in a profession to help other people. Being a Methodist at that time, it seemed appropriate to attend Bronson. The fact that I was born at Bronson in 1934 also influenced my decision.

Patricia Hauke Dahlman '55

Teachers

When I was six years old, I became ill with a kidney disease and spent time in a hospital. I had to stay in bed, get shots, and take terrible tasting medicine. The nurses were all so nice to me, and I was fascinated by what they did. My church emphasized service to others. I attended a two-room school and my teacher for the seventh or eighth grade convinced me that I might be capable of becoming a nurse. As a high school senior, I spent half days in a co-op program working and learning in the hospital. Thanks to the support of nurses and teachers, as well as my parents, I had the courage to apply to Bronson.

Carol Peeks Gunneman '63

My friendship with an eighth-grade teacher, Mary McCormick, influenced me. Eventually she left teaching to seek a career in nursing. She went to Bronson, graduating in the class of 1932 and she encouraged me to attend Bronson. I have always been grateful to her. I received a good education.

Christine Gierman Jarchow '33

Altruism

It was September 1943. World War II had taken our men and we were all doing our best to support our country. We dealt with gas rationing as well as food rationing, and we sang patriotic songs and saluted our American flag. So one very naïve girl, just out of high school, decided to become a nurse and help her fellow men.

Beth Ellinger Jirikovic '46

It never occurred to me to be anything other than a nurse. Oh, there was a brief time when I thought of being a fabulously famous and wealthy archeologist who discovered tombs and treasures in Egypt, but always, it came down to nursing. My mother died of leukemia when I was 14, and I spent quite a bit of time being the home care person, as my father had to work. The idea of being able to help another person in such circumstances was a powerful altruistic motivation. The choice of Bronson was sort of made for me, as a close friend, a year ahead of me in high school, had decided on Bronson and Albion College, and we were going to go together. She went to Albion for a year, waiting for me, and then lasted only the first semester in Bronson. I loved the program.

Katherine "Kit" Bosker Gifford '54

While in the Peace Corps, in Kenya, I had an opportunity to work with a UNESCO researcher on a reading project for hospitalized children. While volunteering, I thought it would be interesting to work as a nurse midwife. I spoke with as many nurses as I could and they all enjoyed their jobs. I applied to three nursing schools from overseas. Two of the schools had a waiting list. Bronson didn't.

Nancy George '89

Other Reasons for Choosing Nursing

Attending Bronson was my second career choice. I was accepted at Western Michigan University with plans for social work. Then, on a whim, I stopped at Bronson with a girlfriend from 4-H. We located Mary B. Anderson's office and I asked for information on applying. It sounded like a challenge—they only accepted applicants from the top one-third of high school graduates. My mother was against the idea. She told me that nurses work too hard and have difficult hours. She was correct for the most part, but my mind was made up. I never regretted it. In retrospect, I think that Sue Barton nurse novels also influenced me. True!

Kay Cook Davidson Hanson '64

In 1963 choices for female higher education were primarily secretary, teacher or nurse. The reasons I chose nursing were three instead of four years of education (I was wrong—33 versus 32 months) and I would always have a job (I was right).

Mary Ann Fink Rebert '66

Motivation to become a nurse was never clear to me—-a skill was necessary for employment and so I pursued nursing. Even so, it did not occur to me that the medical model and pathological approach to health were mindsets for delivering care in a narrowly prescribed way. Exposure to sociology, education outside of the medical model, opened a new perspective for me. I learned that self-empowerment concepts enhanced the healing arts, beginning a process of transformation for me. What a burden it was to "make people well" back then. Was it me or the system? Nurses offered health education but not empowerment. Permitting choices seems more effective. Utilizing my nursing background in another setting, social work, was an interesting process and a mental transition. Fortunately, my career was in a model of practice that made education and theory of both professions very valuable, well beyond a focus on pathology and medical treatment only. Families in crises have all kinds of needs!

Patricia Lingle Kleynenberg '66

When I was in high school I worked as a nurse aide at Bronson. I enjoyed the work and decided nursing should be my career. I picked Bronson as it had the cadet nurse corps. Our class did not receive the uniforms and was the last Bronson class to be part of the corps.

Nancy Willis Shepard '48

I worked as an aide in a small rural hospital. The only anesthesia provider was a nurse anesthetist. I was able to go back to surgery and observe her work a couple of times. I thought, "Wow, what a cool job she has." I decided to go to nursing school and on to become a nurse anesthetist. It was the best decision I ever made.

Debra Ringler Sponseller '77

These stories have different twists. However, they demonstrate the influence adults have on children they touch. Along with a penchant for service, a nursing career most often came to mind in direct relationship to a special nurse in the lives of young women, whether mother, aunt or caregiver.

THE FLORENCE NIGHTINGALE PLEDGE

I solemnly pledge myself before God and in the presence of this assembly to pass my life in purity and to practice my profession faithfully. I will abstain from whatever is deleterious and mischievous, and will not take or knowingly administer any harmful drug.

> *I will do all in my power to maintain and elevate the standards of my profession, and will hold in confidence all personal matters committed to my keeping, and all family affairs coming to my knowledge in the practice of my calling.*
>
> *With loyalty will I endeavor to aid the physician in his work and devote myself to the welfare of those committed to my care.*[36]

CHAPTER 3 NOTES

---

[1] *Bronson Bulletin*, 1962 Winter; 1. "Lighting the path to life of service."

[2] Dossey, B.M. *Florence Nightingale: mystic, visionary, healer.* Springhouse, PA: Springhouse, 2000 p. 23.

[3] Selanders, L.., Florence Nightingale lecture and journey, England, 2003 May 5–16.

[4] Dossey, B.M., *op.cit.*, p.88.

[5] *Webster's new world dictionary, 3rd college edition.* New York: Prentice Hall, 1994. p.898.

[6] Calabria, M.D., and McCrae, J., ed. *Suggestions for thought by Florence Nightingale: selections and commentaries.* Philadelphia: University of Pennsylvania Press, 1994. p.ix.

[7] *Ibid.*, p.30.

[8] *Ibid.*, p.xi.

[9] *Ibid.*, p.33.

[10] *Ibid.*, p.xiii.

[11] *Ibid.*, p.74.

[12] Dossey, B.M., *op. cit.*, p.75.

[13] Dossey, B.M., *op. cit.*, p.87.

[14] Dossey, B.M., *op cit.*, p.87–89.

[15] Dossey, B.M., *op. cit.*, p.87–95.

[16] Selanders, L., *op.cit.*. The lamp often depicted as an Aladdin-type lamp, is disconcerting to nurse historians who know better. The lamp that Nightingale carried was a Turkish lantern, more like a cylindrical Japanese lantern. Some pictures do have the lamp accurately depicted.

---

[17] Dossey, B.M., *op. cit.,* p, 121.

[18] Dossey, B.M., *op. cit.,* p. 129, 153.

[19] Nightingale, F. *Notes on nursing,* New York: D. Appleton, 1894.

[20] Dossey, B.M., *op. cit.,* p. 162

[21] Dossey, B.M., *op. cit.,* p. 163.

[22] Dossey, B.M., *op. cit.,* p. 131.

[23] Dossey, B.M., *op. cit.,* p. 165–166.

[24] Dossey, B.M., *op. cit.,* p. 219–221.

[25] Dossey, B.M., *op. cit.,* p. 221–222.

[26] Dossey, B.M., *op. cit.,* p. 304–306.

[27] Dossey, B.M., *op. cit.,* p.239.

[28] Dossey, B.M., *op. cit.,* p. 248–249.

[29] Bronson added an additional year of training in 1906.

[30] Selanders, L., *op. cit.*

[31] Dossey, B.M., *op.cit.,* p. 381–382.

[32] D'Antonio, Patricia. *Reflections*, 1997 3rd/4th Quarter, pp. 16–17. "Nineteenth century nursing: science and the values of duty, will and power."

[33] Cornelia Veenhuis Cody's 1920s story gives an example of the family physician recommending Cornelia, but not her sister, for nursing school. He said that the sister was too pretty and wouldn't last a year.

[34] Ella Beck Newton was Marilyn E. Newton's mother.

[35] Jane could not recall the name of the nurse. Was it Jane Mayfield?

[36] This "Florence Nightingale Pledge" was formulated, not by Miss Nightingale, but Mrs. Lystra E. Gretter, who chaired the Farrand Training School for Nurses committee at old Harper Hospital in Detroit. It was based on the Hippocratic Oath taken by medical doctors. She wrote the pledge for commencement of its Class of 1893.

CHAPTER 4

THE MONUMENT SURVIVES THE GREAT DEPRESSION, 1930s

The early 1930s found the hospital focused on survival, much as one would expect in post-Depression years. The nursing school and hospital, in order to operate, were dependent on church donations. Receipt of patient's payments continued to fall short of actual costs incurred. Bronson was one of 77 hospitals managed by the Methodist Episcopal Church in 28 states and Washington D.C., with a total of 9,374 beds and 281,778 patients from July 1, 1930 to June 30, 1931.[1] The American White Cross Guild was its service arm, a major source of revenue through donations of money and supplies built on the labors of a volunteer women's force.

Miss Clara Pugsley had a dual role as the Michigan White Cross associate state director and as the superintendent of linen at Bronson. Annual reporting through the decade attested to the need for charity to keep hospitals across the nation from failing. "Bronson Methodist Hospital is a good place to use that sacred thing called 'money' in human service . . . . Hospital work is Christian service. Our hospital [Bronson] receives people of any creed or no creed. The richest and the poorest get the same care."[2]

The local Bronson White Cross Guild (BWCG) was organized in the spring of 1935, and Dr. S.W. Robinson, Bronson superintendent, provided a home for the

BWCG on Pine Street. Its first fundraiser successfully made $1,000 through a production with 60 to 80 entertainers as the draw! A committee of almost 50 guild members sold tickets. Many physicians and their wives were patrons. They needed a healthy hospital in which to practice as much as the community needed inpatient care and staff needed jobs. It took everyone to keep the monument alive.

By January 1936, 250 women participated, according to their interests, in a variety of Guild subcommittees that focused on the nurses and students, children, babies, flowers, and reading. They could work at home on projects, such as sewing needed hospital supplies or fundraising, or outside their homes by volunteering at the hospital. A jelly group was responsible for the gift of 118 glasses of jelly, to be used on patient's trays.[3]

Four hundred people attended the first BWCG luncheon in May 1936, including guests from Kalamazoo, Detroit, Flint, Toledo, Indianapolis and other cities. The luncheon showcased the volunteer resources needed to keep the hospital in the black. Dr. John G. Benson, superintendent of the Indianapolis Methodist Hospital, spoke about women's part in modern hospitalization to the gathered members and guests. Just as women were needed to do a wealth of behind-the-scenes work for Bronson's survival during its first 30 years, the situation still had not changed:

> Dr. Benson stressed two points, first the adventure in cooperative kindness, and second, the creation of a new health consciousness and health mind. In olden days, according to Dr. Benson, people defied disease, but now a new creed has shown health as normal and disease abnormal. He urged women present to catch the spirit of the White Cross and not be blinded by institutionalized social service. He pointed out the challenge: "How can we get the advantage of hospitalization to all persons in a community?" He said he himself did not know the answer. That is up to the people themselves, he concluded.[4]

Sometimes the BWCG called upon nursing students to help with its activities, but mainly the women of the Nurses Guild provided support to the hard-working, dedicated students. Guild members and students each had their roles to play in providing no cost- and low-cost labor to support the hospital system. "Student Nurses Welcomed," was the subtitle of a *Kalamazoo Gazette* article, which stated,

> The principal objective of the Nurses Guild is to contact and help the student nurses of Bronson Hospital. This group has a membership of 50, and during the last year members have given about 600 hours of service. Their year's activities included parties for two classes entering training, flowers furnished for the nurses when they are ill and for the nurses' homes, decorating the nurses' dining room on special occasions, birthday remembrances for each nurse, entertaining the graduating class in the spring, and a Christmas party with tree and gifts for all."[5]

Funds were often raised through the sponsorship of social events similar to those during the first 30 years of the hospital's existence, that is, with variety shows, musical offerings, and book reviews, and, in 1937, cookie parties were inaugurated to fund the Children's Guild activities.

To whom were nurses faithful? Service to others was expected, the martyr archetype often a pattern of women.[6] Paramount was service to the hospital, patients, community and physicians, not necessarily in that order. Stories told in interviews often show that the four were integrated. Service to one was service to all, while taking care of one's self did not seem to be a necessary component of the caring equation.

DORIS GARLOCK CROCKETT '31

When Garlock[7] was seven years old, she decided to become a nurse after her 10-year-old brother's physical condition required a private duty nurse for several months. He had a ruptured appendix, an appendectomy at home, and complications related to the acute abdominal infection. Garlock recalled that many doctors were not available due to the war, and their family doctor had the flu. Her brother had been treated with hot compresses and castor oil, not a favorable treatment for appendicitis. The family did not expect him to live through the day that the World War I armistice was signed in 1917. When he recovered, Garlock knew that she would become a nurse just like the woman who had cared for her brother.

Her strict Methodist family was the reason Garlock chose Bronson. She recalled Ingathering Sunday's when the women of the Methodist Church would bring canned fruits and vegetables, as well as linens, to church to be sent to Bronson Methodist Hospital.

Garlock applied to Bronson in 1929, and was accepted when she was 17. Her eighteenth birthday came in November, but she was allowed to enter two months earlier. She received an apron pattern before school started so she could make several of them to wear over her uniform, which she would be issued at Bronson upon her arrival. Both Garlock and her parents cried when it came time for her to leave home. They lived in a small town, Carson City, a 100–mile trip over gravel roads. Kalamazoo seemed so far away. Her belongings, packed in a travel trunk and sent the previous week by train, arrived before she did.

> Garlock set a slow, steady pace during her book interview. Her tone of voice and manner were matter-of-fact, without inflection, and she projected a sense of being grounded and stable in both her personal and professional life.

Osborne Home, a big house behind the *Kalamazoo Gazette* building on John Street, became her first residence on the Bronson campus. Garlock moved in along with 13 other freshmen. Fourteen girls lived in one large attic with one bathroom equipped with a toilet, washbowl, and tub. A second washbowl was located in the hall outside of the bathroom. She and the other country girls were afraid to light the Humphrey heater for their bath water. They wouldn't attempt a bath unless one of the girls from Kalamazoo was there to light it for them.

Two other homes, North and West, housed students who were expected to be at breakfast at 6:30 A.M. and on the patient-care unit at 7:00 A.M. Students had three hours off for class, either 9:00–noon, 1:00–4:00 P.M., or 3:00–7:00 P.M., sometimes later if patients required attention or other hospital work needed to be done. It was a long 12-hour day and often the students missed class because needed service was the first priority. Could it have been a philosophical decision that experiential learning was more meaningful than sitting for lectures?

The first three months of school were probationary, with time spent scrubbing floors, walls, and cleaning the service rooms. Since Garlock knew how to sew, she didn't have to scrub floors but instead was assigned to the linen room. She mended bed linens, hemmed drapes and curtains, and made breast and surgical binders. One day she was sent to a dry goods store on the corner of Michigan and Burdick to replenish material supplies. Garlock could not recall a worse fear than being sent to the store as a probie[8] who did not know the city. Finding her way back to the hospital seemed overwhelming.

Four or five classmates dropped out within the first three months of school—the rest stayed to graduate, except for one classmate who died suddenly of a kidney problem. Her funeral was held in her family's home in Albion, Michigan, with Garlock and three of her classmates serving, in their uniforms, as honorary pallbearers. Death was commonplace. So many patients died from acute infections—men in their forties who were admitted to the hospital with pneumonia, a young girl with simple blisters on her heel, and women who had "back street abortions." Antibiotics likely would have saved them. Nursing students were expected to objectify incredibly personal experiences and handle their grief because death was common and normal. No formal place existed within the nursing education structure to share one's fears or grief.

Residence rules confined students to campus at 8:00 P.M., Monday through Friday. Curfews for the weekend were 11:00 P.M. on Saturday and 10:00 P.M. on

Sunday when movies were forbidden, except for inspirational films at the Presbyterian Church which met at Central High School after its church building burned. Students would attend, just to get out to see a movie.

Monday evenings meant going to the YWCA on Rose Street for the dreaded, "swim and gym" activity. Most of the students were too tired to enjoy the exercise. Tired as they were, however, they eagerly dashed to the best part of Monday night—the popcorn wagon outside the YWCA. They ate their five-cent bag with delight. When asked what other "fun" activities occurred, Garlock replied that there was no time for them. Occasionally the girls caught an afternoon movie if anyone had ten cents, which was rare. Once in a great while, at the height of America's Great Depression, her family might send Garlock a dollar.

She could not recall anyone dating young men, except for one "rootin' tootin'" heavy-set girl who left the program suddenly, leaving in her wake a rumor that she had had a baby.

Garlock learned that only last names preceded by Miss or Mrs., could be used when addressing other nurses or students. When doctors entered the room, all nurses deferred to them by standing, giving up their chairs, and tending to the physicians' wishes. Students were paid $6.00 a month. Payment for a broken thermometer or syringe was subtracted from the stipend.[9] This misfortune, however, never affected Garlock.

Grandpa R. was the first patient every freshman saw that year. Garlock couldn't recall his diagnosis but knew that he couldn't speak well and that he gestured wildly with his hands and feet to compensate. His four-bed ward cost him $3.00 per day. All patients in wards received baths every other day; their backs were rubbed, and they received a sponge bath before bed. Flowers were removed from patients' rooms and set in the hall each night. In the morning, fresh water was added to the vases and the flowers returned to their respective rooms.

Patient units had small kitchens. A Bunsen burner facilitated needle sterilization. First the students washed the needles, which were then sterilized in the burner's flame for use over and over again. The nurses sharpened needles when they found barbs on reusable ones.[10]

Clinical practice rotations included obstetric nursing with a kind supervisor, Miss Marie Wantz, and operating room nursing with an equally nice supervisor, Miss Dena Wolters. Garlock thought both of these women were excellent role models. Misses Wolters and Wantz lived next to the hospital at this time, and nursing was their life. She found Dr. Boys and the nurse anesthetist, Mrs. Wildermuth, to be most intimidating. "She was a little bitty thing and everyone was scared to death of her."

Mrs. Draher was the nurse administrator. Garlock couldn't recall that she taught or was involved with the students' education. Clinical practice affiliations included three months at Herman Kiefer Hospital in Detroit, with six weeks practicing in the tuberculosis ward and six weeks with contagious diseases such as scarlet fever and diphtheria. While their student colleagues from other programs were allowed to wear white stockings and white shoes during the clinical rotation at Herman Kiefer, the Bronson students were stuck with the hated black shoes and hose! Another rotation in the Bronson diet kitchen introduced them to a dietician who had "funny ideas" and insisted that eggs not be refrigerated. Garlock was also sent to Crystal Springs Church Camp for two weeks to be the camp nurse. She rode with Dr. Meader, the district superintendent of the Methodist Church, and his son. It was a good time, with no bad experiences.

Since Garlock entered school at 17, she was only 20 when she graduated in 1931. At age 21, she could write the state board exam and find a nurse position. During the interim she returned home. With only one graduation ceremony each year in May, both September and February graduates returned to Bronson to be part of the formal event.

Garlock first practiced as a private duty nurse and lived with classmate, Marian Vandenberg[11] at her family's home on Oakland Drive. Marian's father drove Garlock to Oakwood to catch the trolley into Kalamazoo on workdays. She next secured a position with Dr. Homer Stryker. She went with him to deliver babies in homes, scrubbed with him as his surgical assistant, and served as his office nurse. He leaned toward orthopaedics but practiced general medicine in the 1930s. "He did everything," she said. She recalled assisting with a home surgery involving double mastoiditis (most likely an incision and drainage). The patient was also contagious with scarlet fever so he couldn't be moved to the hospital.

RUTH MCLELLAN —STUDENT GROWTH AND PROFESSIONALISM

Miss Ruth McLellan, appointed superintendent of nursing in 1934, was a forward-thinking woman with a vision for nursing that could bring advance practice into the twentieth century. Her speeches to the community seem paradoxical to Dr. John Benson's May 1936 message to the BWCG. McLellan described nurses as professionals, with a place at the table, an egalitarian role driven by collegiate education and remuneration commensurate with their knowledge and skill level. No longer were they simply the physicians' handmaidens, paid low wages to do physician-extender work and to deny nursing science's merits. Even so, McLellan shared her concerns about the movement of nursing education away from hospitals and into higher education. Newspaper articles offer insight into her plan for patient care improvement as well as making nursing an acceptable profession for women and men.[12] One can only conjecture about how her Altrusa Club speech was received: "Nursing is in a transitory stage. We're on our way, but we don't know where we're going. After World War I, schools of nursing made flattering offers to student nurses, but then the Depression came." She closed her remarks with the question: Should schools of nursing belong with a college or university or with a hospital? "On the one hand, the college is apt to forget the actual needs of the nurse and overemphasize theory, while on the other the hospital may exaggerate the practical side and overlook theory."

Her May speech, "Nursing as a Profession," to the monthly general meeting of the Bronson White Cross Guild, included a celebration of National Hospital Day and the birthday of Florence Nightingale (born May 12, 1820). Most likely the topics of her two speeches were similar.

Two changes in the School of Nursing occurred during Miss McLellan's 1934–1937 tenure as superintendent. Both are noted in the August 1, 1935, letter that Gladys Thornburg received after her acceptance to the school. First, "Your white uniforms will be supplied here. You will not wear aprons." This mandate was newsworthy since the message indicated that pinafores and aprons gave nurses the appearance of uneducated housekeepers. The second change was the award of college credit!

> White uniforms, hose and shoes took the place of pinafores, aprons, black stockings and shoes in 1935, a change memorialized and sung to the tune of of Notre Dame's "Victory March,"
>
> **Our Old Black Shoes**
>
> Cheer, cheer for our old black shoes,
> Dirty and worn, and broken down, too,
> Think how they have stood the test,
> Days and nights without a rest!
> Stockings with holes in heel and toe
> With runs we've mended where they show.
> Here's a cheer! Farewell tonight!
> Tomorrow—"hello" to white!

> We are happy to inform you we have arranged to send your class to Western State Teachers College for one subject (Chemistry) a day. At the end of the school year you will have earned a college credit, which we trust will be a stimulus for you to work toward a college degree at some later date. There will be a nominal fee of $2.50 per term for this subject, as well as the textbook needed. You will wear your street clothes rather than your uniform when in attendance at college.[13]

Obviously, these changes were congruent with Miss McLellan's vision of advancing nursing toward professionalism.

Ruth McLellan Remembered by 1930s Graduates

Students often depicted directors of nursing as strict and rigid disciplinarians who made their own rules, or as caring mentors who acted in a kind way when the student was in distress. Perceptions varied within the context of students' experiences. Miss McLellan was not an exception.

Contrasting behaviors are noted in stories about Miss Ruth McLellan during her tenure. Margaret Ruth Martin, graduate of 1938, provides this account:

> I arrived with my parents for the initial interview with her [Miss McLellan]. We were told my grades in high school were not sufficiently high enough to qualify me for admission to the program. My father prevailed upon Miss McLellan to summon the hospital administrator, which she consented to do. Upon his arrival, he reviewed the hospital grades of my sister, Helen, who was in her third year at the school. He stated that her grades were excellent and that I should be granted admission to the program provided that my grades were in the upper third of the high school class.
>
> One of my classmates dropped a sterile instrument on the floor during a surgical procedure, which she picked up and placed on the sterile surgical tray. Miss McLellan, upon learning of this action, immediately sent the girl home. It was rumored that the poor girl committed suicide shortly thereafter.
>
> In our first year, Miss McLellan notified all students that it was mandatory for everyone to have their tonsils out. This demand was a shock to all of us since we were given no choice.
>
> Miss McLellan was exceedingly strict when enforcing the rules and regulations, a perfect match to her seemingly cool and unfriendly attitude. In contrast, I should relate that during my second year I became homesick, and apparently Miss McLellan either observed my condition or was told by a classmate. She called me into her office and, in a kindly manner, told me she had made arrangements for me to return home for a week.

Excerpts from McLellan's Reports

Miss McLellan's monthly reports, September 1934 to August 1937,[14] read at the Administration Committee meetings from when she resigned, start with student enrollment. For example:

> Students, September 1, 1934-------------------66
> Preliminary students admitted------------------25
> Students completing course of nursing-------- 4
> Students in the school, October 1, 1934------87

Another excerpt from September 1934 described an informal system used to welcome and mentor students beginning their first day:

> Upon the day of her arrival, the new student was met by her Big Sister at the School of Nursing Office. She was then under the guidance of the older nurse for the day, to get acquainted [until] an informal welcoming service, which was sponsored by the entire student body, in the parlors of the YWCA. Reverend Ellinger addressed the students.

Dismissal reporting contains details such as:

> Miss . . . , a member of the Class of 1935, was sent home Monday, September 10, because she had disregarded the rules of our school. Saturday evening, September 8, in the company of another student and two gentlemen, she had gone out of town without permission. When she returned to the Nurses' Home, the night supervisor realized that she had been drinking. She was suspended indefinitely."

Tonsillectomies were the operation of the 1930s, supposedly a way to cure contagious throat infections. Miss McLellan stated, in October 1934:

> Fifteen of the twenty-five preliminary students had tonsillectomy operations two weeks after they entered the School of Nursing.

> Inasmuch as the inflamed tonsils were present before they entered the School of Nursing and should have been remedied before they came to us, it was thought wise to ask the parents to assume some responsibility. Each parent was requested to pay $5. The response was excellent.

Miss McLellan included a list of Christmas gifts the students received from three women, ten physicians, the Lovell Café, and a local funeral parlor in her December 1934 report. She stated, "They were also remembered with many Christmas greetings from former patients and graduates of the School of Nursing. Mrs. Draher (the previous director) and Miss Kunkel (Theory of Nursing instructor) each sent greetings." Miss McLellan also described Christmas:

> It was a beautiful day in the hospital. In the early morning the patients were aroused by the familiar carols sung by students as they marched through the corridors, each carrying a lighted candle. As the breakfast tray was carried into the patient's room, each guest was delighted to find a lighted candle upon the tray, bearing a Christmas greeting. The supervisors had arranged this ceremony. At noon the patients were again surprised at finding a tiny begonia plant on their trays, each plant conveying a cheery greeting from the Medical Auxiliary. The night trays were a bit unusual. Each one was interesting because it carried a decorated Christmas cookie.

A similar Christmas 1934 story was told by Marjorie Peck from a student's perspective. The spirit seemed to be catching:

> It was Christmas morning and snow had been falling gently during the night. Rising at 5:30 A.M., we dressed into our uniforms—the blue and white striped dresses with starched white aprons and bibs, put on our hair nets, and fastened our white caps. The ground was white when we dashed out from four different locations: Osborne, North, and West homes and the upstairs of the Annex. Usually we attended chapel before breakfast, but this morning was special. We formed a procession to walk through the halls with lighted candles

> while singing carols and hymns of Christmas. Our repertoire varied from "Jingle Bells" to "O Holy Night," and the patients could see us as well as hear us because the night nurses had opened all the doors.
>
> Completing our singing on the first floor, we climbed the stairs that circled the open elevator shaft to the second floor and then to the third floor. Being one of the taller nurses, I was the last in line. As I started to follow the procession, I looked up through the open grill on the elevator and saw a picture that will forever be etched in my mind. It was the sight of all the nurses in their starched white aprons, holding the lighted candles as they circled up the stairs. It brought tears that couldn't be controlled. I swallowed hard and began to sing as I too climbed those stairs.
>
> I do not remember who originated the Christmas procession of light and song but that person was divinely inspired. My memory is a precious one.

1930s REPORTS AND DOCUMENTS

The Annual Booklet, Bronson Methodist Hospital, 1931, (a report to the American White Cross Hospital Sunday), connected student stories and demographics.[15] Verbatim information has been reproduced in this text on pages 117–119. Four homes accommodated the student nurses. In each home was a supervisor, who was in charge:

- ***West Nurses Home:*** 18 student nurses and the supervisor live here.
- ***Osborne Nurses Home:*** the superintendent of nurses, four supervisors, and 32 student nurses have their rooms here.
- ***North Home:*** this home has 26 student nurses and a supervisor.
- ***School Building:*** the first floor is taken up by the room occupied by the educational director, the classroom, the demonstration room, and a small laboratory. The second floor had room for seven nurses.

Requirements for Admission to the School of Nursing[16]

1. Applicants are requested to make personal application if possible, if not, by letter to the Superintendent of Nurses.
2. Applicants must be at least 18 years of age and not over 35 years.
3. Of average height and good physique.
4. Vaccinated before entering the school.
5. Physical examination by the home doctor and report mailed with the application.
6. Dentist examination, work done, if necessary, before entering, and report mailed with the application.
7. This hospital requires high school graduation.
8. Normal- and college-educated students, and high school students with high marks, will be preferred, provided they meet the requirements in other respects.
9. Applications are not desired from candidates whose personal or family affairs are likely to interfere with the continuity of their training. The work of the hospital and school is of such a character that it should be given uninterrupted attention.

Information about the School of Nursing

The Principal of the Training School [the director of nursing], with the approval of the General Superintendent, decides the fitness of the candidates for the work and the propriety of retaining them or dismissing them at the end of the term of probation or during its course. She may also, with the approval of the general superintendent, terminate the connection of a pupil with the school at any time for misconduct, inefficiency, or neglect of duty.

Bronson Methodist Hospital is an Accredited School[17] and gives a three-year course. Students completing their three years of training are permitted to write the State Board Examinations. The course of instruction is approved by the State Board for Registration of Nurses.

We enter two classes a year, September and March. The exact date of registration is decided later in the year and applicants are notified in plenty of time to complete their arrangements.

The hours of duty vary. We aim to have an eight-hour service. Each student has two half days off each week, one during the week and one on Sunday. Time lost through illness must be made up. Student nurses are taken care of when ill, for a reasonable length of time.

Pupil nurses are allowed $6 per month. This payment begins at the end of the four months' probation period if they are accepted. They receive board, room and laundry from the date of their entrance. They will be permitted to wear the uniform when accepted, and after that they will be required to wear the uniform when on duty.

Students are required to furnish their own textbooks (which are purchased through the hospital at cost), and each student must have her own textbooks, notebooks, pen and ink. Other personal expenses are governed largely by the tastes and habits of the individual.

Registration fee is $55. This fee does not cover the entire expenses for books and uniforms for the three years, but the remaining expenses for books and uniforms are not large. Diploma fee is $3.25, payable at least six months before graduation.

Two weeks' vacation is allowed the first and third years and three weeks the intermediate year. Vacations are allowed during the period when class work is suspended.

McLellan Exonerated

Minutes of the December 21, 1936, Administration Committee stated, "The present nursing situation in the hospital was discussed. No action was taken." Lack of details and minutes of January 18, 1937, would lead one to conclude that the shortage of nurses was serious, compounded by graduate nurse illnesses during an influenza epidemic.

All was not well when the Administration Committee met in the Guild House on Monday, January 18, 1937. Obviously, someone was not happy with Miss McLellan's performance:

> Inasmuch as certain statements were made in the recent trustee meeting to the effect that charges of a serious nature had been made against Miss Ruth McLellan, Superintendent of Nurses, we wish to inform all trustees of the findings of the Administration Committee, which investigated these charges.
>
> This committee has met several times in the past week. We have taken testimony from many witnesses, examined documentary evidence, and thoroughly sifted the charges. Our conclusion is that these charges are wholly without foundation and Miss McLellan is completely exonerated.

McLellan Improves Conditions of Nursing Practice

A shortage of nurses and money was documented, and Miss McLellan recommended ". . . the advisability of retaining the next group of students, who will soon complete their training, as general-duty nurses." A decision was made to pay the new graduates a minimum of $50 [per month]. Remuneration was the issue. The January meeting provided more evidence of the money shortage, in a discussion about the necessity of keeping an executive housekeeper, ". . . the opinion of the committee that we could dispense with her services, thereby making it possible to spread this person's salary over the payroll of the people who at present are working under the executive housekeeper."

The decision to hire new graduates became an annual practice at Bronson over four decades. When students graduated they immediately started to work as GNs, a title that could be used prior to passing the State of Michigan registered nurse licensing examination.

Eight-hour shifts, including classroom time, were approved, ". . . except in an unusual emergency."[18] For the 1930s, students' eight hours per day were multiplied by six clinical practice days for a 48-hour week. Students were still practicing at least 40 hours per week, plus ten classroom hours, throughout the next three decades. On many occasions, swing shifts were assigned so that 16 practice hours could be managed within a 24-hour time frame. Hospital direct-care services continued to depend on the least costly labor available.

McLellan and Robinson Resign

Miss McLellan was employed as the superintendent of nursing in 1934, the same year Dr. William Puffer resigned his position. She and Reverend Samuel W. Robinson were appointed to their positions the same year, most likely McLellan had previous connections with the new hospital superintendent. Their tenures from 1934 to 1937 coincided. The *Kalamazoo Gazette* article of January 8, 1937, notes, "administration difficulties . . . as the general reason for Robinson's resignation." Most likely McLellan's support came from Robinson, and with his resignation she felt the need to resign.

The Reverend Alfred Way, D.D., Secretary of the Michigan State Council of the M.E. Church, was appointed temporary superintendent, which required his relocation from Detroit to Kalamazoo. Bernice Hammond became the new superintendent of nurses.

1930 GRADUATE STORIES

Ena Kraft Jackson '32

In September, 1929, I entered Bronson's three-year nursing program. In 1932, following graduation, I returned to my hometown of Frankfort, Michigan, and worked for a brief time in its small "home hospital." Then I returned to work in 1934 at

Herman Kiefer Hospital, Detroit, where I had spent a three-month affiliation as a Bronson student. I cared for patients with tuberculosis and other communicable diseases. You name it, we had it. However, diphtheria vaccine was taking care of that dreaded disease and a measles vaccine was being developed.

I returned to Frankfort in 1937 and found the small hospital closed, so my parents and I opened our home, which became a very busy source of nursing care during the next 14 years. Four physicians trusted their patients to our care. Before we bought a small anesthesia machine, I don't remember how many cans of ether I poured over people's noses. (Ether was dripped from holes poked into the can over a gauze mask that covered the patient's nose.) Surgeries, mothers and babies, accident victims, and medically treated illnesses kept us busy.

During the mid '40s, the community (and especially my family and I) realized that Frankfort needed a proper hospital. Local donations from natives and our Crystal Lake "summer people," as well as matching funds from the Hill–Burton Act, built a 29-bed hospital on a hill overlooking the harbor. We moved patients, mothers and babies, and equipment into the new facility on November 19, 1951. Paul Oliver Memorial Hospital is now a satellite of Munson Medical Center in Traverse City. I am still (1997) a member of the hospital auxiliary.

Dorothy Armstrong Chase '32

My greatest Bronson joy was bedside care. I also enjoyed associations with students and supervisors, weekly assembly with Dr. Puffer, and the kindness of doctors, especially Dr. Boys. I spent six months in the X-ray Department and remained in charge even when I was assigned to patient care on another unit. It troubled me to leave a patient half-bathed to assist in X-ray, though none complained.

I now marvel at the ease of giving injections with sterilized, wrapped syringes and needles that are disposable. At Bronson, I recall the two-burner gas plate on the three floors and in the diet kitchen. To sterilize the needle we boiled water in the bowl of a large spoon. We then drew the boiling water into the syringe repeatedly, after which, with forceps, we attached the needle to draw in the medication. Both needles and syringes were used repeatedly. We did many tasks that orderlies now do, since we only had one orderly for three floors. At the hospital, we managed with poor equipment so that made home nursing with little equipment easy.

Alethea Mae Crawford Utter '32

Special people I remember at Bronson as a student include Ann Gwinn Draher, superintendent of nurses and Principal; Dr. Puffer, general superintendent; Dena Wolters, surgical supervisor; Marie Wantz, maternity supervisor; and Mother Baird, the house mother. In 1936, I graduated from the University of Michigan School of Anesthesia and became a Certified Registered Nurse Anesthetist the next year.

During World War II, I entered the U.S. Army Nurse Corps and served as a nurse anesthetist for three and one-half years: two and one-half at Stark General Hospital in Charleston, N.C., and one year at the Military Hospital in West Point, N.Y. I was discharged five years later in 1947, and married Marvin E. Utter on December 8, 1956. When he died in 1962, I returned to Kalamazoo to administer anesthesia until I retired in 1975.

Marquita Land Vander Hoef '35

Land was born on Mackinac Island. She was cared for by her paternal grandmother after her mother's death from pneumonia when Land was five years old. She grew up in Cheboygan, Michigan, graduated from high school in 1932, and entered Bronson School of Nursing that fall, accompanied by her sister, Eleanor Land, who graduated from Bronson in 1935. Land remembered her dream of going to nursing school at Massachusetts General Hospital in Boston, but her grandmother said Boston was too far from home. Resources seemed to be a challenge; a nursing student could not get a loan. The money for her to attend Bronson was provided by Pastor Goodrich at Albion College, $65 for three years.

Land described a typical day as a student nurse in 1933. Even breakfast was a ritualized procedure in a world that seemed to be controlled by rituals and rules. Maybe the rituals imparted a sense of conformity that brought a feeling of safety to situations that were in God's hands:

> We are up at 5:00 A.M. to be ready for breakfast at 6:00. We cannot enter the dining room until the superintendent of nurses, the instructor, and six supervisors enter. They are beautiful examples of women in white—very stiffly starched and perfect. We all troop behind them, hungry and eager to start the new day, filled with unforeseen events.
>
> We are seated at five large tables. Two handsome, male college students are assigned to serve us after Mrs. Ann Gwinn Draher, superintendent of nurses, blesses the food.
>
> We may sing hymns for 15 minutes after the meal, and we do so happily and lustily to the accompaniment of the battered upright piano. Our pianist is a classmate of mine whose zeal for speeding up the beat of the music puts joy and great fervor into our hearts. Before I know it, I am whistling the tune instead of singing. Suddenly I realize that this behavior could cause me to be sent into conference with one of the two persons most responsible for our maturing from young high school graduates into respected and honored registered nurses.
>
> The day has officially started, and we march to our respective stations. We gather in a circle in a room assigned and listen to the night report. The head nurse examines our hands for clean, neat, uncolored nails and hair covered with the compulsory hair net. She also inspects our shoes—black "Enna Jetticks"—for a shiny appearance and our uniforms for cleanliness and, of course, the proper right angle of the pride of our lives, our white caps banded with black velvet ribbons. Narrow black ribbons identify second-year students while wide-black ribbons are worn the third year.

The head nurse assigns duties for the day. By this time it is a little past 7:00 A.M. and we know that later we will have an hour or two off duty to either go to class or to our dormitories to rest. Our day does not end until 7:00 P.M. Coffee breaks do not exist so we do not feel cheated or abused. It is the Depression era, and we are all most thankful for a warm place to enjoy three good meals to keep us healthy during our absorption of the medical art of nursing care.

The head nurse assigns me to a young woman in a private room located by the dumbwaiter (the poor section). Admitted during the night with a ruptured appendix, she has already advanced into the dreadful complication of peritonitis. The only ways we have to combat this type of illness are morphine sedation, glucose and saline intravenous, drain tubes in the belly area, and continuous hot turpentine stupes. Good nursing care is part of the treatment for she must be turned every hour to keep her from developing pneumonia. We are really quite modern.

The night nurse has already arranged the electric hot plate on the bedside table and a large basin of water is already boiling. Inside the basin is a large square of wool blanket that had been a gray paper-mill felt.[19] I prepare a new portion of one-quarter turpentine to three-quarters olive oil (if I remember correctly) and mix it well. I have a wooden tongue blade, that I have padded with cotton on one end, and wrap it tightly with a half bandage and tie it securely. I use this blade to spread the turpentine mixture over the woman's abdomen from ribs to pubic area. Then I remove the wool square from a stupe wringer, that is made from two portions of a broom handle, about 12 to 14 inches long, and slipped into the two hemmed ends of a stout piece of canvas-type material about 18 inches long and 10 to 12 inches wide. The two handles have allowed me to wring the hot wool square very dry, and with my two thumbs and forefingers, I pick up the two corners of the wool and cool it slightly by waving it in

> My memories include Wednesday night chapel with Dr. Puffer in charge, our small classroom in West Home, swim nights at the YWCA, curfews of 8:00 P.M. during the week and Saturday night at 11:00 P.M., the good food in our small dining room, and short visits downtown where folks knew we were nurses because they could smell the ether on us.
> ***Nora Thomas Brandeberry '33***

the air. I touch it against the inside of my elbow to test if it is safe for application. I then apply the wool, and cover it with a square of old rubber sheeting and a white bath towel.

I stand by her bed, changing this stupe about every 10 minutes. I watch for evidence of possible blistering of her skin. To my relief, I see none. The olive oil protects her skin, and I have not allowed the hot material to spread out beyond the oiled area. In the meantime, I give her a warm sponge bath and turn her every hour on the hour. I rub her back frequently with exhilaration. The cooling, refreshing alcohol will help reduce the raging fever that is flooding her system. A washcloth dampened often with ice water goes on her forehead at all times. I watch the intravenous bottle and refill it from a flask sitting on the nearby dresser—both very sterile and carefully handled. Neatly arranged butterfly tapes hold in place the dressing on the surgical area. The dressings used are called fluffs and we make all of them in the supply room. They are sterilized in the autoclave in surgery during the night.

Our techniques are excellent for we have no wonder drugs to help fight the battle of infection. I learn by all of the responsibility given to me. I learn how to be a sought-after private duty nurse. Whenever possible the doctor chooses the nurse who cares for his patient. I have already decided that I'm going to be that kind of nurse. I am also learning to observe every little change in the countenance of my patient, the abdominal shape and flaccidity, respiratory reaction, and signs of tremor due to a blood stream infection. I am also learning to stay at my post until I am relieved.

My floor supervisor slips in every so often to encourage me and to see that things are as they should be. The senior nursing student who assists the supervisor comes in every three to four hours with a hypodermic to keep the patient quiet and restful during these crucial hours. I am relieved for dinner and for class attendance, and then, back on duty until 7:00 P.M.

At the bedside, I record everything in good order on the patient's chart. The surgeon comes in at least three times during the day. He has made me feel good inside by commending me for doing a fine job.

> At 7:00 P.M. or a little after, another student, who will carry on during the long night, relieves me. I return to my room, bathe, and study until 9:30 P.M. At 10:00 P.M. the lights must be turned out and I go to sleep, knowing that I have done something beautiful and wonderful for someone.
>
> This young woman was my daily responsibility. She recovered and went home after several weeks. I never saw her again, but will never forget her.

After graduation, Land was invited to work at a hospital in Jackson, Michigan, apparently arranged by Miss Ruth McLellan, the superintendent of nursing at Bronson. Land accepted the position and stayed for six months until she married a man who had been her patient. Her next position was in private duty nursing.

Marjorie Peck Ollila '35

> In the fall of 1936 I left Bronson to study Public Health Nursing at the University of Michigan. I had graduated from Bronson in 1935. While I was at Michigan, I was sent to the Health Department at Midland, Michigan, to do my fieldwork. At the completion of the course, I was offered a job in the Midland Health Department. All the disciplines, all the attention to details, all the minute observations that I had been trained for and learned at Bronson were needed for this field-related position. The tasks, at times, were extremely demanding and I became very appreciative of my training.
>
> One special experience involved one of my high-school classmates who was a dear friend living in Saginaw. She was married, had two little girls, and was expecting a third child. The country was still experiencing the effects of the Great Depression and her husband had been laid off from one of the automobile companies. Thus she planned to deliver the baby at home, and I told her that, if she could arrange to deliver on a weekend, I would travel to Saginaw from Midland to help. The Midland Health Department gave me permission to take a sterile obstetric pack with me. On Saturday morning her husband called to tell me that labor had started. I left Midland in a hurry because the Saginaw River was at flood stage

> and was threatening to block the roads. I arrived in the early afternoon just ahead of the flood and before my friend's labor pains became severe. I asked the husband to go to a pay telephone to call the doctor who had attended her previous deliveries. As the pains increased, I kept sending the husband to call the doctor and to ask him to hurry. He did not come. About 8:00 A.M., I draped my friend with the sterile linen, and she delivered a baby boy. Everything had gone smoothly. At 9:30 A.M, the doctor arrived and I was overjoyed to see him. He examined the mother and baby and then said, "You were luckier than I was, my baby died." He looked at my Bronson pin on my public health uniform and said, "I think Bronson Methodist Hospital trains some mighty fine nurses."
>
> After the doctor had gone, my friend asked, "Do you know what you said when our son was being born?" "No," I replied. She said, "Your words were, 'Dear God, let him breathe.'" I also learned that appeal at the Bronson School of Nursing. It is called humility.

Gladys Thornburg Richards '38

Thornburg's memorabilia included poems with authors cited but no dates. A letter sent to Miss Thornburg on August 1, 1935, detailed a list of tasks to be accomplished prior to her arrival at Bronson in the September Class of 1935, including the purchase of sewing articles that will be "a necessary part of your equipment." Uniforms, supplied at the hospital, were white, a change from the pin stripes mentioned by students prior to 1935:

> A watch with a second hand, a fountain pen, six suits of cotton underwear, and six slips of white cotton fabric with shadow-proof hem, the slips, when completed, to be 11 inches from the floor. Two pairs of plain white oxfords with cushioned rubber heels, six pairs of white stockings, either lisle or silk, one pair of gymnasium shoes, one gymnasium suit, and one dress that will be suitable for a dinner dress or semi-formal party. Your white uniforms will be supplied here. You will not wear aprons. Bring a sufficient number of printed name tapes to mark the belongings that you will purchase after you arrive.

Her reflections on her Bronson experience are excerpted below:

> I entered training in 1935. There were 12 of us in the class. We all lived in one room on the third floor of Osborne Home. We shared one bathroom with one tub and no shower. We took turns bathing and got along very well. An outside exit led to the fire escape, which was seldom used. No one evidently wanted to escape. I remember Lyle Nottingham, our trusted orderly, who often helped put casts on broken arms and legs. He could do anything, it seemed, and was always willing—an excellent role model.
>
> Nine of us graduated in 1938 with a class motto, "Honor lies at labor's gate." The *Kalamazoo Gazette* reported that our Monday evening's graduation, held at the First Methodist Episcopal Church was the smallest class in 12 years. Prior to the graduation, we attended a Sunday baccalaureate service at the Congregational Church. On Tuesday, an open house honored the graduates and alumni with demonstrations of the newer techniques in nursing and an address by Dr. W.O. Jennings, a local surgeon who also lectured to student nurses, concerning the latest advancements in medicine. Later that evening the alumni hosted a banquet at the Gull Lake Country Club.

The Thirties Close

"Kalamazoo now has approximately 150 graduate nurses who are active. Half of these are attached to Borgess, Bronson, Fairmont, the State Hospital, and Pine Crest Sanatorium. The remaining 75 are private duty nurses affiliated with the Nurses Registry at 1329 Hillcrest Avenue."[20] Was this number similar to national demographics in cities the same size? Or did the number represent a shortage? Seventy-five nurses for five hospitals average just 15 to cover 24 hours a day, seven days per week. Borgess, Bronson, and State depended on their nursing student pools to staff their direct patient-care services.

The hospital, as a monument to women, required their dedication and servitude to survive throughout the twentieth century, given the context of the times.

Though nurses often viewed themselves as professionals, the attitudes of physicians, hospital administrators and the general public were not similarly informed. For example, nurses were recognized for following physician orders, not for their clinical expertise. Who called the physician after diagnosing impending medical complications, and who reported patient progress to physicians daily? The nurses. The monument was a heavy one, supported by the women it was meant to celebrate, another paradox that often went unnoticed.

CHAPTER 4 NOTES

---

[1] Bronson Methodist Hospital, *Annual Report, July 1, 1930 to June 30, 1931,* p.5.

[2] Bronson Methodist Hospital, *Annual Report, July 1, 1930 to June 30, 1931,* pp.20–21.

[3] *Kalamazoo Gazette*, 1936 January 1, "White Cross Guild forms to aid Bronson Hospital."

[4] *Kalamazoo Gazette*, 1936 May, "White Cross has first luncheon."

[5] *Kalamazoo Gazette*, 1938 May, "White Cross Guild has a busy year of service."

[6] Pearson, Carol S., *The hero within: six archetypes we live by. New York*: Harper & Row, 1989. pp. 98–115.

[7] Oral interview with Doris Garlock Crockett, by Jackie Wylie, 1997 July 22.

[8] Students, in their first months of training, were on a probationary status. They were called "probies" and wore a starched white band of fabric on their heads in place of the esteemed school nursing cap, which had to be earned by successful completion of probation.

[9] Payment of $0.95 by student, Miss Gladys Thornburg, for a mercury thermometer, confirmed in a statement dated 1936 July 21.

[10] Reusable needles were still being checked for barbs in the 1960s. This was accomplished by inserting the needle into a sterile cotton ball and feeling for smoothness or a catch, the barb.

[11] Marian Vandenberg later became Marian Vanderweele.

[12] *Kalamazoo Gazette*, 1937 January 14 and May 2.

[13] Gladys Thornburg's letter is housed in the Bronson Methodist Hospital School of Nursing Alumni archives.

[14] Monthly reports are part of the Bronson Methodist Hospital and School of Nursing Archives housed at the Western Michigan University Archives. *Passim* over next two pages.

[15] Hospital Sunday was the day that all Methodist churches in Michigan donated to Bronson, based on resolutions adopted by both the Detroit and Michigan Conference, "That the conference considers it the imperative duty of every pastor to support faithfully our Michigan White Cross Sunday, by co-operation with White Cross Chapters and Hospital committees, by faithful efforts to raise at least the cash apportionments, by co-operation in obtaining supplies and interesting people who may make special gifts, and urges upon every pastor such co-operation."

[16] Michigan White Cross, exerpts from its *Annual Report, 1930 June 30 to 1931 June 30.*

[17] "Accredited" was not the appropriate term to use because the school was not accredited by an accrediting organization; however, it was approved by the Michigan State Board of Nursing which was required to operate the school of nursing.

[18] Bronson Methodist Hospital Administration Committee minutes, 1937 January 18.

[19] Paper mill felt was a fabric used on paper rollers in the making of paper. The tan, wool felt had to be replaced periodically. People who worked in the mills took the heavy felt material home to make warm blankets. It could also be used for hot compresses. Marquita Land's mother and grandmother and other relatives worked in the paper mills, and this tan felt was used for winter covers on their beds.

[20] *Kalamazoo Gazette*, 1939 May 4, "Nursing profession in city has a long history."

Section II.

WORKERS

CHAPTER 5
REVVED UP BY WAR, 1940s

World War II changed everything. Military-trained physicians and nurses returned to civilian practice transformed by managing large numbers of casualties in the field. They had learned about patient outcomes and evidence-based practices, revolutionary ideas, never before thought possible, by observing incredibly fast recovery times for wounded soldiers, prompted by the necessities of war. Moving injured soldiers—war casualties from the battlefields—after immediate wound care, through the military hospital system was a real priority. Fractured legs, for example, were quickly stabilized, first by splinting and second by intramedullary nailings in surgery, inserting a long steel rod into the bone canal, or using metal plates screwed to a broken bone to hold it together. Get the patient up and walking on his own as soon as possible!

TRANSFORMATIONS IN PATIENT CARE

Doctors returned from overseas into civilian practice in the mid '40s. In their wartime experience, they had tried many new ways of caring for patients that older doctors on the home front had neither heard about nor had practiced. Nurses and physicians were suddenly thrown into a new, post-war era. The name of the author who wrote this next 1940s story was lost shortly after its submittal, but it is a reminder that once home, the transformed nursing and medical teams faced the old guard.

> One glaring example which occurred while I worked in the 12-bed women's ward was early dangling (sitting the patient on the side of the bed) and walking post-surgical patients early in their postoperative period. It was late in my first year [of training]. All the patients returned to their own beds following surgery because we had no post-anesthesia or surgical recovery rooms. The surgical patients stayed in our unit from admission to discharge, except for their surgical hour(s) in the operating room, unless a change was requested. Occasionally this adjustment occurred since there was a price difference between ward beds and private rooms. Those in the ward beds were less affluent; patients were moved according to their means.
>
> My patient had abdominal surgery and was doing well. Her physician was recently discharged from the military. When she returned to the unit from surgery, her care was routine and comfortable for the time—watch her closely, with TPR[1] and BP frequently, turn her often—no pillows under the knees. We were learning to endorse the importance of deep breathing and coughing.
>
> On day one (the first postoperative day), she had a liquid diet and routine care—a bath, turning, back rub and pain medication as needed. The back rub was given with alcohol then and resulted in dry, itchy, flaky skin. In the long run that treatment added to her discomforts.
>
> Day two after surgery came with this challenge: she was to dangle her legs. That instruction meant the nurse and patient pulled and tugged at each other until the patient was more or less vertical, sitting on the edge of the bed with her legs hanging down. Afterward, the nurse's uniform had usually been pulled askew; her cap (probably caught in the curtain surrounding the patient's bed) was settled over her left ear, and she looked like she was the one

who should be in bed. A whitish-gray patient was not trusting the nurse, hospital or doctor at this point.

Day three after surgery, several orders were given. Among them were some to make sure the digestive system was functioning properly and everything going in the proper direction. Then came the order, "GET THE PATIENT UP TO WALK!" My frame of reference at this point was to dangle patients on day seven or eight and walk on day ten or later depending on the type of surgery. Incisions needed to heal before upright position pressure could be tolerated. This crazy doctor comes home from overseas and orders his patient up on day three following abdominal surgery—unheard of!

I wasn't one to question doctor's orders, especially in my freshman year. I did manage to ask some questions later on. I had heard of patients eviscerating, which means to spontaneously rupture the incision, with bowel contents spilling out of the abdominal cavity. I had, however, never planned on that contingency befalling one of "my" patients.

With knocking knees, cold hands, and a plaintive sound in my voice, I went to my patient's bedside and helped her to dangle. Doing so was somewhat easier than the day before. I put her slippers and robe on her and eased her to a standing position. Actually, her feet were on the floor, her body more in the shape of a "comma." I could not urge her to stand up straight since I was convinced that she was going to fall apart. The poor woman shuffled across the expanse of that ward, hugging her poor, sore tummy. I was half carrying her. We turned around in unison and I returned her to the bed. My patient received no real moral support from me (the nurse, the expert) because I just knew that she would fall apart, the doctor was crazy, and I should have chosen a career in vegetable gardening instead of nursing.

My patient returned to bed. Her incision remained intact. The color returned to her face, and she had the look of victory. She might recover after all and return to her family, more or less intact. I was glad when the day was over. As you read this account of my nursing beginnings, know that I also recovered.

Staffing

"Do without" was the slogan regarding nurses, physicians and hospital equipment. All three were needed in the war effort. Movement of nurses from their communities into the war effort drained 3,000 nurses per month into army and navy medical corps,[2] including some Bronson nursing staff and new graduates. Short of nursing staff, directors coped by supplying the remaining nurses with ancillary staff by building nurse aide programs to meet some of the physical care needs that they believed nurses could safely delegate. No fee was charged to the women 18 to 50 years old who donned aide uniforms and took short, quick courses taught by RNs. Dr. Perdew, hospital superintendent, cited the difficult personnel shortage for direct patient care while the Board of Trustees offered public gratitude to Red Cross and White Cross nurse aides for volunteering about 1,500 hours per month.[3]

High school girls were recruited as volunteers for a 1948 after-school, four- to five-o'clock program to read, sing, play games and talk with hospitalized children, filling the void created by limited visiting hours. Jean Culverwell, superintendent of the pediatric department, managed the program with selection help from Mrs. John Hornbeck, director of public relations. A clue to the problem was this not too patient-friendly quote: "Their parents had to leave the ward and the regular nurses were too busy to pause for the friendly chats which mean so much to sick children." The students, some of whom belonged to the Kalamazoo Central High School Nursing Club,[4] supported the over-burdened nursing staff.

Women of the Bronson White Cross Guild labored behind the scenes, canning 4,442 quarts of peaches and pears in fall 1944 for the hospital's bare fruit cupboards.[5] They were given extra sugar rations especially for canning. Guilds from around the state sent cash, fruit and other supplies. These women often received words of praise for their volunteer work in the monthly *Bronson Bulletin.*

The nursing school was an important part of an interdependent hospital community. Almost every *Bronson Bulletin* during the 40s presented a nursing student's story including pictures. Students, as freshmen, made up the majority of daily, direct-caregivers, performing the least complex patient-care tasks. Their roles included medication management, and scrub and circulating services in the operating room. As juniors, they were responsible for treatment and total patient care within every medical service offered in medical, surgical, pediatrics, and obstetrics. Seniors managed the complexities of clinical judgment and delegated tasks to less educated nurse aides, often with indirect supervision by the nursing staff and house supervisor.

MONUMENT EXPANSION CONTINUES

The Bronson bulletins of the 1940s are full of stories promoting hospital expansion along with the necessary fundraising. "Any Waiting List Is Too Long . . . When Your Family Needs Hospital Care!" The message appeared over and over again.[6]

Actually, building expansion preceded and followed the war, beginning with a six-story addition that was dedicated and opened in September 1940.[7] A bigger hospital meant more inpatients and hospital beds. More beds meant increased need for inexpensive labor and a constant supply of professional nurses. Students previously housed in the original 1906 hospital found their quarters enlarged and more livable after a 1944 remodeling that converted old hospital wards into student nurse wards, a study room, and improved quarters for a housemother. "Nearly 80 nurses and student nurses are housed in the hospital building and in North Home on John and Lovell Streets."[8] By May, 1944, plans were in the making for another 100-bed expansion as well as construction of a real nurses' residence to house 125 students.[9] A new residence was not yet to be, however.

South Home at 430 John Street was purchased in fall 1945 to house 22 students, allowing acceptance of a freshman class of 50 students, the largest ever. A second residence at 426 John Street was also purchased for the use of hospital staff.[10] In July 1949, the nurses' home, on the corner of East Lovell and Henrietta, was moved to a new location on Pine Street.[11] Year after year, "the largest class ever" began a three-year course of study, testimony for the growing need for nurses and students within the expanding hospital enterprise.

Surgical procedures were popular in the late forties with decreased mortality rates and relative safety compared to the days before antibiotics. A fund drive goal to raise $800,000 doubled the number of operating rooms and decreased a waiting list of one month.[12]

By the summer of 1948, expansion became a reality with expenses of at least $1,800,000.[13] When the cornerstone was laid, all hospital services were provided by staff consisting of more than 85 percent women, but male-oriented culture dominated even the hymns sung and prayers offered:

> FOR the Glory of God, Father of all men.
> FOR the relief of suffering and the recovery of health
> without regard to creed, color, or race.
> FOR the advancement of medical science and
> the teaching of the healing arts,
> FOR the uniting of the community and the church,
> and for continuing the healing ministry of Christ,
> WE lay this Corner Stone.[14]

JOYCE SAVAGE '47

When I was about five years old[15], my tonsils were removed at the doctor's office. A boy named John Springs, from Belleville, Michigan, went with me; he was first for the procedure. I can remember the open-drop mask being put over my face for the ether, not an enjoyable experience. When I woke from the anesthesia, my throat was sore, of course, and John Springs was raising Cain. At the foot of my bed, I saw a nurse who was an apparition of absolute beauty. I can't remember her helping me, but she was a beautiful vision. From that time on, I wanted to be a nurse and played hospital with all of my dolls.

If my younger sister wanted to play with me, she had to play hospital. I was pretty dictatorial, but my play hospital was well organized. I had a place for broken legs and arms, a place for diseases, and communicable diseases, and a place for operations. The bathroom was the "surgery," and the linen closet was probably used for storage. I played this game until I was 12 or 13 years old, which would make my sister five or six years old. We had a good time together playing hospital.

The rest of the family were teachers. In the early forties, the only choices for women were nursing, teaching, or secretarial. I certainly did not want to do the latter because I was no good at typing. It's my sister's skill. My folks had no preconceived ideas of what I should be; if I wanted to be a nurse it was all right with them.

I had gone to school in Belleville until the tenth grade, and then I went to Hillsdale High School the last two years. I adjusted to Hillsdale and graduated June 10, 1943. Dad and I returned to Belleville that night so I could work in the Willow Run bomber plant, which I did, so I did not go to school that fall. In order to work, I needed to verify my age as 18 because I looked younger. I was hired as a grease monkey to clean the machine guns on the big B-24 consolidated liberator bombers for the next 15 months. I started work on June 14, 1943, at the defense plant, and enjoyed the work, but some things that I learned there I could have done just as well without knowing. Factory life for this very naïve girl was really extraordinary.

Once I finally got my family's Methodism sorted out, I accepted the church tenets and remained with the United Methodists. I did not go to college or other education institution before enrolling at Bronson. I did visit Henry Ford Hospital in Detroit, but Bronson being a Methodist hospital influenced me to choose it.

In the application process for Bronson, I had to get a physical, of course, with the immunizations, particularly typhoid, and I thought I was going to die from them. They were given intramuscularly three weeks apart. I was working at the defense plant and I went to work one night when I felt more dead than alive. My arm was red and I had a high temperature. I felt absolutely awful, hardly able to move my arm.

Cleaning waste gunk on the B-24s meant moving my arm down the gun and which I couldn't do. I did live through that night, taking the hour or so of sick leave we were allowed.

I started my nurses training on September 19, 1944, as part of the Class of 1947. The first year focused on classroom learning. Every time an inspector (getting inspected is not all bad) or a senior entered the room, we had to stand. That behavior carried over to arriving for hospital duty, listening to report, and standing every time the doctors appeared. Sometimes I felt like a yo-yo, jumping up and down every time somebody came into a room. It was hard to accomplish one's assignments.

Mrs. Groat taught Drugs and Solutions for which I could answer her queries, but couldn't necessarily tell her how to do the math. We went around and around many times on dosage calculations. Compared to now, there weren't many medicines. When we worked in the Central Supply dispensing medications, we were required to write up every medication we gave, why we gave it, the amount, the dosage (not only what we gave, but the regular dosage, too), the symptoms of overdosage, and the side effects. It was a good way to learn about drugs, but now it would be virtually impossible to use this technique.

A sociology assignment at Western Michigan ripped our class apart. We took sides for an assignment, and Jean Blake and I were on opposite sides of some discussion about writing a life story. Something about the assignment was misunderstood by many of us, however. The result was that some of us said we would not write that paper. In the end, Jean was the only one who held out. She never did turn in a paper. She lived by her principles and I admired her for sticking to them.

Not until our senior year did our whole class heal from that sociology "tempest in a teapot." By that time a P.R. person at the hospital, Harriet McDowell, became our class advisor, and somehow she got us working together again and, of course, it was just sad that we had forfeited so much companionship. That common low point, however, helped hold us together over the years. At our fortieth reunion, almost everybody came back and had a marvelous time, a direct result of our freshman year of classes up on the hill.

I didn't have many typical "days" because I worked 3 to11 P.M. and nights most of the time. We worked at least two, sometimes three, or more days or nights of 12-hour shifts, seven to seven. I was so tired I was often sick. I needed a certain amount of sleep that the schedule denied me. It took years of pursuing my nursing career not to feel fatigued.

When we came on duty at 6:55 A.M., we already had been to chapel at 6:00 and then breakfast at 6:30. We would get report from the night nurse and our assignments. In the first days, when I had my band but not my cap, we were assigned to cleaning the beds and units, as well as preparing for new patients. We graduated up to admitting or discharging patients and, eventually, giving baths.

We served cancer patients on the fifth floor, a very nice floor with Mrs. Stell as the head nurse. A private-duty nurse was a drug addict, so we always gave her patients their shots. We never gave her a narcotic key or allowed her to give the shots, a given and never discussed.

March of 1945 we received our caps, and the next day, after I had worked 7–11 A.M. or 5–11 A.M. or whatever, I was in charge of the wards floor, with 11 beds for men and 12 for women. With everyone in war work, we didn't have many extra people so students were enlisted to help. Being in charge of a ward even for a couple of hours was a major responsibility. I became aware of this burden the day I returned to duty after my capping ceremony.

Cadet Nurse Corps

The establishment of the cadet corps when we were in training was a significant event in nursing. Our part in the war effort was important because we released so many people back into the service. All but one of us were cadet nurses then. We wore a cadet nurse uniform: a beautiful gray suit with red epaulets and a heavy winter coat. I believe we had a raincoat too. You might describe the cap as a variation of a tam, worn on an angle. If we had shoe coupons, we were required to wear black shoes and a white blouse with our uniforms. With the cadet program came our uniforms, paid tuition, room and board, and $15 a month the first year, $20 in the second year, and $30 a month in the last six months. Not a great deal of money, but we didn't have time to spend much more. A movie now and then was about all we had time for.

We did pay for shoes and stockings. Great lines would form for nylon stockings, and you had to show your student card or your registered nurse card in order to buy white ones, not nylons, but white rayons that were scarce and hard to come by. I reached the point where I was using cotton stockings, which were fine. Only after they were washed about a hundred times did holes begin to appear. My shoe situation was troublesome to me, partly because I have a very narrow foot. With a shoe coupon, I'd buy white ones for nursing duty that would wear out just as the next coupon was valid, so I never had other new shoes.

By Christmas when I was a junior, in 1945, my folks had moved to Wisconsin and I was a long way from home. Miss Anderson had some reservation about my traveling so far in the middle of winter and almost forbade me to leave. Trains were crowded because soldiers were beginning to return from overseas. I had to take a train from Kalamazoo through Chicago to La Crosse. To assure I could board the train I wore my Cadet Nurse Corps uniform. When I arrived at Chicago's Union Station it was a buzz. All the returned servicemen were in a separate section to access the trains first. Because of my uniform I was able to join them. The next day the radio announced that over a million people had gone through Union Station that day and I was one of them.

Holidays

Patients who were in relatively good condition and minimally mobile were sent home. We didn't keep them over holidays, particularly Christmas, New Year's, and Thanksgiving. Instead of attending chapel on Christmas morning the students sang carols as they descended the fire escape. It is one of the most beautiful memories I have of Christmas.

> **Rotations**
>
> Along with others in my cohort I spent three months at Kalamazoo State Hospital and two months at Sigma Gamma.

Kalamazoo State Hospital

I'm one who has always enjoyed breakfast, a very important meal to me, to be consumed as soon as my feet hit the floor. At the state hospital, we walked about a half-mile to where the meal was served. Since we went on duty at 6:30 we were up early. It was a beautiful fall that year, and as we walked we would shuffle through the falling leaves. By 6:00, I could have eaten anything that hadn't moved for 30 seconds. State hospital food, our student food at least, was particularly good, unlike Bronson's by comparison. The many shortages because of the war meant relinquishing our sugar coupons and meat ration stamps to the hospital, whereas our coffee ration stamps went to our parents. We really ate well. I think I gained ten pounds and Jean gained about 20, mostly due to the fresh air, the walk before breakfast, and good food.

I never was allowed to work in the locked ward, perhaps because I wore glasses. One night we had a horrible thunderstorm during which the lights went out, so all the doctors beamed their car headlights into the locked wards because, with no lights, a tragedy could have resulted.

Another time a very tall man, probably about six foot five, was waiting in "men's receiving" for awhile. All of a sudden, a male attendant brushed by me and grabbed him. The next day this fellow was in the tepid tubs. He must gone off the deep end, and the staff were trying either to control him or help him overcome his trauma. He was in the baths for a couple of days, the therapy that was used in those days.

Michigan at the time was quite advanced in its care of the mentally ill. I helped with electric shock, which was very frightening for the patients. I really don't blame them, thinking back on the process. No pre-shock was available then. Now some anesthetic is administered. I remember holding both a woman's jaw and a half rubber heel as tongue depressor to keep her from fracturing teeth and swallowing or chewing up her tongue.

Interviewing a woman who was in a high manic phase was a fascinating experience. She talked about sitting-room curtains that were bloomers in one of those "back hall" wards. Another patient was a schizophrenic who would pull out her hair that grew no more than a quarter of an inch or so. She was nearly bald most of the time. Many people in these wards had been there for years, and probably would die in them. It was a sad waste of humanity simply because we didn't know what to do for the patients. We didn't have the medication or the instruments, or the nursing personnel for insulin therapy. The knowledgeable personnel in this area were serving with the army or navy nurses.

Sigma Gamma Orthopedic Hospital

Sigma Gamma near Mt. Clemens provided rehabilitation for polio patients using hot packs. Sister Kenney had just begun to implement her theories. Polio was still rampant every year. One of our patients was a well-developed 15-year-old boy named Norman who was post-polio. He had lost use of his arms. It was then that I decided I could handle most any affliction. I could go through life without my legs, but I couldn't do without my arms. I lacked a few social skills at that time, and I hadn't been required to give a pretty boy a shower, him standing there in his "all together" and me clothed. I had to think hard and wash very carefully.

Another time one boy at the pool threw a screaming fit, when a student nurse from another school threw water in his face and corralled him. She had safely managed the boy's behavior. A supervisor scolded the student in front of the boy. Not that she shouldn't have been scolded or reprimanded, but not in front of that boy.

Work Weeks

Working more than the assigned eight hours a day bothered me. Mentioning the violation to a supervisor who expected me work more hours than were technically allowed, with the class load I had at the time, taught me in no uncertain terms not to question authority. Assignments didn't change.

As new graduates in 1948–49, about the time 40-hour weeks were initiated, Jean and I decided that we were underpaid and overworked. We had been on duty upwards of 60 hours a week and didn't always get paid for the extra time. One night, at our two o'clock meal break, we got to talking about this situation, and we decided to strike. We issued an ultimatum that included raises and most of all, a 40-hour week. It probably took not more than three or four days to realize we'd riled up the male superintendent who was very upset. I can't really blame him because nobody thought of striking—of nurses striking—in those days.

At 3:00 in the afternoon on the day we were to strike at 11:00, the superintendent signed a paper that specified a 44-hour week (instead of 40) with a raise in pay. There's always a give and take with this kind of negotiation, but the truth is that, to this day, I don't know if I would have participated in a strike.

Today's Career Choices

I have known some marvelous nurses who had memorable careers. My director of nurses, for one, once was named Nurse of the Year. Other Oregonians were recognized by the state for their service on the first Project Hope ship to travel to Vietnam in 1960, as well as for going to the Sudan and Ethiopia.

Throughout my career, I have been mostly inactive when it comes to participating in nursing groups. Later I realized that if I had problems with professional nursing associations, bellyaching was not the way to solve them. I needed to take action to change what I didn't like and so I became active in these organizations around 1970–71.

The rewards of nursing are wonderful—the satisfaction of helping different people—I loved the work, but I've become overwhelmed by the huge problems which remain, particularly lack of nurses and support money. These deficiencies and many more wear people like me down. Would I choose nursing today? I don't know. I really don't know. Although I've been retired about seven years, I have not looked back to question my career choice.

WHITE CAPS YEARBOOK MAKES ITS DEBUT

The 1942 Senior Class dedicated the first publication of the school yearbook to, "Miss Alberta E. Erhart, Superintendent of Nurses, in appreciation of her interest and understanding of the students and for the youthful spirit she has given to the Training School." Its 29-page annual was created by an editorial staff of 21 students, with Gwen Ramsey as the leader. Dena Wolters was honored as the class advisor.

Insightful comments within the class history tell the collective story of the soon-to-be graduates:

> There were about 30 girls in our class when we started, but one by one they drifted out—some were married, some went to college. People say they couldn't take it, but I just say they didn't like it.
>
> We were examined by the medicos in and about Bronson. We were assigned classes, classes, and more classes. We practiced, practiced, and practiced. We ate and slept at proper intervals, but in more or less of a daze, and once in a while we went for a stroll around town or to a movie. That routine didn't last too long because we became acquainted with the town and its people. From

> then on, several porches of Wayside Home rang with the voices of my classmates and their friends.
>
> We had a trio in our class that was blamed for everything—regardless of what occurred the trio did it. We all lived to tell the tales.
>
> And then it was Christmas and those of us who could not go home were so homesick.
>
> Finally the day we had been waiting for arrived—in the last of February we received our caps. Our dignity had been earned. For a year we went through countless agonies, snubs, tortures, embarrassments, and scoldings. Our contacts with Miss Lane were masterpieces! Remember how she had us walk around the Annex to see if we could observe something that was new or different? And remember our bandaging classes where we tucked in the edges for neatness?
>
> How could we forget—and yet as we look back on these experiences now, it seems they weren't so bad.

Graduate stories often turned into positive memories—the good remembered, the agony buried. Other students to come would be exposed in similar fashion to rather oppressive teaching habits that bordered on right-out abuse—another of those paradoxes where uncaring teaching approaches were supposed to make caring nurses unfold. Junior Class reports for the yearbook once more testified to the difficult environment that students faced:

> On the fateful afternoon of September 2, 1940, a group of 28 girls gathered at old Osborne Home. Little did they know of the joys, sorrows, and heartbreaks in store for them. Little did they care, because they were going to become part of the "Army in White." The probie days were the hardest, I think.

A "Last Will and Testament" complements both the class history and its class prophecy. It carried 21 personal legacies left to lower-class members, along with a general section. From the general section, humor was noted:

> We, of Bronson Methodist Hospital's White Parade, who believe in "Survival of the Fittest," hereby make our last will and testament. We, the Senior Class wish to thank Mother Purvis for the use of her dilapidated laundry cart, in which we had many a thrilling ride. We will to her a bigger and better "box-car" for bigger and better rides.

Senior pictures included a quote describing some meaningful graduate-to-be characteristic, plus nicknames, one for each student. Last names were often modified so that Miss Moffett became "Moffy"; Miss Archer, "Archie"; Miss Peterman, "Pete"; Miss Wilson, "Willie"; and Miss Smith, "Smitty." Long first names were typically shortened so that Alice became Al and Elizabeth was Betty.

Typical topics and pictures appeared in *White Caps,* 1942, depicting student memories: of classmates, hospital staff and scenes, and brief biographies about nursing supervisors and teaching staff, as well as words of wisdom and congratulations from nursing and medical staff. Some wrote their thoughts in poetic formats. W.G. Hoebeke, MD, summed up what was often felt by students and graduates:

> It is human to take good things for granted and so good nursing seldom rates the appreciation that is its due. With this in mind, we extend to the Senior Class our thanks for their willing and efficient services during their years of training.

The class motto was, "Enter here to learn, Go forth to serve." The class mentor, fondly called Suzy (Susan K. Lane, RN), recited a quote that exemplified her message that began with the first day of class:

Do all the good you can
To all the people you can
In all the ways you can
At all the times you can
As long as ever you can.
—John Wesley

Pictures of 20 graduate nurses, 15 second-year students (part of the "Army in White"),[16] and 23 freshmen with caps were part of that first yearbook. Also included was a Rogue's Gallery encompassing an "Anonymous," interesting "Who's Who" caricatures, initials, and comments such as, "Where's that linen key?" Those who trained at that time knew how to decipher these clues.

AFFILIATIONS AND ADMISSION STANDARDS

A statement in the June 1943 *Bronson Bulletin* told how to speed up the training of nurses. The article refers to the School of Nursing at Western Michigan College as part of the reorganization:

> We are now teaching approximately 95 percent of the theoretical work during the first two years . . . leaving the senior year for special affiliations and the small amount of class work necessary. This means students will be away from school six months during the senior year, three months with the Children's Hospital of Michigan, and three months with the Kalamazoo State Hospital for a psychiatric affiliation.[17]

A belief at the time was that affiliations were a State Board of Nursing requirement for beginning RN training as a generalist with knowledge and practice in medical, surgical, obstetric, pediatric, and psychiatric services. The state board RN examination was administered in five separate tests, covering each area. Also the administrators recognized the need for broad training to add personnel diversity to Bronson patient-care services. Since by this time new graduates were often employed at Bronson, the affiliations cut some of the inbreeding, an event related to limited travel or opportunities to move to other geographic locations. However, it is quite amazing how many nurses did have practice opportunities outside of their home communities.

Admission standards were high, a result of the affiliation with Western Michigan College, which offered an opportunity to earn a baccalaureate degree with a major in nursing. Students were chosen from applicants who were in the upper third of their high school class, had one year of high school or college chemistry, could meet college entrance requirements, and had passed a Bronson pre-entrance examination.

INSIGHTFUL MODELS OF BEHAVIOR

Bronson's in-house publication showed appreciation for the perspectives of perhaps fictional patients, visitors and nurses about what it was like to be in the hospital in 1942. The nursing shortage and multi-tasking responsibilities were recognized, although clinical competence often went unnoticed. It was always, and is today, the little things that count—the good and bad *are* remembered.

> **How to be a Model Patient**[18]
> Having recently completed a four-day stay for a second operation, I feel fully authorized to talk (and what patient doesn't) on "How to be A Model Patient." Problem number one is how to influence nurses and get along with people.
>
> It's only normal to think that your pain deserves a great deal of audible sympathy from those who attend you. Our tip is [not to] play for sympathy but, instead, to quickly convince the nurse that you are a reasonable individual who appreciates the little extra service extended to you.
>
> Keep in mind that the nurse has a difficult job. She has to be a combination Florence Nightingale, Jeanne d'Arc, Elsa Maxwell,

and Tillie the Toiler. Try lightening her load during the day (or night) and see how much genuine pleasure it gives you.

How to be a Model Visitor (by One Who Has Learned the Hard Way) [19]

If you're the intuitive type, you'll sense automatically when the nurse wants you to leave the room so routine tasks may be performed. If not, she may have to ask you outright. In either case, do it cheerfully; Bronson, like every hospital, is short of nurses. As the store in Maine said in its sign, "Be kind to our clerks, they're harder to get than customers."

Above all, don't let the list of restrictions and suggestions cramp your style. Try to be natural and cheerful. Or if these qualities are contrary in your nature, then at least, act cheerful.

How to be a Model Nurse by a Mere Patient [20]

Even though her countenance may be unseemly, the ideal nurse is to the patient a thing of beauty and a joy forever! For this is a thing of personality whereof we speak. And personality depends not on good looks nor grace nor social amenities. It is being yourself at your best!

The gal we're thinking of comes into the room crisply, like a clean, fresh breeze off the ocean, not like three cents worth of yesterday's lettuce. She has the happy knack of getting the patient's mind off his physical and mental irritations. And sometimes this takes some knacking! The folks who were born unreasonable and never grew up, she tolerates quietly and efficiently, knowing that in a day or two some kindlier soul will occupy that bed anyway.

She has a good sense of humor and is quick to laugh at a good joke or smile at a poor one. Though she is busy, she never seems to miss an opportunity to drop a word of cheer or do some little thing that will add to the patient's comfort.

Quietly, but firmly if necessary, our ideal young lady in white makes the patient feel that the hospital, like any other good organization, has to have certain rules and regulations and that these must be adhered to if everything is to get done on time for everybody.

> She doesn't gossip. That is, she doesn't repeat things that shouldn't be repeated; the rumor department is strictly out of bounds for her. But then, on the other hand, she usually has a stock of little tidbits of legitimate news for the edification of her patients.
>
> Superwoman? Not a bit of it! She's just like a well-trained, intelligent girl who likes her job and people! There is at least one in every uniform, and sometimes she just forgets to make an appearance, that's all.

HOW THESE BEHAVIORAL MODELS CAME TO BE, 1940–1949

Pauline Munger Neiderlander '40

My mom was our family doctor's assistant in the homes of his patients, acting as his Girl Friday and midwife. She encouraged me to become, as she called it, a real nurse, and so I entered Bronson in 1937 and graduated in 1940. It was the closest school to my home.

My greatest fear was giving medications. I was slow in doing so because I always checked the dosages three times. My great joy was discharging a patient in good health who had been admitted gravely ill and knowing that, in some small way, I had helped.

One evening, after hours (curfew), some of my classmates and I decided to go to the Wayside Hall kitchen to make taffy. We were all pulling the stuff when we heard a knock at the door. The visitor would be our housemother, Mrs. Auld. Sometime passed before one of us finally opened the door. We were sharply reprimanded.

> I loved wearing my cap. Shirley Evans was my idol. I thought she was a wonderful person and a super nurse. I was awed by her. My greatest fear was that I could never become a good enough nurse, and my greatest joy was doing the best that I could. I remember one patient who said, "You don't say much, but what you do say means so much."
>
> ***Ione Bailey Ambrose '49***

No interns or residents worked at Bronson in those days, but the doctors were nice to us and taught us a good deal. I have always remembered bedding down of our patients for the night, only to have them disturbed by crickets under the refrigerator in the hall. Periodic kicks silenced their chirps. I, too, remember being breathless, as we all ran down Lovell Street to catch the trolley to our classes at Western.

Thanks to Bronson and our superintendent of nurses, E.B. Hammond. We entered into school a frightened group and left with confidence, grateful for our education. Our class was small, but we have maintained a close relationship, with a reunion every year since we graduated.

Gwen Ramsey Sheppard '42

Our class was fortunate to have had Susan K. Lane as our nursing arts instructor, although at the time we did gripe about her. Looking back, she was the best thing that happened to us.

Our class was "close knit," and many of our small class of nineteen still keep in touch, like a family with fond memories galore. I can't believe that we are "so far over the hill!" Fifty-five years have passed since our graduation and all those crazy escapades that I was involved in. I feel fortunate that Bronson accepted me. I worked in the Army Nurse Corps as a flight nurse from 1943 to 1945 and was a nursery nurse in 1946 to 1948.

Winifred "Winnie" Gerard Vander Meer '42

In the 1940s, team nursing was considered to be efficient. One treatment nurse was in charge of all treatments, nurse aides were assigned to give baths, and orderlies did what needed to be done.

Between the first and second floors of the Lovell Street addition (1940) was Central Supply and the medication room. Central Supply prepared sterile supplies for use in the operating room and for treatments on patient-care units. All surgical packs were autoclaved there. A blackboard on the wall showcased daily artwork by our own chalk artist, Ship Sherwood. People passed by just to see his creations.

A "med" nurse reconstituted Novocain™ from tablet to liquid form for injection by boiling distilled water and dissolving the tablet, an old practice. Medications were passed from one central location, and one nurse passed all of the medications. To give "hypos" we boiled water in a spoon over an alcohol flame, put a pill in a syringe, drew up the correct amount of water after calculating the dosage, and ejected part of the solution if the dose ordered was less than what we had prepared. We took a special class in Drugs and Solutions.

Mrs. Thelma Groat, a 1924 graduate, taught Material Medica. We learned that tincture of benzoin was placed in a big steamer. It was a round, two-gallon, metal kettle set on legs with castors. It "shot" out medicated steam for respiratory ailments.

The rule, we were admonished, was: if no BM in the P.M. then MOM (Milk of Magnesia) in the A.M. We gave 3-H enemas (high, hot and a hell of a lot).

On nights, the surgery nurses went to the kitchen to make night lunches for all of the staff. The lunches were sent to the patient-care units on dumb waiters. Night crews also made gauze dressings when not busy with patient care.

Probies cleaned the service rooms located in the patient-care areas. There was always a clean and dirty utility room. Students learned about surgical and medical asepsis and keeping clean equipment separate from equipment that had been exposed to patients and was considered contaminated. Probies also passed trays to patients.

The evening supervisor was Eleanor Mengel on 2 West, a new unit, and the good third-floor supervisor was Mrs. Punch. Three private duty nurses I remember were Gertrude Harmon, a 1929 graduate, Helen Rankin, and Adriana Van Boven. Seriously ill and wealthy patients' families often hired their own private duty nurses since not enough RNs and students were available to provide continuous, acute care.

Bronson did not have an anesthesia department until Dr. Armstrong started the anesthesia group in Kalamazoo. General practitioners would give the anesthetic for each other, and some nurses were also trained. Doctors Boys and Jennings had their own nurse anesthetist, Mrs. Edna Wildermuth, who could use the "gas" machine.

Phyllis Pettyjohn Ockerman '43

At a reunion lunch in Kalamazoo, six classmates from the Class of 1943 recalled events that occurred during three years of training—particularly in their probie days.

Our first day on the men's ward—on 2 East—one patient asked for a duck. The probie came to the desk and said, "The patient wants a duck," with a bewildered look on her face, and Helen Punch, the supervisor explained that he was asking for a urinal. Shortly after, another student answered a light in the men's ward, and the patient asked for a vase. Not understanding his request, she asked, "For how big a bouquet?" We couldn't stop laughing. How "green" we were!

In my junior year, working 3–11 P.M. on the first floor, I was about to go off duty when a patient light came on. With a flashlight I answered the call. It was a two-bed room. The man in the first bed had turned on the light. He told me his roommate had retrieved his clothes from the closet, dressed, and exited the room through the window. When his wife had visited him two days after a herniotomy, she relayed that her ex-boyfriend was in town. So, the patient left the ward to check on his wife. It probably frightened her—it sure did me!

Dora Wright remembered so much about those days, and Greta Nidy described many funny experiences. We all remembered Suzy Lane and how often we heard, "Ten points off your bandaging grade."

Elaine Fox Glittenberg '43

What stands out in my memory is that we were required to sign a paper pledging that we would not smoke, drink, or get married during our three years in training.

Bronson was building its first expansion when I went into training, September 2, 1940. Our rooms were situated in Osborne Home, next to the *Gazette* building. I still have my three-year diary that I kept while I was in training. I still read it every so often. It brings back so many memories. The first six months were the hardest. We all cried frequently, but also had fun.

I remember Suzie K. Lane, our Nursing Arts instructor. She was a World War I army nurse, an element of her background we never forgot. She had us all in tears at one time or another. One of her favorite remarks was, "Don't come back without it." We all hated her off and on but, when we all gathered together years later, we agreed that we were lucky to have her as one of our instructors because of all we learned from her.

Martha Sherwood Burrell '44

Probies, can we possibly survive? Are we worthy of this white headpiece? How do you keep these shoes clean? Can we remember to hold the door for a doctor? Can we learn what Miss Sweet is dearly trying to teach us in Nursing Arts class? Will the Diet Kitchen supervisor miss the cookies we so cleverly confiscated? What is the penalty for feeling scared and/or inadequate, being a possible early dropout, a disappointment to our family, a disillusioned nurse hopeful?

Then, there was Miss Erhart—a Bronson graduate, our superintendent of nurses, our role model, so professionally correct as well as human and kind, and, by the way, beautifully representing the spirit of nursing. Her quiet and meaningful reading of devotions from *The Upper Room* started our day.

We survived. We even graduated and were proud to be the Class of '44. We hold deep gratitude for all who were a part of our Bronson Methodist life experience.

Winifred Mein Terpstra '44

It was very early in my life when I first envisioned a career in nursing. As a child, I was always helpful in caring for my siblings. My father always called me his "little nurse." The choice of going to Bronson Methodist Hospital was made because it was close to home and a couple of my classmates were enrolling there. Our family also went to BMH for care and believed it was a great hospital.

The first year five of us shared one room. We slept on old hospital beds, our dressers were shared with a roommate, and we used orange crates for our bedside tables. The entire class, 25 of us, used one bathroom on the third floor of the original BMH. An elevator took us to the third floor. It was the kind that had a gate. If the gate wasn't closed, the elevator would not move, so we had to go down three flights of stairs to close the gate and ride back to the third floor.

The friendship we shared with our roommates and the other coeds was one of our greatest pleasures. Our eyes and ears were open to absorb this new life. We walked every day from BMH to Western Michigan College to attend classes. We had regular study hours from 7:00 to 9:00 P.M., then one "free" hour before lights out, carefully monitored each night by the housemother.

Our probie year of providing care to "real" patients was exciting. Working on our 12-bed wards was so much fun and we learned so much about treating patients. We began to feel like nurses! The greatest joy was learning so many new skills and putting them to practice. Sometimes it all seemed overwhelming, but the more we learned, the more we desired to pursue a career in nursing. The greatest fear, at times, focused on "book learning." We wondered if we could absorb all of this knowledge, remember and apply it. The most memorable lesson admonished us to be compassionate and caring in addressing all of the patients' needs. We were very happy that we could assist people who were ill and watch them improve because of our help.

The person I remember the most was "Precious Miss Sweet," our nursing care instructor. She was so patient and kind and taught us the true meaning of being a good nurse. Miss Wolters was our surgical OR head nurse and had such a positive way of making us want to do our very best, even though we were fearful of working with doctors in the operating room. Miss Erhart was a great role model, with her quiet and personal grace. Many folks helped in molding us for our future years as RNs. We all, of course, prayed so very hard to earn our diplomas and pass our state board exams, sanctioning us as registered nurses.

Marilyn E. Newton '45

Those first few months were a real eye opener for me. I came off the farm for the first time and moved into the "Big City." Whenever I hit rough going, or had doubts of whether I would be able to succeed in our profession, my father would ask, "Are you ready to quit yet?" He was not convinced that I had chosen the right path, but I would not give up.

We began living in the dormitory of the old hospital on John Street. We then spent our final year in North Home on the corner of John and Lovell streets. As we entered our second year, we had the opportunity to join the U.S. Cadet Nurse Corps. It paid our tuition if we agreed to stay in the profession for the duration of World War II and six months beyond. In return, we were issued military uniforms, one each for winter and summer. They consisted of gray, white-and-red trimmed, three-piece suits, including hat, purse, and topcoat. We also received a small monthly stipend (our expenses were minimal). A Kewpie burger and malt on South Street was our main expense.

In our second and third years we received our pediatric training at the Children's Hospital in Detroit. We returned to Kalamazoo for our psychiatric training at the Kalamazoo State Hospital.

We worked hard for long hours, but we also enjoyed many good times and had many close friends. As the son of one of our classmates told us at our fiftieth reunion, "Your class must have been a very special group of gals." His mother, Madonna Kenyon Blakely, later to be an advanced Alzheimer patient, treasured this event as one of the last to hold her interest.

Margaret Edgerton Brown '45

Margaret's story details her "love affair" with surgical nursing practice. After marrying and raising three children, she accepted a position in a new open-heart program in 1971. She then became manager of multiple patient services.

I graduated from Bronson in 1945. We had been Cadets during our training period. Some of us went to the Battle Creek hospital and some joined the Navy for their last six months. I was asked by the hospital to finish my training by serving with the last six months in the OR. I agreed to stay for a year.

My intent was to enroll in a postgraduate operating course. I applied to different schools that offered the programming, and was accepted at New York Hospital, Cornell Medical Center, to enter in January 1947.

The year prior to my enrollment, Dr. Howard Jackson persuaded me to scrub for him and granted me a six months' leave of absence, to pursue my studies. Being in New York was a great experience with great experience for me. I met my future husband in the city and we married in 1949. Meanwhile, Dena Wolters wanted me to return to Bronson to teach, so I put my postgraduate study to work in 1950. I taught and managed the Bronson OR and helped organize the hospital's new Emergency Room.

I was on the inactive list from 1956 to 1969 while raising our family. When the Community Nurse Organization needed help, I tried working for it. I had throughout kept up with OR periodicals in the hope that someday I could again serve in that milieu.

In 1971, an open-heart program was initiated in Appleton, Wisconsin, where we were living. I was hired, even though it had been 20 years since I had worked in an OR. The staff provided wonderful help and patience in my orientation. That next fall I was asked to assume the management of the surgical services, which included OR, Open Heart, Recovery Room, and OP. The assignment was a challenge for me, but I did learn to enjoy the experience. I retired in 1987; even so, I have continued to be active with the hospital and in the community.

Beth Ellinger Jirikovic '46

It was September 1943. No shuttle service was available to us so we walked to college and back, hoping that we would be at the hospital in time to go on duty. Our regimen was very close to a military one. Doctors were God, and we always stepped to the back of the elevator when they entered. Students who were seniors and juniors also took priority. We had very strict hours for leaving the facility in the evening and, should you in any way not adhere to them, you were confined to the dorm for a certain number of weeks or even sent home permanently. Occasionally, we did have a short night out. We went to the YWCA and had a super time jitterbugging with soldiers from Fort Custer. Walking home one night, I saw the largest sewer rat I had ever seen. Believe me, I made it home in record time.

In surgery, I was a second scrub nurse to Dr. Stryker. We used some innovative tools such as a teaspoon. (Common household utensils were sterilized and used as surgical instruments occasionally.) On the hospital floors, as the war was drawing to an end and some physicians were returning from service, we again found ourselves making equipment, such as combining catheters to make a drainage system for a patient with a bowel obstruction. The night shift was always innovative, especially since you were the one-and-only nurse on duty.

We were so proud to receive our uniforms and caps and to start working on the floor with patients. We attended classes during the day and often worked from

7:00 P.M. to 7:00 A.M., a 12-hour night shift. We did every task, from changing patients to soaking and wringing isolation linen and scrubbing diapers on a washboard before sending them to the laundry. We also worked in Central Supply, cleaning and wrapping needles, tubing, and other items before sterilizing them in the autoclave.

We did our affiliation with the TB hospital in Detroit and the psychiatric hospital in Kalamazoo, long before the use of psychotropic drugs. I became the best French hair braider on the staff.

Compared to modern day techniques and equipment, we were somewhat archaic. Yet, in all honesty, I believe we were allowed a more "hands-on" approach, where the patient feels a personal relationship to his or her nurse. We felt their pain, and we cried when we could do no more and they passed on. Some nights were totally insane. We got our own oxygen tanks, we gave hands-on care and back rubs to each patient, and on those nights when a patient died, we washed them, enclosed vital areas, and made them ready for the funeral director.

Now I too am old and waiting for the day when my Maker will take me home. I hope that my good deeds outweigh my youthful, stupid blunders. As they say, "Nothing is forever." I view the closing of Bronson Methodist Hospital's nursing program with sadness, yet I am proud that over the years many well-trained, caring nurses were created in this school. God bless us all. We cherish the memories.

Margaret Gould Carter '47

I never wanted to be anything but a nurse, like an aunt who was one. My greatest joys in nursing school were the friends that I made and being remembered, even still, by patients whom I cared for 37 years ago.

I started my education at the University of Michigan in the fall of 1942. Jean Culverwell, a classmate, had attended the University of Michigan. I got a "D" in Anatomy and could never overcome that deficiency. I think I was close to a breakdown before I left. Leaving was the best decision I could have made because BMH was a much better choice for someone as immature as I was at the time.

The fall of 1944 found me in a room with three strangers: a redhead who had the most engaging giggle, a sophisticate with more clothes that I had ever seen, and a tall, bashful, country girl who was very intriguing. I was a bit older, having left the School of Nursing at the University of Michigan my junior year. Starting over was not easy but, in retrospect, I would not change a thing.

I believe it was Dick Vander Molen's first year of employment at Bronson. Most of us enjoyed his good humor and took advantage of his good nature. Those years were a very happy way to begin a career that lasted 27 years.

I worked a year in the operating room under Miss Wolters and then on to Spokane, Washington, where I took a "temporary" assignment in one of the few civilian recovery rooms in the nation. I enjoyed the work so much that I stayed two and one-half years. January, 1951, found me in Riverside, California, where I did surgical nursing for about eight months. Then in Michigan again I was the first civilian nurse to work in the recovery room at Percy Jones Army Hospital, where I enhanced my education considerably.

In mid 1952, I was invited to join Bronson in organizing and setting up what was to be called PAR, Post Anesthesia Recovery Room. Drs. Marshall and Armstrong, anesthesiologists, and some of the surgeons, including Drs. Weadon and Machin worked with me to establish a protocol: turn, cough and take blood pressure. We were housed on the hospital's second floor across from the elevators. I left the project late in 1954 to return to Spokane, at the request of some anesthesiologists, to create a recovery room at Sacred Heart Hospital.

Nancy L. Willis Shepard '48

When I was in high school, I worked as a nurse's aide at Bronson. I enjoyed the work and decided nursing should be my career choice. I picked Bronson School of Nursing because it had the Cadet Nurse Corps program, although we didn't get the uniforms in this last class of the program.

I enjoyed dorm living and making new friends. One of the most embarrassing experiences happened when I was first put on a floor to work as a student. I put the wrong name on a deceased patient who was sent for an autopsy. I had to go down to the autopsy room and change the name in front of all who were there to observe the autopsy. It never happened again.

My greatest satisfaction was making my patients comfortable. Only once did I seriously consider dropping out of nursing. It was after working a 12-hour shift in pediatrics with ten babies to feed every three hours and caring for other sick children by myself.

My favorite departments in which to work were the delivery room and nursery in the OB department. It is a great joy to see a newborn baby and the happiness that it brings to the parents.

One of the greatest fears a nurse has is the fear of giving the wrong medication or the wrong dosage to a patient. Some of the doctors were difficult to work with and added to the stress of the environment. One of the biggest problems for us in nursing, as either a student or graduate nurse, was never having enough people working at the same time, so you were not able to give as good care to patients as you would like. The problem still exists today.

The skills learned in nursing helped during the rest of my life in raising a family, helping friends, and being a caregiver when needed.

Ellen Emig Gunter '48

When we started school in 1945, we lived in the six-bed room in the old hospital on John Street. It was the old surgical unit. We had bunk beds, a desk, and a locker. We were fitted with uniforms; I think hemlines were 13 inches from the floor. They were washed, starched stiff, and ironed at the hospital. Sometimes we had to use a nail file to open the sleeves, but we were so proud. Classes were held at the hospital in the Nursing Arts lab with Miss Sweet. Medical doctors taught their medical specialty subjects, such as pediatrics, and various medical conditions. Miss Wolters taught operating room nursing, Mrs. Groat, pharmacology.

We were placed on the patient-care units early in our career to pass water and wash patients for meals. We worked before class and after class. We walked to Western for classes, taking the trolley up the hill.

When we were capped, our parents sent food. I think we had three cherry pies in our room, but we lost two of our roommates and felt bad for them. Ours was the last class to be admitted to the Cadet Nurse Corps, which paid $20 a month. When Bronson was adding the current building, Reverend Perdew, who presided over morning chapel, convinced us to pledge money for the new addition.

As juniors we started our affiliations. Our pediatric affiliation was near Detroit. We had a chicken-pox epidemic with several sick children, and one of my classmates succumbed. The children had cerebral palsy and post-polio disabilities. They were away from their parents and needed TLC as well as therapy—mostly physical.

We spent three months at Kalamazoo State Hospital for our mental health affiliation. We worked in Admitting where hydrotherapy was performed. We watched three people in tubs, with a sheet over the tub, only their head visible, with water running in and out for four hours. I'll never forget the day I was alone, and a woman loosened the sheet enough so that she could lower her head into the water. I grabbed her hair to pull her up and tried to tighten the sheet enough so that she wouldn't drown. Scared!

Two of us applied for an affiliation in surgery at Cook County Hospital in Illinois. We were accepted and had a very interesting experience. The set up was entirely different set up than Bronson's and patients with more extensive surgery.

Surgery on a "blue baby" was even performed, a first in the country to have heart surgery.

While living at East Home, I worked nights and slept days in the center room upstairs. Dick would call, "Man overboard." I don't think I even opened an eye. At times everyone likely walked through that room. I slept on. When I finished my shift, planning to go straight to bed, our housemother sometimes would greet me with the news that an autopsy was scheduled. I'm sure I was the first to see the seven required. I also lived in North Home on the first floor with a window. Classmates came in and went out after hours. We liked movies.

As seniors we had more responsibility on the units, taking charge on evenings and nights with a registered nurse supervising us. They were wonderful, knew what was happening on each unit, and who needed help. (Nursing) staff was spread thin in those days. One lesson I learned the hard way related to drugs and medications dispensed from Central Supply. My one drug error involved sulfa. The pills were put in an envelope for us to dispense at night. The patient should have had two pills and I gave one. I was mortified when in the morning I had pills left over. I had read the dose on the envelope but thought it equaled one pill.

We did have a wonderful three years with friendships that lasted a lifetime.

Janet Macgrayne Camery '48

I grew up wanting to be a nurse. My mother was a nurse. She graduated from Bronson Hospital School of Nursing in 1913. Her name was Mina Weber. I chose Bronson for several reasons. My mother was a graduate, we lived in Kalamazoo, and I had attended Western Michigan College, riding the bus for one year, where I heard about the five-year nursing program.

I have many happy memories from my three years at Bronson. They include, the probie cap, the narrow velvet band (black) on our nurse's cap when we were juniors, and then the wide velvet band on our cap when we were seniors, as well as the blue cape and the gold lining. Starched white student uniforms—when I walked, my knees hitting the skirt would make a sound—I still have the one I wore the last day as a student. Many friends and fellow students had signed it. Our two affiliations—three months at Kalamazoo State Hospital and two months at Children's Orthopedic Hospital in Mt. Clemens, Michigan. Our instructors who were so understanding—Miss Sweet, Mrs. Groat, and many others whose names I've forgotten. Our beautiful capping ceremony at the United Methodist Church. I still have the Nightingale candle that I was given.

Bertha Spitters Olin '48

Remember bed check every night at 9:00 P.M. by the dorm mother or some other appointed checker? One of my classmates had met a young man whom she very soon began to date quite regularly. Once in a while she would stay out later than nine and would be queried about not being in her room. She answered by saying she was on the first floor visiting me. Her room was on the second floor, and the monitors never seemed to doubt her excuse. They would also check with me, and I would go along with her story (with my fingers crossed). Finally, I told her, after her excuse passed muster a couple of times, that her luck might soon run out and perhaps she could come up with another plan. We discussed ways in which she might try to fool the staff.

One night when she knew that she would be staying out after nine, she tucked pillows under the covers of her top bunk bed and placed a wig on the head pillow facing the wall. That evening, when it was time for bed check, the dorm mother stuck her head in the door, saw the filled bed, and went on to the next room. The prank worked, but in the end it didn't make much difference because she quit school to get married.

Joan Vander Linde Phillips '48

My fondest remembrance is the freshman class choir. We practiced faithfully. Early one bright, cool, Easter morning in 1946, wearing our crisp white uniforms and caps—oh yes, we had been capped by the time Easter came—with polished white shoes and hose and our navy capes with the gold linings, we walked briskly to the Kalamazoo College chapel to sing in a sunrise service. "Low in the Grave He Lay" was the hymn that has remained a favorite all of my life. I still hear the deeper alto and lighter soprano voices. The melody is ingrained in my mind. On our return to the hospital, I was subdued and refreshed, a moment that has been with me for over 50 years, long after my nurses training culminated with lifelong friendships that solidified forever on August 16, 1948, graduation day.

Betty Tageson Schumacher and Ruth Cardiff Matteson '49

Thirty students enrolled in September 1946, and a total of six of us were in room 301, the third-floor dorm remodeled in the old hospital. This arrangement caused a hardship when trying to study since we were all used to being alone with our books. As a class, we were very close. The class congregated in our large room (it was large enough to accommodate everyone) or in the hallway. We were homesick at times, and our first Christmas was a sea of tears—while singing carols. Unfortunately, we lost two "roomies" at capping, and four of our other classmates. Now our large room held only four.

Tageson's most memorable lesson related to giving a man an oil enema. She was told by her instructor to use glycerin but soon found out that mineral oil was the oil of choice. Cardiff's worst experience with enemas involved emptying the bedpan. She vomited profusely and thought she would never be able to be a nurse. Also a 90-year old man was the subject of her first bed bath. He thought she was too young to wash his "impossible."

Early in the spring of 1947, Tageson and Cardiff went to Chicago to see Sonja Henie's Ice Revue and stay at the YWCA. They sneaked out early to catch the bus but missed it coming back. It was 2:00 or 3:00 A.M. when they returned, but Cardiff's mom saved their necks by calling Mrs. Wright to say they'd be late.

Each morning Monday to Friday, we were required to go to chapel for a prayer and a Bible reading. None of us was really awake until we stormed down the stairs to breakfast. This meal consisted of cereal and soggy toast, except twice a week we had sweet rolls.

Our junior year, two more of our roomies left. Tommi got married (a real no-no), and joined her Marine husband. Mary Rapp was diagnosed with possible TB so was told to go home and "recover"; happily, she came back the next year and graduated.

Now we were two and our class had shrunk to 20. We felt badly about loosing our roomies, but our last year was looming on the horizon. Our senior year, we were kept busy. Cile Kraft had married in April 1948. Then Cardiff pulled a no-no and got married. Everyone in the class knew but kept a tight lip, for which Cardiff was grateful.

We spent two months at a very rewarding place to work, Sigma Gamma in Mt. Clemens. It was a rehabilitation center for children suffering from many ailments such as polio, congenital hips, and cerebral palsy.

As graduating seniors, we were well entertained by everyone. The doctors gave us a formal dinner dance at the Gull Lake Country Club and escorted us to and from the party. The faculty hosted a breakfast, and the freshmen and juniors also gave us a party.

The most wonderful news came a few months later when we all passed our boards on the first try. Even though we were told that we were the worst class ever, we were also the first class in Bronson's history to accomplish this feat. We were all PROUD.

Marjorie Bouws Cole '49

Nursing was a choice I made in high school. When it became necessary to select a school, I narrowed the field to Bronson or Michael Reese in Chicago. Cost was the reason I decided on Bronson.

I remember the day that over half of my class and I left a class at Western Michigan College because the professor was late as usual. That day we waited 20 minutes after the hour. I had NEVER skipped school before. We wiled away the afternoon and returned to the dorm to find Miss Anderson waiting. We were only mildly disciplined. From this experience, I can honestly say that, as a professor, I have never been late to a class that I was teaching.

Miss Anderson and Miss Wolters were people from whom I learned the art of supporting your staff and students. They intervened for us often. Overall, I have always felt that I was given an excellent, broad nursing education. As I pursued additional degrees, never did I feel that I lacked basic nursing knowledge.

Florence G. Clementz Manning '49

I earned the money for tuition and my parents gave me personal expense money. My total expense for three years was $300. My journal for the first year shows bus fare was five or ten cents; a movie, fifty-five cents; a coke, five cents; a sundae, twenty-one cents; saddle shoes, $5.14; and white shoes, $6.18.

On my arrival at the dorm, I was greeted by my big sister, Nancy Willis, with a welcome gift. This experience was meaningful, and we remain friends today. Four of us occupied the room to which I was assigned. It was next to the snack room and also looked out on the emergency room entrance. We could watch Mr. Hall arrive with his ambulance. Dr. Machin had been stationed in India during the war and had brought back Indian tea in wooden boxes.

We soon met Miss Sweet and Miss Shirley Evans, our Nursing Arts instructors. We worked on the floors under the supervision of Wanda Grauman, Betty

Madden, and Margaret Gould, third-year students (Class of 1947). They were special people. Another special person was Dick Vander Molen, who would arrive at the dorm after his school day. His cheery shout, "Man on the floor." (According to Dick, he changed his announcement from "Man Overboard," mentioned in an earlier story, to the more apropos, "Man on the Floor.") His warning alerted us to his arrival to buff the floors and do other chores or favors for us.

Many adjustments were required. My parents had raised me to think for myself. They allowed me to express my views on different issues and make appropriate decisions. I found it difficult at first never to question the why of doing things certain ways. I was now in a very regimented lifestyle. We were required to hold doors open for doctors and hop off of our stools, while recording, when physicians appeared at the nursing stations. I really struggled with these changes in my life. When things got rough, my parents were there to encourage me.

The capping ceremony took place at the end of a six-month probationary period. We lost seven of our classmates. In a very impressive ceremony, we received our white caps and our Florence Nightingale lamps. How proud we were.

To end my first vacation, my roommate and I took the bus to South Haven for a day of relaxing on the beach and swimming. In spite of covering up with a beach towel when out of the water, I got a severe sunburn. When I went back to the hospital to work, large blisters broke out on my back and the back of my legs. My legs became swollen and stiff, and I could barely walk. I was sent to the infirmary where I spent several days. I remember Miss Wantz coming to see me and saying, "Miss Clementz, I don't know if we have a lobster or a nurse." Even though I got the sunburn on my vacation, I still had double time to make up before I could graduate!

The comradeship and closeness we experienced as classmates were especially meaningful and continue even now. When we assemble we still reminisce about our lives together at the old nurses dorm and the North Home.

UNFORGETTABLE STAFF

Mary B. Anderson, Nurse Administrator

Mary B. Anderson, a person of authority, became acting director of nursing in June 1944, following the resignation of Alberta Erhart.[21] Miss Anderson was a 1935 graduate of Copley Hospital, Aurora, Illinois, who first came to Bronson as head nurse on the maternity unit for one year, then moved to Rockford, Illinois, in May of 1937. She returned to Bronson in December of 1940 as educational director of the School of Nursing. She belonged to several professional organizations including the Kalamazoo District Nurses Association of which she was president, 1941 to 1943.[22]

Memories of Miss Anderson included that she wore her nursing cap proudly while walking tall and straight with her white starched uniform and a tall collar fitted tightly around her neck. Always looking professional, she wanted all of the nursing staff to look the same. The skills she taught in nursing helped in raising a family, helping friends, and being a caregiver when needed.

Miss Anderson lived in the nursing staff home, located at the back of the hospital on Cedar Street, with Dena Wolters, Marie Wantz and their dog, Cinder. In 1945 she hired 15-year-old Dick Vander Molen, becoming a surrogate mother to him while the nursing students became his big sisters. Dick's early story is connected with hers and a lifelong friendship that ensued.

Dr. Perdew granted Miss Anderson a leave of absence in the early fifties to further her knowledge on building and architectural design. On return to Bronson, she directed much of her energy to hospital expansion and to the building of Truesdale Hall later in that decade.

Dick Vander Molen, Jack of All Trades, Sole Recipient of an Honorary BMH School of Nursing Diploma

I was 15 years old and the youngest Bronson employee in the spring of 1945 when I went to work for Dr. Hazel Prentice for 35 cents an hour in the laboratory, feeding the rabbits and guinea pigs and cleaning their cages. I thought I was a failure because so many of the rabbits died.[23]

That summer Mary B. Anderson asked me if I would like to transfer to the nursing department and work in the nurses' dorm. I accepted the job change eagerly, and for the next three years I was known as Dick the Buffer, an adopted teen for the student classes of the late forties.

I never will forget the Cadet Corps nurses marching in formation to the First Methodist Church and the soldiers who dated them. In August 1945, the hospital buzzed with the dropping of the atomic bomb on Japan, and we wondered how soon the war would end. Still, work continued as usual—nurses worked 12-hour shifts and many employees worked nine hours a day, six days a week. The personnel department, bonus pay, personal days, and birthday holidays were still years away. Our dedication to humanity was our reward.

The war did end that August and the nurses were all excited about their boyfriends coming home and about getting married. Nurses I had not yet met returned from student affiliations in Detroit and Mayberry. They talked about their September graduation at the First Methodist Church, the first of 32 that I attended. Mrs. Kirk informed me that a new class would soon arrive. It was exciting for me—new girls to meet—and I wondered if I would ever again see all the seniors that I loved.

I turned 16 and was back in school with a sense each day that 3:30 P.M. would never arrive when I could go to work. I would practically run from Central High School to Bronson and the job I loved. How exciting it was to ring the man bell and yell, "Man overboard," and later, "Man on the floor," and to begin buffing student rooms and hallways. Of course, to make things look good, I had to buff Mrs. Moffet's room on the third floor and Miss Sweet's room on the second floor. Each floor had one phone and I loved to answer it when the students were in class.

One of the joys of my job was pushing a four-wheeled cart to deliver milk, bread, crackers and peanut butter, along with 100-pound cakes of ice, to North and South homes. Mrs. Wright always wondered what took me so long. The errand gave me a chance to visit with Mrs. Howell, the maid, and Mrs. Ellis, as well as the juniors and seniors who always seemed to be hungry and waiting for me. I spent much of my time visiting. Between chats, I managed to buff and wax floors in the big dorm, help Herman (who worked in the kitchen) store all of the donated jars of fruit in the fruit cellar, move furniture, and retrieve luggage from the attic which, on occasion, housed a hidden boyfriend for a night or two.

North Home was my favorite dorm of all the houses that the hospital owned. It stood on the corner of John and Lovell streets until it was moved to Pine Street, becoming known for many years as Pine Home. It was big and beautiful with a large front porch. I sat on the porch many nights with Mrs. Ellis or student nurses, watching people and cars traveling along Lovell Street. As you entered the front door you faced a wide staircase leading to the second floor, and dividing the rooms on the east and west. In the back of the house were two stairwells with a big attic accessible from either stair. A beautiful, huge fireplace graced the living room. I could never explain the feeling that I had years later, watching the house demolished by a bulldozer to make room for hospital expansion.

The Class of 1948 arrived that September (1945) in my sixteenth year. What better way to meet them than to carry in their heavy luggage, which I didn't mind, and show them to their rooms. I wanted to know all of their names.

The hospital was still comparatively small and most of the 175 employees knew each other by name. Housekeeping consisted of three janitors and five maids. Maintenance had two mechanics and three firemen. Support services for nursing included two orderlies and a handful of nurse aides. There was Amos the iceman who delivered 100-pound ice cakes throughout the hospital that were made on site. I'll never forget Lyle in surgery, Jack the wall washer, Floyd the engineer, Tillie in the cafeteria, Evelyn the cook, Mrs. Kirk the housemother, Miss Noble in Purchasing, Dorothy in Laundry, Superintendent Dr. Perdew, Herman in X-ray, the RNs and student nurses, Mrs. Stell on Hall 5, Shirley Evans on 2 West, doctors home from the war, volunteers, and the rest of the employees who helped to make the slogan on Bronson's letterhead, "Where Skill and Sympathy Meet."

G. Ray Hall drove his ambulance to the back of the hospital with sirens screaming. He would ring the emergency bell and not so patiently wait for the nurse assigned to the ER to ride the elevator from the fifth floor operating rooms or to run down the five flights of stairs to unlock the ER door.

With blood pulsating out of my leg in 1946, several students living on the third floor of the dorm accompanied me to the emergency room. I accidentally stabbed myself in the leg and cut an artery. They rang the bell and waited for the nurse assigned to ER to arrive. The next six days I was a patient on 3 West with Mrs. Miller, the supervisor, keeping traffic to a minimum. Dr. Howard Jackson, who always wore a bow tie, was my doctor. Mary B. Anderson visited me and wanted to know how and why I could be so stupid as to stab myself. I must admit I really enjoyed my stay in the hospital and all the attention received from the student nurses.

I volunteered to work all of the holidays, not because I got paid ten cents more an hour but because it was a special time for me. I cheered up homesick students who could not afford to go home or had to work as part of training. Turkey and all the trimmings were always served in the cafeteria by Tillie, Grace, and Lois. By Christmas I knew the new freshmen by name, as well as all of the juniors and seniors. Everyone gave me candy and cookies and wondered why I stayed so thin. Mistletoe hung over the sign-out book but nobody wanted to kiss a 16-year-old. Mrs. Howell, the South Home housemother, and the seniors invited me to their Christmas dinner in 1946. It was another special memory for me.

The kitchens on the second and third floors were favorite places to gather and talk about the Tigers, Mary B., politics, and the grapevine stories that Jack Tribe and I did well in keeping alive. Mrs. Wright would catch me talking with the students and would ask, What was I doing? I always had some feeble excuse.

The faithful Methodist women will always be remembered delivering jars loaded with pears, peaches and plums to be served to patients and employees. Each year the White Cross Guild worked for weeks preparing to stage its annual lawn festival to raise money for the hospital. And who could forget the two beautiful, big oak trees that had to come down as the hospital expanded? The lumber was saved and used to construct the hospital chapel.

Senior nursing students in South Home were displaced on May 27, 1947, with a written message from Miss Mary B. Anderson informing them that Dr. Robinson, a new surgical resident, would be arriving and moving into first floor quarters, while lab students would take over the second floor. Nursing students had the option of moving next door to 426 John Street (an old dark-brown house) or finding an apartment for a couple of months.

During 1947, my last summer as Dick the Buffer, I helped Jack Tribe wash all the walls in the big dorm. I believe it was the first time that they were ever washed. Jack, with his numerous funny jokes, was one of my favorites, Floyd Rothwell, chief engineer, hired me to be the hospital electrician and was my boss for several years. Floyd took me under his wing when I was 18 years old and taught me everything that I could digest about being an electrician. Floyd also taught fire safety to the student nurses.

I began working in the maintenance department as the hospital electrician in 1948 but continued to be a friend to the student nurses through 41 years of employment and eventually becoming the director of plant operations. I fell in love not only with my work but also with most of the students, and I finally met the love of my life, Betty Lou Gosling from the Class of 1951.

The completion of Truesdale Hall was a big 1957 event! The new furnishings were stored in the basement of the hospital. Dr. Perdew, Mary B. Anderson, Miss Wolters and Miss Wantz, along with other employees and students, volunteered their time, from 5:00 to 10:00 many evenings, to move chairs, tables, lamps, beds, mattresses, and other furnishings through the tunnel to Truesdale Hall. It was a labor of love, fun and exciting, knowing that the long-awaited, full-fledged nurses dorm was finally a reality. For those of us who worked long hours each night putting together new furnishings and arranging rooms, it was a time of excitement tempered with sadness. We were excited about a beautiful new dorm but saddened that Pine and East homes, where students were housed for years, would be torn down.

I have always been proud of and have considered it a privilege to be a friend to student nurses: to listen, encourage, and be helpful during their three years of training. I know that, in some small way, I was a part of their life at Bronson. Those were special teen years for me when students in the classes of '45, '46, '47, '48 and '49 treated me every day with kindness and care. Their care inspired my wife and me to give the same kind of support to students in the years that followed. The good times will last for a lifetime.

The Senior Class of 1959 proudly dedicated its *White Caps* yearbook to a true Bronson family. "Besides providing a home away from home, Dick and Betty have unselfishly helped guide us to our goal. Betty, always capable and dependable, setting a professional example on 3 to 11 P.M. Dick, a sincere friend, always wishing to lend a helping hand or an extra word of encouragement." The honor was never forgotten and was one of the nicest tributes that Dick and Betty believed they received at Bronson. Students befriended by the Vander Molens maintained their relationships for years.

Dick Vander Molen is the sole recipient of an Honorary BMH School of Nursing Diploma.[24]

CHAPTER 5 NOTES

---

[1] TPR is the abbreviation for temperature, pulse and respirations.

[2] *Bronson Bulletin*, 1942 November, "Hospitals asked to sacrifice at war conference."

[3] *Bronson Bulletin,* 1942 November, "Nurses' aides supplement hard pressed regulars."

[4] *Kalamazoo Gazette*, 1949 January 4, "Bright eyes, happy laughter greet 15 girl entertainers."

[5] *Bronson Bulletin*, 1944 October, "Many hands cooperate to can 4,442 quarts of peaches, pears."

[6] *Bronson Bulletin*, 1946 April, "Any waiting list is too long . . . When your family needs hospital care! The superintendent looks ahead."

[7] *Kalamazoo Gazette*, 1940 September 1, "Bronson Hospital's new six-story addition to be dedicated September 8."

[8] *Kalamazoo Gazette*, 1944 February 8, "Rest, recreation, and study center provided Bronson Hospital nurses."

[9] *Kalamazoo Gazette*, 1944 May 18, "Study adding 100 beds, home for Bronson nurses."

[10] *Kalamazoo Gazette*, 1945 April 28, "Bronson Hospital adds property for dormitories."

[11] *Kalamazoo Gazette*, 1949 July 20, "Moving big house draws many curious spectators."

[12] *Kalamazoo Gazette*, 1946 May 12, "Post in Bronson campaign taken by Turbeville."

[13] *Bronson Bulletin*, 1948 Summer, "Expansion begins."

[14] *Bronson Bulletin*, 1949 Summer, "Larger buildings—new services."

[15] Self-taped interview by Joyce Savage, 1989 March 29–30.

[16] *White Caps,* 1942, ". . . September 2, 1940, 28 girls gathered in Osborne Home . . . On March 5, 1941, this same group, now numbering 24, received their caps and capes." Later alumni records list 20 graduates.

[17] *Bronson Bulletin*, 1943 June, "Nurses school plays vital role at Bronson: broad training helps maintain important patient services."

[18] *Bronson Bulletin*, 1942 November, "How to be a model patient."

[19] *Bronson Bulletin*, 1943 March, "How to be a model visitor."

[20] *Bronson Bulletin*, 1943 June, "How to be a model nurse by a mere patient"

[21] *Kalamazoo Gazette*, 1944 June 28, "Mary Anderson heads Bronson Hospital nurses."

[22] *Ibid.*

[23] The rabbits were used for pregnancy tests. If the test was positive, the rabbit died.

[24] Dick Vander Molen's story is a compilation of shared memories and Bronson publications including the *Catalyst*, 1980 November, and "Dick's Digest", a part of the Alumni Association of BMH School

of Nursing *Bulletin* during the 1980s and 1990s. His book, *The Bronson I Knew, Gone but not Forgotten,* was published by the Alumni Association in 2005.

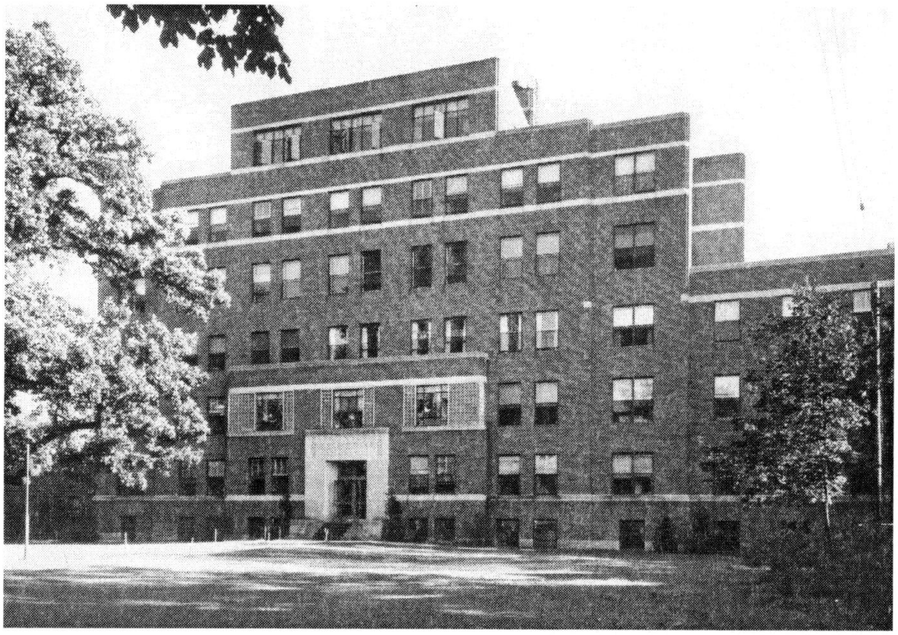

43. In the 1940s, Bronson's main entrance from Lovell Street.

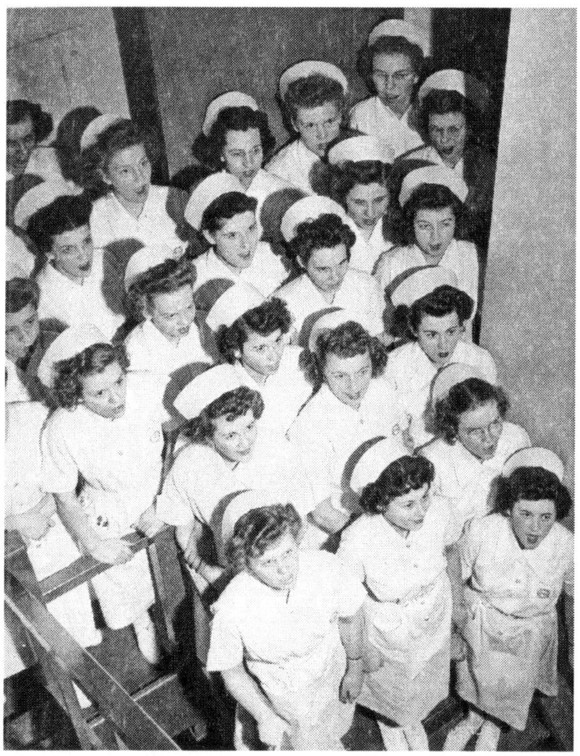

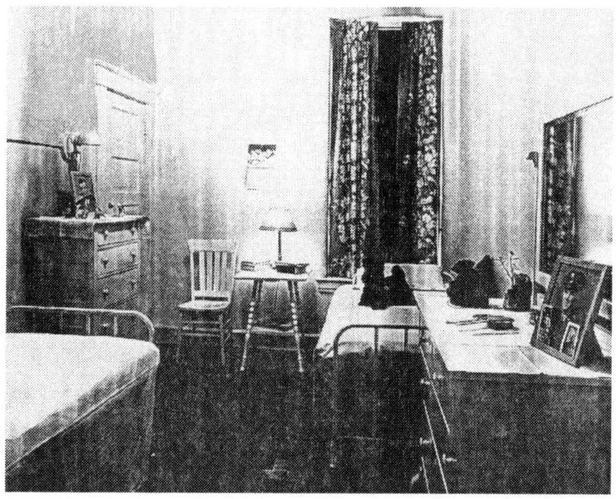

44. (above) Typical student room in dormitory, 1944.

45. (left) Christmas morning at Bronson Methodist Hospital, 1946. Freshmen student nurses wearing probie bands started on the sixth floor and worked their way down through every floor singing Christmas carols and songs. Patients who felt well enough joined in the singing. Christmas was truly a special day for the patients who enjoyed the harmony and joy of the music.

Form 52
DIVISION OF NURSE EDUCATION

BUDGET BUREAU No. 68-R-121
APPROVAL EXPIRES AUGUST 31, 1945

APPLICATION FOR MEMBERSHIP IN UNITED STATES CADET NURSE CORPS

I hereby apply for membership in the U. S. Cadet Nurse Corps established under the Regulations of the Surgeon General of the U. S. Public Health Service, promulgated pursuant to the Act approved June 15, 1943 (Public Law 74—78th Congress) entitled "An Act—To provide for the training of nurses for the armed forces, governmental and civilian hospitals, health agencies, and war industries, through grants to institutions providing such training, and for other purposes," and

for enrollment in the BRONSON METHODIST HOSPITAL SCHOOL OF NURSING
(School of nursing)

at KALAMAZOO, MICHIGAN
(Address of school)

under the plan approved by the Surgeon General in accordance with the said Act.

In consideration of the training, payments, and other benefits which will be provided me if I am accepted as a member of the U. S. Cadet Nurse Corps, I agree that, if accepted, I will be available for military or other Federal governmental or essential civilian services for the duration of the present war.

(Signature) Joyce E. Savage

Date September 17, 1944

John F. Savage
(Parent or legal guardian (see over))

To applicants for membership in the U. S. Cadet Nurse Corps:

Your country offers you financial aid to complete your preparation for nursing because nurses are such a vital part of the activities of a nation at war.

Your signature on this form constitutes a pledge to remain active in nursing, in *either* military or civilian service, health permitting, throughout the war.

The pledge to serve throughout the war does not prohibit marriage. Many essential nursing services, including Army nursing, are open to married nurses. An increasing number of nursing schools are enrolling married students.

If you have not reached the age of majority under State law, the signature of your parent or legal guardian is also required on this application.

4407—FEDERAL SECURITY AGENCY—U. S. PUBLIC HEALTH SERVICE—August 1943. 16—38437-1 U. S. GOVERNMENT PRINTING OFFICE

46. During World War II many students signed an application like this one for membership in the Cadet Nurse Corps, 1944.

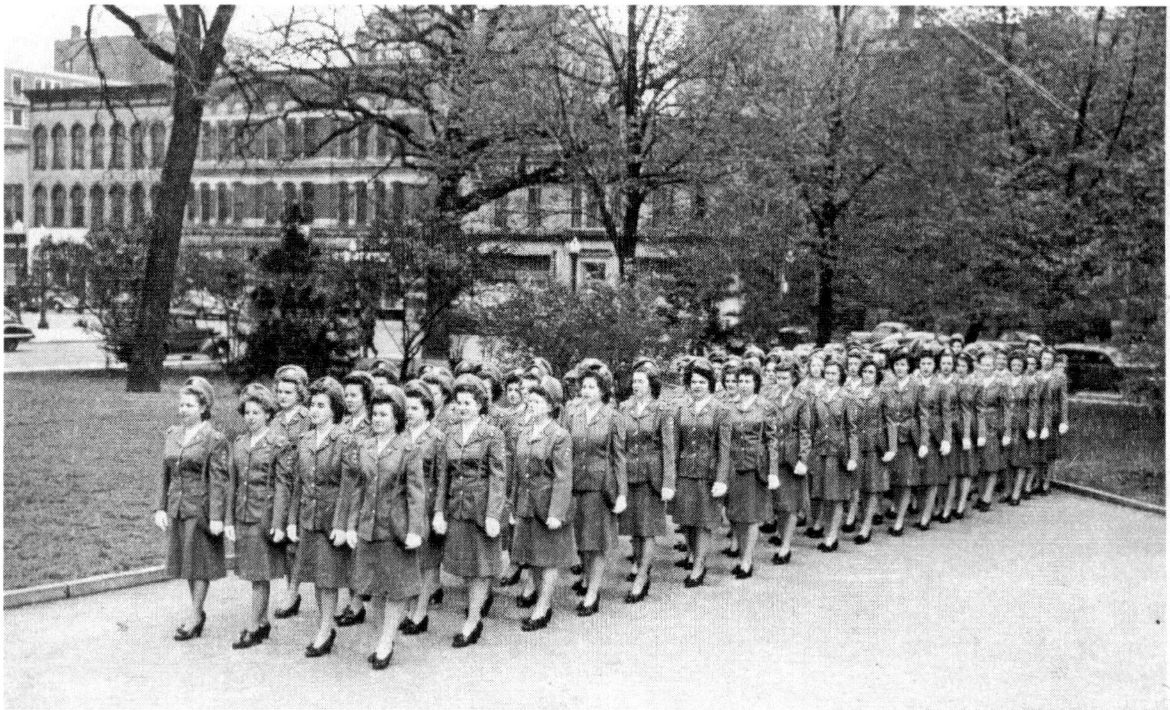

47. Official photograph, Bronson School of Nursing Cadets, 1947.

48. Senior Cadet Nurses leaving to take their final six months of training under auspices of Army and Navy, 1945 (left to right): Cecile VanEyk, Gladys Kamps, Alta Fowle, Phidora Terwilliger and Veronica Rimkus.

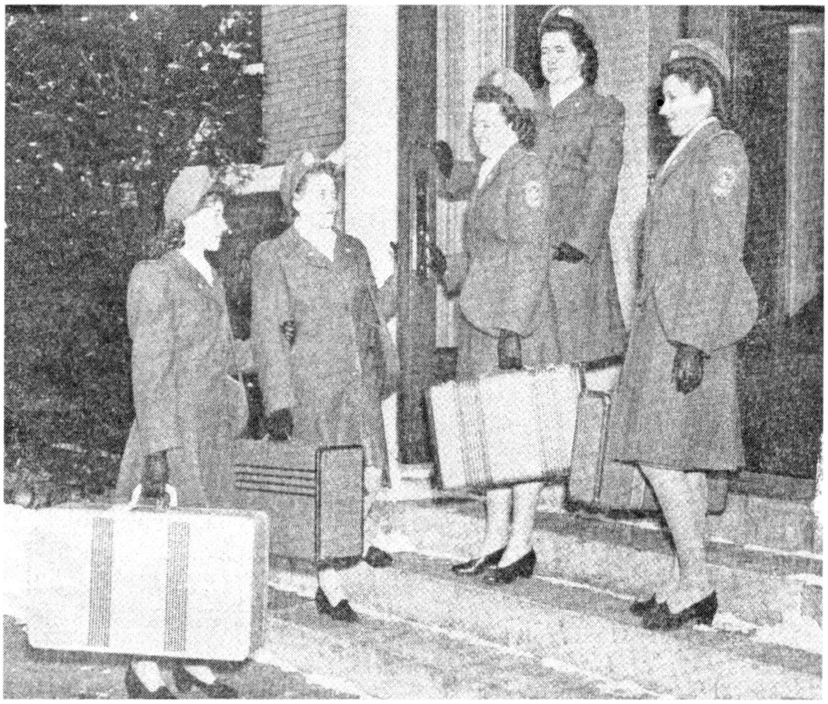

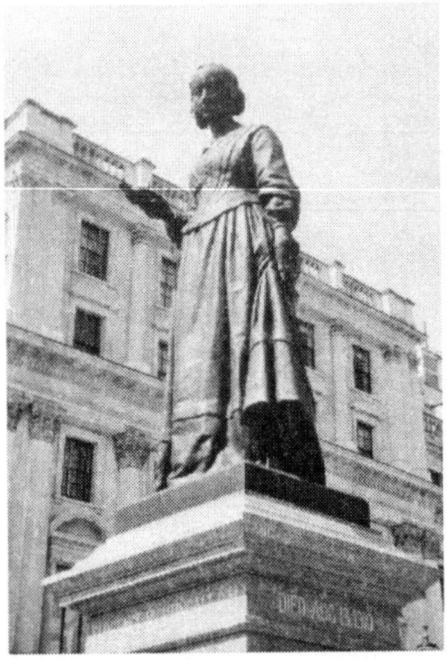

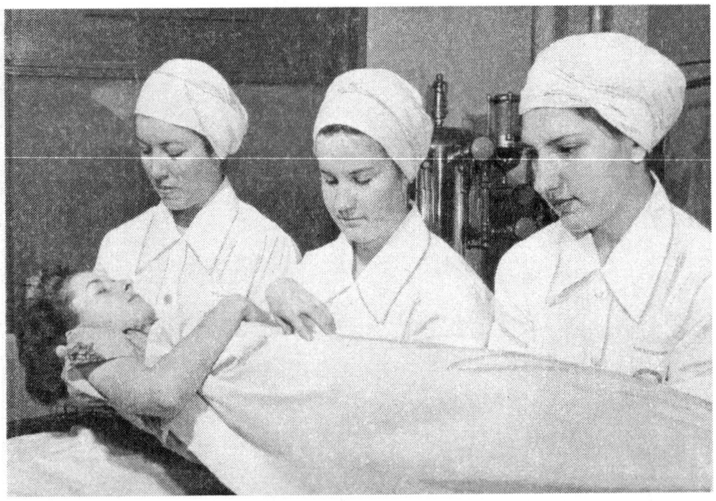

49. (above) Florence Nightingale memorial in Waterloo Place, London.

50. (top right) Student nurses in operating room demonstrate proper transfer technique (left to right) Grace Swigart, unidentified, Beth Ellinger. Patient is unidentified, mid 1940s.

51. (middle right) Mary B. Anderson leading daily chapel service, 1943. Notice upperclassmen in front and students with probie bands in back.

52. (bottom right) Unidentified student performs wound irrigation under the watchful eye of Miss Perry, 1944.

53. (below) Lt. Gerda Bouwhuis '40 was one of 24 American flight nurses in the first contingent sent to the South Pacific. She was the second white woman to set foot on Guadalcanal, and was later awarded the U.S. Army Air Medal.

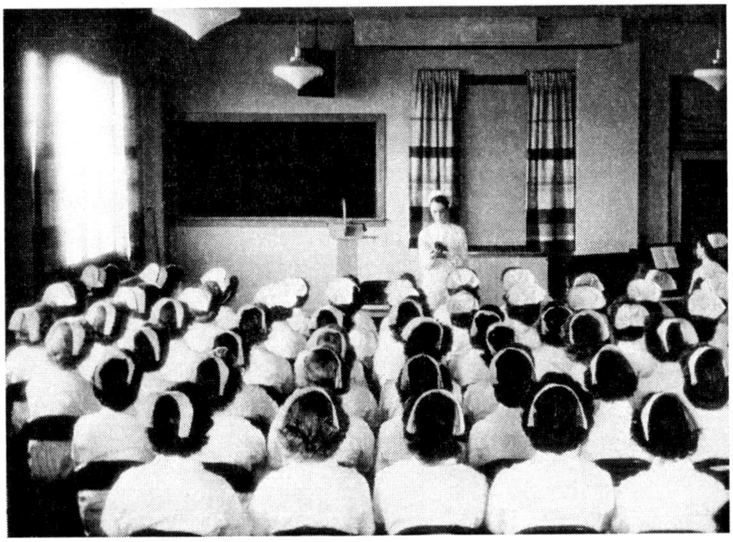

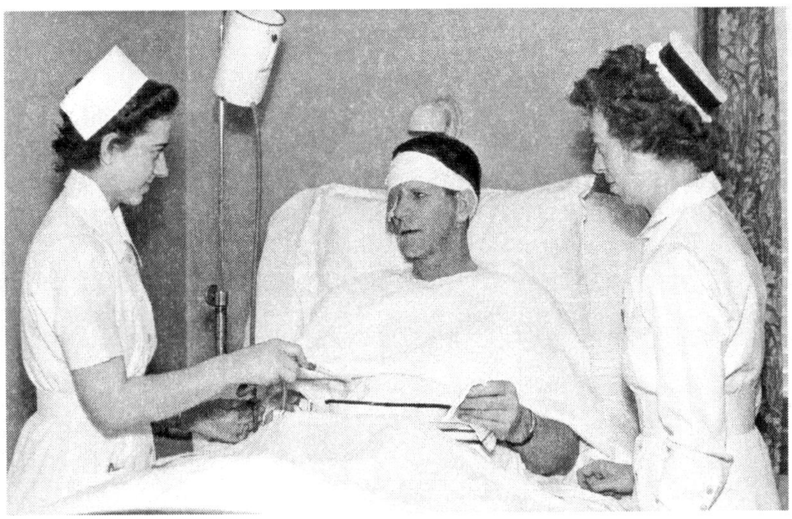

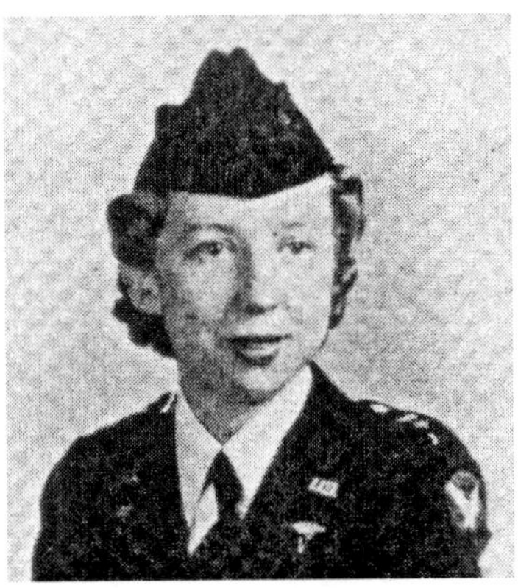

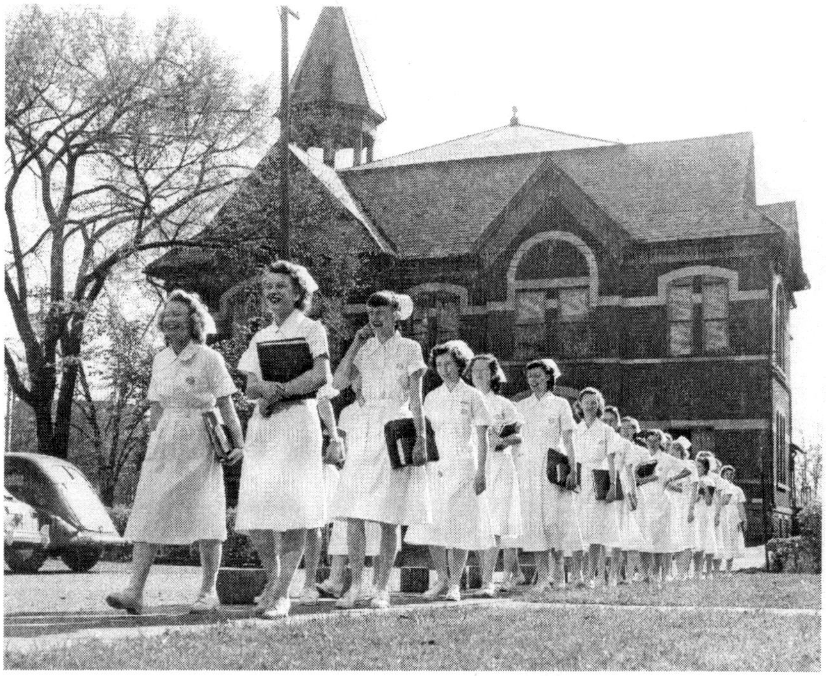

54. Freshmen students walking to class with Kalamazoo Public Schools administration building in the background, 1948.

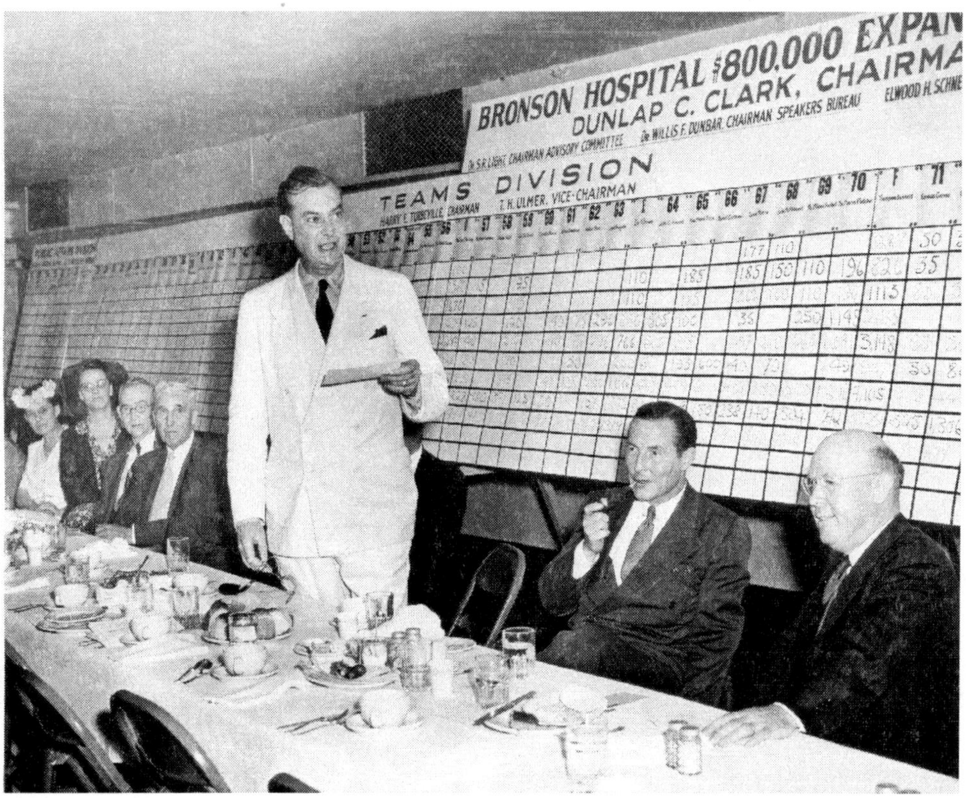

55. Bronson fund drive victory dinner held in Harding Auditorium, June 1946 (left to right): Unidentified, Mary B. Anderson, Dr. Albert Way, Charles Campbell, speaker Dunlap C. Clark, unidentified, Dr. Perdew.

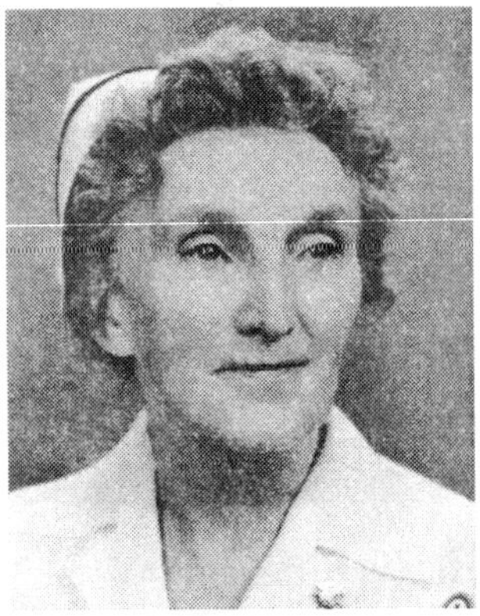

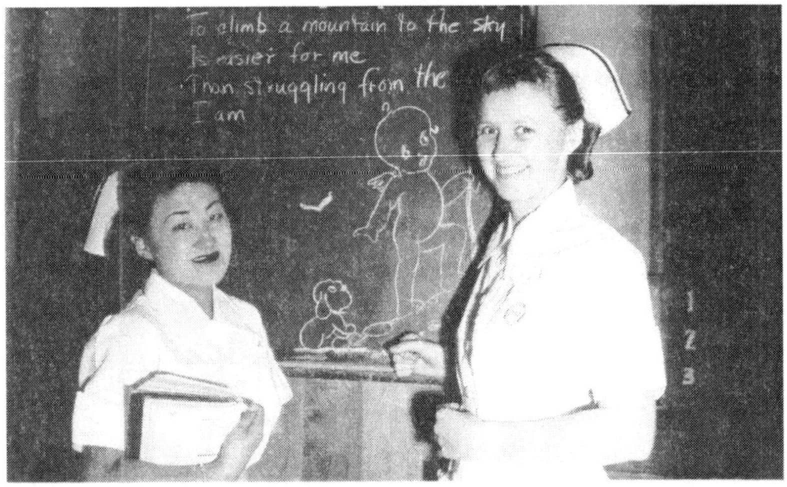

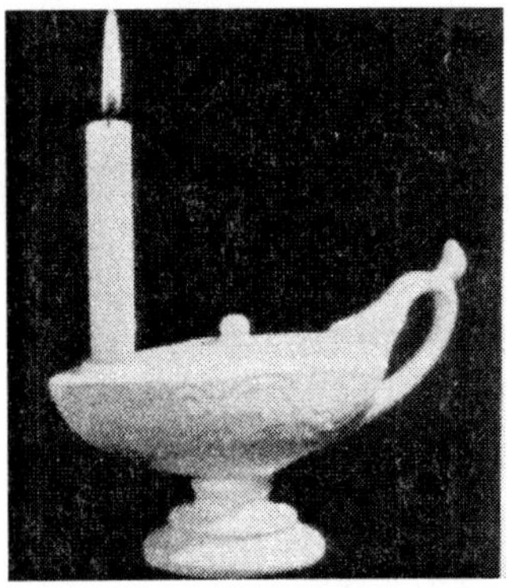

56. Miss Leone Sweet, Nursing Arts Instructor, taught many the true meaning of being a good nurse, as photographed ca 1948–1949.

57. (above, left to right) Tomo Hamamura and Gwen Motyer copying a little verse and drawing for the amusement of all who come and go, 1948. Thelma Groat started this pleasant Bronson custom by every day assigning a second shift senior student to "blackboard duty." This bright spot increased traffic on the stairs that saved wear and tear on the elevators.

58. Florence Nightingale's actual lamp was a six-sided cylindrical lantern. A Lamp of Knowledge (left) was used in Bronson capping ceremonies.

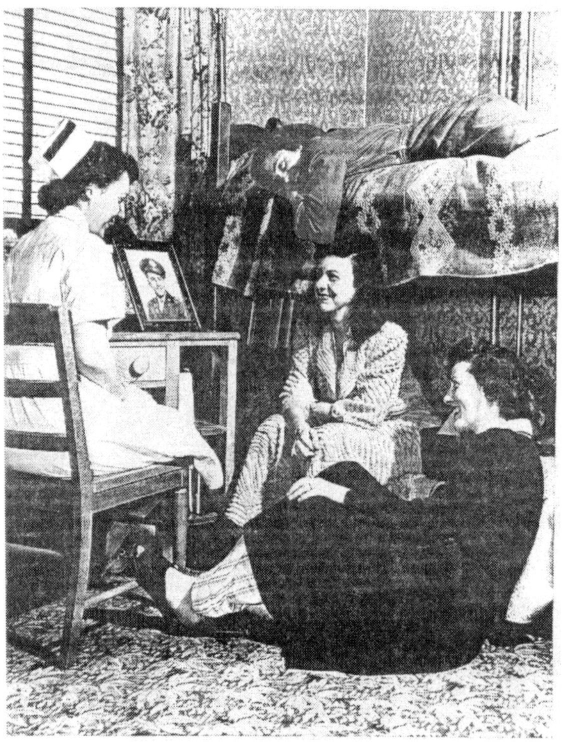

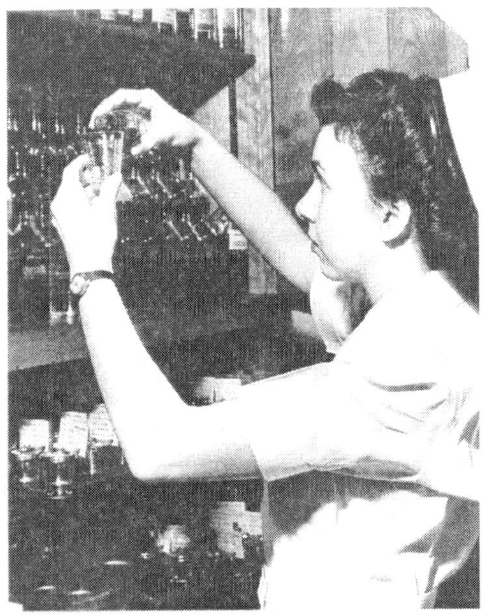

59. (above) Mary Luedders preparing medications for dispensing to patients, 1948.

60. (left, left to right) Ellen Griner, Betty Lou Tageson, Mary Luedders, and Lucille Kraft chatting in a student's room, 1948.

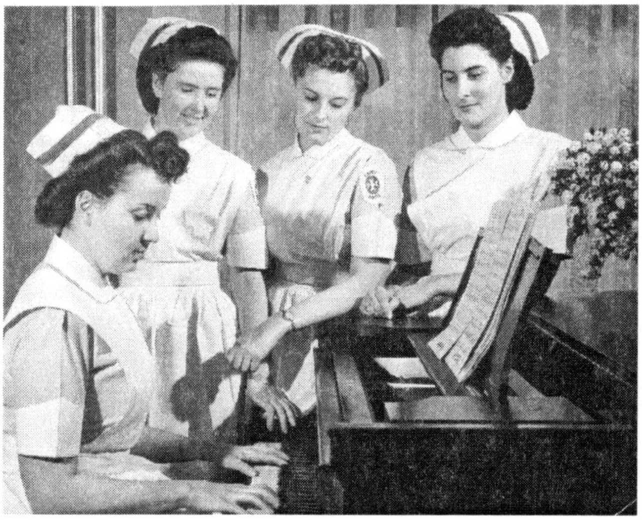

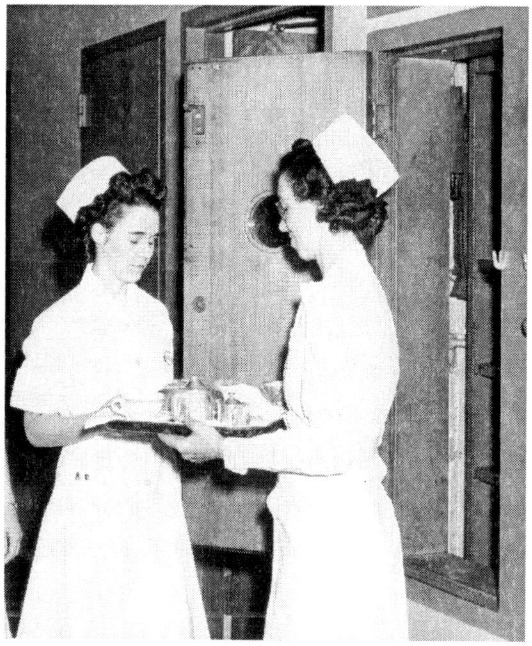

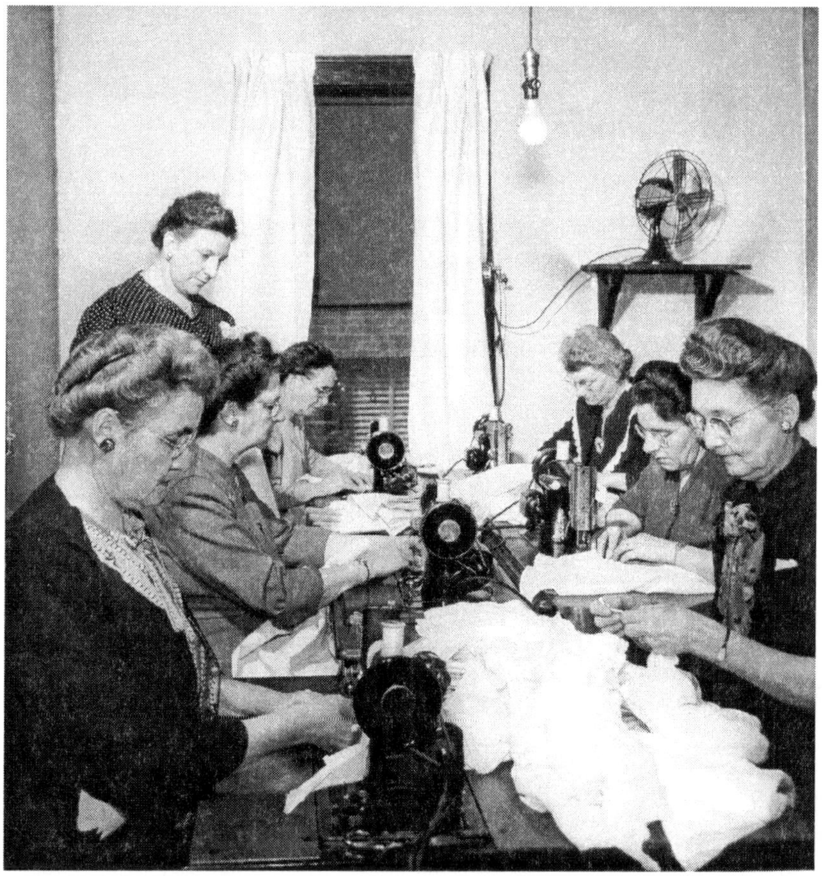

61. Cadet nurses enjoy some time for relaxation, 1940s.

62. Mabel Stell takes a patient tray from the dumb waiter and gives it to student Marcia Ward who delivers it to the patient's room, 1946.

63. Berean Class, First Baptist Church, sewing supplies for the hospital. (Seated, left to right) Mrs. L.C.Bramble, Mrs. L. Scott, Mrs. George H. Martin, Mrs. Don Thayer, Mrs. Forrest C. Thompson, and Mrs. C.H. Robinson, (standing) Mrs. Donald Lowden, 1948.

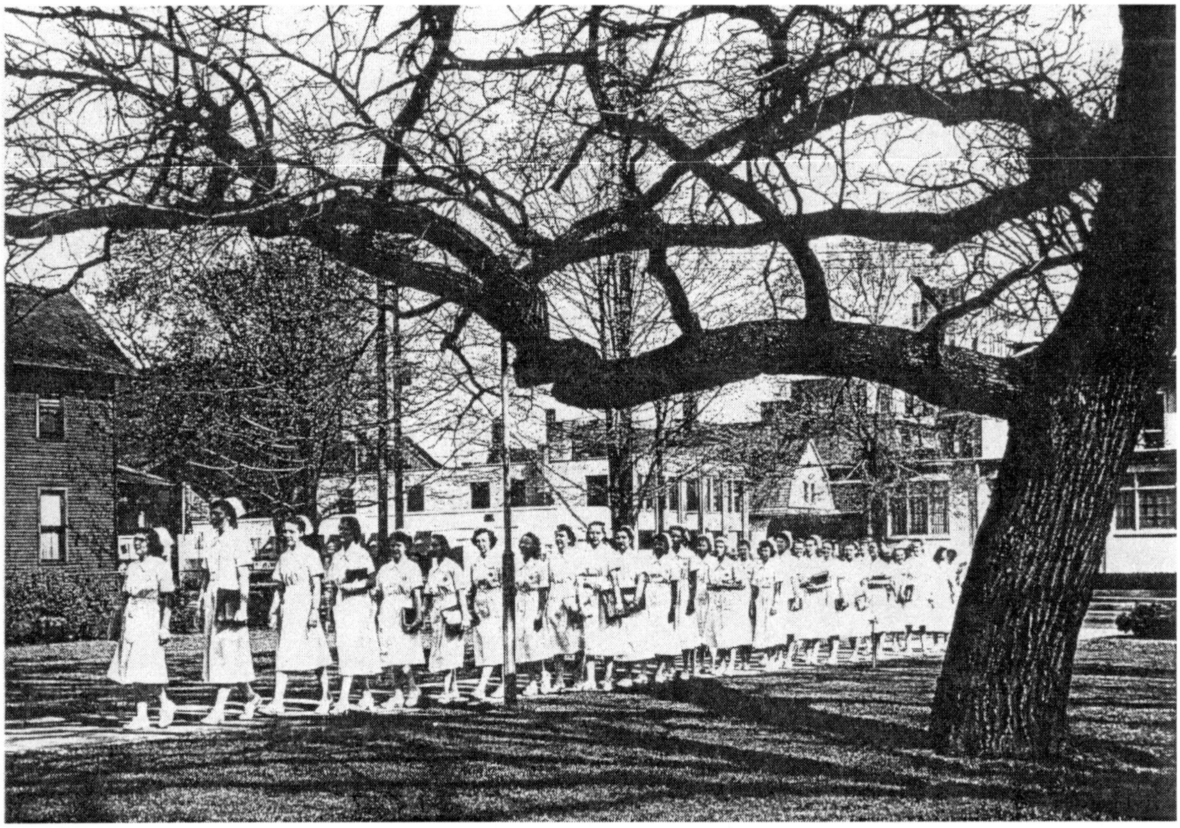

64. Class of 1950 walking from Lovell Street to the front entrance of Bronson Methodist Hospital. Notice American National Bank building in background and the Philip's residence on far left.

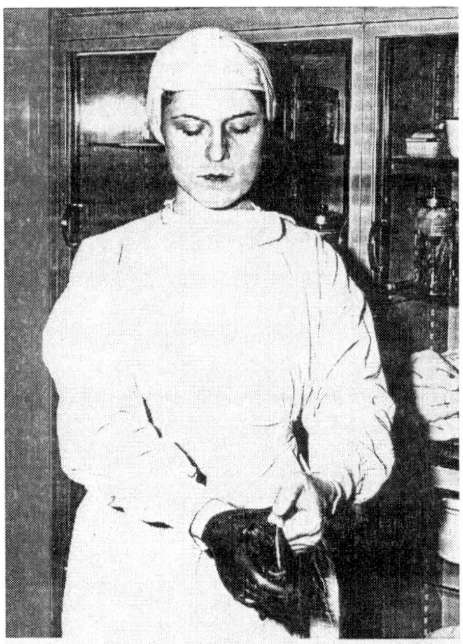

65. Norma Lee Carpenter removing gloves after surgery, 1947.

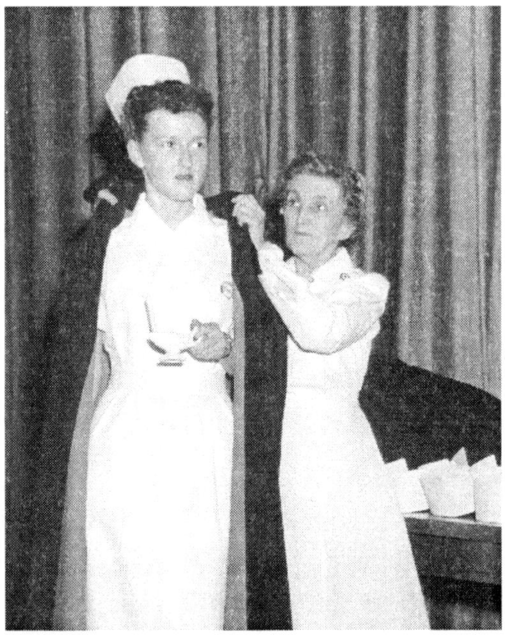

66. L. Sweet cloaking student nurse Shirley Motyer during capping ceremony, 1950.

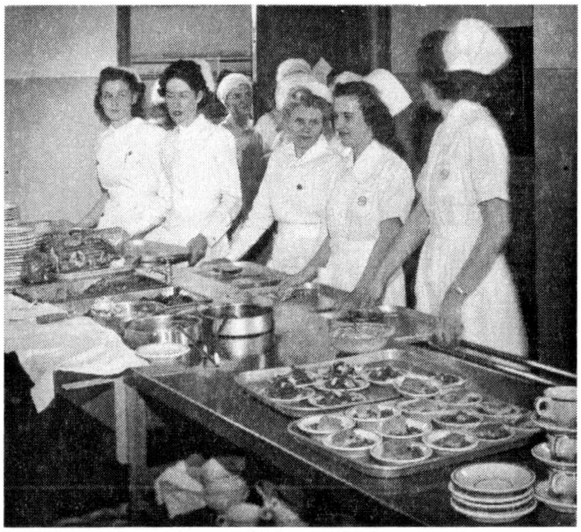

67. Hospital cafeteria line, ca 1940s

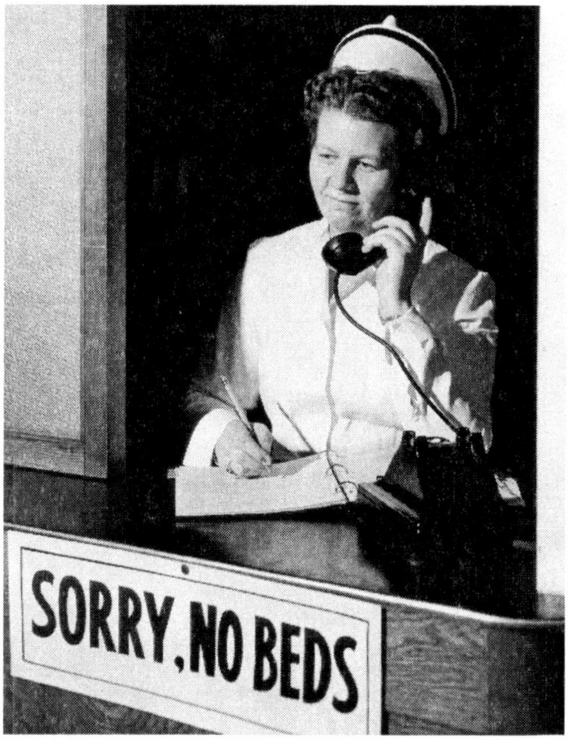

68. Louise Huffman, House Supervisor, during time when there was not enough room in the hospital for everyone who needed care, December 1949.

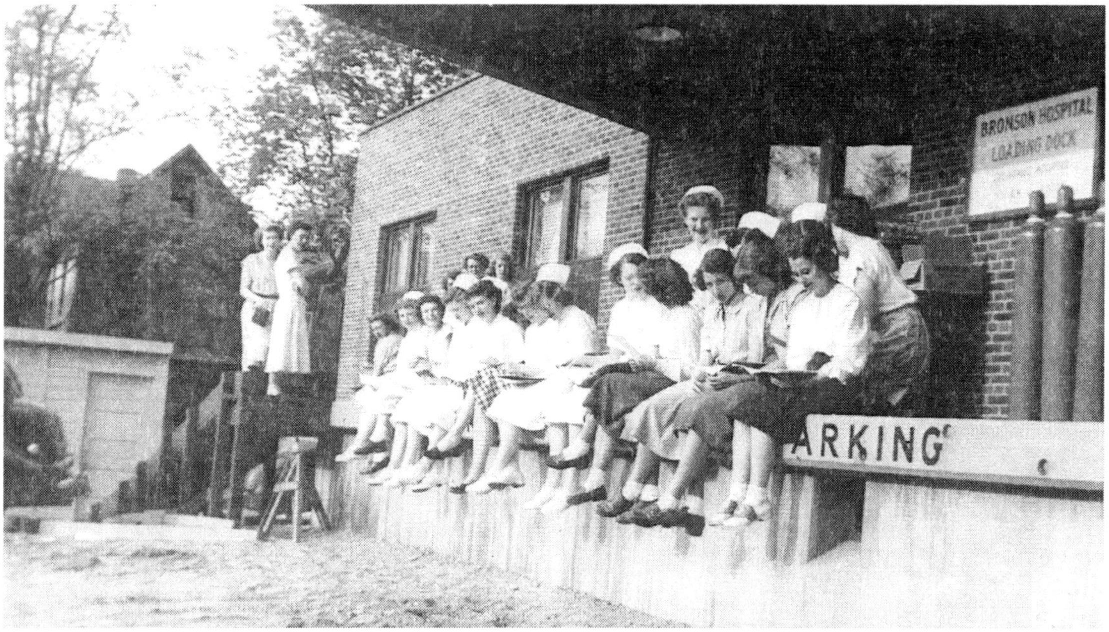

69. Freshmen take a break from Nursing Arts Lab on the dock off the Cedar Street Service Building, ca 1948–1949 (left to right): Esther Ryefield, Doris Allen, Sue Berkey, Maxine Woker, Joane Baulch, Betty Gosling, Ruth Spriggs, Nancy Burgess, Joyce Phares, Sally Shaffer, Mildred Dipert, Ruth Fox, Gladys Goss, Beverly Butler. Above: Jacqueline Schultz, Betty Rogers, Ruth Rosemurgy, Caroline Casler.

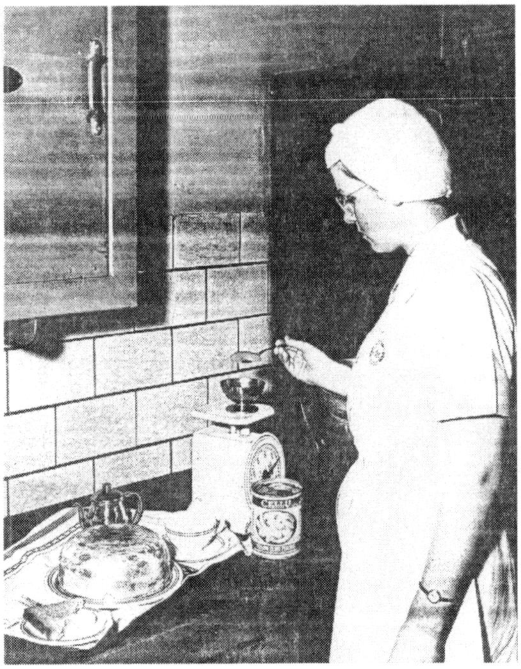

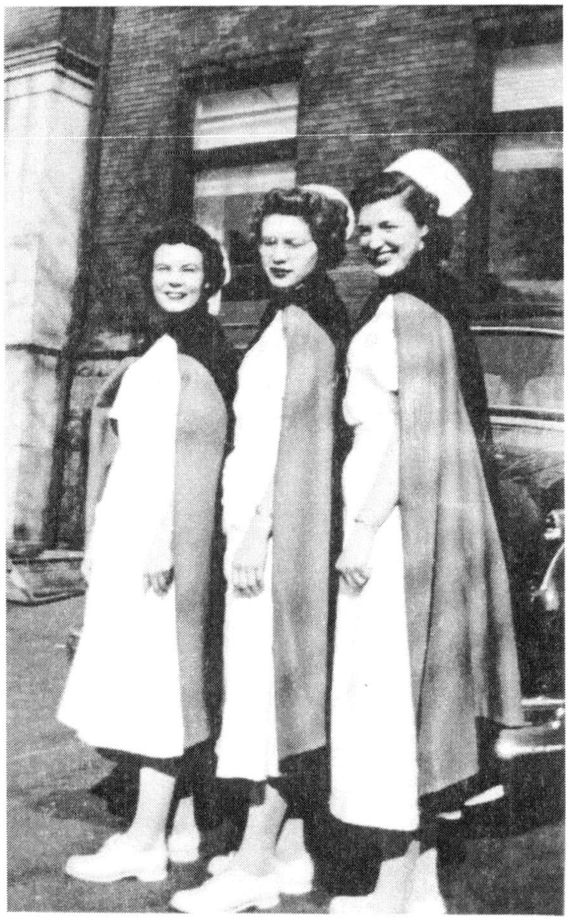

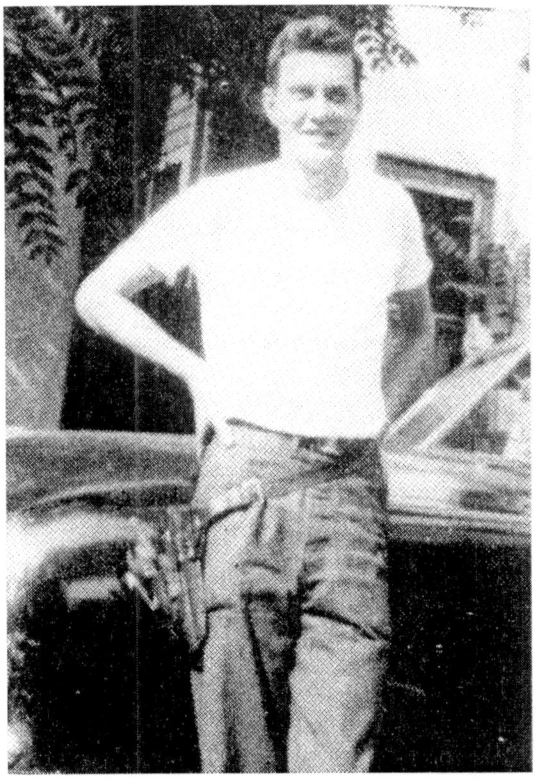

70. (above, left to right): Joane Baulch, Shirley Arendsen and Betty Gosling in front of dorm, proudly wear their uniforms and capes, ca 1949.

71. (top left) Kathleen Chute in diet kitchen weighs a tray in grams, assuring that one of the 40–50 patients on special diets receive a meal that is not only tasty, but nutritious, and designed for his own needs, 1949.

72. (bottom left) Dick Vander Molen, was the "Man On The Floor," friend and confidante of students from the late 1940s. He is the only Honorary Member of the Alumni Association of Bronson Methodist Hospital School of Nursing.

OUR FRIENDSHIPS

Of all the gifts by which we are blessed,
Surely our friends are among the best.
Were it not for light of friendly faces,
The world would have many lonesome places.

Without the kind deeds and cheery smiles,
How could we travel life's weary miles?
The helpful words of the spoken praise
May brighten some sky for days and days.

Have you told your friend across the way
How you would miss him if he went away?
Your kindly cheer would give him a lift
And make in his clouds a silver rift.

Remember, hands in their last repose
Can't hold the gift of a lovely rose;
Ears that are silent to noise of earth
Will not hear the praise of spoken worth.

Of all the great ships that cross the sea,
The "Friendships" seem the best to me;
Others are loaded for war and strife;
Friendships, with healing for the hurts of life.

We are hoping the time soon may be,
When all the ships of air and sea
Will carry supplies of our good will
And not machines to maim and kill.

—Dr. Alfred Way

CHAPTER 6
AT THE HALF CENTURY, 1950s

Nursing careers were childhood dreams that Bronson Methodist Hospital School of Nursing turned into real-world choices because of the school's affordability, *e.g.*, $500 for a full three-year program, and its excellent reputation. Like F. Marilyn Newcombe Bryant '54, young women were influenced by crisp images of starched white uniforms and smart blue capes on older students they saw in the community and by their own imaginations as they listened to that old radio program, "Dr. Christian," with his nurse June, played by Rosemary DeCamp. They chose Bronson over other schools in the fifties, sometimes because they had been born there, had grown up in Methodist families, had encountered role models in summer camp nurses, or because it was a smaller training school than those at Henry Ford and Harper hospitals in Detroit.

CLASS CHARACTERISTICS

In a welcoming orientation the earliest class was told that its members represented the "cream of the crop" of that years' applicants and that they would mature much faster than others in their age bracket because they would experience new life and death firsthand. They would also see much joy, suffering, and sorrow.

Betty Gosling Vander Molen '51 found these remarks to be accurate in her case because of her naïveté at that time.

It's the special, lifelong friendships that epitomize the graduates of the 1950s:

- ***'50,*** Our class has remained very close, and special friendships have developed and remained over the years.
- ***'52,*** All the good friends I made, all the fun times, tough times, trying to make the grade.
- ***'53,*** Friends I made, my closest sisters and friends for life.
- ***'54,*** Many lifelong friendships, my dearest friends yet today.
- ***'55,*** The camaraderie of classmates who lived, studied, and worked together for 36 months straight, establishing lifelong friendships.
- **'56,** My greatest joy is the lifelong friends I made.
- ***'59,*** Extra-ordinary women gathered together in a dormitory lounge—many of them away from home for the first time—to receive directions and to make friendships, many of which would last for a lifetime. I think we call that "bonding" now.

In the beginning, Phyllis Weenink Ossewaarde '50 felt like she was entering a convent, isolated from the real world, but it was all those "firsts" . . . first bed bath, first cath, first injection, first birth, the first death (even if expected) and caring for the body before the undertaker arrived, first day of a new rotation or affiliation, first day scrubbing in the OR, first day "in charge," and on and on and on, that grounded reality. "The first time I gave an enema the tubing came apart, squirting water all over Miss Campbell's feet. Was anyone else terrified of trachs and iron lungs during that post-polio era?"

Esther L. Wyman '57 remembered giving her first "hypo" medications under the supervision of Mrs. Irene Cripe. They were "prelims" for a patient on 2 East who was going to surgery later in the morning:

> Mrs. Cripe watched me draw up the medications (a mixture of morphine sulphate or Demerol® and scopolamine, as I recall). I can still see us walking down the 300 numbered hall toward my patient's room. I was nervous and excited at the same time. I cleansed the area on the upper arm, inserted the needle, and pushed in the plunger. As soon as I charted the medication on the work part of my split shift, I rushed to class.
>
> Sitting in class, I relived giving my first shot. All of a sudden it came to me—I hadn't attempted to aspirate before pushing in the plunger! I was sure I must have hit a vein or an artery and expected to be summoned from class any minute. It was one of the longest class periods I ever had. When the class was dismissed, I literally ran to 2 East and asked about the patient. The nurses said she went to surgery and assured me everything was just fine.
>
> From that day on, I never forgot the aspiration step in giving SubQ or IM injections. Actually, on many occasions an IV was needed, and I wished finding a vein was as easy as I had imagined early in my nursing school days.

Fears

Fifties' grads came to realize that their greatest initial fears turned into confidence about their own abilities as time went by. Fear of failure, whether in meeting high expectations of teachers, or in manually replacing machines critical to patient survival under electrical brownout conditions, or at following stringent rules, was high on their lists. As Patricia Ann Hauke Dahlman '55 responded during an interview, "Fear of not being able to survive our probationary period (when we wore imitation nurse's caps called 'probie bands') proved justified, as only one-half of my original class completed the course."

At first some eventual colleagues, deservedly or not, were also feared, *e.g.,* "I had a healthy fear of each hall and house supervisor, of my first Nursing Arts or clinical instructors and some doctors, especially surgeons and particularly neurosurgeons, for whom respect bordered on fear. As a scrub nurse, I would shake in my boots, I was scared to death of them, Having to scrub at night for the neurosurgeons like Dr. W. . . , who frequently yelled and threw instruments at the regular scrub nurses, petrified me. I goofed, of course, catching his finger with a clamp."

A whole range of fears, some less critical than others, affected this decade. How "creepy" it was to return to your room through the hospital with all the night sounds from patients' rooms. Not knowing who might come out of a room, Gwendolyn Rosser Calkins '53, hurried to her own. For Patricia Robertson Bigelow '50 and Betty Gosling Vander Molen, their ". . . greatest fear, probably like many other people, was making a mistake that would harm a patient." They knew that people's lives were entrusted to them and that a mistake could be fatal. Ethical dilemmas sometimes intertwined with their fear of harming others.

Ethics

One of the areas Bronson stressed was ethics. Virginia Culver Brouse '56 and Marlene Juday Kracko '55 both remarked that Bronson helped develop a strong ethical base that has stayed with them. It influenced their careers by enabling expanded roles.

An ethical issue surfaced when Marilyn Newcombe Bryant '54, was head nurse on a general surgical floor, 3 East, in the late fifties or early sixties. A patient in a Thomas splint had been improperly positioned in the splint, and his skin condition on the injured leg was severely deteriorated. She had called the condition to the attention of the attending physician a few times and, when nothing was done about the problem, reported it to the Chief of Staff. An orthopedic doctor was promptly called to correct the situation, and Marilyn was much relieved for the patient! On another occasion she was filled with, " . . . profound anger and sadness when, as a student on Peds, I witnessed the death of a baby. A physician had pumped too much blood into the child's body against the rule to infuse no more than 10cc per pound, and this amount was significantly exceeded."

Monitoring other professionals as well as themselves, nurses like Janice McClellan Duryea '53 witnessed a registered nurse who one morning could hardly hold her head up, let alone walk or talk. She was addicted to Demerol® and had used it all night while working the 11–7 shift, signing it out to her patients and taking it herself. Here was a case of losing one's license and the privilege to work as a registered nurse.

Elizabeth VanVoorhees Bower '59 remembers capping. The capping ceremony was accompanied by gifts—new testaments and lamps that symbolized the one Florence Nightingale carried when making night rounds on wounded soldiers in the Crimean War. This pledge was pasted inside the Bible:

> I solemnly pledge myself before God and in the presence of this assembly to pass my life in purity and to practice my profession faithfully. I will abstain from whatever is deleterious and mischievous, and will not take or knowingly administer any harmful drug.
>
> I will do all in my power to maintain and elevate the standards of my profession, and will hold in confidence all personal matters committed to my keeping, and all family affairs coming to my knowledge in the practice of my calling.
>
> With loyalty will I endeavor to aid the physician in his work and devote myself to the welfare of those committed to my care.

This "Florence Nightingale Pledge" was formulated, not by Miss Nightingale but by someone else more than 30 years after Nightingale began an institution for the training of nurses. Mrs. Lystra E. Gretter, who chaired the Farrand Training School for Nurses Committee at old Harper Hospital in Detroit, based the pledge on the Hippocratic Oath taken by medical doctors for the commencement of the hospital's Class of 1893.[1]

Memorable Lessons

From the pens of the fifties came indelible lessons learned during Bronson training: including that the patient always comes first and that helping others with kindness and honesty, nurses are Angels of Mercy who relieve pain and suffering and, if possible, save lives. What a discovery that a half-grain morphine dosage, given frequently to relieve the patient's suffering, wouldn't kill a dying patient!

Children and teenagers at Sigma Gamma in Mt. Clemens, afflicted with cerebral palsy, TB of the spine, *etc.,* presented a true lesson in courage. "I was always awed and inspired by the spiritual strength and intestinal fortitude of many of my patients, adults and children alike," wrote Suzanne Berkey Esenwein '51, and she continued, "The greatest insight we can have about our patients is to have been one ourselves, for better or worse."

> Taught that all staff and doctors were to be shown respect by standing each time a doctor approaches the nurses station, we also learned that the ER was not the place to take sick students, when my roommates panicked at my 104° fever and rushed me there. The night supervisor chewed us out severely but later came to the dorm with ginger ale and to see how I was.

Beth Simpson Fletcher '59 described another occasion: when,

> Coming home, I think from Mrs. Beatty's who had a dog, my roommate's eyes began swelling. Liz couldn't see and we had to

> study, so we took her to the ER (we had been warned!). "Couldn't you give her something that will reduce the swelling, but won't make her sleepy, because we have to study?" brought a physician's order, I.M. Benadryl® and an aminophylline suppository. I swear I saw the intern wink as we started back to the dorm, a trip I'm sure Liz doesn't remember.
>
> One of Miss Huffman's much remembered phrases is, "Don't pat the linens," when making a bed, but we learned and never forgot her instructions or those of Mrs. Cripe for the aspiration step in giving SubQ or IM injections.

Fletcher also wrote about the first time she cared for a patient who had expired. She and Carrie Lewis had to replace the patient's false teeth. "Looking back now, I can't imagine assigning that chore to my daughter."

A few weeks before graduation, Patricia Hauke Dahlman '55 was one of the senior students selected to serve a two-week stint as camp nurse at Lake Louise Methodist Camp near Petoskey. The experience made her realize what a responsibility nurses carry. Virginia Culver Brouse '56 acquired the ability to be objective and have compassion, yet retain the capacity to problem solve and function with her values and beliefs intact at Bronson. Discipline has remained an invaluable tool throughout Suzanne Berkey Esenwein's '51 professional and personal life, and Betty Hoogstraten Smith Kaub '52 adds, "Many times while practicing my specialty, psychiatric nursing, I had to make decisions and always was able to do so."

Although it sometimes was difficult to go to lunch after attending an autopsy, as time went on students learned, to some extent, to separate their nursing experiences from their personal lives:

> We were nurses who had to sell our abilities and ourselves. We had to convince and educate people to make decisions for their best well-being. Taught always to look our best, do our best, act professionally, be proud of our profession, and to wear our caps

> proudly, these lessons set the direction of our lives. How could anyone be a mother without training to be a nurse?

HOW THE ALMA MATER CAME TO BE

During the first nearly 52 years of its existence, the Bronson Methodist Hospital School of Nursing never had an official song. At its September 1955 assembly, the first of a new academic/clinical year, Dr. Perdew offered $100, $50, and $25 prizes for the three best poems. All students, faculty, and Alumni were eligible to participate.[2] Once an alma mater was selected, it would be set to music that was chosen in a parallel contest open to any person in Michigan. Linda Smith DeLand '57 won first prize, and 47 years later she reflected on how she wrote the winning entry:

> Sometime earlier that fall I saw a poetry contest notice posted on the infamous student bulletin board, across from the mailboxes and Mrs. Brown's[3] office. The deadline was shortly after Thanksgiving. My interest was piqued, although a poet I was not, and I did not put pen to paper until the Sunday night after Thanksgiving.
>
> As I had done many times in my three years at Bronson, on that Sunday night I rode the Indian Trails bus from Charlotte to Kalamazoo. I was reminded of the contest and impending deadline as we covered the miles back to school. I recalled the few school songs with which I was familiar and then focused on the highlights of my early life at Bronson. Our uniforms, capes, caps, pin, faith, loyalty, joys and sorrows, golden memories, and the Nightingale Pledge seemed like the core of our lives then and still do as I look back today.
>
> When I got to my room in the dorm (a house on Pine Street), I wrote down the ideas that had come to me as I traveled. There was little time for editing so I submitted my poem the next day. The rest is history.

Here is the text Linda submitted:

Oh, here we are together
    All Bronson nurses true,
In uniforms of white
    And capes of loyal blue.
Our heritage we hold
    In love that's always just,
Faithful to tradition
    And to the nursing trust.

Each golden memory lingers
    Of days beyond recall;
With bygone joys and sorrows
    We build a mighty wall.
Our pin and cap declare
    The PLEDGE we'll not forget
For days at dear old Bronson
    Have been the happiest yet!

DAILY SCHEDULES

Blue wool capes and student uniforms hardly compensated for the swing shifts, for example, on Hall 6, 11 P.M.–7 A.M. Saturday, 3–11 P.M. Sunday, and 7 A.M.–3 P.M. Monday, or the "split shift" 7–11 A.M. work, 11 A.M.–3 P.M. class, and 3–7 P.M. work again.

Having worked the first week on nights, at the end of her freshman year, Erlene Williams Kimber was fine Monday and Tuesday. Then came Wednesday evening. Williams Kimber's alarm had been set for 2 P.M., but when she woke up it was dark and her roommates were out. A search of the quiet John Street freshman dorm found four students in a room playing cards, so she asked, "Is it 10:30 P.M. on Wednesday?" Upon their reply, she thought, Oh, oh, she'd been asleep since 8 A.M. and was a little late for her 3-11 P.M. shift. Then, "the kind staff fed me and mused about how I had managed to sleep for over 14 hours."

While students' memories of Bronson are mostly pleasant ones, fifties grads recall being very tired most of the time. The schedule was frenetic: night shifts on duty and then class work during the day. The students were immersed in attending Western Michigan College and Bronson classes, observing autopsies at the morgue and funeral homes, floor duty, and getting enough sleep. What kept many of them going was a never-ending supply of peanut butter and bread.

Quite overwhelmed by the vastness of Western, they were always together as a group, taking a chartered bus to and from classes. When time permitted, they walked that long trek back to Bronson. Some even felt like guinea pigs when Upjohn delivered the "newest" vitamin pills, put them in huge bowls, and requested that nurses in training take one each day. A hospital couldn't be run with sick students, right?

Everything was not sweetness and light, of course. A very short litany of worst experiences included getting up in the mornings, coming down with the measles in Miss Sweet's Communicable Disease class (great timing!), and "I hated doing those Sub-Q infusions—are they ever done anymore?"

Looking back, it became plain how valuable daily chapel was during the freshman year. Their varied schedules the following two years did not accommodate chapel services. Later, Patricia Hauke Dahlman '55 realized how important chapel and prayer had been in her spiritual growth, "Asking God for strength and help as we began our day of study and/or work aided me in persevering, no doubt about it." She also recalls the restrictive dormitory hours that young people today cannot comprehend: three 1:30 A.M. curfews per year??!! In 1955, Marlene Gabriel '58 remembered, freshman students had a curfew of 8:30 P.M. As 18-year olds, however, they were still full of energy and not ready to settle down to study. Otherwise, 9 P.M. weeknights and 11 P.M. weekends were "sign-in times."

ROTATIONS

Apprehension ruled over the first day of three-month assignments to a new rotation or affiliation—OR, OB, a "Rural Affiliation" in Marshall, Psych at

Kalamazoo State Hospital, *etc.* Central Service duty, in addition to the diet kitchen and formula room, was part of the junior year. Near the end of those assignments, confidence replaced tentativeness as each student gained experience.

Surgical Nursing

Hall 6 was a surgical floor used for the freshman-year clinical practice rotation, although it was not limited to surgical patients since some doctors preferred it for their patients. Its popularity may have had something to do with the attention the patients received from the head nurse and staff or the excellent care provided by these nurses. Some patients were recovering from cataract surgery and required absolute bed rest, with sandbags to keep them from turning their heads. They were in the hospital for at least seven days and two people were required to turn them, "log fashion" every so often. Others were men with "TURs" with all their apparatus for flushing the catheters. The treatment seemed so complicated—all that tubing, clamping, and bags of solutions. Women with radium implants were off limits to most student nurses, although sometimes they had to answer the call light and assist staff. It seemed that community leaders, doctors' family members, and physicians were placed on Hall 6 when they required hospitalization. Esther L. Wyman '57 remembers one long-term patient on Hall 6.

> Mrs. P., who most all of us cared for during our rotation, required a complete bed bath every day. She was a patient for so long, she knew what we were to do and how we should do it. Mrs. P. had high expectations for the care she received, and Mrs. Stell made sure she got it. The room was expected to be clean, tidy, and everything in its correct place.
>
> Mrs. P. asked for me to be her nurse. Evidently she liked the way I cleaned and trimmed her toenails after soaking her feet in the wash basin. Everytime I used my bandage scissors thereafter, I was reminded of her.

Obstetrics

Service on OB had Pat Hurd coming out of the admitting room in tears, "But Mrs. Hinkel said she wouldn't have it in the shower!!"

Is the sign that used to be on the wall still in the Fathers' Waiting Room—the one that read something like: "Every time a baby is born, it is a sign that God has not lost faith in mankind."

The three-month rural affiliation was one of the best learning experiences, however, because it stressed skills that small hospitals without a Central Supply needed you to do, according to Gwendolyn Rosser Calkins '53 and Shirley Martin Moffatt '55.

The State Hospital

Tenure at the State Hospital taught much that was not in textbooks. It brought Rosser Calkins into a world that she had never known. There she found that the people who appeared the most sane and stable were the patients.

When a Grand Rapids student nurse was killed by an inmate, Marlene Juday Kracko '55 went to the rotation with some reservations, but she followed the rules to the letter, locking and unlocking doors according to protocol. Her classmate, Shirley Martin Moffatt, however, left the rotation with a lifelong discomfort with psychiatric patients.

A first encounter with nuns—they were Borgess students—occurred during rotational time at the state hospital. To her delight, Beth Simpson Fletcher '59 found the nuns to be just like the rest of us (or did she delude herself into thinking she was nun-like?).

"One time we saw a fire at the state college from the hospital lounge. Most of us were watching the fire, but Sue Mindrum was looking out the window on the other side of the room. We'd been told about the type of people who set fires, and Sue was looking for the arsonist."

DIRECTOR OF THE SCHOOL, 1950–1978

Over the years no one influenced as many aspiring nurses as Helen Weber. More frequently mentioned by fifties' students than anyone else, she stands out. Marlene Gabriel '58 remembers that, when she was a student, Mrs. Weber was director of education, a savvy woman who, understood students and was very long on patience. She took us aside one day and told us, "Just keep that housemother out of my hair." Some recalled her Pharmacology class or looked to her as a role model for professionalism, while others just plain revered and respected her. To Sharon Martin Daniels '59, she was professional, fair, stern yet kind, caring, and always interested and ready to listen to her students, professionally and personally. She was a superb role model because she lived and practiced integrity. "How lucky we were to have had her for guidance," as illustrated by this story:

> When our class received our junior's black bands during an appropriate evening ceremony, with friends, family, faculty, and other classes attending, Mrs. Weber called my name, "Shirley Martin." As I accepted my band, I quietly said, "Mrs. Weber, I'm Sharon Martin, not Shirley."
>
> She was embarrassed and said to the audience, "I'm so sorry. I misspoke and called Sharon, Shirley. You see, we have a Bronson grad—Shirley Martin, Class of 1955—who is on the staff at the hospital, but lest you think I don't know the correct names in this junior class, I assure you I do."
>
> She then looked at our class and the audience and proceeded to recite each first, middle, and last name in correct alphabetical order, omitting none! The audience applauded and she replied, "Thank you, but I still must apologize for my error."[4] We all knew she cared for us on an individual basis.

Mrs. Weber, a graduate of Butterworth Hospital School of Nursing in Grand Rapids and the University of Minnesota, served the School of Nursing for 28 years.

She joined Bronson in 1950 as associate director of the School of Nursing and was promoted to director in 1966. When Mrs. Weber retired in 1979, nearly 1,500 students had graduated under her tenure. She was instrumental in raising the quality of education and facilities at the school, and it was under her direction that the school was first accredited in 1956 by the National League for Nursing. Mrs. Weber also secured federal financial aid for students, maintained an affiliation with Western Michigan University, and encouraged faculty to return to college by arranging for tuition reimbursement and modifying their schedules.[5]

During Mrs. Weber's time at the school, enrollment increased and the attrition rate significantly decreased. She was responsible for implementing a realistic nursing program aimed at meeting the changing health needs of society. In 1957, for example, students were allowed to marry and, if they became pregnant, they were required to take a 12-month leave of absence. Prior to that time, students were not allowed to marry before the last six months of school, and pregnant students were dismissed without the opportunity to complete their nursing education.

Further, as a mentor, Mrs. Weber shaped the lessons learned by Jackie Clark Wylie '62 as recounted below:

Helen E. Weber, Director of Education

My respect for Mrs. Weber grew in increments as more of her many human, caring characteristics gradually sank into my brain. I probably took her for granted as a student. I can't remember caring what a director did or what decisions she made, though Mrs. Weber always looked in control and able to determine who lived and who died, who passed, who failed. I figured the only time you saw administrators was when a problem surfaced, and I tried hard to avoid having the "problem" label attached to me.

She was not the warm and fuzzy type, and I wasn't bright enough to know that other caring characteristics might lie concealed under a cool, professional demeanor.

Her strengths became obvious to me when, in 1965, I accepted a position as the Operating Room Instructor. I had left a position in which the recent supervisor found it necessary to control—she could hardly attend meetings and thus allow the OR staff nurses to be in charge for a few hours—not a position I wanted to be in. I had known a more open supervisor who encouraged staff nurse decision-making, and I looked for that kind of opportunity again. I found it with Mrs. Weber. Thank goodness! I was back in an environment of trust, with the expectation that I had a brain and could manage my practice.

Mrs. Weber was a listener, quiet and reflective, yet witty and always protective of students. She took their stories to heart and protected them within her power. She never shared information that someone might later hold against a student. For this reason, and for her own protection, she developed the habit of being somewhat aloof. This characteristic never bothered me since I believed she knew that she was doing exactly the right thing. She always accepted staff innovations and listened hard to hear any new ideas for curriculum development. Admissions was a process she controlled to keep the process fair for every person who applied.

My next incremental learning came when she offered me the director's job about six months before she retired, although she wasn't precisely in a position to do so. Bronson often promoted its staff nurses and middle managers to higher positions. As I recall, positions were not posted in those days, or, at least, not all of them. She must have offered a suggestion to the administrator to whom she reported. We met with Mr. William Johnson to confirm my appointment since he would become my boss. I accepted her summer 1978 offer to become the associate director to learn the director's role that I would begin in December when Mrs. Weber would leave after 28 years in this leadership position. She taught me what directors do, responsibilities I could never have imagined as a student or instructor.

The first day after she retired, I sat at her desk for the first time and I felt like the great imposter—or as better described—a not-so-great imposter. People would surely see right through me. How could I have thought I could manage? Had I lost my mind when I agreed to accept the position? It was an anxiety-producing first week as I waited for calls and consultations that I thought I would not be able to handle; Mrs. Weber, though, was a good mentor.

The second week seemed less threatening and slowly I conquered my fear as I realized that I really was ready for the job! It quickly became fun as well as challenging, and I remembered Mrs. Weber's words of wisdom—where to get help when I needed it. Particularly, she had given me names of people to call, like the School of Nursing directors in Grand Rapids, Flint, and Detroit. They were experts and could further mentor me as needed. Mrs. Weber had prepared me well!

I have never forgotten that she said, "You know, you and I are different people." I thought she was referring mainly to her introverted and my extroverted ways. "You will not behave as I have and you should not expect to." She shared with me a piece of her history. As a young nursing administrator, in order to feel in control, Mrs. Weber chose never to socialize with the people she managed. The strategy developed into a conscious pattern that often appeared exclusionary to others. Students and staff, however, were never excluded in her planning and acceptance, only in social situations. She helped me learn to accept my own style and not to try to emulate her. She gave students and staff permission to be themselves and to become more than they thought they could be, a true mentor to all.

Many of the policies set by Mrs. Weber never changed throughout the remaining life of the school. I always asked myself: what were her reasons for adopting them? Why did she employ this procedure or evoke that principle? Why was a policy written a certain way? I would try hard to follow her logic which, I believe to this day, was in the best interests of the students, staff, and the hospital at that time.

We may have had different personal characteristics, but our bottom line was the same: advocacy for students, staff and, indirectly, the patients served. One of Mrs. Weber's sayings, when some nit-picking occurrence tried her patience, was, "I can handle the elephants; God save me from the gnats." Could this imagery have been foretold by her mind set during her own pre-entrance interview that she experienced in 1931? "The director [of Butterworth] was a petite lady who asked me how tall I was. When I told her I was six feet tall, she said 'Are you in good health otherwise?'" In retrospect, Mrs. Weber's response would have been, "Yes, Miss DeVries, I am in good health. I have survived."[6]

Precursor to Accreditation—Top 25% Nationally

The National Committee for the Improvement of Nursing Services, affiliated with the National League of Nursing Education,[7] invited schools of nursing to participate in a survey intended to provide " . . . relative national standing of your basic program and six of its component factors."[8] Bronson complied and began the process for meeting national nursing-education standards under the direction of Miss Mary B. Anderson, who hired Mrs. Helen Weber in 1950.

The survey compared and rated a national sample of schools of nursing in six areas: student health, curriculum, clinical facilities and experience; library facilities; qualifications and size of teaching staff; and instructional salaries. Building upon identified strengths and correcting weaknesses served as preparations for a next step, voluntary NLN Accreditation.

The results of the survey were to be published in the *American Journal of Nursing* in the fall of 1949 if schools gave their approval. The work was cosponsored by the American Nurses Association, the Association of Collegiate Schools of Nursing, the American Association of Industrial Nurses, the National Association of Colored Graduate Nurses, the National Organization for Public Health Nursing and the National League of Nursing Education.

No doubt Bronson was pleased with the outcome. "The profile indicates that your school has been included in the Interim Classification of Institutions Offering

Basic Programs in Nursing,"[9] and was ranked ". . . among the top 25% of the nation's basic programs in nursing." Those ranked in the lowest 25% would not be included.

Bronson's best three strengths were curriculum, qualifications and size of teaching staff, and instructional salaries. Ranked second were library facilities, and third its weak points, were student health and clinical facilities and experiences. Student health referred mainly to the overcrowded living conditions and safety of the junior and senior students living in four wood-framed homes adjacent to the hospital. Additionally, too many clinical experiences were scheduled on evening and night shifts, indications of shortages in nurse staffing and the necessity for student labor to provide patient care outside of planned curriculum experiences.

Most likely the in-house feelings of superiority were dashed when, five years later, a NLN accreditation body stipulated that all factors in the survey had to meet standards at the highest level, not just three of the six. Again, in 1954, lack of adequate housing and the length of evening and night assignments would not meet the standard.

Meeting National League of Nursing Education Standards

Mrs. Weber was introduced to collegiate nursing education standards during her enrollment at the University of Minnesota. Her Bronson Methodist Hospital position provided a venue for building the educational arm of the nursing department (the school of nursing) and later separating the school leadership from nursing service, with the philosophical adjustment from student nurse as worker to student as learner.

As assistant director of Bronson Nursing Education, in 1955 Weber oversaw the faculty and hospital administration efforts in achieving NLN temporary accreditation, with recommendations for improvements that would ultimately gain full approval.

Bronson administration understood the value of nursing students and was cognizant of past difficulties with recruitment. What resources could draw more young women to apply? A national organization's stamp of approval was one answer, with program changes that benefited students and the hospital culture. It responded by addressing the NLN standards[10] which focused on school of nursing administration—the school philosophy and policies, curriculum, faculty credentials, students services, library resources and periodic self-evaluation. Some of the faculty's practice time had to be devoted to the improvement of the student learning environment and outcomes designated by national nursing education standards set by the NLN.

Bronson first submitted an application for full accreditation in May 1954 for review by the NLN Board of Review for Diploma and Associate Degree Programs. Often a submitted application was a way of determining program strengths and weaknesses. When the NLN Board encouraged Bronson administrators to better articulate program strengths in several areas before requesting the final accreditation step, an on-site visit by an expert nurse educator was planned to verify, clarify and amplify the submitted application, and to offer recommendations. Obviously the NLN Review Board supported programs that were upgrading their educational standards. Strengths that made accreditation achievement a strong possibility were identified as well as areas that did not meet NLN standards. It was an evolutionary process for the nursing department, with subsequent development of the School of Nursing and a department of continuing education for nurses.

Florence E. Elliott, NLN assistant director from the Department of Diploma and Associate Degree Programs and nursing education consultant, visited Bronson on March 14, 15, and 16, 1955, to meet with the Bronson Board of Trustees Nursing Education Committee, administration, faculty and the Library Committee. A nine-page, single-spaced report, voicing her observations and recommendations was forwarded that April.

First, "It appears that an educational philosophy has not been formulated."[11] Ms. Elliott observed that development of individual students was voiced by the faculty but not written in a philosophical statement and included in the school bulletin. Also, the nursing staff perceived students as workers, not learners. Ms. Elliott suggested that nursing staff be included in the formulation of the educational philosophy in order to reframe their thinking about the needs of students in clinical practice.

Second, "The stated aim of the school would be of little value as a guide for planning the educational program." Educational objectives were needed to specify ". . . the kind of nurse the school expects to graduate,"[12] and then provide to students the nursing theory and practices to attain desired outcomes. Awareness of faculty and staff, who they were, and what was important in nursing practice and education were prerequisites to what nursing students needed to learn.

Third, was the goal to improve "Instructional Personnel."[13] Full-time and part-time instructor educational credentials were limited. Mary B. Anderson, Director of Nursing had an MS degree and Helen Weber, Assistant Director of Nursing Education, had a BS degree majoring in nursing education. The nursing arts instructor had an MA degree and the medical nursing instructor a BS degree. Bronson often hired its brightest young nurse leaders into instructor positions without advancing their education. Other strengths included the backgrounds of the dietician and librarian who had appropriate credentials and the WMU faculty who taught nursing students in their science courses. Ms. Elliott suggested that a committee be appointed to prepare for the inclusion of the WMU faculty in curriculum development.

A compelling argument promoted a plan for advancing the education of Bronson graduates since few continued their education to degree levels. Elliott's comments provide insight into the nursing practice culture surrounding the Bronson nurses:

> There are two very obvious complicating factors to such a plan, which must be faced. One is the fact that nursing remains primarily a woman's profession, and matrimony and motherhood are apt to upset the best-laid plans. One less likely to be considered is the fact that apparently only a very small number of graduates of this school have in the past gone on to continued study in the field of nursing education. Thus there would be the need to formulate positive plans to motivate nurses (either individually or as a group) in such a way as to create a desire for graduate study in those graduates who appear to have this potential for advanced positions.[14]

Ongoing instructor in-service education was required if the program was to become accredited since hiring of qualified nurse educators was viewed as impossible in southwest Michigan. Clinical instruction was considered a weak area and could be enhanced by more instructor supervision and less dependence on nursing staff.

A faculty organization was needed ". . . to assume responsibilities for the program . . . "[15] beyond the committee structure that was in place and so the Faculty Association was developed.

Fourth, "The preclinical period is very short and includes a heavy classload."[16] In response to this observation, WMU freshmen science courses were repositioned to be taught the first two semesters instead of compressed into one. At the same time instructors began the process of managing freshmen clinical assignments. Previously unit nurse managers had assigned student work hours.

Fifth, "No plans for clinical instruction appear to have been formulated."[17] It was necessary to connect classroom content with concurrent clinical practice within the three-year program of study and to base it on program philosophy, goals and objectives.

Sixth, "Less than one hour a week of clinical instruction is given to major critical services."[18] Elliott suggested that classroom activities be reframed into a patient-centered focus. Her assessment reflected her observation that both instructors and nursing staff thought in terms of the care of diseases rather than care of patients. It was further noted that content presented by guest resource persons such as dieticians, physicians, social workers and special therapists should be part of the instructor's clinical instruction plan.

1. Medical-surgical instructors carry a heavy teaching and supervisory load.
2. The assignment of students to the medical-surgical units is done on such a hit or miss pattern that efforts to plan for comparable learning experiences as well as patient-centered conferences are extremely difficult if not impossible.
3. The head nurse group appears to have limited understanding of the part clinical experience plays in the education of students.
4. Students often spent a disproportionate amount of time on evening and night assignments when supervision and instruction is limited.

To correct the shortcomings, Mrs. Weber designed elaborate practice schedules to designate students' clinical practice hours in selected patient-care areas so that their nursing practice was comparable in length and service. Anna Stryd '61 recalled knowing her practice schedule up front for the three years in which she was enrolled.

Seventh, "A four-week assignment for administration of medications is questioned."[19] Though faculty defended the practice as essential, Elliott pointed out the value of teaching, not only a functional model of practice but also the case method, a more patient-centered approach.

Eighth, "The evening and night assignment is excessive."[20] Questioned was the finding that some students spent nine months of their 36-month experience working evenings and nights. Elliott recommended that nursing service plan for redistribution of RNs, LPNs and nurses aides on the day, evening and night shifts, ". . . so that the need to use students would be reduced."[21] She suggested that learning experiences unique to evenings and nights be identified for the benefit of students, staff and the school. Educational value had to clearly connect clinical practice to nursing theory. Once again the message was that students needed to be identified as learners.

Ninth, "A record of state board performance reveals a rather high number of failures."[22] Elliott noted that recent records demonstrated scores that were "well above the national mean," and that ". . . scores as seen would appear to compare favorably if they are typical." [23] Possibly Elliott had noted that earlier state board scores had not been as favorable but were evidently not an issue at this point.

Tenth, "Students are housed in rooms which have three or four students. Bunk beds are used."[24] Noted was the fact that a new residence hall was in the planning stages.

Eleventh, "The library holdings appear limited for a school of this size."[25] Book volume numbered 562 for 100 students. Recommended were learning strategies to encourage student use of the library and policies for selecting new references, as well as maintaining the effective deletion policy that had kept references current.

The summary statement listed visible program strengths. Desire to improve the quality of student education was obvious within the Board of Trustees Nursing Education Committee and the hospital administrators. They wanted a sound educational program built on national standards and felt confident that they could meet the criteria to achieve accreditation. Faculty were stable, hospital physical facilities were excellent and the college course affiliation represented program strengths.

On the other hand, the number of faculty with appropriate credentials was limited, and they managed the program of study in an informal way, without policies and procedures for building curriculum ". . . as an integrated whole,"[26] attending to student services and to their own lifelong learning. Patient-centered nursing practice and student as learner required a paradigm shift similar to the expectation of collegiate programs. Mrs. Weber was the positive force in creating a healthy learning environment during her Bronson tenure.

Mrs. Weber's Brief Autobiography upon Retirement

This winter I will complete 47 years of daily contact with the nursing profession in an institutional setting.[27] I use this forum to express appreciation for the privileges these years have brought to me personally and professionally.

I entered Butterworth Hospital School of Nursing in 1932, vaguely aware of the immensity of the financial depression but unprepared for the stark reality of a hospital whose patients were there only because the severity of their illness made it impossible to survive otherwise and where people who appeared at the emergency entrance to ask for food were actually hungry. My 1,095 days (quite literally) as a student confirmed my belief that nursing was my calling, introduced me to some unforgettable patients, and gave me a healthy respect for my blessings.

Upon graduation, I had the good fortune to be one of two persons selected for employment. I had a job! And it was a job tailored in heaven for a person who enjoyed patient contacts and who was a little bossy by nature. I became head nurse of Men's Surgical, a 26-bed unit including a 16-bed ward. "Staff" consisted of several students and an orderly, and the census was regulated solely by gender and a surgical diagnosis. There being no PAR or ICU, a room euphemistically titled "recovery" was used for life-threatening conditions or patients disruptive to the ward and occasionally for its intended use—recovery from anesthesia. I learned something of organization, improvisation, and the value of teamwork. In the spirit of the times, I saved half of each paycheck toward a goal. After ten years I departed for the University of Minnesota.

Maintenance was the least expensive compensation the University Hospital could offer and the most expensive item in a student's budget. We worked 24 hours a week and no money changed hands. We lived on campus and had flexibility in arranging our hours each quarter to accommodate class needs. I worked as a scrub nurse for some outstanding surgeons and spent my cash for tuition, textbooks, and five-cent Cokes with conversation at the corner drugstore, solving men's greatest problems (Phi Beta Kappa, Rexall Chapter).

That year was followed by 13 years at St. Barnabas Hospital. Here my reflections turn to the "family" orientation of institutions of the era. There was a spirit of unity among employees, regardless of the contribution made by the individual. St. B was "our" hospital and we had a shared pride in it. Our service staff was largely composed of Scandinavian-born people, long-term employees, many of whom still spoke with that delightful upward inflection. One day, following a school inspection by the State Board of Nursing, I met our carpenter, Albert, who asked, "Did ve pass?" Yes, we did. Thank you, Albert, for the pleasure of having been part of the family with you.

Those years extended through the Second World War. Suddenly everyone was not only working but also working overtime. People wanted to have all of their postponed medical needs taken care of at once, and half the medical and nursing professionals were in the armed services. The United States Cadet Nurse Corps came into being and most students belonged to that federally subsidized program—complete with a commitment to spend the last six months of their programs in an armed service or underserved medical facility. I had the "opportunity" to chair the Minnesota League for Nursing committee that planned that senior-cadet experience for Minnesota schools. Meetings convened on Saturday afternoons, especially football Saturdays.

In a metropolitan area with 22 private hospitals, institutions are chosen for various reasons. Our patients tended to come from the high-income segment of society. I learned that some of the busiest, most influential people became the faithful corps of volunteers who were the dependable staff supplements for the duration of the war, while also learning a measure of diplomacy in coping with chauffeurs who delivered favorite dishes prepared by the family cook but not consistent with the patient's prescribed diet. Most of all I learned that my greatest satisfaction lay in working with students.

And so I have indulged myself for 28 years by association with Bronson Methodist Hospital School of Nursing. I take pride in the growth and quality of the hospital, the services it provides, the enthusiasm and dedication of faculty members, and the professional contributions made by the graduates of the school.

Those were the years, but the memories are of the people who made it a joy: Boards of Trustees, supportive administration, loyal faculties, helpful coworkers, students individually and collectively. On some occasions I have regretted my sharp teeth! Thank you for accepting me as I am.

OTHER UNFORGETTABLE PEOPLE

Hazel Latondress (Smitty)

Hazel Latondress[28] was a constant presence on the nursing service side, especially visible in patient-care areas and in administration, with a long line of promotions that were hard to avoid because of her skills in managing both people and a complex system. She managed patient-care services for 35 years.

Hazel Latondress arrived in Kalamazoo in March, 1949, expecting to work for Dr. Burrell, a resident physician whom she had met at Kansas City General Hospital two years after she had graduated from its School of Nursing. Dr. Burrell was planning to open a practice in Kalamazoo, and he was recruiting a young, bright nurse to manage his office. Hazel accepted his offer, arriving in Kalamazoo three months before the office was ready to open.

Hazel needed a job in the interim so she worked at Bronson for three months before moving into the office practice where she had been promised a percentage of the annual income. She worked from 7:00 A.M. to 5:00 P.M. and at Bronson from 5:00 to 11:00 P.M. as the polio emergency nurse, reporting to Shirley Evans.

> I just walked across the street from the office to Bronson. The nursing office would call me when a new patient was admitted. After two to three days, when the patient was moved to a polio ward, I was told that I could have the night off. I would get a call a few hours later, and the nurse would say that she was sorry, a new patient was arriving and I'd be back to work. I worked long days—that's how I paid for my car.
>
> Office nursing wasn't for me. I returned to Bronson full time in 1950 as the relief house supervisor, filling in on all three shifts. House supervisors managed all admissions to patient rooms and the surgery schedule. They also juggled the staff to fit patient numbers. It was the best job I ever had, making rounds on all units during the shift, and staying close to patients and staff. I especially liked rotating between all three shifts. Occasionally, when a unit was really short staffed, I'd stay and give direct patient care, providing most functions except baths. For example, one day a LPN was stewing and fretting—she had special plans after work and still had treatments to do. She said, "I can't leave, I still have to do a cath." So I said, "You go ahead and I'll do the cath for you." She never forgot that gesture. If a nurse had trouble starting an IV or was having trouble managing some other treatment, I would help her.
>
> Louise Huffman, my second supervisor, was a typical rule-oriented army nurse. We called her Lou. If you didn't follow the rules you were chewed out and, if you did, you were complimented. If we happened to work a day shift together, she'd ship me out to a floor to float for four hours. I'd be assigned to five to seven patients, then return to the nursing office. Miss Huffman would help Miss Wantz, and I'd return to the house-supervisor role for the afternoon. I did a little bit of everything.
>
> Next, I reported to Miss Wantz, the assistant director of nursing—a sweet little lady who could chew you out like nobody's business; but the next time she needed help or wanted some task done, she could be sweet again. She'd say, "Now honey, you were the only

> one I could chew out. I had to chew somebody out so I had to chew you out." Then came an apology. Then again she laid me low and said, "I just had to bawl someone out. Now you can go back to work."
>
> For awhile I reported to Mary B. Anderson, the director of nursing. She was most interested in the census. "Keep the numbers up!" she would admonish, and I'd say, "What do you want me to do? The census is low. I can't go out and beat people over the head." She would shake her head and say, "Well, just don't refuse anybody."
>
> Then Dr. Perdew called me on the carpet because I refused a "big wheel." I didn't know the big wheels in Kalamazoo and I treated everyone alike. One day I said, "Dr. Perdew, I'm down here so much I'm wearing out your carpet." He just looked at me and grinned. Dr. Perdew was a close-to-the-front-line administrator. He knew what was going on and followed up. I always felt that he listened to me.
>
> My title changed to associate director but the role was similar to what I did as house supervisor, and in the early 1960s my title changed again to director of patient care, and I reported to Virginia McPhail. She left me alone to make decisions, even when I asked for her input. She would reply that she would think about one issue, but she always gave me the power to make the decision.
>
> Manuals became popular in the sixties because of state requirements. For awhile my job was to assist each department in writing its plan in the event of disaster. I wrote most of them.

To sum up Hazel's story, her words are quoted from the *Catalyst*[29]:

> In my job, I meet each day with an open mind. I want to accomplish more than I can do. To continuously work toward innovations that promote better patient care is my greatest challenge. I must also be flexible and willing to accept change. This advice is good for new nurses because, if you don't accept change, you will get lost in the shuffle.

Mrs. Latondress had 800 professional and nonprofessional people working for her—the largest department in the hospital. Her work force included nurses, technicians, attendants, clerks, coordinators, transport messengers, and aides—the people who were closest to the patients. Vivian Ryan, a nurse who reported to H. L. said, "She always has time to listen to you—no problem is too little, and she is open to suggestions."

To list her accomplishments, said Connie Hubbell, RN, Assistant Director of Nursing Service, was an endless task built on hours of working, reading and motivating those leery of change.[30]

Many Remembrances—Named and Nameless Caring People

Who could forget the many LPNs, orderlies, maintenance workers, kitchen and housekeeping staff, switchboard operators, supervisors, doctors—some who hadn't forgotten what it was like to be students themselves—all connected to and a very large part of the success and history of the hospital's School of Nursing?

Mrs. Martha Beatty, social/recreation director, devotedly gave of herself and opened her home to all student nurses. Her house was a "home away from home," especially the parties and picnics she arranged for hundreds of students. Memories of five graduates have her planning Friday dances and directing the choir.

Beth Simpson Fletcher '59 recalls their housekeeper who, taught us to speak a little German, for our trips to Woods Lake where we talked about our "maid," in hopes the guys there would overhear us and be impressed." Erlene Williams Kimber '57 remembers, "Margaret at the Pine Home who made my bed many mornings when I got up late and raced to work or class." Also, she wrote, the housemothers were, 'old' (like I am now!)."

Stories of housemothers like Mrs. Lewis and the missing couch, as well as Mrs. Lyons who made so many trips up to the second floor to find the sources of so much noise, come from other students. "When Mrs. Lyons did room check, she couldn't find us at first, "Girls, girls, girls, girls, girls, girls! What will you think of next?" She shouldn't have asked, and how did she know about a cat in the dorm?

The interest, encouragement, and friendship of our unofficial Big Brother, Dick Vander Molen, the hospital's electrician, who much later became the hospital's chief maintenance engineer, and who married a Bronson graduate, cannot ever be forgotten. The Class of 1955 gave a surprise baby shower for them when they were expecting their first child. He has long been the editor of the Bronson *Retirees' Newsletter,* received by so many who were touched by him and his continuing dedication to Bronson. Loved then and even now, he recorded all the many memories for everyone to enjoy. How thankful the students were for their many reprieves at the Vander Molens'—what a godsend Betty and Dick were—and still are.

Favorite Instructors

The housemothers and so many neat, excellent instructors really cared about the student nurses and wanted them to do well in their chosen profession. Besides multiple remembrances of Mrs. Weber, the special people mentioned more than once in mail solicited from this decade's alumni were Miss Louise Huffman, Mrs. Mabel Stell, Mary B. Anderson, Miss Leone Sweet, Dr. Hazel Prentice, and Miss Shirley Evans.

Miss Huffman was a stern taskmaster, house supervisor, clinical instructor, and an excellent nurse who was not appreciated at the time, but became a friend and role model who expected the highest quality of nursing care. Patricia Hauke Dahlman '55 recalls that, "Reassuring Miss Huffman, whom we eventually came to revere, [was] at my side while I endured the entrance physical exam. We became grateful to her for instilling in us the highest professional standards." Later Dahlman felt "sad at times about the lack of professionalism in nurses at work in doctors' offices, clinics, hospitals, and nursing homes around the country, telling myself, 'Miss Huffman would turn over in her grave,' if she knew of a particular situation I had observed or heard about."

The head nurse, Mabel Stell, presented a former military demeanor, and she wrote evaluations of the students. She is remembered for saying that she gave C to the freshmen, B to the juniors, and A to the seniors because, if she gave A's to the freshmen, "What would they have to work toward?" Esther L. Wyman '57 continued, "Mrs. Stell made sure the patient who had high expectations for the care he or she received, got it. She helped us gain the experiences we needed to become nurses." Mrs. Stell, supervisor of Hall 6, became role model and friend to Betty Gosling Vander Molen '51, and she too expected to learn the highest quality of nursing care. Her influence also stayed with Barbara Gardner Henry '50.

Four alumni were impressed by Mary Anderson who was imposing but friendly. Her dedication to professionalism and that of Miss Sweet encouraged perfection in nursing procedures. Miss Sweet graduated from Battle Creek Sanitarium in 1903, joined the Bronson Methodist Hospital School of Nursing in 1941, and retired in 1952. She is remembered by Winifred Mein Terpstra '44 as patient and kind, an instructor who, "taught us the true meaning of being a good nurse." It was Miss Sweet who taught Patricia Robertson Bigelow '50 "how to make a patient comfortable with tender, loving care."

Dr. Prentice did autopsies so gently and with such respect, it made having to attend them a tolerable experience for Erlene Williams Kimber '57. She performed the first autopsy Esther L. Wyman '57 had observed:

> She was skillful. She took the "knife" and made a huge incision from sternum to pubis in one quick smooth stroke. The abdomen was opened wide. I felt really lightheaded for a short period of time. Fortunately, I was able to stand straight and be attentive despite my churning stomach. Anatomy became reality during autopsy observations. Miss Tina Boomgaarden, surgical nursing instructor, insisted that, in order to receive credit for attending the

> autopsy, we had to write a complete review of all systems. A certain number could be "partial," *e.g.,* if cause of death was determined after examination of one or more systems/organs and the pathologist didn't proceed with the rest of the body, we might receive credit for attending. A number of times, when a complete autopsy was anticipated and one or more students attended, only the chest or abdomen was examined, so no credit was given. Writing autopsy reviews helped us later to serve as pathologists' scribes.

Miss Shirley Evans, head nurse on Hall I, was the absolute ideal—her manner, poise, and professionalism made her an exemplary nurse—according to Patricia Robertson Bigelow '50 and Suzanne Barrett Van Dyken '53.

Other fond recollections related to Miss Campbell and Mrs. Cripe, "who had a kind of soft hum as she observed us" (Wyman didn't know if the hum calmed her or her students). Mrs. Short, was exceptionally nice and soft-spoken, Miss Ione Bailey and Miss Ellen Emig, were both Bronson graduates and assistant instructors. All three contributed their highly professional skills and attributes to the students' educational experiences. Even Miss Heneveld laughed when students were learning to place patients on and remove them from their bedpans. Miss Nellie Koster was the Marshall hospital administrator who meticulously supervised in an informative and kind way. Eunice Maatman deserved the dedication that appeared in the 1957 yearbook. Miss Dorothy McGinnis administered our pre-admission aptitude testing and taught the Psychology for Nurses class, and Miss Virginia McPhail was the clinical instructor for Medical Nursing under whom a care study was written.

"Fine, professional women" were Miss Marie Wantz and Miss Dena Wolters, along with those admired as role models: Mrs. King and Mrs. Fieberkorn (shift supervisors), May Hideman, Miss Wolters, and Mrs. Van Vranken who later became Mrs. Lord.

And the Doctors, with Patients or Not

Remember the interns who used to help us? Dr. Lubavs taught us how to start IVs because, at that time, the procedure wasn't taught to student nurses. Many fine physicians were on staff at the time: Doctors Boys and Jennings, Conrad and Hanson, Jackson, Cooper and Callandar, Heersma and Dew, Hoebeke, Birch and Peake, to name a few.

The techniques of Drs. Birch and May, whom Barbara Gardner Henry '50 believes are great men, were worth watching, and Janice McClellan Duryea '53, "will never forget the first and only time I saw a doctor cry large tears. Dr. William Birch at Bronson was delivering a full-term baby and he delivered a 'monstrosity.'" Other stories about him leave different impressions, like the one about a nervous student named Schmidt who greeted him in the utility room with, "Good morning, Dr. Bitch." The next morning she found Dr. Birch in the room again and, without hesitation, he exclaimed, "Why, good morning, Miss Shit!"

Certainly the recipient could not forget the resident Dr. Victor Berglund's kiss under the mistletoe on Peds or having the *handsome* Dr. Cooper do your appendectomy when you were a junior. Then, Dr. Glaser, the pathologist who was very systematic in his approach to the entire autopsy procedure, was so respectful of the body. He insisted that everyone in attendance do as well and gave the impression that he liked to teach, being very good about explaining his observations. Doctors as teachers also included the surgeon, Dr. Weadon, who named his instruments as he selected them for the laminectomy Janice McClellan Duryea '53 assisted him with, or during the outpatient circumcision of a blue-eyed, 21-year-old from Kalamazoo College that left an impression she never forgot! —"the things that doctor had me do."

Earlene Williams Kimber '57 remembers at least two doctor–patient stories. The first one involved an AWOL patient. An inebriated diabetic had woken up, dressed, and gone home. After a search, Kimber called the patients home and was told by her husband, "Sure, she's here." Then Kimber called Dr. Herbert who discharged the patient. The second story involved an extra body that she discovered in one of the beds when she was a young, new grad working on Hall 3, 11–7. It was the patient's husband! "I woke him and told him that visiting hours were over, then spent the rest of the night blushing (much to the delight of the intern on duty and the rest of the staff)."

Some nurses in this period saw hospital staff and physicians as a functional family. (Recall Mrs. Weber's comment about hospitals during this era.) Lois Hoyt Brown Richmond was one loyal Bronson nurse who fit well in the Bronson family. Her responsibilities grew, as evidenced by the cumulative list of her administrative titles, and she adapted well to the system in a long period of technological expansion. The parting comment in her story (below), captured more than 40 years later, demonstrates her love for nursing within the hospital setting and the feeling that the patient comes first. Changes were made to better patient care.

LOIS IRENE HOYT (BROWN) RICHMOND '56

I was born and raised in the rural agricultural community of Richland, Michigan. We lived on a small farm, had some animals and a garden, two loving parents, one brother, one sister, and lots of relatives. We didn't have many fears day to day. The crime rate wasn't often discussed. Going into Kalamazoo was a big deal that we did infrequently.

My decision to go into nursing was made about eighth grade. I really don't know why. I never considered any other professions. Nursing was my choice for as long as I can remember. Women in the fifties seemed to opt either for teaching or nursing, and I did not want to teach. My maternal grandmother was a self-taught midwife. We do not have any other medical people in the family. My paternal grandmother was a teacher and attended what was then called Western Normal Teacher's College (now Western Michigan University).

I had my first summer job in the tenth grade. I clerked and did the stocking in the local grocery store. Many migrants worked for the truck gardens, and these people were our main customers. In the eleventh grade and until graduation, I worked for a private family (owners of the Kalamazoo Laundry), cleaning, cooking, shopping, and running their household in general. I worked full time during the summer and after school and weekends as needed.

Attending the local school, my upbringing was very typical. Our school activities were fun and enjoyed by most of the students. I was active in school and we always seemed to have many activities to pursue. I played tennis, softball, and basketball and then was a cheerleader for the school's first football team. I took part in most activities: school plays, yearbook preparation, choir, *etc.* Our school was small compared to today's schools. Thirty-two students made up my graduating class of 1953.

I met and started dating my first husband in the eleventh grade. When he decided to join the military, he tried very hard to convince me to marry him and forget about nursing school. I never abandoned my plans. He went into the army, and I prepared to go to Bronson. My parents planned to pay for my schooling. Even so, I applied for a scholarship. I was awarded the Marie C. Wantz Scholarship, which was helpful. I think it paid $200 toward my tuition.

My brother and sister did not attend college, so it was different when I packed up to leave for school. My parents obviously approved of this decision. Entering the School of Nursing was an exciting experience for me. I didn't have any problem adjusting to dorm life; perhaps having attended summer camps helped.

Some of the classes at Western Michigan University were hard for me, especially chemistry. I thought my rural school had not prepared me for college chemistry. As I recall I passed with a "C." I weathered the storm and progressed through the curriculum. I enjoyed school. Some experiences I remember well. On campus at Western, we looked so obvious in our white starched uniforms and caps and our navy capes, which were nice and warm because they were made of wool. As a group going to class, we appeared to be rather regimented. Our schedules were busy; we didn't have time to get bored or have much time to spare.

I started smoking while in my senior year of high school and so I continued to smoke in nursing training. I remember so well studying in the elevator of Wesley Hall (the oldest part of the hospital facing John Street) where I could also smoke. Some classmates would be in their rooms saying prayers for those of us who smoked!!

It was fun to sneak out and go for Kewpie burgers late at night. I remember one student who stayed out late most nights and who would arrange with someone to open the door for her, but the late-night student left training before the end of the freshmen year. Our rules were very strict compared to today's, and we lost many students, especially during freshmen year, because they could not adjust to the rule demands. Though the hospital food was good, I enjoyed eating at my parents' home whenever possible and, since I was from Richland, it was easy for me to go home frequently.

Time went fast. We moved to the "John Street Houses" during our second year. I had three roommates: Betsy Hanna, Ethelyn McClure, and Katy Shoemaker. We slept in bunk beds and had two desks to share. The four of us got along well, with each of us picking up after herself and pretty much following the rules. I don't remember anyone getting into any major problems.

We had one clinical instructor that all of us will remember for the rest of our lives. She was Louise Huffman, a tough army drill instructor who carried military techniques with her into teaching at Bronson. If you were not afraid of doing a procedure, you would be after she was finished with you. She really put the fear of God into us, which made all of us reluctant to be around her. We also knew she had the power to fail us so we took her threats seriously.

A big hurdle was attending the first autopsy. As if it were yesterday, I can still remember losing sleep over this assignment. The room was poorly lit and small, and the formaldehyde odor was so strong we almost passed out. The instructor was Dr. Hazel Prentice who was also rather threatening. She loudly kept asking everyone to move closer to observe. It was not exactly what we wanted to do!! Taking care of those who died never became any easier but remained a task that was necessary to perform. I respected death and had to reconcile myself to the inevitable, not easy for a young student.

We worked rigorous schedules consisting of classes and floor duty. The kitchen presented a special treat for us. We learned creative ways to enter after hours and help ourselves to yummy baked goods and steaks that were delicious. I can't believe we were so devious, but I remember this escapade well. I also remember that we kept some wine to go with the steaks in a peanut butter jar that we submerged in the water tank on the back of the toilet.

Numerous and humorous incidents, as well as sad ones, took place during day-to-day activities. Daily discussions in the dorm highlighted the events. Old 2 West was a polio ward, and the sound of iron lungs is a familiar memory for me. On night duty, we would circulate among the patients with a flashlight, checking each one while these massive machines forced their breathing while they slept. The fear of power failure was always with me. The machines could be hand-operated, but that procedure would be very labor intensive.

My boyfriend came home on leave before going to Germany. He convinced me that, if we secretly married, I would receive a wife's government stipend and we could save the money for a house. I finally agreed and Betsy, my roommate, and her boyfriend went with us to Angola, Indiana, where we were married in a little chapel. All within 24 hours, we married and returned to Kalamazoo, and my husband boarded the train for Kansas and Fort Leonard Wood. When my checks came by mail, I always cashed them at Louie's Restaurant on the north side of town. The owner there knew my in-laws and was aware of the situation.

I was always a little fearful that someone would discover that I was married. Helen Weber was in charge of the school and I often thought, what if? I guess I was too busy to really worry about consequences. My husband came home for a brief visit and though it certainly wasn't planned, I became pregnant. I knew I would be about five months along when we graduated, and I assumed I could probably fit into my uniform.

We did an affiliation at Oakland Hospital in Marshall. I went with Joyce Kreiger to live in a private home. Two incidents occurred in Marshall that I will never forget. First, I delivered a baby with forceps, and the process was really hard to do. My feet almost slid under the delivery table because of the strength necessary to extract the baby. The baby was healthy, with some evidence of forceps marks. The second incident took place when I was in charge of a rehabilitation unit. An elderly gentleman got up in the middle of the night. He thought he was going to the "wine cellar." Instead he fell and broke his hip. I felt sadly responsible for a number of days.

Before returning to Kalamazoo, Joyce and I took a few days off to camp up north. We decided to dye our hair blond while we were there and almost ruined our hair with the peroxide. It really looked awful so we bought some Nestles color capsules. What a mess! I can remember breaking the plastic capsule and putting this terrible looking dye on our hair. Our hair was a brown/henna color when we returned to Kalamazoo.

We did a second affiliation at Kalamazoo State Hospital. Several incidents stand out in my mind. I worked many hours overtime for extra money. One day I remember well. I was with two patients who were in water tubs for therapy. Only their heads protruded from canvas covers that were fastened over the tubs. The patients continually tried to drown themselves so I constantly had to keep their heads above the canvas. It was a very tense assignment. Another time I worked the ward that housed many schizophrenics. One of them grabbed my nursing cap and flushed it down the toilet! Then she danced and laughed and laughed. This trick had been played on others before.

I remember well some of the patients who suffered from catatonic schizophrenia, an amazing condition that was improved with medication in the years that followed. For me, it was like walking down an art gallery hallway and looking at sculptures along the walls. Sometimes I would stop and stare into their non-expressive faces that didn't change with any kind of stimulation.

I spent one weekend working in the acute-care area where tar ointment was being applied to the entire bodies of two of my patients. It was the biggest mess I have ever seen. The mixture was black, smelled terrible, and found its way onto every thing. We applied it with wooden tongue blades. Of course a visit to Kalamazoo State Hospital was not complete without a stint in the "shock lab." My brain shudders when I think about these treatments. After the electrical current was administered, the patient would shake and convulse while about four staff held him or her to the table. The treatment seemed so gruesome, and I really don't know if it ever helped anyone.

Our training at Bronson was tough and very task-oriented. We graduated in 1956, and I started working nights in the Emergency Room. I know we performed many treatments and did many procedures that we probably were not prepared to do, but ignorance is bliss. We had been taught to make decisions and work efficiently. I always felt that we were trying to respond in the best interest of the patient, so I have no regrets. The tasks were many with only a few of us to do them. My career gave me many rewards and much satisfaction. Many times students operated the hospital, with only a few registered nurses on duty in very specific areas. My career continued at Bronson for 31 years. I worked in many different capacities with many titles and various jobs, for example, head nurse, supervisor, assistant director, *etc.*

The best part of the job was the people I worked with because the hospital functioned like a big family. I often felt like it was my second home, having spent so much time within its confines. Cohesiveness and camaraderie of the employees and doctors made it an enjoyable place to be.

I have never regretted that I pursued nursing. Since Bronson Methodist Hospital School of Nursing was a diploma school, I went back to Western Michigan University and completed a BS degree in Health Studies. Many times I considered going to other geographical areas to work, but the facts were that I really liked Kalamazoo and my work at the hospital with my family so close. I could not think of any good reason to leave this area. I elected to take early retirement in 1987 after an administrative shakeup. My job at that time was assistant vice-president, Nursing Administration.

Memoirs of Bronson students in the early 1950s include those that originated in other countries and tell different stories of common student experiences. Clearly, perception is highly individualized.

KATHERINE "KIT" BOSKER GIFFORD '54

It never occurred to me to be anything other than a nurse when I grew up, except for the brief time I was going to be a fabulously famous and wealthy archeologist who discovered tombs and treasures in Egypt. My mother had died of leukemia when I was 14, and I spent quite a bit of time being the home-care person as my father had to work. The idea of helping another person in such circumstances was motivated by a powerful sense of altruism.

The choice of Bronson was to some extent made for me, as a close friend, a year ahead of me in high school, had decided on Bronson, and we planned to attend together. She spent a year at Albion, waiting for me, and then lasted only the first semester at Bronson, which I loved. My roommates were and still are good friends, and the education has been invaluable, although I have not been actively involved in nursing for nearly 40 years.

The most valuable lessons I learned in nursing school were to "do it right the first time," that panic gets you nowhere, and that caring and compassion are invaluable gifts to give patients, family, and friends. In a few episodes of being "the patient" in hospitals that were not necessarily so dedicated to the tenet that the patient comes first, I learned that we were truly given training to be envied. It was a wonderful base for compassionate and contented living, whether or not we stayed with formal nursing. Living for nearly 30 years in a bit of Canadian wilderness, the lessons I learned at Bronson have been a constant help in taking care of husband and daughter, of loggers injured in work accidents and requiring private duty care behind a log on the beach waiting for a small plane to take the patient to a hospital, of a succession of domestic and wild animals, and of my own good health and physical condition.

We were, in those years, blessed with many wonderful examples of what it meant to be a nurse: capable, gentle Helen Weber—strong, stern, very capable, and a fine bedside nurse; Mary B. Anderson, who was, I think, greatly under appreciated; and, for me, Louise Huffman, in the Nursing Education Department, who was our main nursing arts instructor. She was an army veteran, stout, and slightly exophthalmic, with a very unsmiling, rough exterior. Yet when, as a very green probie, my first patient died in the middle of the procedure—taking a rectal temperature, and I am not kidding—Miss Huffman put her arms around me and hugged me. She comforted me more than I probably needed, and went to great pains to convince me that I hadn't caused the death. I can still hear her rumbling, as she shook her head firmly, "Miss Bosker! Those who cannot work with their heads are forced to work with their feet. *Think* first, and then do your walking only once."

Certainly the person from Bronson who has had the most lasting influence on my life was Dr. Hazel Prentice. She was head of the Pathology Department and performed many of the autopsies, both for the hospital and for the county. I came to know her well through her lifelong companion and friend, Jerry Marvin, who I often had as a patient on 2 East. Jerry liked me, not always the case with her nurses, and she and Dr. Prentice virtually took me into their family. Frequently Dr. Hazel would take me along at night for company when she had to drive to outlying towns to perform postmortems. As I was the only other person there, she gave me marvelous personalized teaching lectures on human anatomy. She and Jerry loved Bruce, my then fiancé and still beloved husband, and they bought my wedding dress with my parents' permission when we married three days after graduation. We grieved when both Hazel and Jerry died.

STUDENT LIFE

For memories of the class activities in which students participated together and the plain fun times they had, Barbara Gardner Henry '50 remembers the parties and picnics, the first one at Gull Lake. Classmate Phyllis Weenink Ossewaarde mentioned that the students were all herded into a Hybels Produce truck for transport to the lake. Planned social activities included Friday night mixers with invited Western students, in the dorm recreation room in the old Cedar and Pine homes. Many college guys showed up and that's how many got dates. A much-anticipated formal event took place at the Kalamazoo Country Club, where the senior students were entertained by the medical staff at a doctors' dinner dance. During that same time, the safety-pin chains worn on senior uniforms were shortened every day marking the days until graduation.

> Just being one of many members of the fine nurses' choir was an enjoyable respite. One time the choir appeared on WKZO (now WWMT) TV when the station was in the Burdick Hotel downtown. Maybe the appearance was on the "Feminine Fancies" show. With little time to stay abreast of current events, the coronation of Queen Elizabeth II, shown on television (a medium that was still a novelty to some) in the Junior–Senior House basement recreation room, was a big event.
>
> We also made the float for Western's homecoming depicting the big hunk of cheese, the mice, and the cat behind bars. We won an

award for our effort. A year or so later, after getting off a strenuous 3–11 shift, I wondered where those mouse heads were. The next day, sitting in the cafeteria and listening to conversation, I heard someone say, "I had the weirdest dream last night. I dreamt these giant mice came into my room." I had had the same dream!

In correspondence, Beth Simpson Fletcher '59, asked "How many remember the huge bonfire at WMU at the time Sputnik was launched?" Or this poem Simpson wrote for her roommate, Liz Van Voorhees Bower '59:

A NURSE

What enters your mind when you hear the word, nurse?
A hospital with siren, an ambulance, a hearse?

Do you think of a young girl all dressed up in white,
Who'll come when you call, be it morn, noon or night?
Do you picture an elderly lady whose air
Is highly superior? Who talks with her stare?

Or maybe that word brings the thought to your mind
Of someone you've met who is gentle and kind!

So you know what I see? I'll reveal it to you.
I picture a person who's honest and true.

One who'll give up her bed in the still of the night
To eagerly join in a life-saving fight.

Who constantly wears such a welcoming smile
You can't help but return it once in a while!

One with confident hands and warm glowing heart,
Who works tirelessly to give your life a renewed start.

And not only will listen but will actually hear
Who'll give reassurance with a word of good cheer,
And simply her interest makes your "blues" disappear.

With one glance it's not at all hard to see
She is blessed with the virtue we term "charity."

And after her work and her duty are done,
Goes home and relaxes—Sleeps! Studies! Has fun!

She's pleasant to live with and makes life a pleasure
Her company you'll enjoy. Her memory you'll treasure.

These traits I consider and put into verse.
And I think I'm describing an excellent nurse.

However, this type doesn't come with the sun.
But I've got it soft. Why? I'm living with one.

High jinks notwithstanding, the hands-on preparation for nursing careers continued unabated during the fifties. Simpson Fletcher had a way with words and composed this tribute about the fifties' students' practice on 2 East:

2 EAST

This is a poem I would like you to note
I'll never reveal how it ever got wrote.
It's about student nurses who work on 2 East,
And though they may like it, they like it the least.
The main thing about it, they don't like the best
Is the fact they can't stop to get no sort of rest!

To see you complete each minute little thing,
There's a Schneider, a Damvelt, and often a King.
If at one time you think you have everything done,
Don't stop, cause you've probably done the wrong one.
"Are your baths done? Your beds made? That water
needs changing."
"And this room is a mess, it could stand rearranging."
"Those clinitests! Haven't you taken them yet?"
"You're the most slowest person that ever I've met!"
"Be sure that you go down to eat when you should."
After all, if you don't, you might miss the good food.
Then when you return and each feed has been fed,

You can get a clean sheet and change that wet bed.
There are enemas to give and I.V.s to be started,
And then when you're through they all must be charted.

When you finish with that, there's a cath to be done—
A foley on the patient in twenty-one one.
If you need help there's always somebody around—
I'm saying they're here, but now, can they be found?
Mr. Whozit would like you to apply a clean dressing,
The place it's applied is determined by guessing.

Would you like to help in isolation with that spinal?
Would you like to!?! The answer's already quite final.
The I&O sheets, the G.U. bottles too,
Must be picked up and emptied—then distribute the new.
Then before you leave, you're as sure as can be
That each one is supplied with that great T.L.C.

So you're ready to leave—a complete total wreck
When somebody remarks, "The narcotics don't check!"
Well, that's the last straw! You give forth a curse
Then turn face to face with that dreaded head nurse.
So you check the charts over on Team One and Team Two
'Til you find the dumb dimwit who did it was you.
You trudge wearily dormward, feeling next to deceased,
You can't wait 'til it's morning and you're back on 2 East.

"'Man on the floor!' calls and 8–10 P.M. study times when the housemother checked to make sure we were studying," were mentioned by Dolores Bos Heath '54, while Simpson Fletcher maintains that, "The skeleton we found in the attic really did help us to learn the bones of the body." Erlene Williams Kimber '57 recalls that Hell Week involved OR "scrubbing" while blindfolded, with lampblack and mineral oil on our arms.

Extracurricular Life

We were noted for trying the patience of our saintly housemothers by engaging in "no-nos," such as popping corn in our rooms or eating popcorn after lights out (10 P.M.), with the aid of flashlights, according to Suzanne Berkey Esenwein '51 and Dolores Bos Heath '54. Ways of making life miserable for the housemother, Mrs. Lyons, were not hard. She made so many trips up to the second floor to find the sources of so much noise, and upon arriving she would always find us in our rooms diligently studying. After she left, the pranks would begin again.

> Does anyone remember the soapsuds in the Kalamazoo mall fountain? Water fights, the cat we rescued and brought back to the dorm, the time three of us went to Chicago with my cousin and his friends to return after curfew. We thought how clever we were creeping back into the dormitory NOT! The word "sneak" seemed to define the three student classes at the end of the decade, perhaps throughout: sneaking down the deck steps to movies at night, feeling scared but smug; sneaking into the State Theater and the time the cop caught us; and sneaking through the tunnel to the hospital kitchen, where we discovered how good the ice-cream was and the little janitor who used to stand guard for us.
>
> Students were often wound up after finishing the 3–11 P.M. shift and, just to wind down one evening, decided to unscrew all the florescent light fixtures on two of the floors. The next day the electrician had to be called. It took Dick all of ten seconds to discover what the problem was.

"No smoking" was allowed while in uniform (unless in the cafeteria) and removal of our nurses' cap when doing so was mandatory. The policy, "No married students," was in effect for all classes until the last six months of training through 1957. It was changed for the Class of 1958: Marguerite Harris Aukerman was the first married student graduate under the new school policy.

"Many memories come flooding back, still fresh in my mind, even after 38 years: friendships that endure because of all we shared, the lessons we learned, the mistakes we made, the tears we shed, and the great fun we had," wrote Sharon Martin Daniels '59.

Joys Recounted

Family and friends figured large in nursing school. For one, "after having two brothers at home, what a pleasure and joy it was being among so many girls," and for another, "Living with young ladies near in age to mine, especially because my sisters were much older than I," the feeling of classmate closeness was strong. "We were like a big family then, and my nursing classmates are like extended family to this day." Among the greatest joys in nursing school were the many lifelong friendships made there.

New Births

Another great joy was the thrill of being present and seeing the birth of a baby for the very first time. Janice McClellan Duryea '53 remembered, "while on Obstetrics affiliation, seeing my first delivery and thinking to myself and later relating to my mother, 'If there is someone who does not believe in God, then they should witness the delivery of a newborn!' I really enjoyed working with the preemie babies." Others wrote that, "Nothing has given me goose bumps as much as a birth of a newborn," and, "I never got over the thrill and awe at each birth I attended."

Recoveries

During the polio epidemic we worked as volunteers with iron lungs and hot pack machines—a whole new concept for us—and the endless exercises, but the joy in seeing some recover made it worthwhile. Another time staff was elated when a 16-year-old accident victim emerged from a coma after six weeks and later went home with very little residual damage. Then, a burn patient was confined to his room for nearly four months. How we cried when he took his first steps out of his room, long before Bronson was equipped with a special burn unit.

And "Making It!"

Why did we all drag our mattresses to the third floor lounge prior to Christmas break? That single event marked two milestones: our "final" get together, and celebration of a triumphant victory over finals. Several mentioned their greatest joy was the fact that they succeeded and graduated, or being relieved to be one of the 36 students remaining for capping ceremony. Out of the 52 students who started, we graduates in the Class of '55 surely did feel a sense of accomplishment. How proud we were to learn that all of us passed State Boards, taken the following October. We were Registered Nurses!!!

LIVING QUARTERS BEFORE TRUESDALE

Prior to 1957 students and their supervisors lived in houses close to the hospital. One of the first homes, known as the Hospital House in the 1920s and later, was purchased by the women's auxiliary and rented to the hospital.

In a taped interview[31] Betty Reed Searles, born 1920, shared recollections from her childhood when she lived in a big square, two-family house across from the hospital during the summers of 1923 to 1927. The house was on the corner of Lovell and John streets, facing Lovell (now corner of Lovell and Henrietta). Mrs. Searles lived there with her uncle, aunt, mother, father, brother, and sister. Her father worked at the hospital from June to August, filling in for her uncle while he was on vacation. Her uncle did hospital maintenance work, including electrical and plumbing, and was also the fireman, shoveling coal for heat and hot water production. Her family lived in the west half of the home. Up to 16 student nurses plus a nursing supervisor lived in the east half. She recalled a long porch, a big front hall with two stairways, living room, dining room, full bath on the main floor, and two stairways leading to three bedrooms. Whether Reed Searles' house was also known as The Hospital House, rented by the women's auxiliary to the hospital, is unclear; however, it later became known as the North Home.

Mrs. Searles also reported that students lived in two other houses on Lovell Street. In fact, nurses lived in several houses along the street. At the time it was common for laborers to live close to their work since ready transportation was not available to the common folks on a daily basis. She remembered the nurses' white starched uniforms hanging on clotheslines and recalled that they were ironed before they became completely dry. She visited the hospital many times as a child.

On properties that joined each other at some point were four homes used for lodging students in the late 1920s: Osborne Home on Lovell Street, and North Home, West Home, and the School Building (all on John Street).[32]

"With our housing condition as it now is with students living in four different homes," wrote an early 1930s superintendent, having them take on some management through their newly formed student government seemed advisable. "It is at least worthy of a trial."[33] Apparently, because these young women were perceived to need an authority figure to keep rules and order, this decision was vetoed at some point by the school's administration. Housemothers, later called "residence directors," were deemed preferable to maintain law and order as well as curfews in students' living quarters.

Margaret Martin Correll '37 remembers, "During our first year we were housed in Osborne Home. Our rooms were all located on the second floor, along with Miss Wantz, the O.B. RN supervisor. The superintendent of nurses, Miss McLellan's accommodations were on the first floor. The second year we were moved to the third floor, which was a large attic dormitory with one bathroom and one large walk-in closet. Each student nurse had her own bed, dresser, and chair. Running lengthwise down the center of the room were several long tables with chairs, intended for use in connection with our studies. Upon entering our third and final year we were relocated in a hospital-owned house approximately one half block away, which we found to be more comfortable and which offered more privacy." Bronson's 1930-31 annual report states that four supervisors and 32 student nurses roomed in the Osborne Home, which also contained a piano, donated by A.J. Stock and J. Henry Ling.

The School Building was renamed the Annex in 1934, most likely because it began to be used for functions other than nursing education. It was "used by the students who are on night duty, in order that they may sleep undisturbed during the day. It has proven to be a most satisfactory arrangement."[34] Bronson's first medical residents, Drs. May and Herbert, occupied the Annex when they arrived. Dick Vander Molen recalled that, in 1945, the Annex was still used for classrooms and, for one year only, when South Home was closed temporarily, students once again lived on the second floor. He also remembered helping seniors Wanda Grauman, Jean Blake, and Phyllis Schultz move out when they graduated in the Class of 1947. The Annex contained electroencephalogram equipment, operated by Mr. McAlpine and set up by Dr. Hazel Prentice in 1950.

A long-term patient care center would be created with the remodeling of student living quarters in the oldest section of the hospital, and it was named Wesley Hall, while one of the other homes, West Home, was closed in August 1937. Miss McLellan also reported that, "New students will be housed at 139 E. Lovell, known as Wayside Hall." Several students in 1940 were moved into a part of the original 1905 hospital, and only four years later was it made more livable. It also included a suite for the house director, Mrs. Hazel Kirk.[35]

In the 1940s Bronson student nurses occupied the East Home, at Pine and Cedar Streets, part of the hospital's "campus." The house, recently remodeled, was not 100 percent complete when the girls moved in—a typical sign of the times. Mrs. M.E. Reusch joined the staff of housemothers to supervise the new dormitory. This upgrade gave Bronson four homes close to the main building, and four housemothers:

Mrs. C. H. Ellis of North Home, Mrs. George Ervine Wright of the main dormitory, and Mrs. Reusch and Mrs. E. Clay Howell of South Home.[36] The South Home was at 430 John Street. In September, 1945, it housed 22 students and a housemother for a class of 50 freshmen, the largest in the history of the school.[37]

Once more the school could expand with housing for more young women.[38] A record class of nurses in 1947 was partly due to an expanded hospital, which had places for 60 students, and students continued to be housed at Osborne Home and the Annex. Patricia Hauke Dahlman '55 mentions moving into the John Street Freshmen Dormitory. Whether that dorm had a name cannot be determined.

If You Can Dream It, You Can Do It—A Five-Story New Residence

Dreams of a real nurses' home were in the minds of the community and first hospital administrators in 1900. But the priority for it remained low on the list until hospital expansion created a need for more student nurses to give direct patient care. The forties marked the beginning of a public plea for funding to build a residence.

WANTED: SUGGESTIONS
From *Bronson Bulletin,* March 1943, p.3

> One of the outstanding needs of Bronson Hospital is a nurses' home. We cannot, of course, in these days of material and manpower shortages, hope to remedy this situation immediately. However, we can gather material and plans toward the day when a united nations victory makes this longstanding dream possible.
>
> If such a home could be built, it would release 50 more hospital beds in the hospital proper. In addition to thus making the full facilities of Bronson available for use by patients, the home would provide a great stimulus to the nurse-training program.
>
> Let's have your ideas! Just drop a line to the Office of the Superintendent.

The dream was always there. The need and the money came together ten years later.

WHERE DID THE MONEY COME FROM?

The dormitory and a special unit for long-term patient care were granted federal aid totaling $329,700, based on a Hill-Burton Act rule that the community would provide the balance of the funds locally. So, in a bequest, the George and Nina Truesdale family[39] donated $255,044, which left a balance of $704,900 to raise from the community campaign.[40] The campaign was well supported by the *Kalamazoo Gazette* coverage of the fund-raising progress. "Florence Nightingale Sabbath, a tribute to the most famous of all nurses, will be observed in all churches of all faiths in Kalamazoo Sunday, with special emphasis on the need to support the Bronson Hospital new nurses' home drive."[41]

A gift of time and loyalty was the major contribution by 275 volunteers challenged to begin the public phase of the building campaign.[42] A complete list of dollar donors to the nurses' home became part of the cornerstone contents, for example the pledges of these organizations:

The Upjohn Company[43]	$150,000
Kresge Foundation	$100,000
Sutherland Paper Company	$ 55,000
White Cross Guild[44]	$ 25,000

The good news, victory was sweet! The campaign resulted in $1,419,502 and $35,905 over the goal! The bad news: The actual bids to build the dormitory came in $85,000 over the estimate.[45]

ARCHITECTS SELECTED FOR $1,000,000 NURSES' HOME

Excerpted from *Bronson Bulletin,* vol.12: 4, Fall 1954

Planning is already well under way for construction of a $1,000,000 home for student nurses at Bronson Methodist Hospital.

At a meeting of the Board of Trustees Sept. 1 at the hospital, the Kalamazoo firm of Stapert, Pratt, Bulthuis and Sprau, Inc. was selected to provide the architectural work for the project.

Plans to construct the new building were announced by Dr. William C. Perdew at the Golden Anniversary Dinner of the Bronson School of Nursing on August 26.

The five-story, college dormitory-style residence, which will house 200 student nurses, will be located on the east side of Pine Street, south of the hospital. It will be connected to the hospital by a tunnel.

The new structure will permit a 50-percent increase in the School of Nursing enrollment, Dr. Perdew reported.

The relationship between hospitals, their schools of nursing, and young women wanting (or needing) an inexpensive education, seemed to be symbiotic. A growing hospital needed the students practicing in a work–study format. The enlarged school could recruit more potential nurses.

PLANS FOR NURSES' HOME MOVE AHEAD
SITE FOR DORMITORY TO HOUSE 200 STUDENTS PURCHASED

Excerpted from *Bronson Bulletin,* vol. 13:2, Spring 1955

The preliminary architectural drawing for the new dormitory for 200 student nurses has been completed and submitted to the State Office of Hospital Survey and Construction for review. Many people have been consulted in developing these plans, including student nurses, school of nursing faculty and directors of other student dormitories.

In addition to the student rooms, the dormitory will contain two large classrooms, faculty offices, public lounge, recreation room,

> health office and infirmary, student laundry, uniform room and many other special features. Steam will be supplied from the hospital power plant.
>
> The hospital has purchased a site on the east side of Pine Street extending from the Harding School grounds southward to and including the Zion Lutheran Church property. The church building, seating 375, will eventually be used as the hospital auditorium, inasmuch as the present auditorium on the 7th floor is no longer large enough to accommodate the school of nursing assembly and other hospital meetings.
>
> About half of the cost of this project is already in sight. On January 26, 1955, the Trustees approved the plans and authorized a campaign . . . in November 1955 to raise $635,000 the balance of the funds needed.

A formal ground breaking ceremony was held at the building site on Sunday afternoon, April 8, 1956, at 3:45, to which the public was invited.[46] Students recalled many visits to the construction site, watching Truesdale being built. Mrs. Clara Lewis was the first residence director at Truesdale Hall.[47]

Truesdale's Early Days

Fanfare greeted the residence hall opening on August 25, 1957. The building would house over 200 students at any given time over the next 30 years. Beth Simpson Fletcher '59 remembers, "Moving to the newly completed Truesdale Hall from Wesley Hall was a dream come true!—More space, later curfews, and even dances to which Western students were invited. I think my homesickness was even beginning to ebb."

Truesdale Hall was dedicated at a public ceremony on August 25, 1957, at 3:00 P.M. with Elwood H. Schneider, president of the Board of Trustees presiding. Also participating in the ceremony were: Rev. Charles E. Bennison, president, Kalamazoo Ministerial Alliance; Rev. W. C. Perdew, Bronson Methodist Hospital administrator; Bishop Marshall R. Reed, Michigan Area, Methodist Church; Garret

Van Haaften, chairman of the Building Committee; and Bronson School of Nursing Choir, which sang, "I'll Walk With God" and "Bless This House."

Garret Van Haaften and Bishop Reed presided at the "Presentation and Naming of the Building" with these words:

> *Chairman:* We present this building to be dedicated to the glory of God and the education of young women in the knowledge and skill of the nursing profession for the care of the sick and injured.
>
> *Bishop:* By what name shall the building henceforth be known?
>
> *Chairman:* It shall be called Truesdale Hall in memory of George and Nina Truesdale, whose bequest provided the first funds for its erection.[48]

Three of four pages of the Fall 1957 *Bronson Bulletin* were a pictorial (the same pictures were displayed in the *Kalamazoo Gazette)* of the modern residence hall and, on the fourth, this editorial[49] by Dr. W.C. Perdew:

RESIDENCE MAY INSPIRE STUDENTS

> The opening of Truesdale Hall was a day of rejoicing for us all. It is a beautiful building with every provision for the comfort of the student nurses. But in the dedication ceremony we lifted our vision beyond the structure itself to the purpose it was designed to fulfill.
>
> One of the phrases of the Nightingale pledge, taken by every nurse, says, "With loyalty will I endeavor to aid the physician in his work." As the Bronson nurses go from their school into lives of service, we trust that their experiences here will enable them not only to aid the physicians of this modern day but also that Great Physician whose compassionate and healing ministry continues wherever there is human need.

It was a beautiful residence that served as a recruitment tool and offered many amenities to students from rural areas and families without material wealth. Parents and their daughters were impressed by the conveniences which went two ways: Second to the beautiful living quarters, it was very convenient to have a 200-person staff waiting to be called at any moment and only five minutes away. The following contribution from Beth Simpson Fletcher '59 is a story of the early Truesdale period after 1957:

> The new freshmen were coming, and now we were the Big Sisters. How lucky I was. At that time housekeepers were cleaning the lounge at Truesdale and had all the furniture in the hallway. A couple of students surreptitiously carried a couch upstairs via the elevator but when they arrived, they couldn't maneuver it into their room so took it to a room at the end of the hall. It just so happened that those students were on vacation. How nice it would be for them to return and find a couch in their room—even if it didn't have cushions. Such was not to be. Unbeknown to the thieves—but made quite clear to them after their apprehension—a room-to-room search had been conducted. Mrs. Lewis, the housemother, was later to tell them, "We didn't know if someone from the outside had taken it, so we called Miss Anderson, and she called the police. We kept the housekeepers here an extra hour looking for it, and they had to be paid for their time."
>
> Fortunately, the thieves weren't fined though they could have been. Later, when one of them was unjustifiably expelled from Peds class and had to have a permit from Mrs. Weber to return, Mrs. Weber (who had already been visited by the student who caused the distraction—we really did stick up for one another) said, with a twinkle in her eye, "I'd be a little careful if I were you, Miss . . . Miss Anderson's still pretty upset about the sofa." I can say with great honesty that that student never stole another couch.

Jackie Clark Wylie '62 moved into Truesdale in the fall of 1959, after living in a college dormitory room with two roommates, three beds, three dressers, and three desks—old, tight living quarters with a community bathroom at the far end of a long, dark hall.

Truesdale looked like a spacious, new hotel to her, with five floors and a sixth walkout lower-level patio and yard. Four students shared a suite of four rooms, two bedrooms, two study-living rooms and bath. Two kitchens and living rooms were available on all but the first floor, which had fewer student suites and more common rooms and staff offices. In terms of student residence halls it was posh! (Note: at peak enrollment, five senior students shared a suite with an added bunk bed. One of the seniors was usually on a three-month affiliation so was actually living at Linda Richards Hall at the Kalamazoo State Hospital, later called the Kalamazoo Regional Psychiatric Hospital.)

Compared to other college-type residences, Truesdale Hall was a quiet place for classes, clinical practice, study, and sleep—activities which accounted for the majority of time, not necessarily in that order. Students did not own TVs, phones, or other equipment that connected one with the outside world. Two hall phones were placed on each floor. In the '50s and '60s the only two TVs, to Clark Wylie's knowledge, were situated in a television room on the first floor and in a lower level recreation room. Truesdale's amenities extended beyond the building itself. Kitchens were supplied with milk and snack foods, such as peanut butter, jelly, and bread.

> Our once worn student uniforms went down a laundry chute only to turn up freshly washed, starched, and ironed, all hung in alphabetical order and waiting for us to retrieve them from the uniform storage room on the lower level. Our seven uniforms, one for every day of the week, were easily identified by our name, handsewn on the pockets along and appearing with the School of Nursing logos. Our freshly laundered and starched caps were kept in a bureau.

QUALITY OF NURSING EDUCATION

How do graduates assess their education at Bronson Methodist Hospital School of Nursing? Sometimes it seemed like they could never satisfy their instructors, "but those times of instruction, experience, and responsibilities held me in good stead many a time throughout the years," wrote Betty Hoogstraten Smith Kaub '52. Their own words say it best:

- Bronson provided me with the tools and skills that I needed to successfully complete 32 years of practice. *Suzanne Berkey Esenwein '51*
- It enabled me to "climb the ladder." *Carolyn A. Herndon '50*
- The education was *excellent,* a superb base on which to build a career and further education. *Dolores Bos Heath '54*
- I was exceptionally well prepared for three positions I eventually took as a registered nurse in Ann Arbor and Lansing and at BMH. *Patricia Hauke Dahlman '55*
- I sincerely believe I could not have accomplished all that I have without the excellent training I received at Bronson. *Marlene Juday Kracko '55*
- Professional skills and attributes of Bronson-trained nurses were well known in other areas of Michigan! *Patricia Hauke Dahlman '55*
- One of the nurses on the unit where I recently had to have some tests done at a hospital in New Jersey was a Bronson grad, Class of '70. I'm proud to say she stood out. *Beth Simpson Fletcher '59*

CHAPTER 6 NOTES

---

[1] Websites identified 2003 August 18, http://www.accd.edu/sac/nursing/honors.html, http://www.countryjoe.com/nightingale/pledge.htm; and September 3, http://www.nursingnetwork.com/florencepledge.htm, http://www.nursingworld.org/pressrel/nnw/nnwpled.htm

[2] *Kalamazoo Gazette*, late 1955.

[3] Mrs. Lucille Brown was Helen Weber's secretary.

[4] Sharon Martin Daniels '59 tells this story related to her public encounter with Mrs. Weber: My roommate and best friend was Sheila Robinson. A few days before graduation, a group of us were

returning from supper and were walking through the dorm lobby. One of the switchboard operators on whom, we had played a few pranks, came to us and said, "I'll be sorry to see you girls leave. There are so many names here that I can't remember each first name, but those of you that I *really* like, I know your first names. As she turned directly to me, "I'll never forget your name, Sheila." Well, no one laughed or missed a beat. I replied, "Thank you very much," and we all strolled into the elevator and when the door closed, we collapsed in laughter! As my dear friend, Beth Simpson, wrote in my annual, ". . . and another thing, I'll never forget you Sheila or is it Shirley!?"

[5] From material printed in Bronson Methodist Hospital's *Catalyst*, 1982 August.

[6] *Catalyst,* 1979; 10.

[7] The National League of Nursing Education was later renamed the National League for Nursing (NLN) and was the name on stationery sent in a 1954 correspondence to Bronson.

[8] National Committee for the Improvement of Nursing Services, 1949 September 6, letter sent to Mary B. Anderson.

[9] *Ibid.*

[10] Elliott, Florence E. Report of Consultation Visit to Bronson Methodist Hospital School of Nursing Kalamazoo Michigan, 1955 April 11. New York: National League for Nursing Department of Diploma and Associate Degree Programs.

[11] *Ibid,* p. 1.

[12] *Ibid,* p. 2.

[13] *Ibid.*

[14] *Ibid,* p. 4.

[15] *Ibid.*

[16] *Ibid, p. 6.*

[17] *Ibid.*

[18] *Ibid.*

[19] *Ibid.*

[20] *Ibid, p. 7.*

[21] *Ibid.*

[22] *Ibid.*

[23] *Ibid.*

[24] *Ibid.*

[25] *Ibid, p.8.*

---

[26] *Ibid.*

[27] *Catalyst,* 1978 November.

[28] Hazel Latondress' maiden name was Smith. Nurses often called each other by their last name or a variation of their last name. Years later, nurses called her H.L.

[29] *Catalyst*, 1978 September; 7, "Hazel Latondress—the best of two worlds."

[30] *Ibid.*

[31] Tape in Bronson archives; interviewer not identified

[32] Bronson Methodist Hospital, *Annual Report 1930–1931,* p. 35, documented the purchase of Dr. H.B. Osborne's property in 1921 for $20,000 and included a photograph of its parlor. It also pictured the four homes, including the purchased Dewing home adjacent to Osborne's, that became West Home on John Street.

[33] Miss Ruth McLellan, 1934 Oct, re housing conditions.

[34] Miss McLellan, 1934 Dec, re the Annex.

[35] *Kalamazoo Gazette,* 1944 Feb 8, "Bronson completes nurses' retreat; rest recreation and study center provided Bronson Hospital nurses."

[36] *Bronson Bulletin*, 5(1): 1947 Jan; 4. "Four students' homes, four 'mothers,'" with picture and article.

[37] *Kalamazoo Gazette,* 1945 April 28.

[38] *Bronson Bulletin,* 5(1): 1947 April, "Record class of nurses offered training in 1947: Expanding hospital has places for sixty girls."

[39] *Kalamazoo Gazette,* 1954 Aug 27, "Plans $1-million home for nurses: announcement of project highlight of Bronson golden year dinner."

[40] *Kalamazoo Gazette*, 1955 Sept 15, "Bronson to get $329,700 federal aid."

[41] *Kalamazoo Gazette*, 1955 Nov 24. "All faiths to honor famed nurse."

[42] A *Kalamazoo Gazette* article of 1955 Dec 2, pictures the volunteers at their kick-off dinner.

[43] *Kalamazoo Gazette,* 1955 Nov 11, re nurses' home pledges.

[44] *Kalamazoo Gazette,* 1955 Nov 18, re nurses' home pledges.

[45] *Kalamazoo Gazette,* 1956 Feb 29, re nurses' home pledges vs. bids.

[46] Dr. W. C. Perdew's press release to press and radio on 1956 Mar 28.

[47] *Kalamazoo Gazette,* 1957 Aug 25; 8. "Open house today: Preview glimpse of $1,355,000 Truesdale Hall."

[48] Dedication and Public Opening Program, Sunday, 1957 August 25.

[49] *Bronson Bulletin*, 15(4): 1957 Fall. "Residence may inspire students."

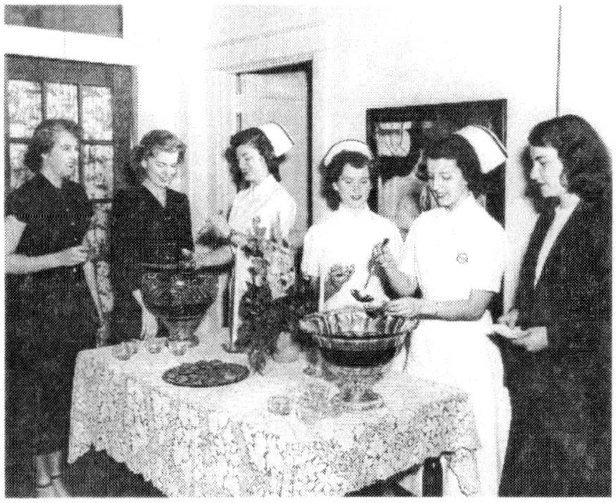

73. Welcoming tea for Freshman class given by upperclassmen in Wesley Hall, 1950 (left to right): Donna Cook, Joan Prause, Betty Gosling, Maxine Woker, Ruth Fox, Barbara Kent.

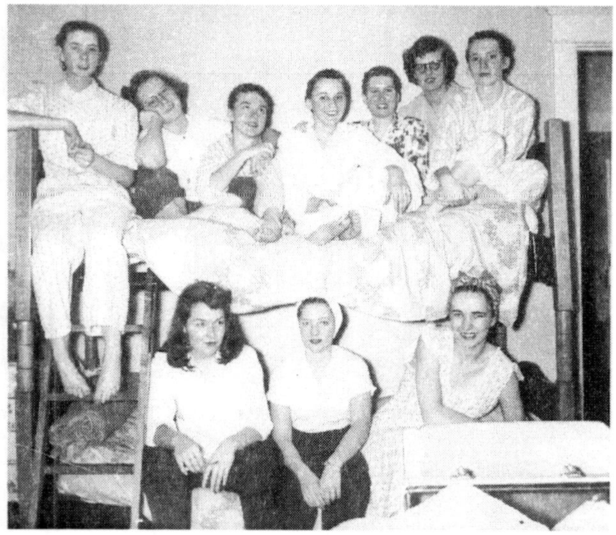

74. Freshmen students on bunk bed at "Big Dorm," 319 John St., Wesley Hall, 1950 (left to right, front row): Marge Hanshew, Darlene Hapham, Marie Dent; (top row) Laura Stephenson, Nancy Burgess, Ruth Spriggs, Bev Soule, Maxine Woker, Joyce Phares, unidentified.

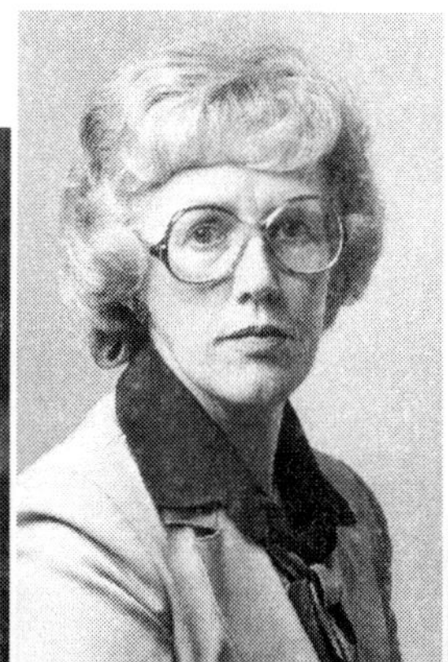

75. (left) Lois Hoyt Richmond, class of 1956, held various administrative positions at the hospital before her retirement in 1987.

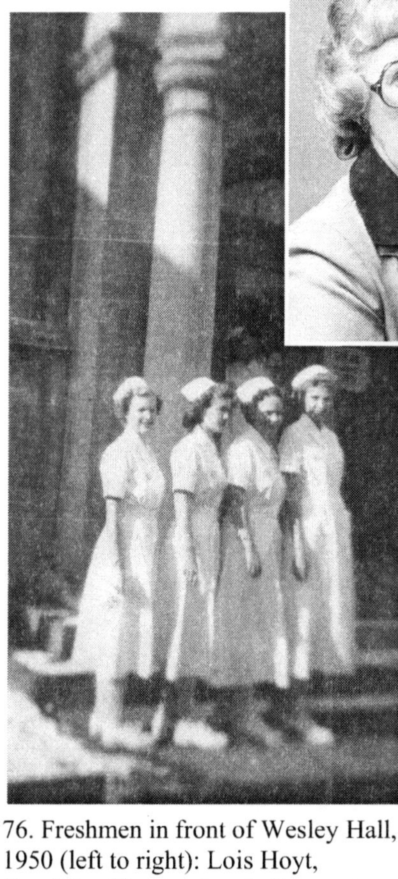

76. Freshmen in front of Wesley Hall, 1950 (left to right): Lois Hoyt, Geraldine Hargan, Jennie Rasmussen, Betty Hoogstraten.

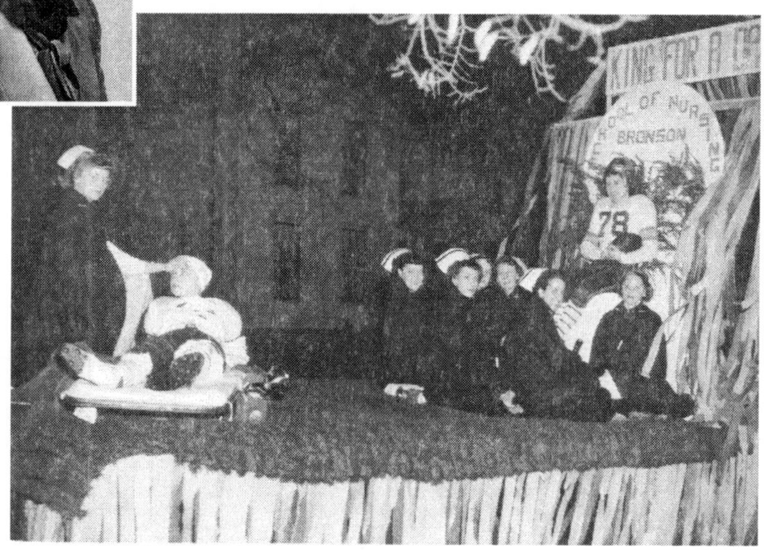

77. Western Michigan College Homecoming Parade float, fall 1950. Football hero, Phyllis LeCronier; injured player, Joan Orr; attending nurse; Lois Bradley. In front of hero (left to right): Bertha Bennett, Donna Kriser, unidentified, unidentified, Peggy Hall.

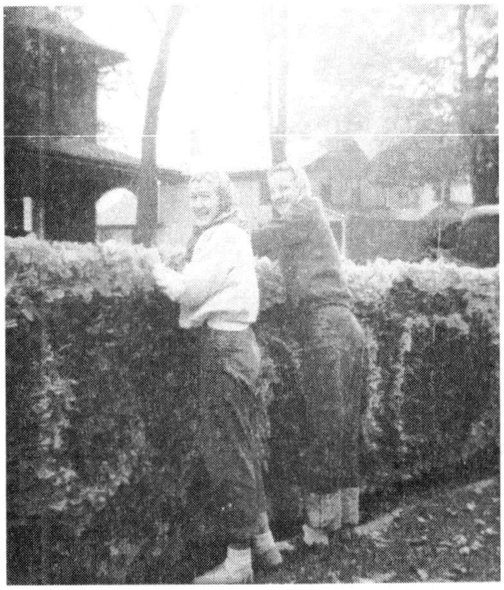

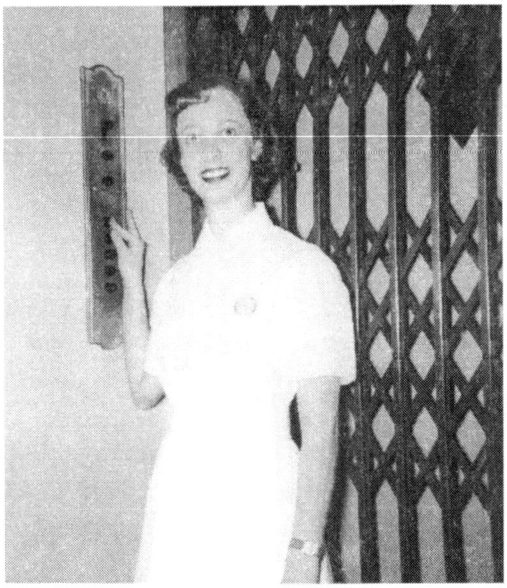

78. Joan McNally and Marlene Waite (above left) worked on the prize-winning BMH School of Nursing float for Western Michigan College's homecoming parade, 1951. Students were active in Western's activities, going to ball games and dances.

79. Freshman Ruth Webb (above right) punched the elevator in John Street Home, 1951. "We freshmen knew how to turn it on after hours and sneak down to the basement and back. There was a hole in the wall due to construction near the old ambulance entrance where we escaped. As probies we were to be in at 7:00 p.m. weekdays. Our housemother must have been hard of hearing because it made so much noise."

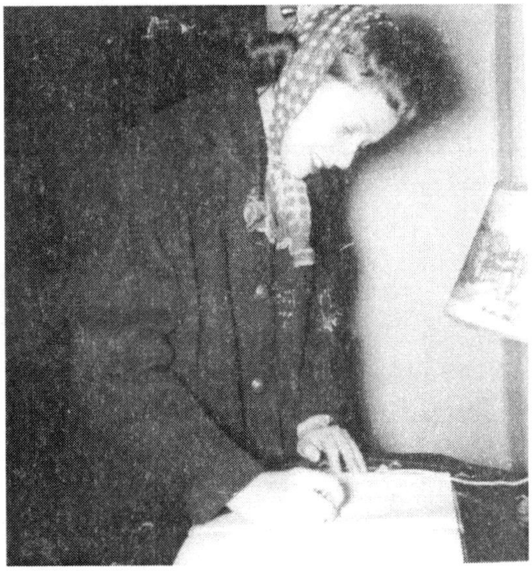

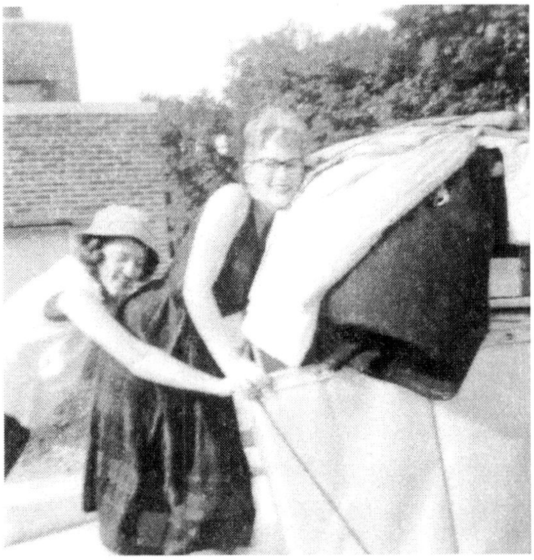

80. Ruth Webb (left) signed out at John St. freshman dorm, 1951. "We were well cared for in those days. Maybe not then, but now I appreciate the concern for us single young ladies, some of whom were away from parental control for the first time."

81. Suzanne Terry and Beverly Pearson (above right) moved from John St. freshman dorm to Junior Home on Cedar St., 1952.

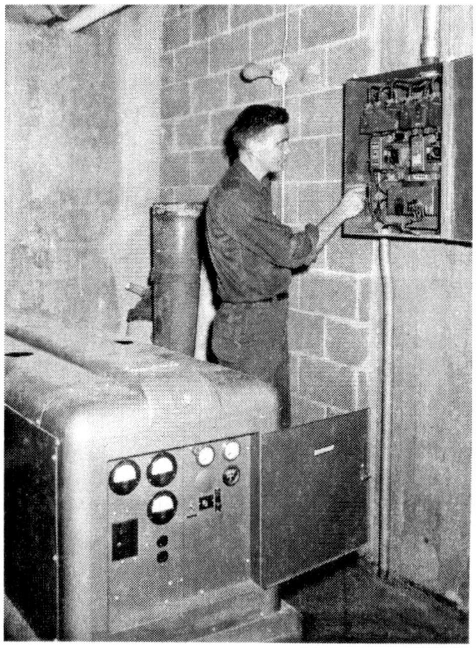

82. (left) Dick Vander Molen as an all-around handyman, was best known as the hospital electrician, 1959.

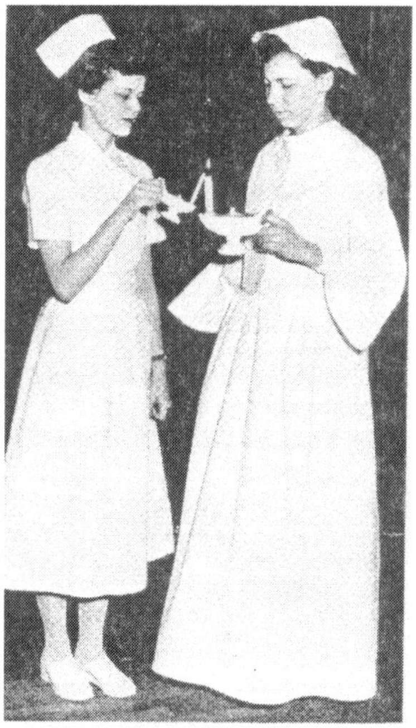

83. (right) Nancy Aldridge, senior class president who represented Florence Nightingale, lit the symbolic lamp of service held by freshman Gwendolyn Jackson, spring 1952.

84. Below left, Mary Tuck's search for the missing piece of a jigsaw puzzle occupied her big sister Janet Cribbs in the comfortable atmosphere of the Bronson junior dorm's recreation room, 1952. Others in the foreground were Lee Harrison (Janet's senior sister) and freshman Ruth Webb.

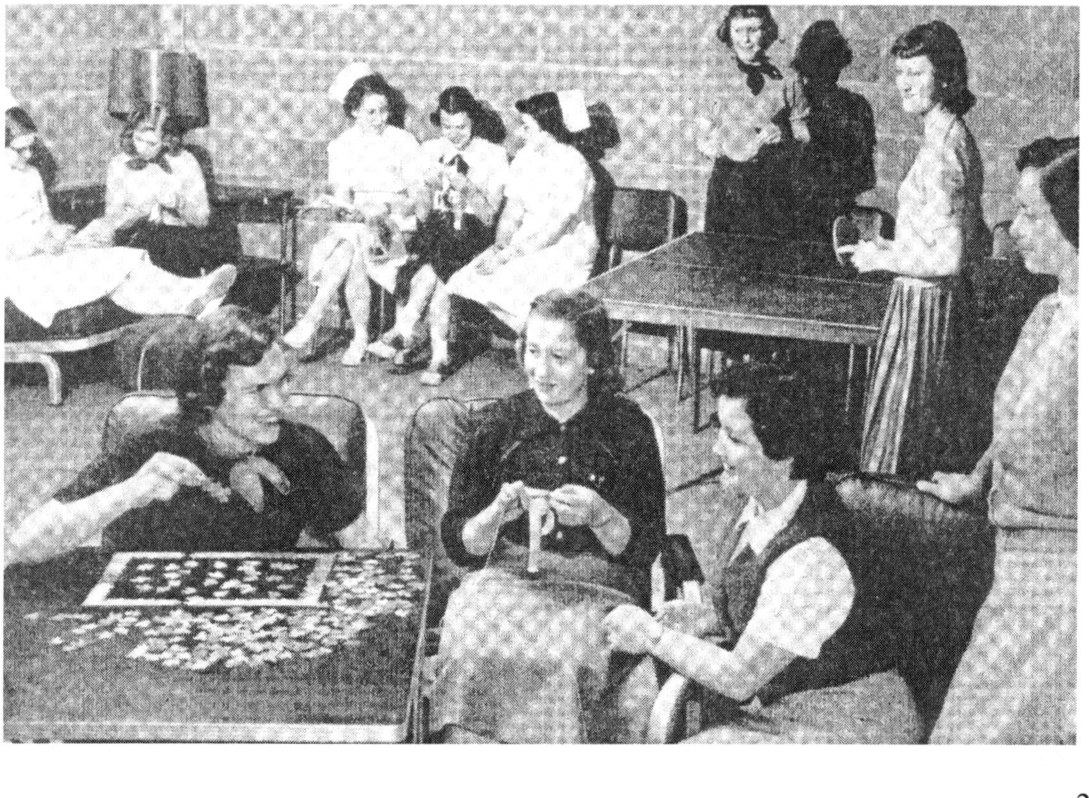

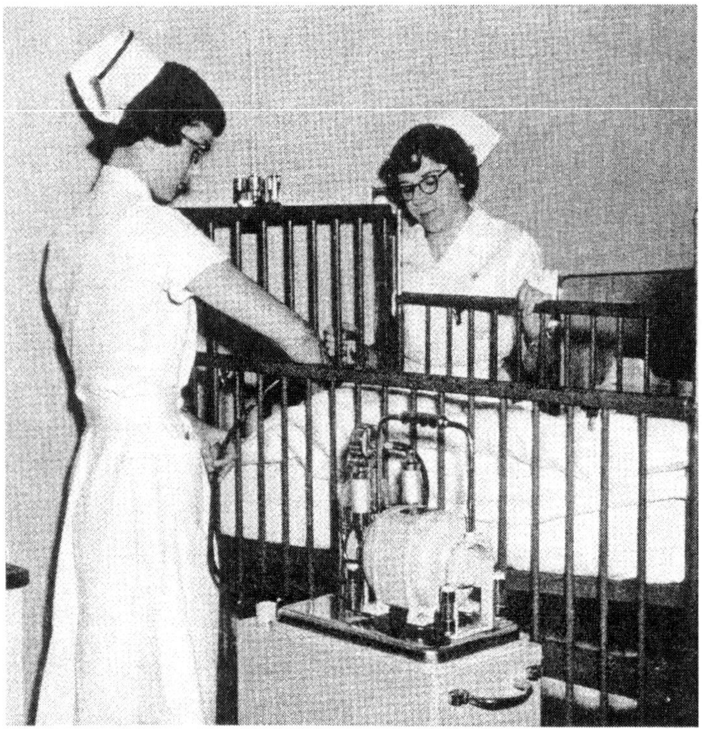

85. The PAR (Post-Anesthesia Recovery) room was opened in 1952. Jane Van Hartesevelt (left) suctioned a patient under the watchful eye of Margaret Gould, supervisor of the room.

86. Bronson nurses' choir rehearsed for the Easter sunrise service, 1952. Gathered around the piano were (below, left to right) Lorraine McCarty, Roxanne Larsen, Joan Moffatt, Mary Lee Moyer, Betty Baker, Eunice "Chick" Thibedeau, Gloryann Fridwall, Phyllis LeCronier, Jennie Rasmussen and Beverly Barker. At the piano was Betty Swigart.

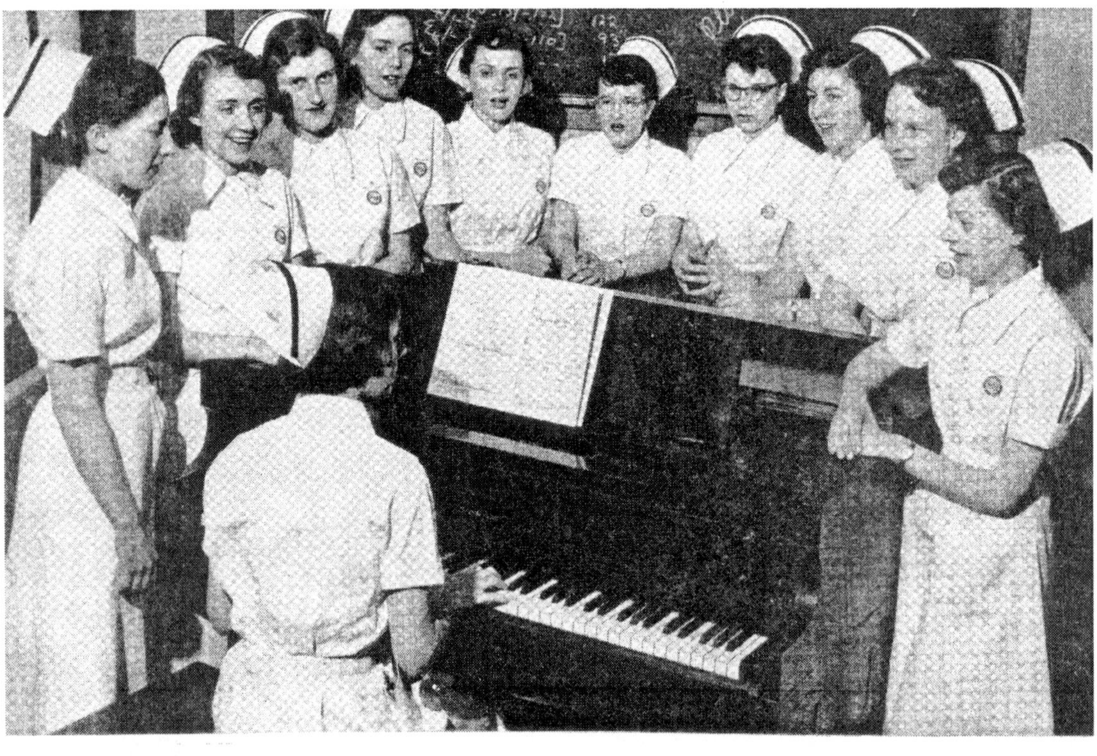

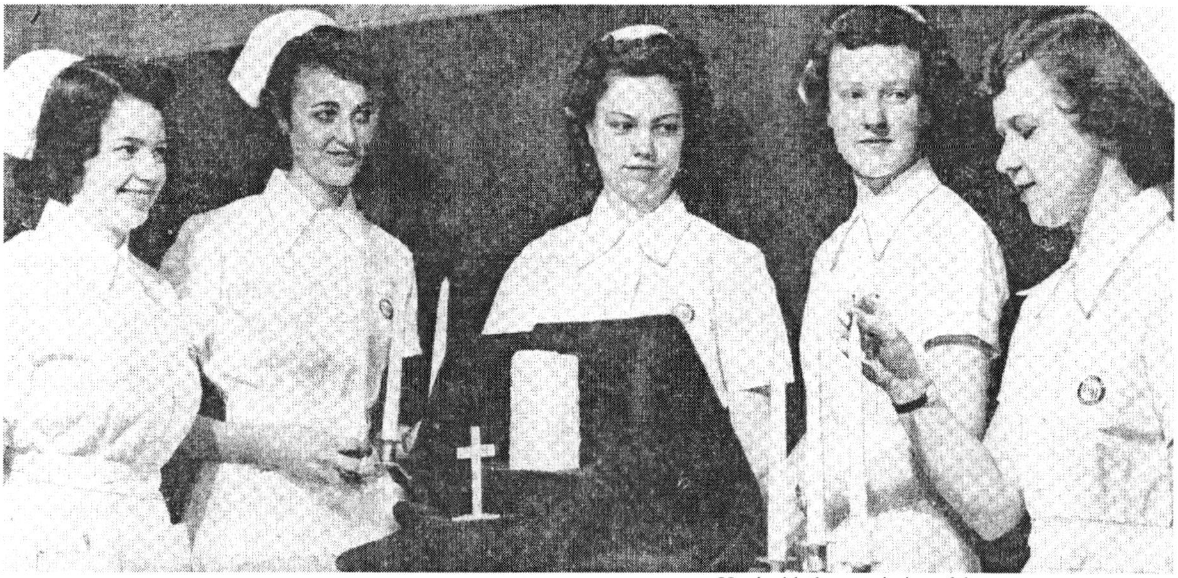

– Used with the permission of the KALAMAZOO GAZETTE.

87. Chapel began the day for Bronson freshmen, 1952. The simple classroom altar was arranged by (left to right) Peggy Haight, Marlene Wolfle, Marilyn Lundstrum, Marlene Waite, and Lauretta Fleming.

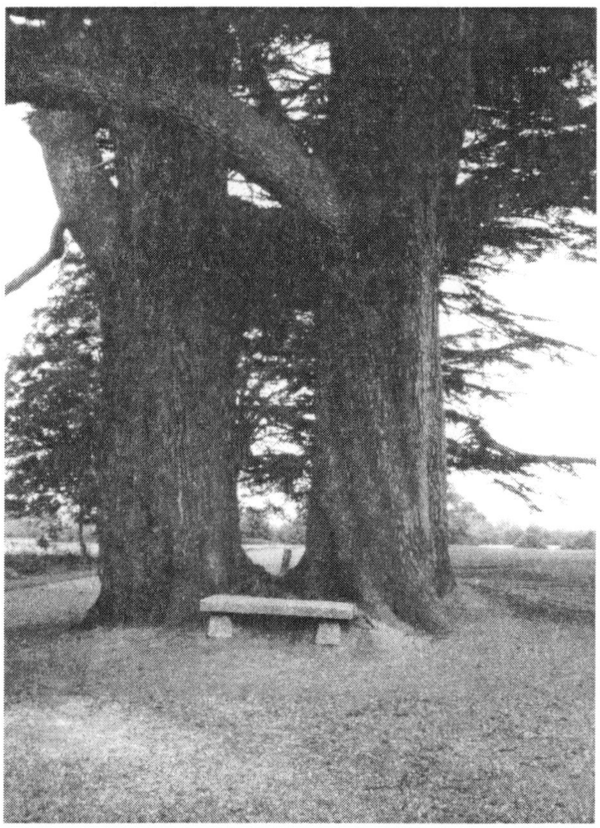

88. Bench, where Florence Nightingale received her command from God, behind Embley Park Estates.

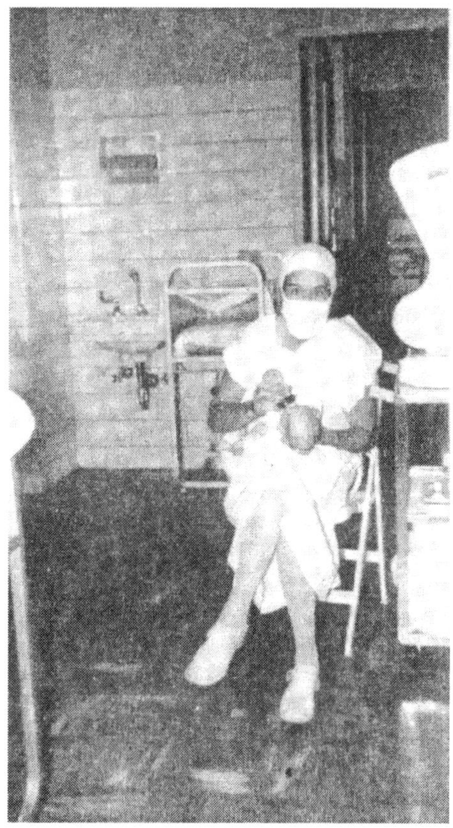

89. Donna Cook fed a newborn at 2 A.M., ca early 1950s.

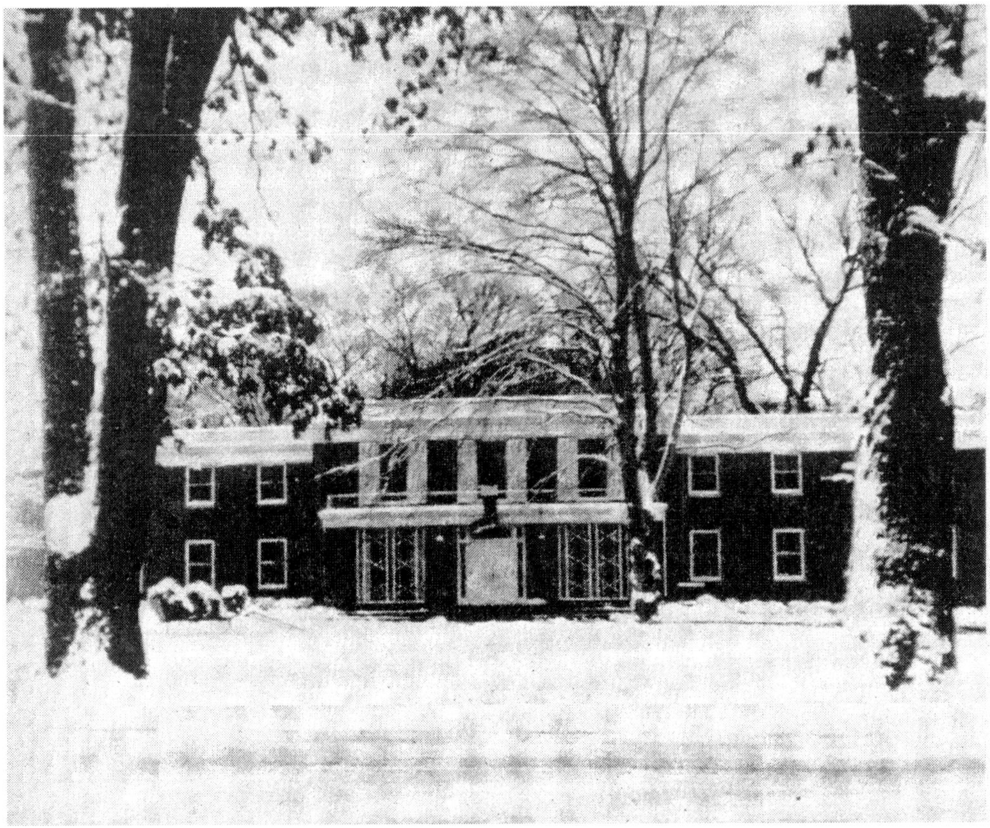

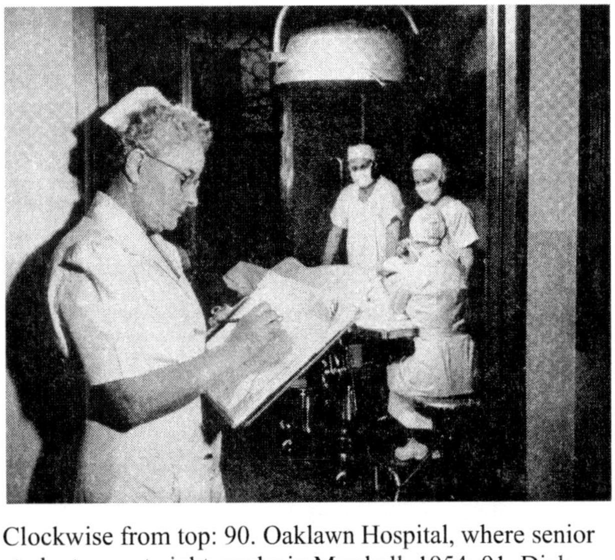

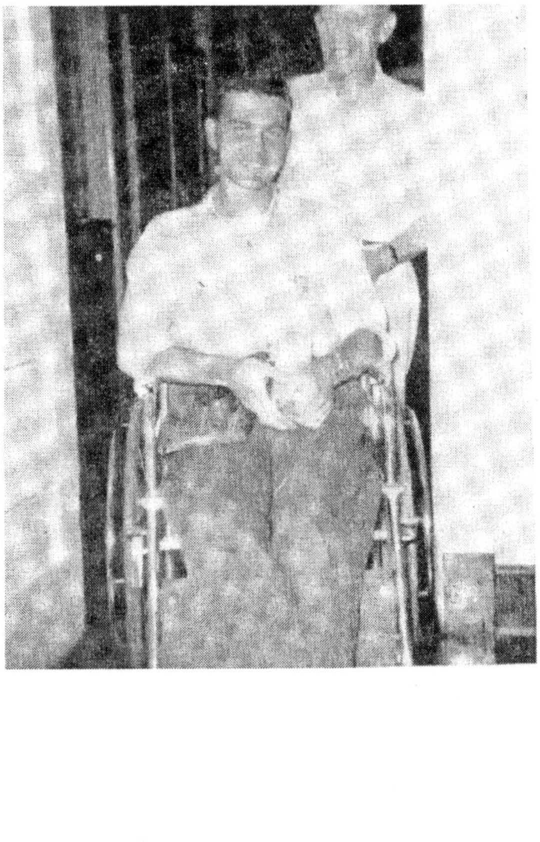

Clockwise from top: 90. Oaklawn Hospital, where senior students spent eight weeks in Marshall, 1954; 91. Dick "Jeff" Vander Molen pushed by Clark "Mutt" Sheldon, 1953; and 92. Dena Wolters, surgery supervisor, stood at the entrance of the new operating room, 1953.

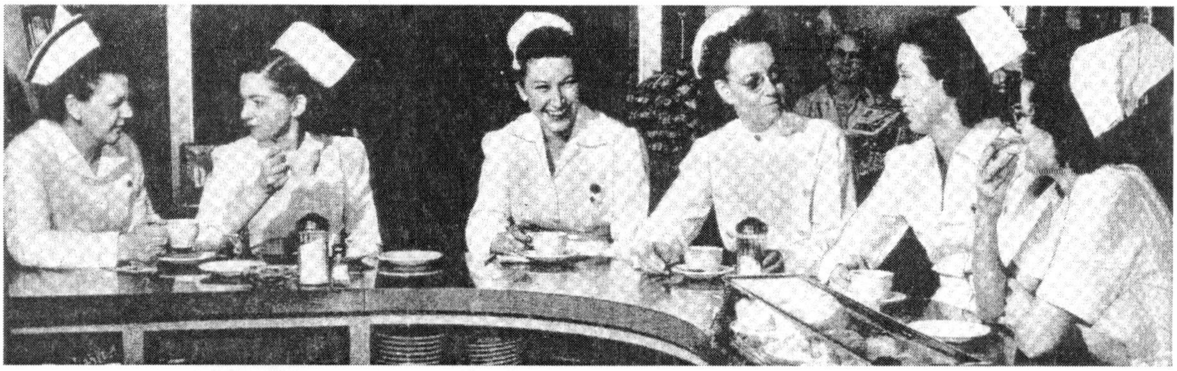

93. Instructors enjoyed coffee at the coffee shop in Bronson Methodist Hospital, 1954. Left to right: Louise Huffman, Nursing Arts Instructor; Virginia McPhail, Medical and Surgical Instructor; Hazel Latondress, Assistant Director of Nursing Service; Mary B. Anderson, Director of Nurses; Ellen Emig, Surgical Clinical Instructor; and, Winifred Gerard, Operating Room Instructor.

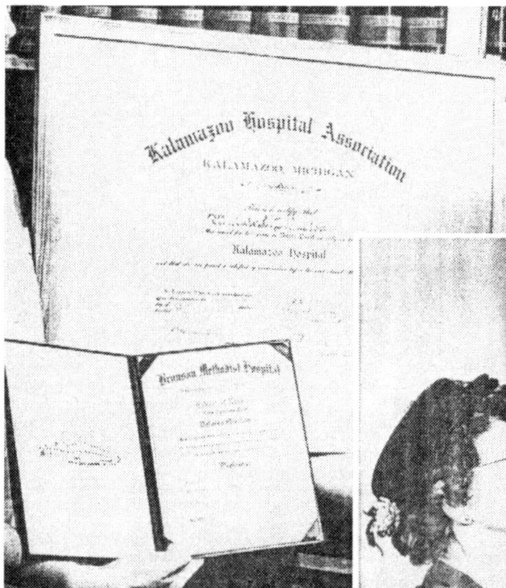

94. Old and new diplomas were featured at the 50th anniversary of the School of Nursing, August 26, 1954.

95. Sophia VanHartesvelt Jacobs gave her Bronson School of Nursing pin to her grandniece, Jane VanHartesvelt, August 1954.

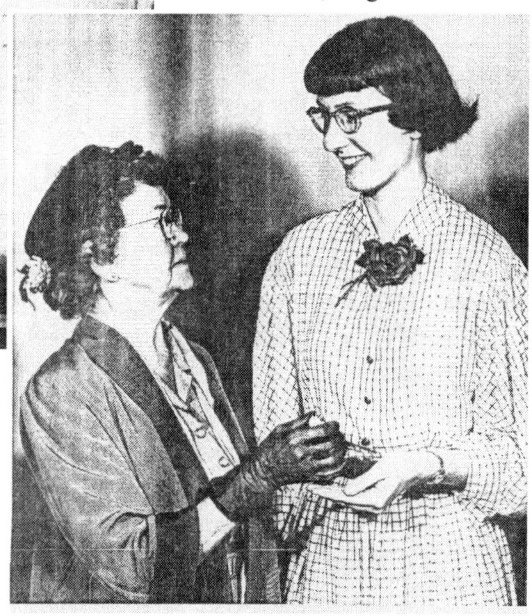

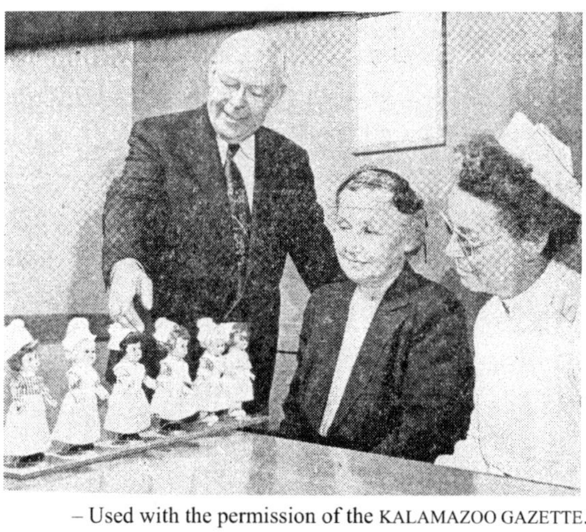

– Used with the permission of the KALAMAZOO GAZETTE.

96. (left) Dr. W.C. Perdew, hospital superintendent; Mina Weber Macgrayne, chairman of the celebration and Mary B. Anderson, Director of Nurses, looked at dolls showing the transition of uniforms' appearance, August 1954.

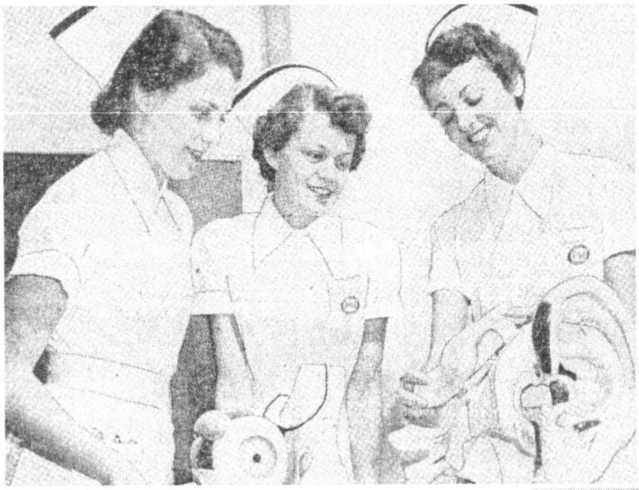

– Used with the permission of the KALAMAZOO GAZETTE.

97. (left to right) Dixie Crane, Gwen Jackson, and Marlene Wolfle studied modern eye and ear models, 1954.

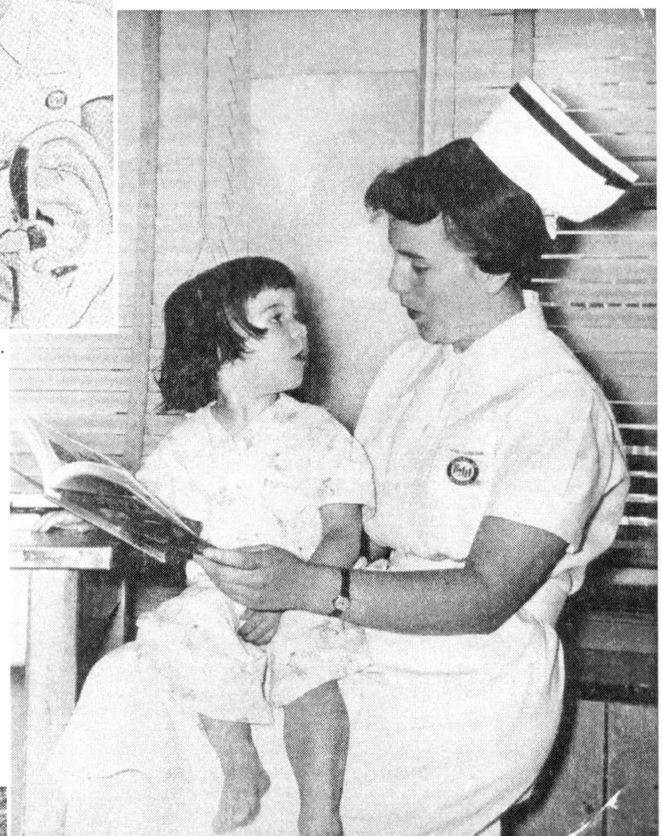

98. Joan Osborn, during her senior year Peds affiliation, read to a patient, ca. 1954–55.

99. (below) Linda Smith received a $100 bill from Dr. W.C. Perdew as first prize for the lyrics of the alma mater. Second prize of $50 went to Helen Weber (left) and third prize of $25 to Clarice Harper, 1955.

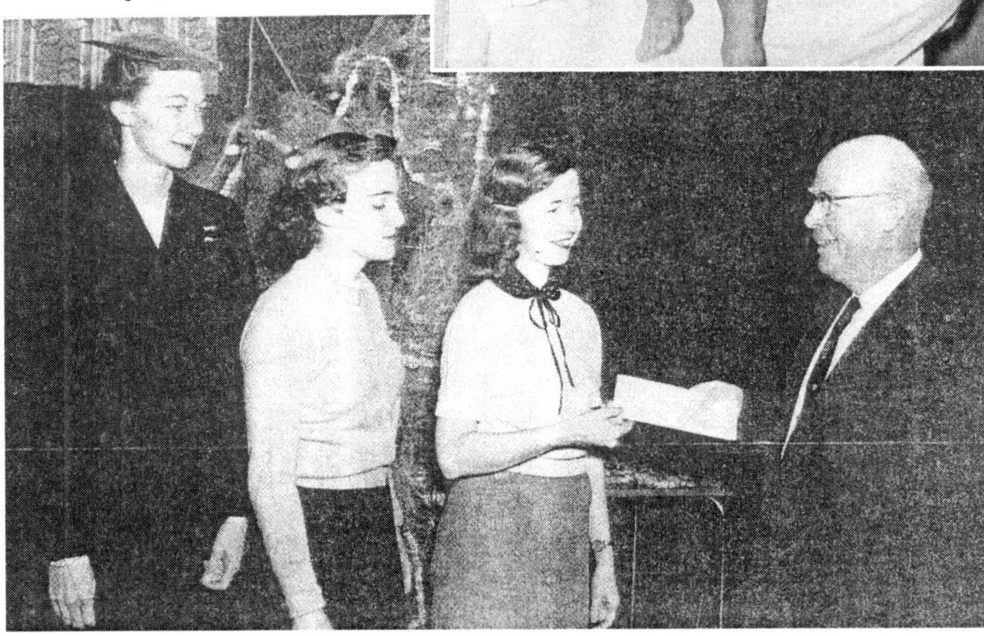

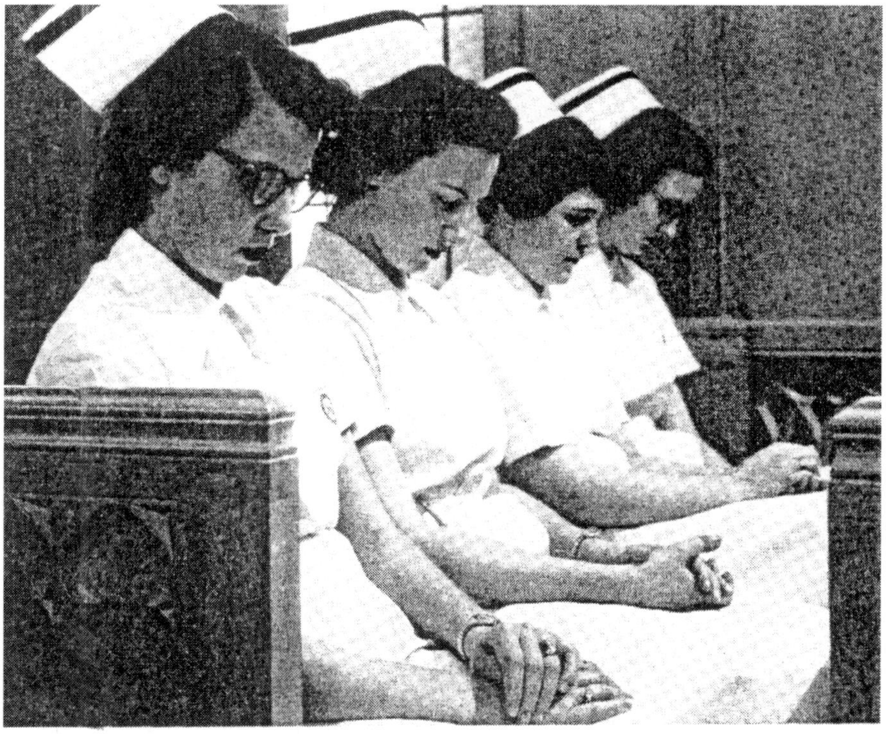

100. Chapel pew, 1955

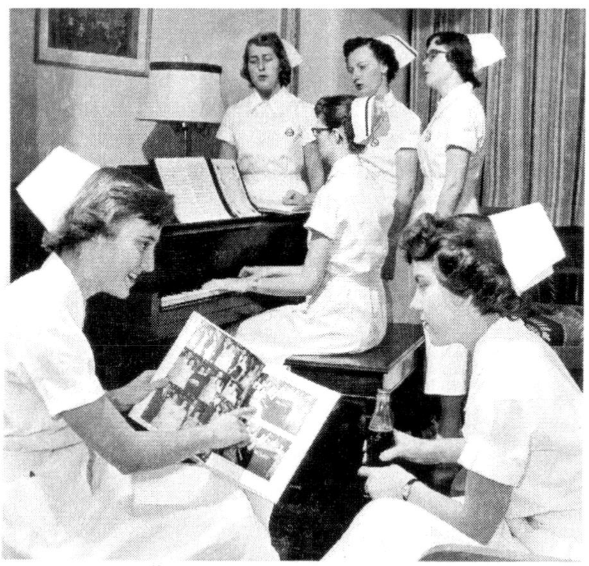

101. Choir members enjoyed the recreational facilities, 1954. Clarice Harper (left) and Mercy Revesz looked at the yearbook while (left to right) Helen Dietz , Shirley Martin, and Sandra Youker gathered around the piano. Rosalee Truax was at the keyboard.

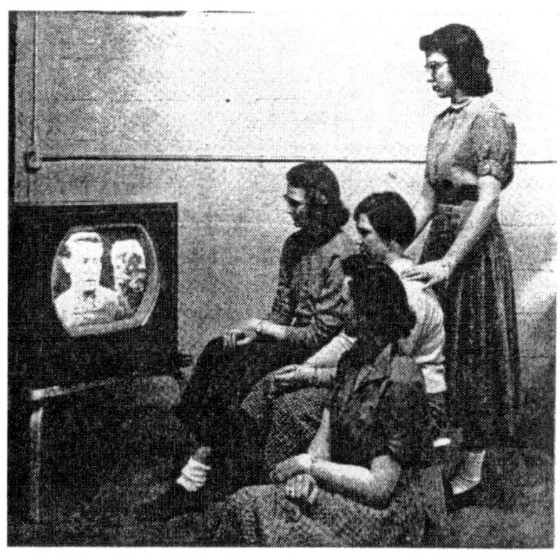

102. Patricia Rogers (standing) and three of her classmates, Rosalee Truax, Marjorie Speers, and Shirley Martin watched one of their favorite TV programs, May 1955.

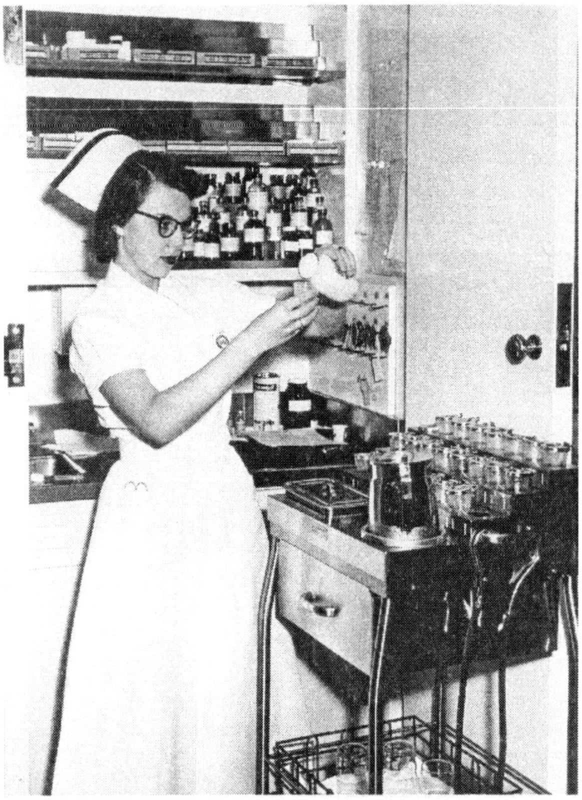

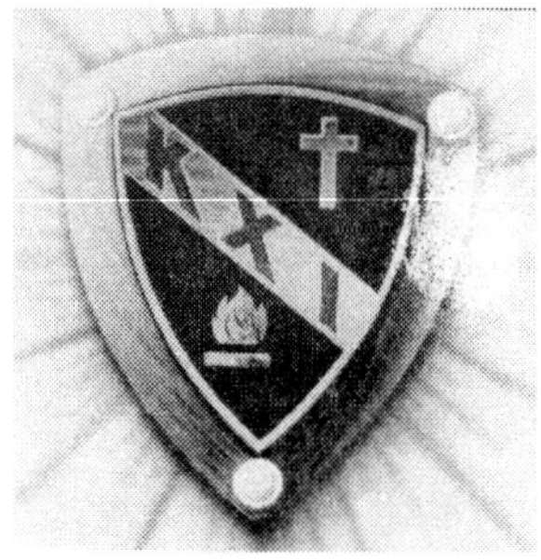

Clockwise from left: 103. Senior student, Patricia Rogers puts her study to good use in the measuring of medicines, 1955; 104. Kappa Chi Iota pin of the nursing sorority founded at Bronson Methodist Hospital, 1956. Its purpose was to promote the religious welfare of student nurses through worship and Christian service; 105. Groundbreaking at Truesdale Hall, 1956. (left to right) Mr. Pratt, Mr. Stapert, Dr. Perdew, Mr. Southon, Elwood Schneider, Mary B. Anderson, Miss Shoemaker, Mrs. Helen Weber, Mrs. Dorothy Dunn.

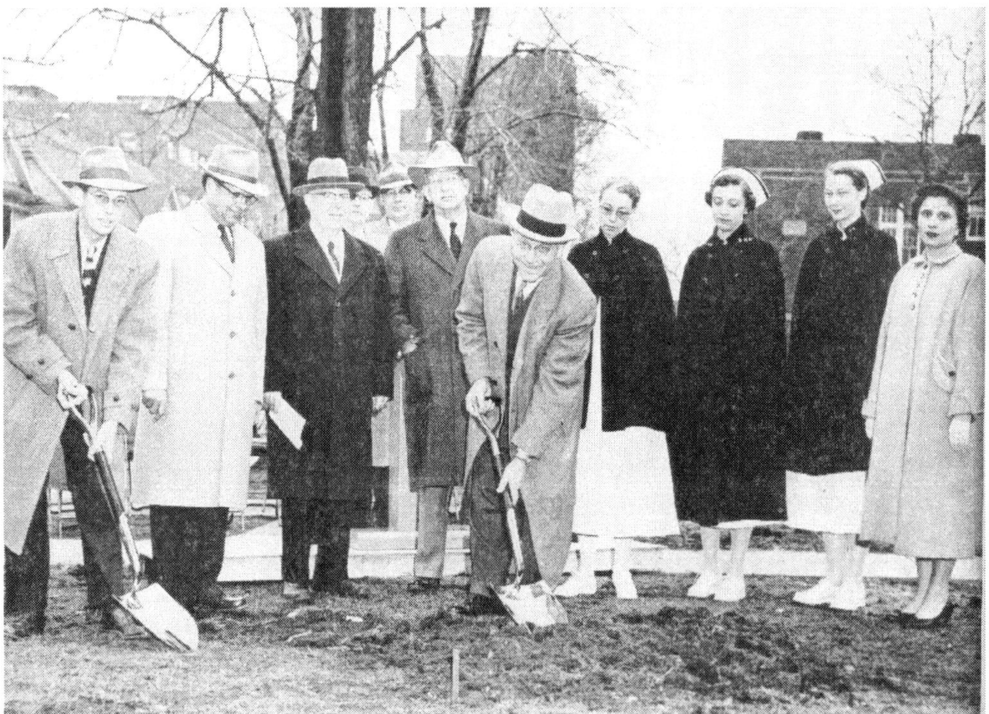

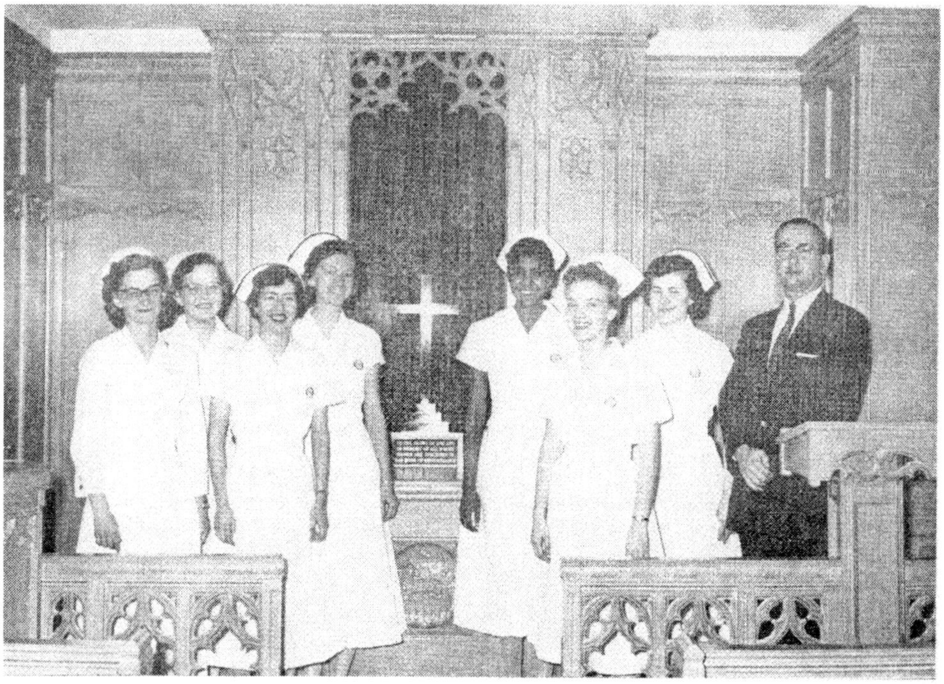

106. (above) Officers of Kappa Chi Iota, spring 1957. (left to right) Virginia McPhail, Sandra Cooke, Loretta Laurin, Darlene Rupp, Carrie Lewis, Stephanie Albrecht, Ruth Weller, and Chaplain Robert Trenery. 107. (below) Directed by Mrs. Beatty, the School of Nursing Choir in their royal blue capes performed at the groundbreaking ceremony for Truesdale Hall, 1957.

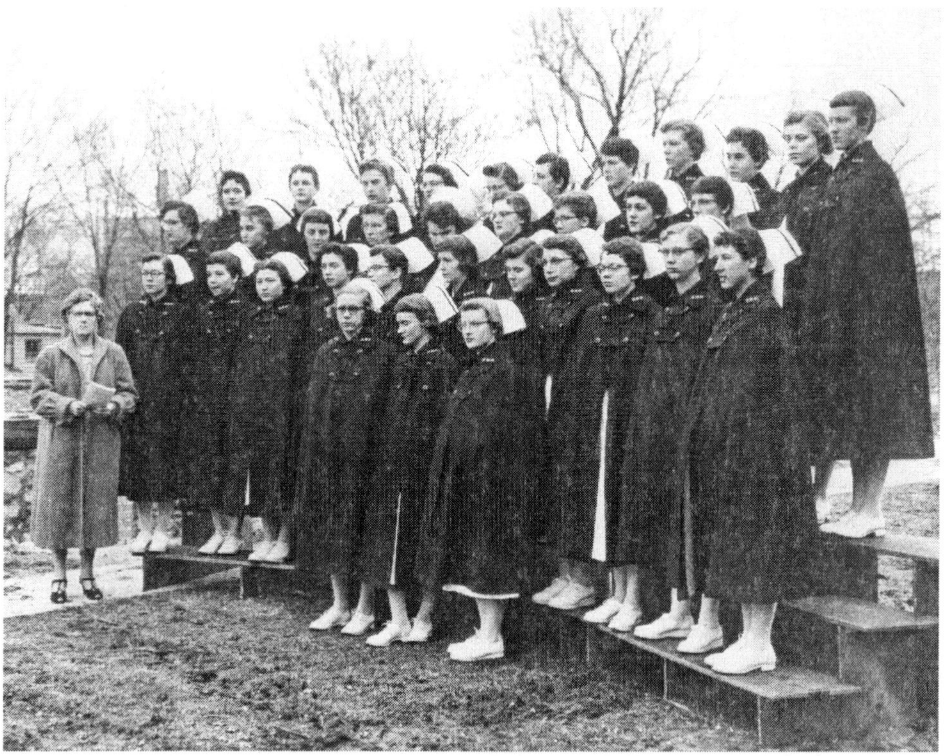

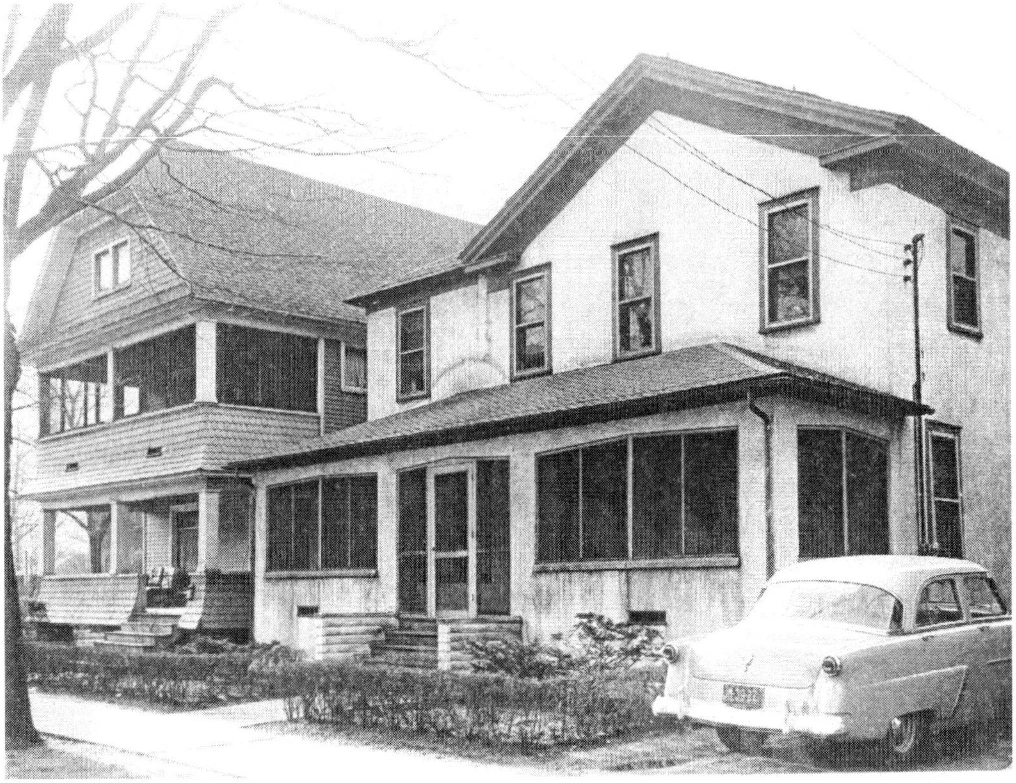

108. East Home (left) in the late 50's was in later years called Cedar Home. The home on the right was connected to East Home with an enclosed walkway. Students lived in both homes until Truesdale Hall was built.

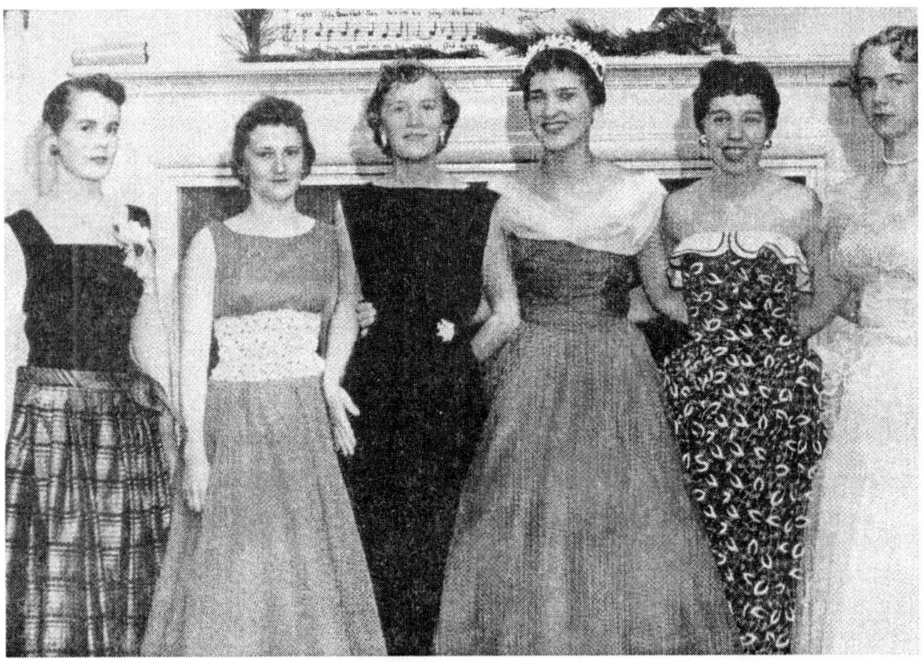

109. Christmas Formal at Hoben Hall, Kalamazoo College, 1956. (left to right) Avis Reichert, Carol McGregor, Esther Wyman, Queen Karmena Lubavs, Carol Keirman, Audrey Russeau.

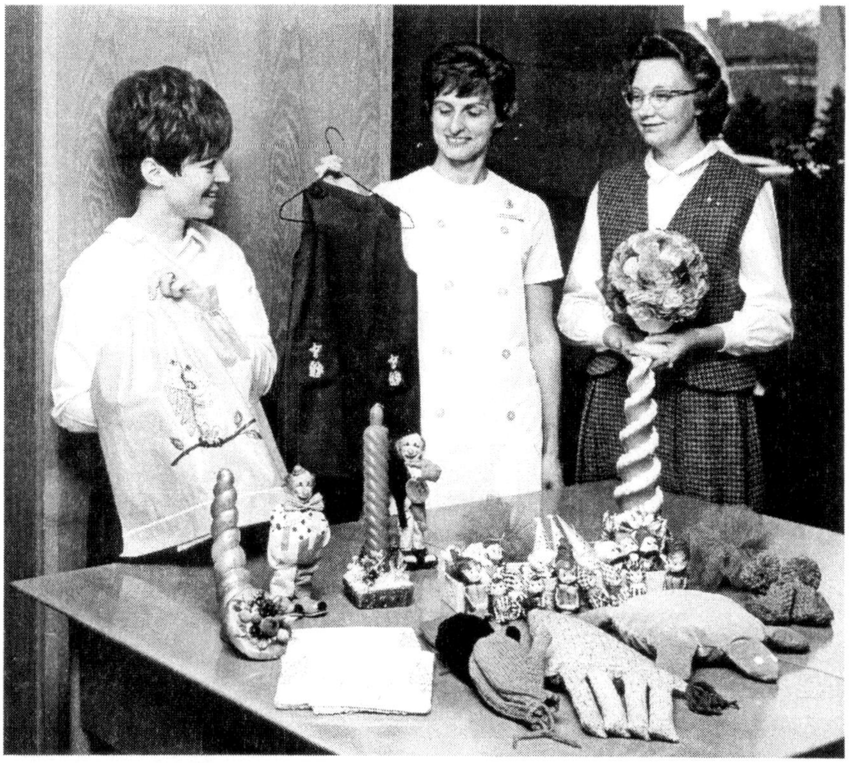

110. Alumni Holiday Bazaar was an important fundraiser for scholarships (left to right) (unidentified student), Beverly Klimp Bloomquist, and Ellen Dixon Weston, ca 1954.

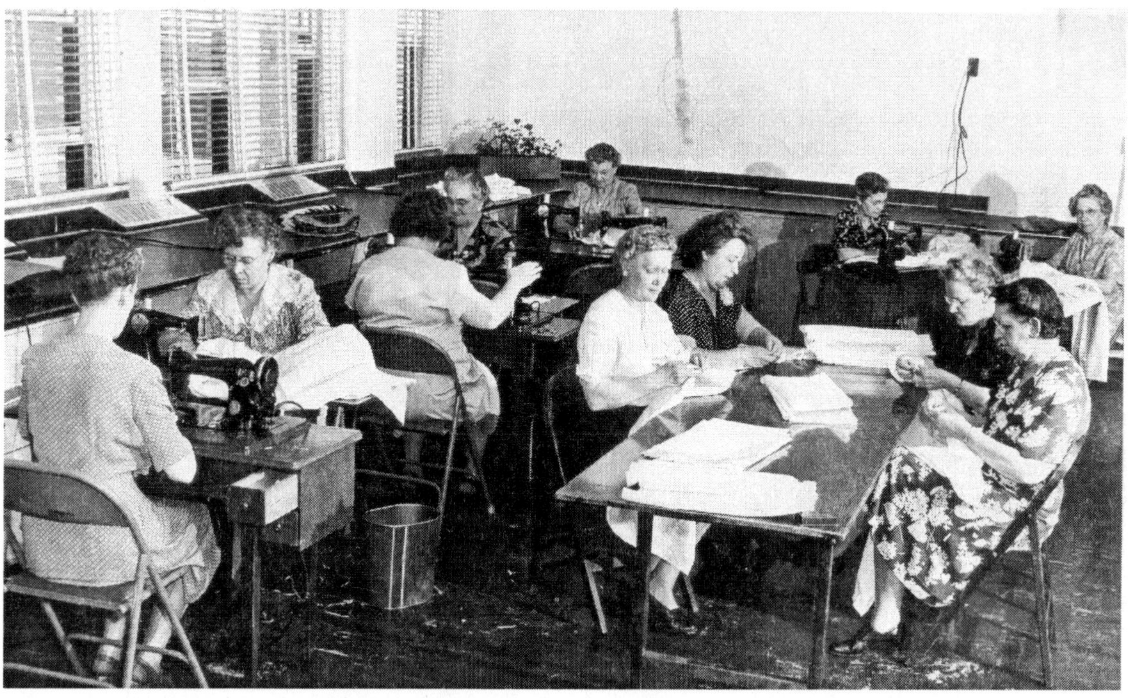

111. The hospital women's auxiliary was divided into a number of groups or guilds, each with its own field of endeavor. This White Cross Guild sewed and folded dressings in the hospital Volunteer Service room.

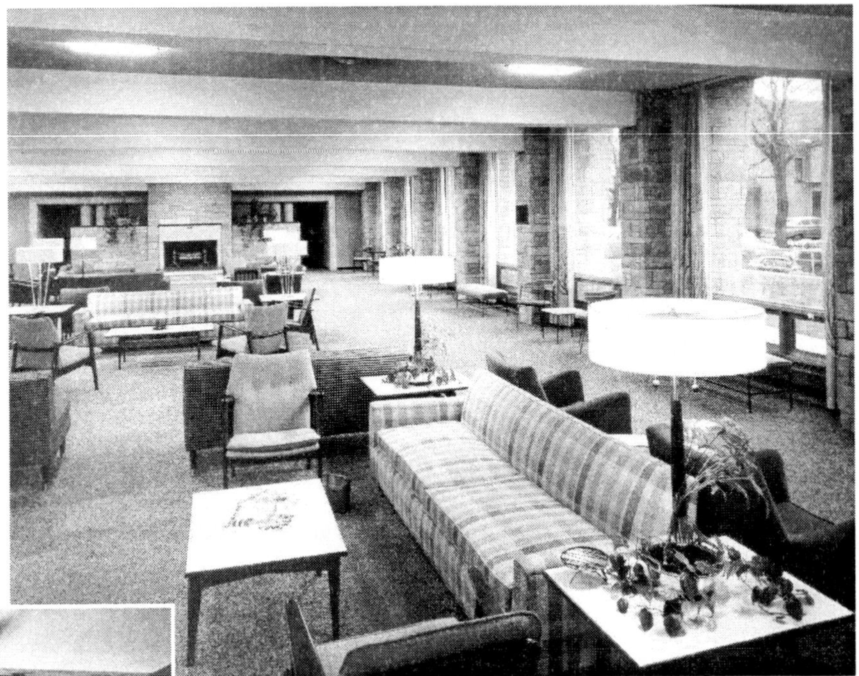

112. (right) Lobby in new Truesdale Hall, 1957.

113. (below) Bronson's annual Christmas formal was held in Truesdale's rec room, December 15, 1957.

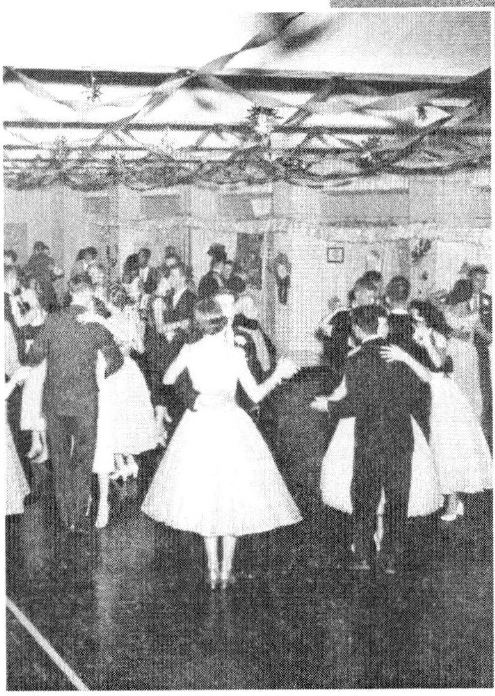

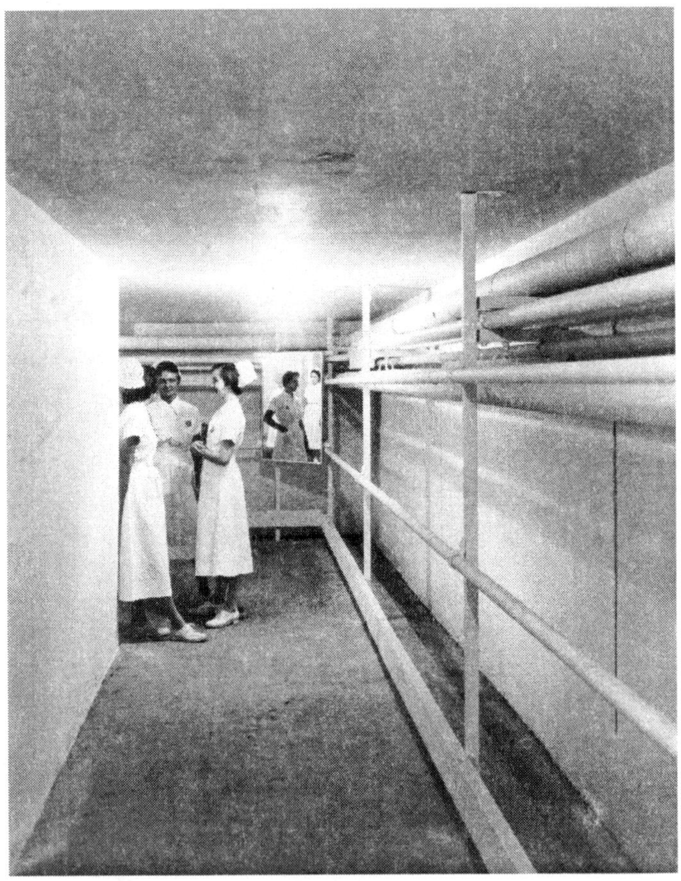

114. (right) The tunnel connecting Truesdale Hall to Bronson required student ID to unlock the door, 1957. It provided a safe and dry passageway especially for students working evenings and nights.

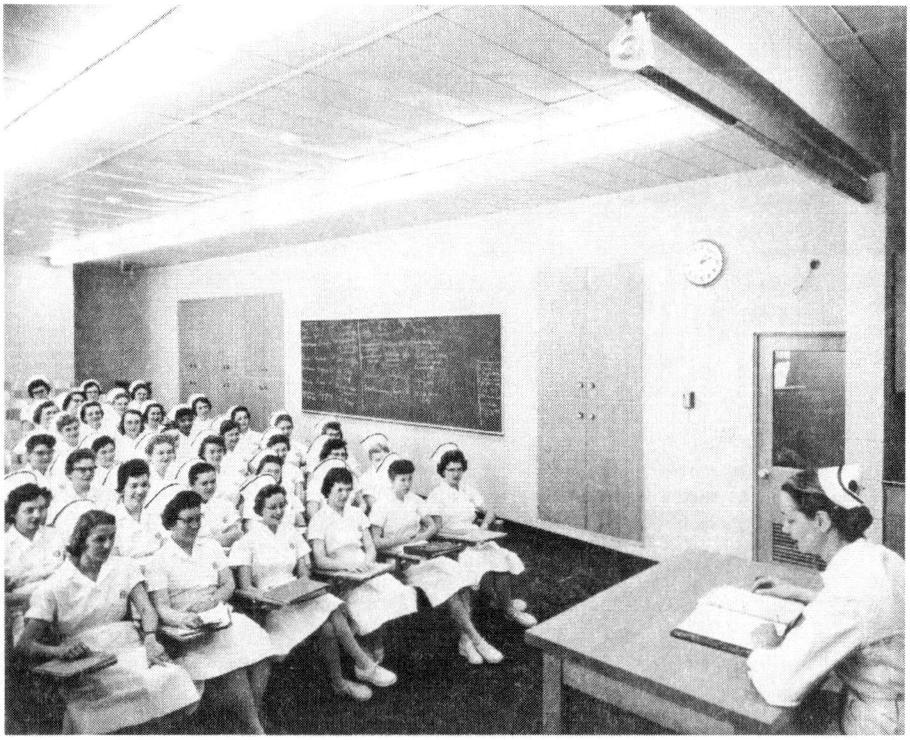

115. (above) Junior students in new Truesdale Hall classroom, shown with Helen Weber at front desk,1958. (left to right) First row: Kathleen Hunt, Elizabeth Van Voorhees, Doris Johnson, unidentified, Pat Hurd, Gaydene Klock; second row: Carol Crookes, Joyce Poll, Barbara Wespinter, remainder unidentified.

116. Looking northwest from the corner of Cedar St. and Pine St. showed construction to complete the east wing floors 4, 5, and 6, known by the students as the 30's wing, 1958.

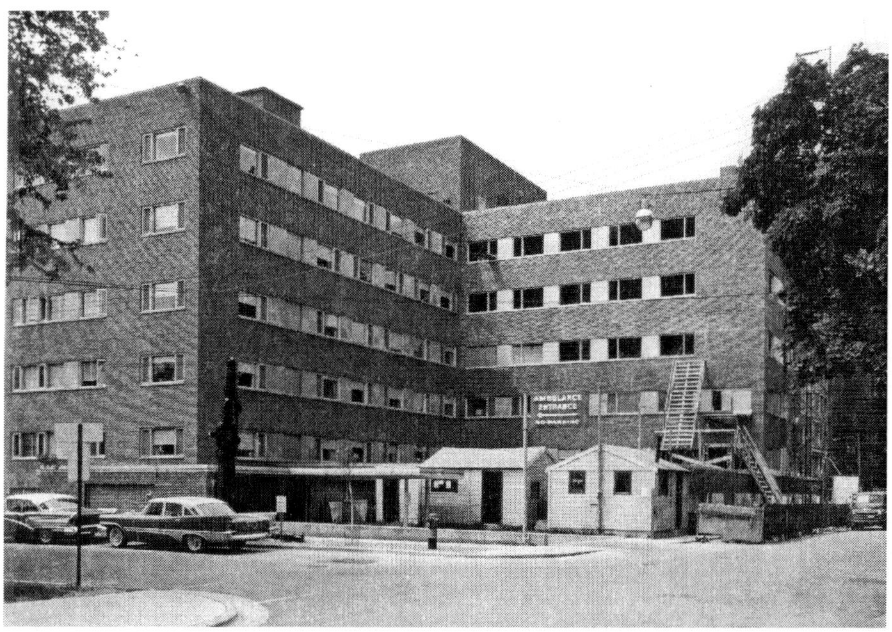

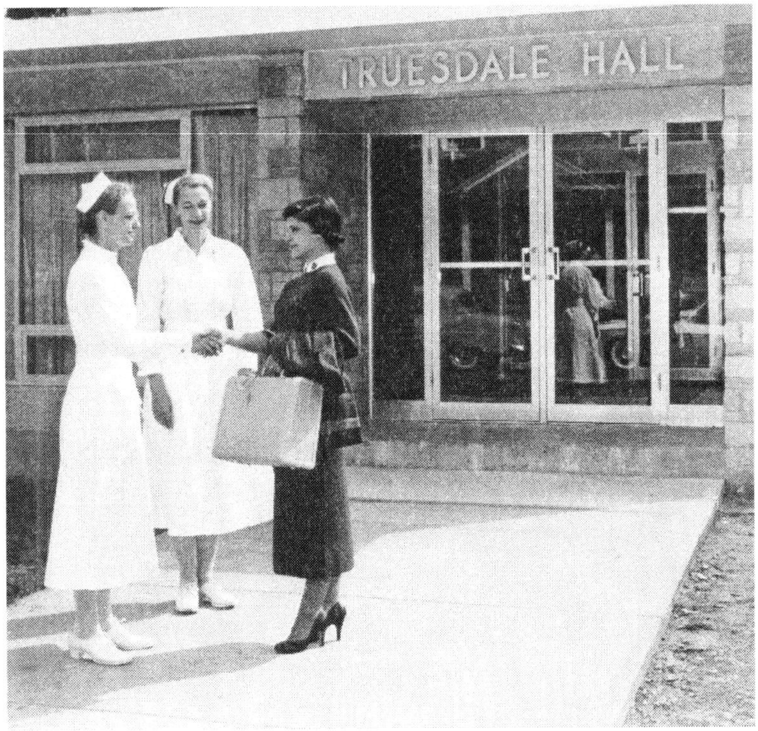

117. (left) Director of Nursing Mary B. Anderson and Assistant Director of Nursing Helen Weber, welcomed Shirley Laurie to Truesdale Hall, spring 1958.

118. (bottom) Class of 1959 shown in Truesdale Hall lobby after graduation ceremonies. Traditionally graduates joined hands in a circle and sang one last song together; frequently it was,"God Be With You Till We Meet Again."

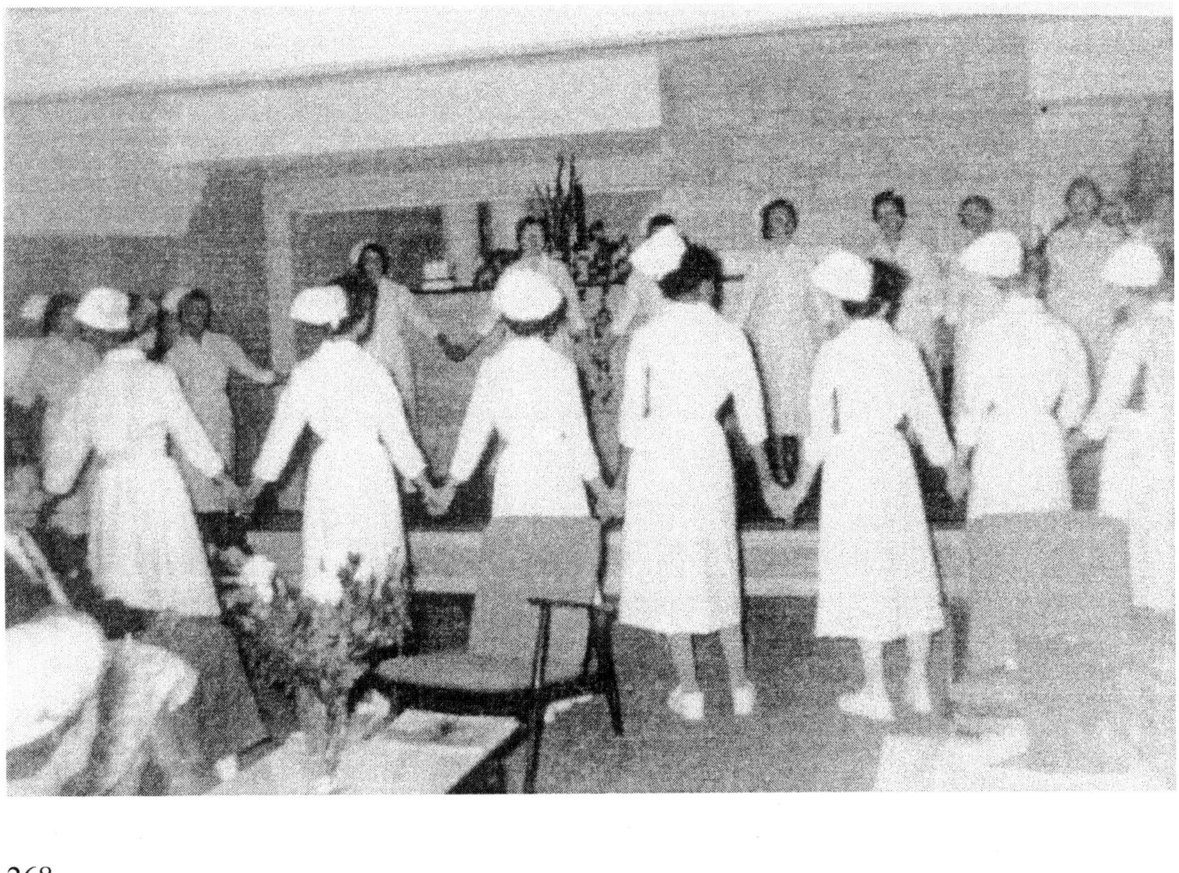

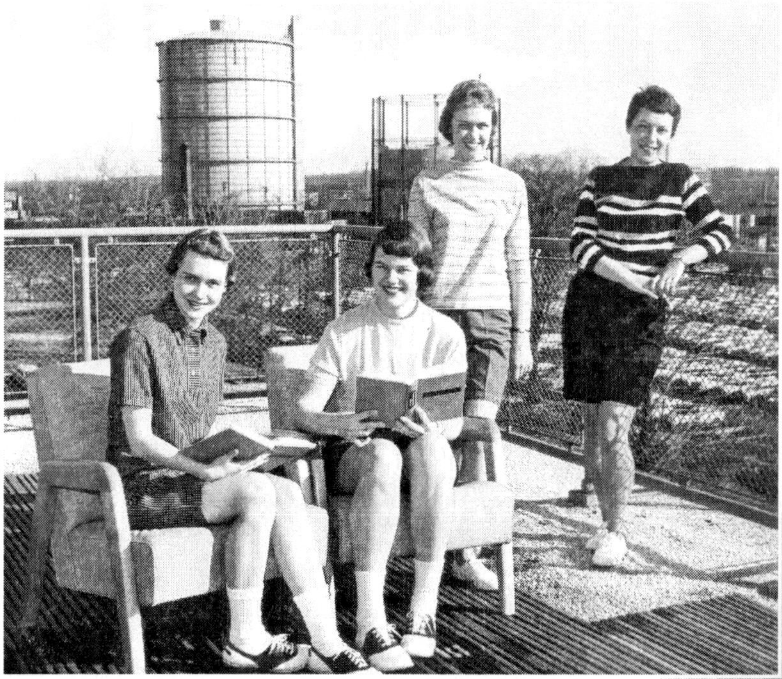

119. (left) Students (left to right) Carolyn B. Lewis, Marilyn Brink, Sheila Robinson and Susan Mindrum enjoyed the sun roof on the 5th floor of Truesdale Hall, spring 1958.

120. (below) Lincoln Junior High School was the site of hospital basketball games, 1959. Top row: Miss Wolters, Miss Wantz and Miss Mary B. Anderson were supportive of hospital sports activities.

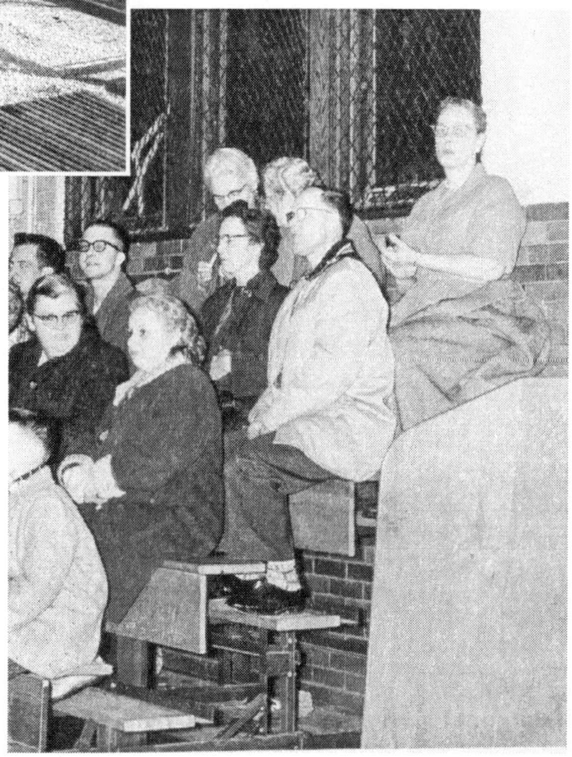

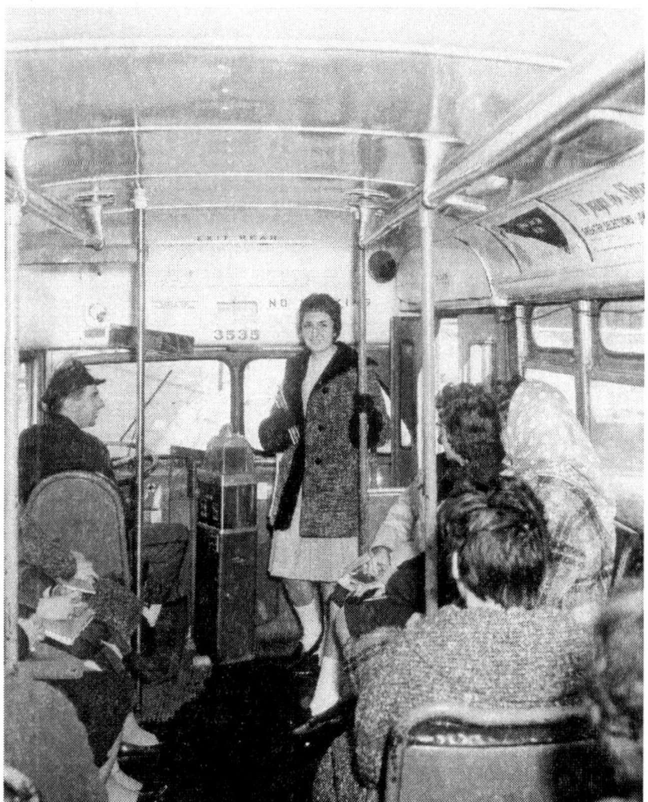

121. (left) Nancy Bumstead boarded a Kalamazoo city bus for WMU classes, 1958–59.

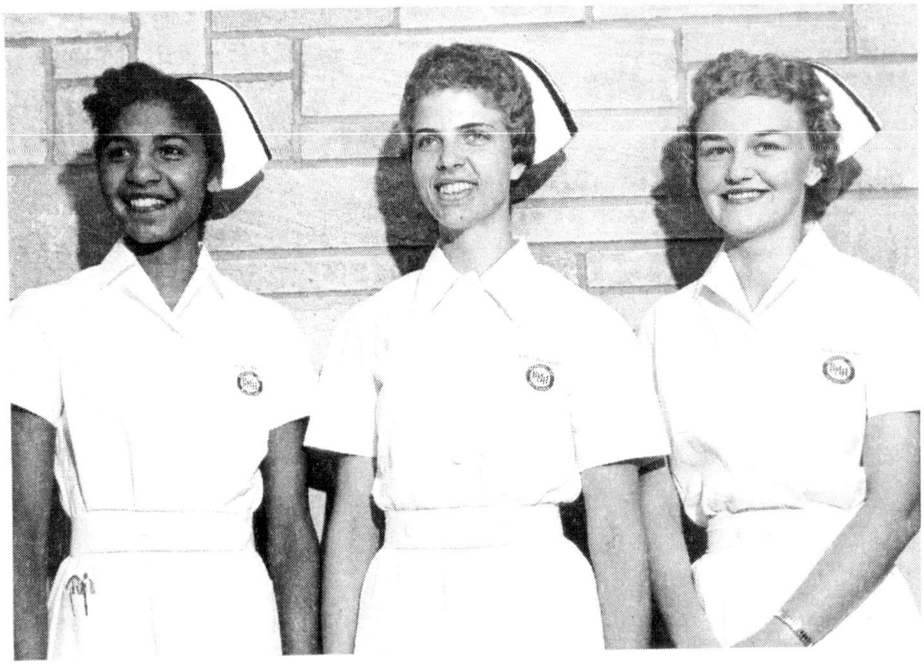

122. Bronson Nurses of the Year, 1958. (left to right) Carrie Lewis, third honors; Joanne VanNaarden, first honors; Juliene Wykstra, second honors.

123. Faculty-Student Planning Committee, National League for Nursing (NLN) Accreditation process. (left to right) Beverly Bradley, Margaret Shepard, Clarice Harper, Lois Brown, Helen Meaker, Mrs. Leonhart, Betty Fitzpatrick.

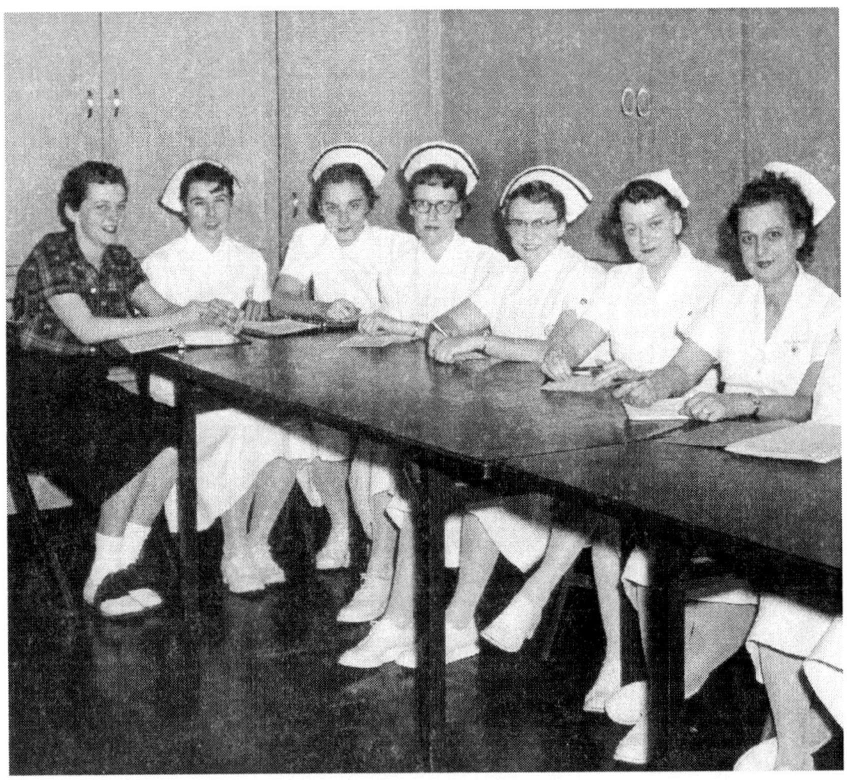

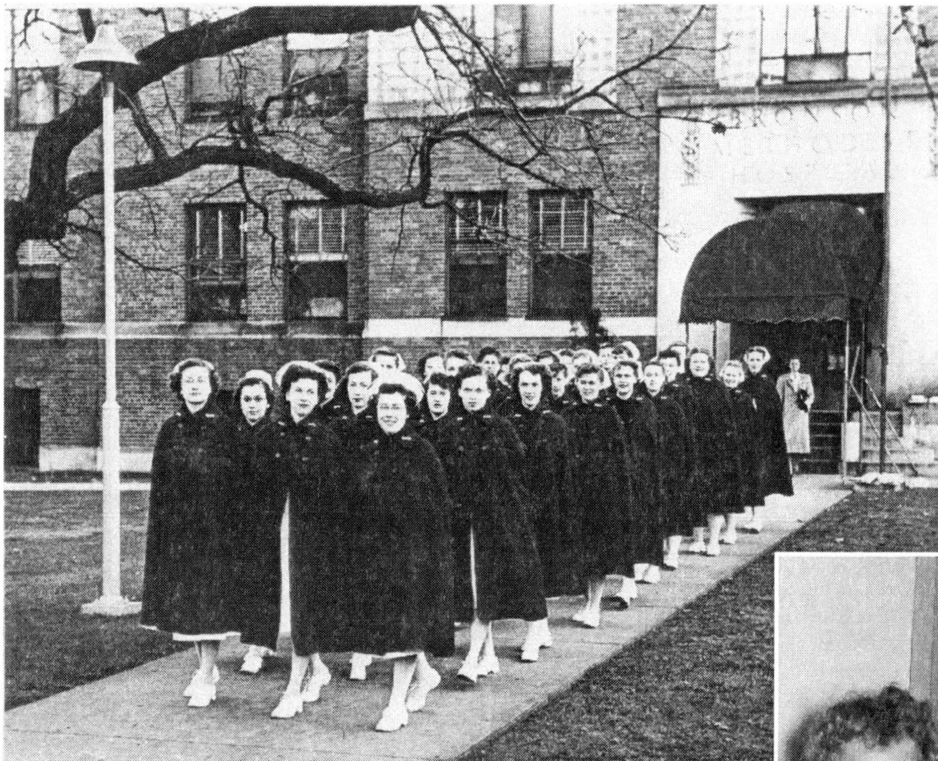

124. Entire class of 1950 leaving hospital.

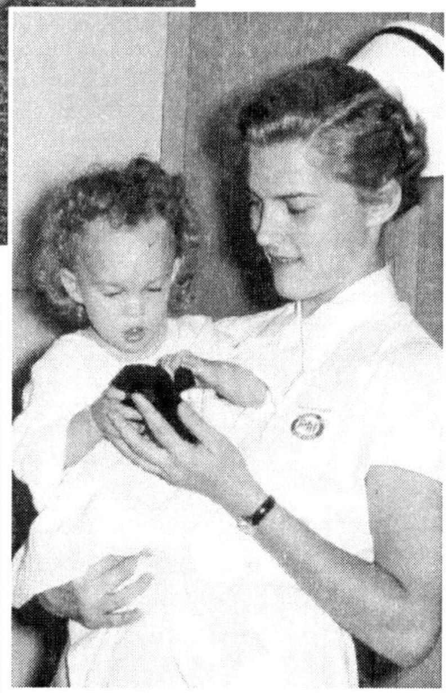

125. Sue Graber and toddler, 1958.

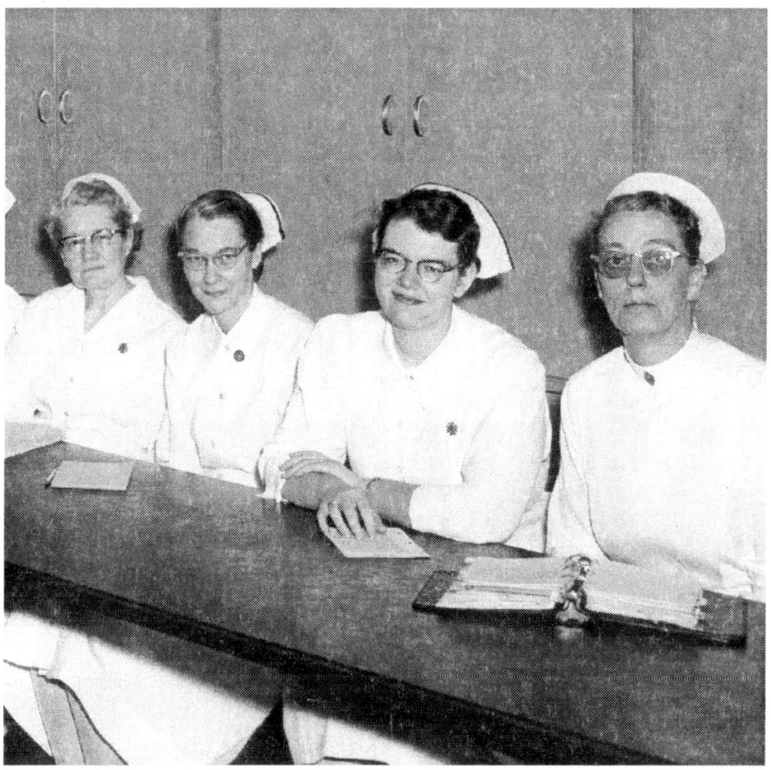

126. Faculty-Student Planning Committee, NLN Accreditation process, (continued, left to right) Miss Marie Wantz, Helen Weber, Miss Parren, Mary B. Anderson. Student input on curriculum was part of this process.

CHAPTER 7
MONUMENT EXPANSION CONTINUES, 1960s

President Kennedy's assassination on November 22, 1963, resonated with early sixties nursing students, "Where were you when Kennedy was shot?" The shock was followed by the Vietnam conflict, which forced most young men to choose college, marriage, or the draft. One other choice was to be a CO (conscientious objector). Several young Amish men from northern Indiana chose that route and were assigned to work duty at Bronson. Senior students Diana Dwan and Marian DeFeyter enlisted in the U.S. Army and spent tours of duty in Vietnam.

THE SIXTIES ERA

Diana Dwan Poole '67

Diana Dwan Poole[1], Class of 1967, was one of 10,000 women who served in Vietnam. Eight thousand of them were nurses. When Dwan was a senior in nursing school, an army recruiter visited, offering a salary, rank, and a chance to live, ". . . anywhere I wanted. I wanted to go to San Francisco and I needed the money to pay my senior year tuition."

Although Dwan had a stereotypical image of women in the military, she was impressed with the petite recruiter who encouraged her along with Bronson classmates Marian DeFeyter and Sandra Sievers to join the army. The three students enlisted. Immediately after graduation, DeFeyter and Dwan drove to Fort Sam Houston in Texas for basic training, then on to Walter Reed Hospital in Washington, D.C., and Letterman Hospital in San Francisco, respectively. Dwan and DeFeyter never communicated with each other again, though they both had tours of duty in Vietnam.

> The day JFK was assassinated, Jeanne Teusink pounded on my door to wake me. I'd worked nights . . .Watching live on TV, Jack Ruby being shot.
>
> ***Gail Taylor Wilson '64***
>
> When President Kennedy was shot, the bus ride back to Bronson was in silence punctuated with sobs.
>
> ***Mary Ann Fink Rebert '66***
>
> Our class was at WMU studying in the anatomy and physiology lab when we got the news. Then we went "home" to Truesdale Hall and huddled around the TV and learned the details. We experienced the loss together as a "family."
>
> ***Helen Sheperd '66***
>
> The saddest event occurred during my senior year on November 22, 1963, when news came of President Kennedy's assassination. I was in the community health rotation, working in the clinics in the Harding Building.
>
> ***Kay Cook Hanson '64***

Dwan spent her first two army years serving at Letterman Hospital. Twice she received orders to ship out for Vietnam. Twice she refused, since women were not required to serve in combat areas, "The third time around, my younger brother had received a low draft number. I knew that no two members of the same family could serve in combat so I went. I also realized I would be missing out on a big chunk of history. I volunteered."

"I was in San Francisco during the hippie, Haight-Ashbury days. When I volunteered for Vietnam, all of my friends suddenly weren't my friends anymore. I took a lot of crap for getting involved in a political war. I felt it was okay, however, because I wasn't going to carry a gun, and I was going to put the boys back together again." Just days later, Dwan disembarked from a military transport in Qui Nhon, where she would spend 12 hours a day, seven days a week, on duty for the next year and a half. "When I arrived, everyone knew I was fresh from the states. I walked into a war clothed in my dress uniform and heels," she said.

Her captain status, at 23 years old, made her the head nurse, first in an orthopedic unit during her first year, and then, upon volunteering for a second tour of duty in Vietnam, in charge of a casualty receiving and trauma unit, supervising the staff nurses who were younger and had less rank, medical corpsmen, and patients.

One of Dwan's first patients was a seven-year old who told her his detached foot was in his boot and then asked if she could sew it back on. "I thought he was kidding, until I looked into his boot. It was then I decided that I could deal with most anything," she said. But she internalized the shock of all the human devastation committed to her care.

Injured soldiers came straight from the field to her unit, still in their uniforms and their amputated limbs lying on top of their bodies. The most difficult situation of all was triaging—those who were expected to die were placed in the corner and screened from view, "We had no time even to hold their hands." This scenario occurred day after day, 75 times a day. "I put it out of my mind. After a while, I didn't hear the mortars falling in the hills surrounding the hospital." In spite of the constant threat of death, Dwan said morale among American soldiers remained high, and at 23 Captain Dwan grew up quickly.

"I made myself tough. All of my nurses thought I was hard because I refused to let them cry in front of the men. Those boys were dealing with enough. They didn't need to see the people in charge around them falling apart too." She said she only fell apart once during her time in Vietnam:

> "I was called and asked if I knew the men in the Medivac helicopter," she said. "I told them they were all my buddies and

> that we had been partying together the night before. That's when I was asked to identify the bodies. They had been shot down and burned by the Viet Cong. I didn't cry then, either. I just started to shake all over. I was given a shot and put to bed for the rest of the day."

When, in 1971, she returned from her Vietnam service, Dwan faced casual or disbelieving attitudes, "On a subconscious level it bothers me." She has suffered the nightmares characteristic of severe post-traumatic stress disorder (PTSD). Recently she participated in a research project that explored the impact of PTSD on nurses who practiced during wartime—a continuing study by the Veterans Administration and Harvard Medical School. PTDS has been studied extensively in combat troops, but its effect on women who were on the ground and experienced the same condition was initially ignored. When others listened and had empathy for the horrendous toll of war on young people on the military front lines and civilians in its way, healing often came, so Dwan Poole tells her story.

Marian DeFeyter Chavez '67

Marian DeFeyter brought to mind that all of the nursing students received frequent recruitment brochures from the armed services. She filled out the request-for-more-information form on one and sent it back. She was at the Kalamazoo State Hospital when she was told that she had a phone call. She couldn't imagine who might call her at this location. It was an army recruiter from Detroit, saying that she was coming to Kalamazoo and would like to meet with DeFeyter, even though DeFeyter tried to convince the recruiter that she had changed her mind and was not interested in an army nurse career. The persistent recruiter won, however, and made an appointment to meet with her. DeFeyter brought two of her classmates to the appointment with her, Diana Dwan and Sandra Sievers. All three enlisted, though later Sievers was allowed out of the commitment due to a family illness. The other two new graduates drove to Fort Sam Houston together, then were assigned to different army hospitals.

It was an exciting first year for DeFeyter who was assigned to a recovery room unit at Walter Reed in Washington D.C. Rioting over civil rights was rampant, and Martin Luther King and Robert Kennedy were assassinated. She saw many government and army officials, to name a few: Senator Robert Kennedy before his death, past-president Dwight D. Eisenhower, Maime Eisenhower, Richard Nixon, and WWII General McCullough who was a patient on her ward. She also cared for many people returning from Vietnam.

> We were at the State Hospital when RFK and Dr. King were shot, and so I remember it even more vividly.
> ***Carolyn Tennant Farthing '69***

Vietnam was the destination of her second tour of duty from October 1968 to September 1969. She was assigned to the 71st Evacuation Hospital at Pleiku in a recovery/intensive care unit. The army had constructed the hospital—nothing like an American hospital existed. Most of the patients were G.I.s, but the army staff also took care of Vietnamese civilians and even the Viet Cong on occasion. They likewise fed the Vietnamese families who came to the hospital with their wounded relatives who often slept on mats in the hallways.

DeFeyter recalled caring for a pregnant woman with shrapnel in her abdomen. Although she died, her baby lived and was cared for to eventually be sent home with relatives. DeFeyter also remembered a G.I. who constantly wrote messages to the nurses with the name of his hometown on them. This bit of information stuck in her mind. He had lost his left arm, and had a fractured leg and mandible. Back in the states in later years, when he was interviewed on TV, DeFeyter wrote to him. He wrote back to thank her for the care that she had given him.

DeFeyter did not sign up for another tour of duty. She served her two years as promised when she enlisted, moved back to Michigan, practiced in Paw Paw at

Lakeview Hospital for a short time, and then accepted a position at St. John's Hospital in Detroit.

CHANGING TIMES NATIONALLY AND LOCALLY

Civil rights issues embroiled the South on what seemed like another planet, while John Glenn put the U.S.A. in orbit. Dr. Kildare and Ben Casey were popularizing medicine on TV and, "We did the twist."

Kay Cook Hanson recalled that she and her classmates weren't exactly role models for healthy habits, with continuous sleep deprivation and poor stress management. It was a smoker's era. "Unfortunately, many of the instructors and doctors smoked, but not while lecturing, thank God. We had to tolerate smoking everywhere—patients, doctors, nurses, families, and our classmates—almost everyone then. The medical profession still has a way to go on this subject."

Chapel was no longer a required student activity. Students went to work without formal prayers and blessings. Some joined KXI, Kappa Chi Iota, a Christian-focused nursing student society, to meet their spiritual needs. Most were grateful not to have one more daily commitment, though the reflective time chapel afforded may well have been one of the keys for self care and comfort.

> My roommate, Jan Johnson, and I raced downstairs to the TV room each time John Glenn was to orbit the Earth. We were both fascinated by the space program.
>
> ***Gail Taylor Wilson '64***
>
> "Dr. Kildare" was the show to watch, and I had started to embroider, and had made two sets of pillowcases, each in three weeks. So I decided I needed a bigger project. I bought a blue and white quilt with a cross-stitch design, which took me five years to finish, and it's on my bed right now.
>
> ***Linda Wigent Burr '63***

Women Who Gave and Gave and Gave

The Bronson Methodist Hospital Auxiliary, dedicated women who continued the White Cross Guild work and a slender Methodist connection, provided hours of volunteer service. In December 1960, they gave their 1957 pledge of $25,000 to the hospital building fund. The money was destined to pay for the tunnel that connected the hospital to Truesdale Hall.[2] Working as volunteers without wages, the ladies were managing a fairly lucrative gift shop. Coffers grew until the hospital decided it would manage the gift shop, taking away one of the best auxiliary funding mechanisms and great support from the community! Auxiliary responded directly to hospital requests and all proceeds benefited Bronson.

The Nurses Guild of the BMH Auxiliary gifted two silver tea services to the students and held a Valentine tea at Truesdale Hall, a newsworthy event in 1963.[3] The tea sets and a silver punch bowl were used for receptions over the next 20 years.

Finances

Hospital financing mechanisms shifted from the church, philanthropists, and direct fee-for-service payers to health insurance from large business employers and taxpayers via the government's health plan. Major church donations must have slowly dissipated somewhere in the 1950s, along with required student chapel attendance. Third-party payer expansion provided insurance benefits for some working men, women, and their families. Medicare and Medicaid legislation of 1965 was meant to complete the benefit-for-all, illness-care package covering those without employee benefits: the elderly and the poor. Medicare became effective in July 1966 and Medicaid, six months later. Gaps still existed for the working poor and their children without access to the insurance benefit or government entitlement or church donations, a situation that has not changed in 40 years.

Government planners underestimated the numbers of people who were without access to health care because of its high costs. Medicare and Medicaid opened the hospital and physicians' office doors to some Americans living with chronic illnesses. They were prepared to treat acute and chronic disease, not to offer paths toward health promotion, disease prevention, and self-health management. No one predicted the burden of suffering and financial expense due to a system that gave incredible power to one group of providers, the dominant medical culture, with its focus on treatment of the sick, including high tech diagnostics and expensive hospitalization involving surgical and medical care. Public health department budgets limped along with resources mainly aimed toward prevention of the spread of communicable diseases, with less attention to healthy lifestyle development or to pollution and a growing toxic environment that fed expensive illness care.

Nationwide, private industry was recognizing the impact of the cost of healthcare. Company executives began to encourage employees to participate in preventive health maintenance programs and to develop healthy lifestyles, in the effort to decrease the cost of providing medical care for illness and injury. They also monitored the employee population exposed to hazardous or toxic materials for related health changes. Employee health services staffed primarily by nurses, and assisted by other healthcare professionals administered these programs.

The imbalance in the system was simply not recognized and no one anticipated the devastating impact it would have on society over the next 40 years. As a response, hospital clinics for "medically indigent patients" increased from one orthopedic service, established in 1945, to eight services in 1960. These clinics also served as part of the training ground for nursing students, interns, and residents,[4] who gave back service to citizens in return for the support of medical education tax dollars.

The paperwork associated with the new federally organized programs overwhelmed the hospitals' business departments. Expected payment reimbursements were slow and were considered to be inadequate compared to rising costs. Not all employers could conceptualize how employee health insurance coverage could be folded into their budgets while still maintaining a perceived level of adequate profits.

Rising costs were a concern, but ways to reframe health care to a model less costly than the dominant medical model were not. Hospitalization, medications, and high-tech invasive procedures were expensive when the medical care was paid for by the young, third-party payer system. Less expensive options, supporting self-care and self-health management as the first line of defense, could have helped everyone to recognize cause and effect. More medical care was not better and often did not make a difference in untreatable cases or in end-of-life outcomes. Medicine and hospital care were not universally connected to healthy outcomes; instead the philosophy was that every life could be saved if every possible effort and resource were devoted to the cause. The medical community tried to fix the unfixable and remove the human mortality factor. Pediatric practices were an exception. They emphasized well-child visits with immunizations and paid attention to growth and development patterns in children. Their approach, however, did not seem to influence the overall high-tech preference in medicine. High technology and hospital expansion went hand in hand.

Public concern was noted in a *Kalamazoo Gazette* article touting increasing costs[5] followed by an editorial[6] asking, "Why can a for-profit nursing home operate with six dollars per patient day while hospitals need $20?"

> The new minimum adult rate will be $20 a day for ward accommodations, $22 for semi-private and $25 for private. The rate changes will finance salary increases and additional fringe benefits for employees. The salary changes have been made necessary by the constantly increasing cost of living, while the additional fringe benefits will make hospital personnel benefits more comparable with those offered in the industry. [7]

It looked like the beginning of a vicious cycle. Unaffordable costs continued to fuel local discussions with Mr. Finch, the newly named Bronson administrator, who defended rising budgets. He pointed out a public incongruency—its desire for state-of-the-art technology, ready at a moment's notice, for no increase in cost.[8] He was right. People wanted a paternalistic system with quick cures, not advice about living healthier lifestyles. The price was high in terms of public health and dollars.

Hospitalization, technological advances, and an ever-growing number of discrete pharmaceuticals helped drive the dominant medical model of illness care. Hospitalization was the favored way physicians managed patients, and it was becoming more expensive every day. The number of older adults who could be hospitalized with Medicare funding required hospital expansion or new ways to practice health care in the community. Less invasive approaches to disease management were not reimbursed. In retrospect, we were heading into an expensive high-tech system imbalance with non-invasive, high-touch care being seen as a thing of the past. The latter was no longer the right approach to take, like shooting oneself in the foot. Resources continued to pour into hospital expansion, fueled by medical-practice domination of health care and the public's love for increasing technology.[9] Given the American mind-set, the demise of non-invasive care was the only possible outcome. Most nurses were employed in hospitals where the focus often was an extension of invasive medical care.

Demise of Private Duty Nursing Practice

Private-duty nurses needed more money, too, to offset inflation and the need to pay their own Social Security taxes, income taxes, and benefits not covered by employers. A $17–19 dollar a day increase was announced by the 43-member, local private-duty nurses organization.[10] Its numbers were dwindling. Few private-duty nurses were hired for either home care or hospitalized patients. It was a rarity to see a private-duty nurse in the hospital. Reliance on a technologically skilled, hospital-financed RN staff was increasing, and expert clinical judgment required on-going continuing education and increasing years of practice for nurses and physicians.

Job opportunities were plentiful for nurses. It was easy to be hired into challenging, hospital short-staffed work situations. Another nursing shortage became obvious—one seemed to occur in cycles of every 15 to 20 years. The shortage meant that students carried a fair share of the load, while being held accountable to professional nursing practice standards with guidance from their RN mentors. The nursing deficits continued to fuel delegation of traditional nursing functions to unlicensed personnel. For example, one concern focused on whether unlicensed personnel could be adequately trained to safely give medications under the supervision of registered nurses, licensed physicians, or dentists. The practice was often sanctioned in agencies managing the care of chronically ill patients in extended care and in the armed services but not in civilian acute-care settings. This nursing concern caught the attention of the public and Michigan legislators.[11] Administering medications required expert clinical judgment beyond the technical skills.

William C. Perdew, DD, Dies—Methodist Rescue Ends

Tribute to Dr. Perdew was paid by the Bronson Board of Trustees after his acute heart attack and untimely death on November 24, 1960, "The nurses' home . . . was a special project of his and reflected his interest and concern in the student nurses who trained at Bronson."[12] He was the last Methodist minister to serve as the chief hospital administrator. His interaction with late 1950 nursing students, in the author's memory, was limited, typically involving a handshake and presentation of diplomas at graduation. Chapel was no longer part of his schedule, although a chaplain was hired to maintain the Methodist connection. Before his death, Dr. Perdew had moved into an administrative role that would become familiar—less contact with the nursing staff and patients—less of a family approach. The Bronson family was no different than traditional American families. We were losing our sense of interdependence and connection.

Dr. Perdew had been appointed as superintendent in 1943, following Dr. Alfred E. Way. During 17 years of Dr. Perdew's leadership, the hospital grew from a 140-bed capacity and a net worth estimated at $900,000, to 310 beds and a net worth of $8,758,000. Women remained the hospital's strong working force, representing 85-90 percent of all employees; this predominance has never changed. Expansion planning continued to be the focus of the administrator, favoring medical care, not nursing, self-care or self-health management. Health insurance and government plans focused dollars on medical management and hospitalization.

First Sectarian Administrator Brings A Business Approach

Daniel Finch became the first administrator with a graduate degree in hospital administration, assuming his role in June 1961. Nationally, managing hospitals was a big business and, at Bronson too, it was no longer a family affair or a religious calling. In a fall speech to the Percolator Club, Mr. Finch pointed out:

> . . . today hospitals must compete with other industries and businesses . . . for employees. They must pay the going rate for comparable jobs and they must provide competitive fringe benefits. This is somewhat of a new concept for hospitals. It is the main reason that 70 percent of each operating dollar goes for wages and benefits, leaving very little for capital expenses.[13]

Hospital nursing wages never compared to the job demands; many nursing hours were required to care for over 300 hospitalized patients. Capital fund-raising campaigns provided matching dollars for the federal Hill–Burton Act that continued to fuel hospital growth.

The School of Nursing's operating expenses for the year ending March, 1960, were reported to be $219,887,[14] a labor value when considering the numbers of faculty and students involved in around-the-clock direct patient care! Additionally, most of the Bronson graduates were immediately hired to support hospital expansion and remedy high turnover rates.

Miss Virginia McPhail Becomes Director of Nurses

Virginia McPhail, Class of 1948, was the third Bronson graduate to become a nursing service director in January 1962. She had served as a Bronson instructor starting in 1949 and returned in 1960 with a Master of Science in Nursing from the University of Colorado. Her title was assistant director of nursing education, and she was the only nurse Wylie knew with a MSN.

She was small in stature, and her quiet voice and demeanor fit her tiny frame. Classes she taught covered medical-surgical nursing, including pathophysiology, and she gave assignments on the content and process of interpersonal relationships (IPR). Some of the class of 1962 called her "IPR Ginny." Wylie loved the knowledge that she shared and enjoyed her organized lectures, feeling comfortable and safe in her classroom, although she couldn't say her enamored view matched those of most of classmates. McPhail respected and liked her and in return she gained Wylie's respect. Hours of study paid off with good grades and a sense of security that built a healthy relationship with this instructor.

Virginia McPhail quickly advanced to the director of nursing position with the 1961 resignation and departure of Mary B. Anderson, and in 1966 she became a hospital assistant administrator, the only woman to hold this rank for a tenure of several years.

CHANGES IN NURSING EDUCATION

Changes in nursing education brought a degree of autonomy to the school on October 17, 1966,[15] when Mrs. Weber's title changed from an associate director of education who reported to the director of nursing services to that of an independent school of nursing director with the school as its own hospital department. Weber's relationship with the director of nursing service became one of partnership. Such change was required to maintain the desired National League for Nursing (NLN) Accreditation that brought status and qualified the school for participation in government grant programs and entry into degree-granting collegiate nursing education. The expectation was that students would no longer be counted in nurse-staff ratios to meet NLN accreditation standards. It took years to actually separate student learning needs from hospital staffing plans.

A shift in educational balance between theoretical knowledge and experiential clinical practice was in process. Still the 1960s students often were assigned to 40-hour practice weeks on all shifts, including weekends, plus class time. When students had an unscheduled day, they often worked extra hours for pay, juniors earning $1.00 and seniors $2.00 per hour for an eight-hour shift. Most students came from working class families and contributed to payment of their educational expenses by, what they called, "working for pay," as a way to differentiate the role as paid staff from their nursing care that was the clinical practice part of the curriculum.

Movement toward a different hospital educational system continued for three decades, with educators trying to decide how to balance theory within academia and experiential on-the-job training. Were nurses being educated or trained? "Training" became a dirty word. A dog could be trained. Nurses were educated for professional practice roles.

Formal Orientation to Staff Nursing

Less than a year after Wylie became a staff nurse, the first Bronson employee orientation was held on June 3, 1963, " . . . designed primarily to acquaint new employees with the hospital."[16] Hospital orientation and continuing education for nurses mushroomed over the next four decades. Students spent more time learning nursing theory and numerous ways to deliver patient care, not simply the Bronson way. Nursing service administrators, directors, managers, and staff nurses complained about unprepared novice graduates who required more and more orientation. New technologies required new kinds of clinical judgment.

Continuing education programs followed the first employee orientation. Nursing staff supplemented their nursing expertise and general medical knowledge with specialty medical care, increasing physician-extender expectations. Nurses needed to constantly grow their competencies to manage complex clinical judgments. They needed to know what they could do to support a healthy healing path for the patient and when to call physicians into action to help manage "turns for the worse." Nurses diagnosed impending patient complications. Expert nursing surveillance became second nature over time but never seemed to be acknowledged unless an untoward outcome occurred. Best patient outcomes resulted from expert nurses who identified impending adverse patient events and were able to avert a patient loss. Wylie can't remember staff nurses and their managers ever saying, "Hey look at us. We saved the day for X patients today, this week, this month, this year. . . ." They were the ones who called physicians into action. Sometimes it seemed as if nurses were only recognized when things went wrong, an issue of accountability without authority to make needed system and cultural changes in hospital practice.

First Intensive Care Units and Outpatient Clinic Expansion

Services and parking lots increased. The Harding School was purchased for $900,000 and remodeled for outpatient clinics and a nursing and medical library. The U.S. Department of Health, Education and Welfare granted $102,685 of the expected $476,000 remodeling cost.[17]

Expansion plans detailed a future decade of construction priorities that were presented at the Kalamazoo City Commission on March 16, 1960. New ground-floor service facilities, construction of a 220-car parking lot built on the site where the Kalamazoo School Administration building had been razed, a remodeled Harding

Building, and four more patient-care floors (seventh to tenth floor), were intended to increase patient capacity from 310 to 500 beds.[18]

A 1964 Bronson–Borgess expansion fund drive provided money for Bronson to add a seventh floor with 50 more beds,[19] and a critical-care unit opened in the fall of 1967.[20] The eighth, ninth and tenth floors were added immediately and were opened in 1968.

A cobalt unit was added to the Radiology Department for the increasing demand in treating cancer and other diseases, with an expectation that the Hill–Burton Act would help pay the cost.[21] The first southwest Michigan hemodialysis unit to care for people with chronic kidney failure (end-stage renal disease) opened in a six-room suite of Wesley Hall. Patricia McDonald, 1961 Bronson graduate, supervised that unit.

Pediatrics could house 61 children, including 12 premature babies, in the four-room "Preemie" Nursery. A new pediatric building was to be added in 1967, with an adolescent wing that would be constructed on the south side of the existing hospital. This addition was to be financed by a cash gift from Mr. and Mrs. Donald S. Gilmore and funds other than the joint Bronson–Borgess fund drive.[22] Cedar Street, between John and Pine, was relocated about 300 feet south in the process.[23]

Technological Advances Accompanied Caring Losses

Where was caring in the 1960s version of intensive care? It took on a different appearance at first glance, with monster-like machines intimidating to patients and families if they were not familiar with high-tech treatment. Intensive care units distanced families from the plan of care, as well as isolated groups of caregivers from each other. It seemed as if staff rarely left the units, even for breaks. Ability to build caring relationships with families and include them in decision-making was often limited.

What were caregivers thinking of? How could we ever think that separating patients from their families was part of a caring, total patient-care practice model or healing environment, especially at times of most critical, life-threatening injury or illness? All of us needed the support of each other, but it was hard to come by. Nurses helped with the inception of intensive-care units. The question remains, why were families not considered to be part of the healing process? It has taken 40 years to bring their involvement back into the caring environment, and at times the value of family presence as equally important to invasive technology is still questioned.

Administrators were insulated from clinical practitioners and practitioners from families. Patients were to be treated objectively (as objects?). Objective caring did not feel right to Wylie. But, she couldn't remember having the courage to suggest a model of care inclusive of family. Staff could not do for the patient what needed to be done by a supportive family. Cognitive dissonance resulted. We cared and did our best, inconsistently with healing family inclusion and often without. Wylie remembered times when she felt uncomfortable expressing warmth, which a supervisor would view as an unacceptable response. It was not viewed as objective. This quote from an in-house publication captures the family exclusion policy:

> At times it is necessary to keep the patient a long period of time and the family is informed of the patient's progress [from a distance] in order to prevent them from worrying. The family is also informed of the strict rules applying to visitors.... Only in extremely critical situations [this meaning expected death] will the family be allowed special consideration, then only for a short time. Routine visiting hours are permitted at seven P.M., and only two people for five minutes.[24]

It took years to regain a sense of family importance, especially at the end of life. Dying has a more honored place, no longer seen as failure on the part of the healthcare team but more as a fact, and Mark Twain's comment that nobody gets out [of life] alive seems to be more of an accepted reality. Only major system changes could integrate family to a level in which family-centered care could be provided but the sixties' culture still could not allow for that result.

LITTLE RECOGNITION OF NURSING INNOVATIONS

Nursing qualities of humility, loyalty, and martyrdom, along with a medically dominant model, kept both big and small nursing ideas and innovations quiet. Though for different reasons, Florence Nightingale had faced opposition when bringing her revolutionary healing and life-saving ideas to light during the nineteenth century. She had physician friends to carry her healthcare message to Parliament and into hospital circles.

Seemingly insignificant changes often brought improved care and monetary savings at Bronson, and nurses quietly tell stories about changes they made. Their ideas were hidden treasures, but digging to find them was hard and deep, stories most often not found, not told, or even recognized for the gift they were—passed on in the sixties to dominant authority, not only physicians, but to a growing hospital administration becoming more separate from the medical model and more aligned with third-party payment systems.

Kathryn VanBruggen '40, received two innovation awards, reported in the December 1963 *Catalyst*. One was a patient convenience, removing the curb to street level for wheelchair access and egress at the hospital exit to the visitors' parking lot from the Harding Building. "Patients can now be discharged from that location relieving the congestion at the emergency entrance." The other, to prevent infections, was the use of nylon pull-string cords on isolation bags to make them easier to use and better to isolate contaminated contents from patients, nurses, and laundry staff.

Helen W. Frazier, RN, became $50 richer for the padded arm board that she designed to increase patient comfort and save the hospital an estimated $1,800 a year. The shorter ". . . padded arm board allows a patient to move his arm during intravenous injection therapy . . . [it] is covered with reusable toweling that's easily cleaned and much easier to use"[25] than the longer, unpadded one that required wrapping with towels.

REFLECTIONS ON BEGINNING NURSING CAREERS

Reasons for being a nurse did not change in the sixties. Many always wanted to be nurses and weren't sure why, while others were exposed to personal illness themselves or the illness of a family member, or they followed a role model.

In the ninth grade Jackie Wylie had explored the idea of becoming a physician. My class had the opportunity to job-shadow professionals and I chose to follow a physician—I don't remember his name or anything about his practice. He talked me out of pursuing a physician career. He told me that medicine would be too hard for a woman, its hours too long, leaving no time for family, *etc.* His assessment made sense to me. The curriculum looked like it took forever and I could not imagine being in college that many years after high school, although my mother said the family would help me. She wasn't impressed with the physician's opinion, but I was. I figured he knew more than my mother did so I chose a nursing program. It looked like a program I could manage, a more realistic goal than medical school. I discovered that, though the curriculum might have been shorter, the hours were long, and often there was little time for family, no different than in medicine.

Suffering with Patients

As a student, I never overcame my discomfort at seeing fear, pain and grief in patients' and their families' eyes, in every body movement and in their words. When patients suffered, I suffered. That sense of connectedness and empathy for patients and families often left me feeling inadequate as the caregiver. Never could I give enough to make it all better. I observed less suffering in obstetrics and the operating room—staff nurse positions that held promise when I graduated in late August of 1962. I believed I could manage caring for families giving birth or people under a form of anesthesia, the best form of pain management in my way of thinking then. Birthing babies was a healthy, happy event with short-lived discomfort and only occasional complications or heart-breaking outcomes.

My first love was family birthing, but I found the staff too intimidating, so I chose the operating room instead, with nurse mentors who seemed more empathic to students and new graduate nurses. By accepting a position in the operating room, assured of a team approach and just one patient at a time, I felt fairly safe and cared for and, in turn, I could comfortably care for others. The smallest team was composed of a circulating nurse, scrub nurse, nurse anesthetist or anesthesiologist, and the surgeon.

New graduates were expected to be competent, autonomous practitioners, able to manage patients, technology, and delegation to unlicensed staff. The newcomers worked the off-shifts and weekends when the least expert support was available. This unrealistic expectation was one of the reasons for high turnover rates and movement into less stressful work environments; it was called "burnout." For some novice nurses, the experience was the beginning of post-traumatic stress disorders that would remind them in following days and years of what it felt like when one was expected to do the impossible, to meet unrealistic cure goals when death was inevitable. Healing sometimes occurred when mortality was accepted and caring for each other took place.[26]

It took years for me to accept the quote, "To every thing there is a season, a time to be born and a time to die. . . ." We did not have the life or death control or impact that we were taught to believe we possessed. Not everyone could be rescued. Caring relationships were what made the difference in the ability of patients, families, nurses and others to accept our inevitable mortality. It didn't matter how many costly medications we gave or how long we resuscitated the dying patient, death was inevitable. Knowing that miracles do happen, we always held out for what, most of the time, was not meant to be. I stepped further away from the suffering that came more from being deprived of the inclusiveness of relationships than anything else, by moving out of the hospital and into nursing education, still in the operating room as the School of Nursing instructor.

Mutuality and Caring Saved Us

As a student, I relived the caring moments and outcomes at the end of each shift, and my reflections produced mixed feelings of joy, anxiety, fear, and grief over outcome possibilities. Caring moments kept student nurses going. Sometimes patients or families sent little notes to let us know what our care meant to them. A young woman, for example, who miscarried and did not appear to have a support system—no one came to visit. Mainly, I was simply present for her, accepting her plight, empathizing without words, not asking questions. After her discharge, I received a thank you for the special care. I wasn't sure at that time what I had done.

Patients were generally supportive and often demonstrated their care for students, prefaced by comments like, "You remind me of my daughter . . . my grandmother . . . my cousin," *etc.* We cared for them and, in turn, we could do no wrong. They cared for us in reciprocal ways. Patients would intervene when a critical instructor or nurse supervisor made rounds to check on our progress; they shared their praise or chided the instructor not to be "too hard" on us. Patients watched over us, and it was mutual caring that benefited each side of the caring equation. Everyone felt better for being in a healthy relationship, though I always thought the instructors were skeptical about patients' positive evaluations of our work.

I learned caring through positive and negative examples—what to do and what not to do. Often I observed situations in which patients or students were treated without a sense of caring concern for feelings or beliefs. I vowed never to treat another as if his or her feelings did not matter or influence outcome overall. We had responsibility without authority. Still, we were able to make a major impact on patient outcomes with our caring presence, our strong desire to heal, and learned technical competencies. Patients told us so.

Many times I attempted to will patients to live or, at least, not to die during my shift, more for my benefit than theirs. It took time to learn to cope with such gravity and, for some reason, I thought that it would be my fault if they died—very egocentric of me when witnessing the end of life. I was a product of that sixties environment and learned the lesson well—we failed whenever a patient died. The message was a part of the powerful, informal, unwritten curriculum. We were led to believe that we had more control over life and death than we really had.

I made a vow at the time of enrollment, "I will finish this program if I hate it or die trying." It was a negative statement, in retrospect, but one that caused me to never consider quitting, even at the possibility of failure. To prevent that outcome, I studied and worked hard to please instructors, nurse managers, other staff, and patients.

It worked! When feelings of fear and anxiety overrode logical thought, my vow kicked in. I had to tough it out. The program was structured, and the rules were clear. I didn't have to like them, just abide by them or not get caught in any infraction. Honestly, I cannot remember intentionally breaking the rules. Students were dismissed at times for what seemed to be small rule infractions and I didn't want to be dispensed with in that fashion.

Actually, a year of college had prepared me well for the Bronson course of study—its science courses at Western Michigan University combined with nursing theory and practice at Bronson. I had the advantage of taking some courses twice because of my previous year at U of M and Western. It never occurred to me to ask for transfer credit, and I don't recall being asked to submit a transcript on the application or in an interview. Maybe my earlier "C" grades testified to the fact that a second time around was healthy. Most students entered Bronson immediately after graduation from high school, and it was a struggle for them to succeed. All class members were enrolled in every course; no one was exempt. In retrospect, the repeated classes strengthened my base knowledge and allowed time to study unfamiliar concepts missed the first time. The schedule was busy! I watched classmates fight their way through their first weeks of transition: homesick, overwhelmed by it all, and in a kind of anticlimactic distress. I secretly felt grateful for the preceding year of preparation.

Friendships formed quickly among those who gained strength through connection. Roommates and suitemates bonded or, if that didn't happen, sought out those with whom to bond, care, and commiserate. We cared for each other very well. Self-care and care for peers happened out of our mutual human needs.

The transition for me, from some romanticized images of who nurses were and what they did to the reality of human and hospital suffering and smells never to be forgotten, was not an easy one. Romanticized notions did not come from my only overnight hospital stay, a tonsillectomy experience when I felt lonely, in pain, and couldn't wait to go home. I can't remember any nurses who were especially endeared to me. One other miserable childhood experience related to a school visit by the public health nurse who checked heads and bodies for lice and ringworm. I lived in fear of contracting ringworm and having my head shaved as happened to some of the girls in my grade-school class.

Expectations at the School of Nursing were clear: study, pass exams, and show up on time both for class and clinical practice to care for patients. All attention was focused on that end. We were a homogenous group—late adolescent to young adult. We lived in close quarters and followed similar daily patterns on which we built a structured relationship in accepting what was to come, and patterns served us well. We often referred to the residence hall as the convent.

Caring, Comforting, and Objectivity

Clinical practice responsibilities in the early 1960s continued to be the learning venue it was in earlier decades. Caring and scary experiences on patient-care units went hand in hand. Senior students functioned as team leaders, having had occasional management experiences as early as the freshman second semester and later in a senior course in management. Supervisory assignments were commonly expected for senior students, and we felt slighted if given the lesser responsibility of direct patient care. Registered nurse supervisors were readily available on weekdays but not so plentiful on evening, and night shifts and on weekends. Often the house supervisor was the expert link for students and novice graduates. We called her when we could not manage impending patient complications. One instructor sometimes covered the whole hospital for the evening or night shift, and often she was not readily available to help when a crisis occurred. Often we were grateful to have less instructor supervision since they were more watchful and critical of student practice than house supervisors and staff nurses, or so we believed.

Staff-nurse mentorship was the expectation—some were kind and excellent teachers. With that support, the shift went well. Nothing could go wrong with kind guiding hands, hearts, and minds. Others were less than thrilled to be preceptors, making it painful to ask a question or for help. Because Wylie needed to strengthen her confidence, often she would dare to ask even if the query solicited a condescending stare. Wylie always wondered if the less supportive preceptors had been reincarnated. Or perhaps they had sprung fully formed from the head of Zeus and had not gone through the clinical-judgment learning curve.

Years later it occurred to me that most patients recovered no matter what they endured. Healing came from within, an internal process, and God was on everyone's side: the patient, student, nursing staff, and physician. If only earlier I had internalized Florence Nightingale's philosophy. We students all learned and most often recovered from stressful experiences. Flashbacks to past traumatic experiences were not uncommon for nurses—we lived with that reality—probably not different for all health-care providers who found themselves supporting people in crises.

Still, objectivity was an expectation that seemed to go beyond one's ability to objectify intimate caring experiences. Feelings were not to be shown, and Wylie never could understand how to be caring and objective—they seemed so dichotomous. She realized that personal boundary recognition within the nurse's role was important, but caring could not be objectified. How to be both caring and able to make a logical clinical decision seemed intertwined. Options and choices for best decision making resided within the context of family and caregiver biases.

Freshmen began their studies in late August or early September, similar to the local college schedule, and seniors graduated three years later, also in September, unlike college schedules. Seniors couldn't graduate in the spring since they were needed to cover summer staffing hours until the juniors became the new seniors and the school year cycle repeated itself. Basically, school was in session seven days a week, 24 hours a day, with 32–40 hours weekly of nursing practice for junior and senior students. Their minds and hands were needed for patient care and frontline management. Freshmen often worked split shifts to cover labor intensive times, like 7:00–10:00 A.M. morning routines, *i.e.*, to monitor vital signs and help with breakfast and baths, then 4:00–7:00 P.M. evening care, and an entire shift on weekends.

> Demands placed on us by the instructors were strict and detail oriented, and this rigor was very important in health care. The innumerable hours in clinical experience, working the evening or night shifts, and being team leaders prepared us for the real world of nursing. We were ready for our professional responsibilities. I have always been able to organize my workload, a skill among many that I learned at Bronson.
>
> ***—Linda Wigent Burr '63***

On the lighter side, little gold safety pins were a favorite gift from upperclassmen big sisters to little-sister freshmen on arrival—1095 days in all—one pin for each day at Bronson. One was removed each day from the golf-tee pegboard on our individual study room walls—a daily milestone acknowledged. The last three months the little gold pins adorned student uniforms—90 of them to count down to that final day when we celebrated by roaming the hospital hallways and inviting classmates, staff, and physicians to sign our uniforms in most interesting places.

> I'll never forget arriving at Bronson on September 11, 1960, and the beautiful, almost new Truesdale Hall. It came with a price—the blue cards—signing out and in for three solid years every time I left and returned to the building.
>
> ***Linda Wigent Burr '63***
>
> Our dorm was better than any Western dorm.
>
> ***Kay Cook Hanson '64***

TRUESDALE HALL

The jump in student admissions in 1960 fit with Truesdale Hall bed numbers.[27, 28] Twenty-six students graduated that fall and 84 freshmen were admitted, with a fall total student population enrollment of 189!

It was expected that single students would live at Truesdale Hall. Tuition included room and board. The only married students were a few seniors, although marriage became more common by 1962, a pattern that coincided with the advent of birth control pills. Signing in and out with exact times and following curfew rules matched those of dorm life at many colleges. Truesdale Hall, with its famous tunnel connected to the hospital, kept students out of harms way.

Kay Taylor '68

I toured Truesdale Hall prior to starting school in 1965. I had liked the idea of a roommate, the suite of rooms, and sharing the bathroom with another two-person suite. I was excited about the prospect of having a roomie and suitemates. This attitude was a contradiction in that I'd always shared a room with one or two sisters and sometimes didn't enjoy that kind of togetherness. Having a roommate, however, was to be different!

I stood in utter dismay and disappointment, with some anger, as I saw my room that first day. It was situated at the end of the hall on the first floor and was one of the private rooms! I hadn't been aware that private rooms were available, and thought it was unfair to have been assigned one without having asked about my preference.

I adjusted and by second semester I was in the "suite of my dreams." I enjoyed the friendship of two different roommates and suitemates. I learned to loosen up a bit and greatly appreciated the acceptance of my classmates.

But, as Frances Burke Kakabeeke '66 pointed out,

> It seemed we had a lot of restrictions compared to WMU students. We were in class or working in the hospital all the time. The housemothers would inspect our rooms, we had to sign in and out each time we left or entered the dorm, and needed permission for girlfriends to stay overnight. Our curfew was 10 P.M. on weeknights, 12 midnight on weekends, and once per month at 1:30 A.M. Twelve months constituted the school year with a one-week break in December and two weeks in June. Our classes after freshman year were held on the hospital campus, so then we only interacted with other nursing students and hospital employees. We sang of the school as a "nunnery."

STUDENT NURSE CHOIR

Miss Judy Smith, Class of 1961, was chosen, in competition among nine soloists, to sing obbligato in a 387-voice choir at the Southwestern Michigan Schools of Nursing Choir Festival, held in Lansing, April 22, 1960.[29] The following spring Bronson's 80-voice choir, directed by Mr. Raymond Jolly, participated in the eighth annual Michigan Student Nurse Choral Festival in Muskegon, with co-hosts Hackley Hospital and Mercy Central schools of nursing.[30]

Phyllis Triezenberg Stapert '64

> I have many memories of my days at Truesdale and BMH, but the one I want to share involve the nursing student choir. We had about 65 members and Mary Lou Van Dyke, one of our instructors, was the very capable and fun-oriented director.
>
> Our choir was very active. We went to the annual Student Nurses' Choir Festival in Grand Rapids where we competed with other student nurse choirs. We even placed first, at least one time. We sang at BMH's annual employee's Christmas party. (What good food and good times!) We even appeared once on "Feminine Fancies," a WKZO-TV day program. We always sang many upbeat songs. One began, "Let there be peace on earth and let it begin with me."
>
> Our practice sessions were as much fun as the performances. It was the most enjoyable choir in which I've participated. I wonder how many years this choir was active. It was just one of the many ways we students shared a real togetherness.

STUDENT NURSES ASSOCIATION

A line formed just inside the door of Truesdale Hall, on Jackie Clark's first day in the fall of 1959, as students collected $10 from each newly admitted student. The amount paid for three years of membership in the Michigan State Student Nurses Association (MSSNA), covering dues until graduation. Joining was an expectation, not a choice. Later, when meeting with other nursing schools, they all marveled at Bronson's 100 percent membership. What a wonderful professional achievement! It occurred to me that the reason for our great showing was not all that professional—we didn't have a clue what we were joining when we paid the dues upfront.

Though political and organizational involvement was limited for most students, Mary Jo Rosa '61, was elected vice president and president elect of the MSSNA in 1960, while senior Nancy Peterson '60, became president of the Kalamazoo District and Dixie Ladd '61, chair of membership.

The local district nurses of Michigan Nurses Association celebrated graduation by inviting the senior class to dinner and encouraging them to join with the American Nurses Association. Clark '62 joined, although it did not seem the popular thing to do. Nurses often felt that the dues were too high and the commitment would not pay off for them personally. Apparently they had not listened to JFK's, "Ask not what your country can do for you, ask what you can do for your country."

CURRICULUM

Use of humor was a great outlet. Carolyn Tennant Farthing provided this 1966 poem (*see* sidebar next page) that helps readers quickly know the students' minds. "It was written while taking courses at Western, but not by me and I can't remember who wrote it."

Faith Abel Huizenga '64

> Freshmen orientation was a blur, except for the time I was blindfolded and told to experience various objects related to nursing, one of which was a peanut butter/banana mixture placed in a stainless steel bedpan like the ones used on patient units.
>
> New practice rotations always started with panic and anxiety with my heart pounding and a sleepless night for fear of sleeping past the alarm clock warning and being late to report. On the other side were the joy, excitement and fulfillment when bringing a newborn from the nursery to the thrilled parents.
>
> And what other occupation provided guidelines to good posture and body mechanics with an instructor reminding you to suck in your stomach and tuck in your butt?

The program of studies was almost impossible for even the best students! Admission criteria were designed to admit only students with above-average high school performance, including science and math courses as a basis for the practice of nursing science. It's amazing that masochistic tendencies were not listed as part of the admission criteria. If freshmen year was meant to weed and downsize classes, it succeeded very well. The message was clear—you will probably be out of here in a few months, just another expected failure. Later in the decade, attrition became a weakness and an accreditation issue, not a sign of curriculum excellence but, more simply, of an unrealistic course of study. Mrs. Weber led the faculty in drafting a program that could be attained by the bright, motivated students traditionally admitted to the program.

A Bronson Nurse's Prayer

Now I lay me down to sleep,
My homework piled up
in a heap
If I should die before I wake,
I have these four requests
to make:
Lay my Anatomy book
at my feet,
Tell Dr. Lawrence it's got
me beat.
Lay my Chemistry book
by my hand,
Tell Dr. Stenesh I don't
UNDERSTAND.
Lay my Sociology book
at my side,
Tell Dr. Horton I'm glad
I died.
Lay my Nursing I book
at my head,
Tell Mrs. K. that's why
I'm dead.

—Anonymous

Applications grew throughout the sixties; it was easy to fill classes with qualified applicants. What was the magic number for total enrollment? Eighty-four seats in "Big T," classroom 1, the biggest auditorium-style classroom in Truesdale Hall, determined the number of freshmen, and all fit into one bus on the daily journey to Western for chemistry, anatomy and physiology, sociology, psychology, and nutrition—all first semester courses, and not counting nursing history, theory, laboratory and clinical practice.

Nursing Fundamentals, lecture and lab, led us into hospital assignments by midterm, two weekends on with the third weekend off. "We learned volumes in the Nursing Arts Lab—first how to wash our hands and the importance of doing so—medical asepsis! Yes!" wrote Kay Cook Hanson '64 who is now an infection control nurse at Bronson. "To this day hand washing is still the best way to contain communicable disease—to prevent contamination of whole populations—and we learned to do it without re-contaminating our hands and arms on dirty sink handles."

Linda Ann Wigent Burr '63

Classes were hard, and I was sure I would flunk the first semester. If one course was failed, there was no second chance. Our big sisters, and even Helen Weber, told us that one-third of us would not graduate. The talk made me nervous the entire first semester since our big sisters told us horrifying stories. This intimidation influenced me to be much more supportive and encouraging when I became the "big sister."

I dreaded my chemistry and microbiology labs. My chemistry experiments always failed—now that I've done them a second time, I know my preparation had something to do with that outcome. I could never see anything under the microscope except an oil blob. Dr. Elizabeth Tuller drank water from a glass beaker while lecturing. We went to class at WMU on a "grade school bus." Often I wore my red-striped flannel PJ's under my coat so I could go back to bed when we returned to the dorm. My yellow calico cat in A&P lab was certainly stiff.

Edna Lord and Elizabeth Heneveld, both wore stiffly starched, long-sleeved white uniforms and perfectly polished white shoes. I loved them both, but hated the Communicable Disease course. I remember becoming quite an expert bridge player and was good at the game of hearts. The bridge came in handy on my psychiatric affiliation—thank God I was on the "male side." I never could have tolerated the women, having to help them set their hair and painting their nails while I tried to provide therapeutic communication. The best part of Kalamazoo State Hospital was the home-baked bread. It made great French toast.

I always liked 2 East patients. Pat Hurd, RN, was my idol. I took care of patients in isolation rooms with the iodophore, Wescodyne® solution for decontamination. Mrs. Damvelt checked to be sure that I changed the solution each morning. The patient's china dishes were washed in the bathroom sink, then Wescodyned before being returned to the kitchen.

We used non-disposable equipment, such as glass syringes, needles, and treatment trays, which all required special equipment to wash, package, and re-sterilize. On an Easter Sunday morning, before inserting my first Foley catheter, I contaminated three of them. I was so nervous about performing this procedure, and I didn't put the catheter into the right orifice on the first try. We carried a book with us so that we could be "signed off" on each and every procedure. The nursing instructors were at our elbow at 7:05 A.M., informing us when a special procedure was being performed on a patient (not yours) at the other end of the hall or even on another floor, like 2 West, and how nice it would be if I could add that activity to my morning schedule. All the baths had to be completed by 11:00 A.M., the beds made with the open end of the pillowcase facing away from the open door, and the sheet seams away from the patient's skin. We counted narcotics to the drop.

My OR experience was scheduled during the summer of my junior year. I worked a split shift, 7:00 A.M. until noon and then 3:00–7:00 P.M. I raced up to the roof of Truesdale Hall to tan from noon to three. I had the best tan ever that summer. I read *Hawaii* the week I worked nights in the OR. We had one case the whole week but lots of cleaning and setting up of sterile tables for morning cases.

An Uncommon Curriculum Activity

Writing legislators to protest proposed mental health cuts in Michigan was one skill that students who had affiliated with Kalamazoo State Hospital practiced in the summer of 1960. "We feel that a preventive program and early treatment of mental illness are the answer to the present-day mental health problem and that with such a plan the ultimate cost of institutionalization will be greatly reduced."[31] The students' letters were mentioned in a *Kalamazoo Gazette* story, with commentary by

Dr. Perdew regarding adequate compensation for nurses and other nursing service personnel, as if the state budget cuts would impact remuneration of nurses.

Political activity was not part of the formal curriculum so the lesson in letter writing most likely was seen as a ploy to appeal to the public. It's a skill that may have benefited health care and nurse assertiveness training that still did not exist in the 60s.

COMMENTARY ON INSTRUCTORS

Mary L. Mason was famous for "Nursing the Art of Origami."[32] The Bird of Happiness was her favorite, she explained, " . . . Buddhist priests receive special blessing for their patience every time they fold 1,000 birds as gifts for children."[33] Miss Mason taught patience to students. She often gave them time needed to think through decisions and to know that the answers were often inside the self, to trust one's own judgment. She didn't seem to follow students as closely as most of the instructors did—a better way to build self-confidence and critical thinking.

> One of the funny memories from BMH was of Miss Mason, who taught us Neurological Nursing, giving us a lecture on cerebrovascular accidents. What she taught through using humor I've never forgotten and probably never will. To demonstrate that damage can affect only one side of the brain yet affect the opposite side of the body, she would hit herself on the side of the head and awkwardly fly across the room, showing how damage to the opposite side of her body occurred. Explaining the process on paper doesn't make the incident seem profound but, if you knew Miss Mason and could visualize this solidly built nurse acting out this symptom, you would probably think it was funny, too.
>
> ***Helen Sheperd '66***

Other instructors and nurse mentors were unforgettable as well: among many others, Mrs. Bestervelt, "Jackson," Mrs. King, and Mrs. Rice stand out. And who can forget Mrs. Stell or instructor Tebina Boomgaarden in OB?

Students were expected to take on increasing responsibilities during my three years in training. Toward the end of my freshman year I was working 3 to11 P.M. on the sixth floor and was put in charge of the 50 and 60 wing, with the support of the instructor, Miss Maatman. Was I surprised when I went to ask a question and was told that she was at dinner. She said going to dinner was OK because I was in charge. Managing the unit was the way we learned in the past! Miss Maatman was an unforgettable 3:00 to 11: 00 P. M. clinical instructor. She was always there for us, expected the best from us and usually received it! She was one of the most compassionate instructors I remember. She seemed to understand that we were students and made judgments with limited knowledge and experience, and was always there to encourage us with a kind and understanding word, with a lesson attached.

Anna van't Zelfde Stryd '61

Organic Chemistry was perhaps the hardest class. (I secretly liked Organic Chem. so much more than high school chem.) Dr. Tuller, our WMU professor, came to the dorm to tutor us as a group. What a great thing to do! We all sat on the floor of the rec. room (basement of Truesdale). I really liked anatomy and physiology. Another superior professor was Dr. Lawrence. No one should forget our anatomy and physiology lab times with her and the dissection of smelly (formaldehyde) cats. Many cats were named after our psychology professor, Charlotte, not a favorite instructor. Some of my classmates were downright rude to Charlotte the professor, not the dead cat.

Kay Cook Hanson '64

My most memorable instructors were: Ruth Kingsley (the epitome of what I thought a nurse should look like and be), Dorothy Kavalhuna, Mary Mason, Barb Damvelt, Jackie Wylie, Mrs. VanBruggen—all of whom were positive role models as nurses, people, and friends.

Lynne Gamble Raseman '66

After a difficult start I fainted just prior to my first case in the O.R. Mrs. Wylie was so positive and encouraging that I spent two-thirds of my career in the O.R. I have always been grateful to Mrs. Wylie and all of our instructors. They made us learn.

Jane Sny Hartman '67

I remember Jackie Wylie and how it was such a pleasure to have her as one of my leaders, teachers and mentors. Nursing school was hard enough without people getting on your case all of the time and she didn't. I remember her as willing to help and always with a smile.

Sandy Starks Winzenz '69

My training at Bronson helped me to meet challenges I never imagined and, in doing so, I gained confidence in myself that has stayed with me forever. It also set a standard of excellence that I have maintained, and made me a champion for the patients in all I do, and gave me excellent role models of strong, successful women like Jackie Wylie. I worked in the Bronson O.R. for a short time after I graduated while my husband finished his education at Western.

Doris Whitbeck Bartell '65

An instructor who made a great impression on me was Anna Mae Spaniolo. She was the picture of a professional nurse as she respectfully dealt with each person, be he or she student, patient, co-worker, or patient family member. Not only was she an instructor of mine but later I had the privilege of being a coworker. Her caring spirit was always noticeable and I appreciate the impact that she has had in my life.

Kay L. Taylor '68

Mrs. Forsythe was a great influence. She demonstrated competence, warmth, intelligence, and compassion. I remember her bustling style and I can still hear her say certain things. Her attention to the whole patient was ahead of its time. There were other memorable faculty and head nurses. Mrs. Rice and Mrs. Meyle influenced me, each in a different manner. I remember Miss Mason as an individual who had an impact on me.

Carolyn Tennant Farthing '69

LINDA VAN DYKE '61

Linda Van Dyke was one of the few students[34] who married in 1960, the year before she graduated. Some of her married classmates became pregnant, had to take a pregnancy leave early in their pregnancies, and could not return to school for a year.

When Linda learned that she was pregnant and due to deliver in November, she worried that she would have to drop out of school for a year. Dr. Peake, a popular obstetrician, assured her that he would support a delivery date that would ensure her graduation in September 1961. The custom-fitted school uniforms allowed for changes in girth, and weight loss or gain, a practical solution to potential student weight changes over three years of practice. The garments were unfitted through the waist but cinched by a belt that was adjustable. Though not the intention, the uniform did accommodate early pregnancy body changes.

By April 1961, Van Dyke completed all program requirements except unassigned time. Unassigned time provided Bronson nursing staff support and often gave students a choice to practice in a clinical specialty in which they had interest and to choose a shift, especially if they chose evenings (3:00 to 11:30 P.M.) or nights (11:00 P.M. to 7:30 A.M.). Since Van Dyke's husband worked a 3 to 11 P.M. shift at the Upjohn Company, Linda chose and was given the evening shift for both unassigned time and her first real work position on 2-East and 3-East. These were the medical and surgical units that she had liked as a freshman when the curriculum introduced several hospital units and fundamentals of nursing practice.

Unassigned time was an informal way to engage students in an early orientation process, and recruiting student nurses into staff nurse roles. Students migrated to practice areas that appealed to them. Once integrated into a nursing team, it was comfortable to simply transfer from student to work status without applying and interviewing elsewhere for a job. There were certainty and stability in staying at Bronson. The practice was abandoned some years later when the NLN recommended deletion of this program requirement.

Van Dyke's love for the care of medical patients won her over. She practiced on 2-East from April to September 1961, received her diploma the end of the week, and went to work the next Monday. The only difference was that she, as a well-oriented graduate who knew medical staff nurse responsibilities, was paid for her services. Her skill competencies extended beyond the novice nurse status, and she was immediately a valued member of the 2-East nursing team leaders.

Physician and staff signing of students' uniforms was traditionally a last practice-day event that began the rite of passage. Van Dyke still has the signed uniform, laughingly sharing how the pattern of signing focused on her extended abdomen.

Her graduation uniform had been altered to accommodate her maternal body shape. Culmination of her three years of loyalty and hard work was to be graduation at the First United Methodist Church with her family in attendance. However, Mrs. Weber called her into her office the day before graduation to tell her that she could not be present at graduation in an altered uniform but could attend the Truesdale Hall reception after graduation. Receiving her diploma unceremoniously at that meeting was an emotional anticlimax to her dream and achievement. Van Dyke was dismayed and disappointed at not being allowed to march and participate in the graduation ceremony. Her feelings were hurt, and denying her involvement in the graduation rite was never forgotten. The rationale for the denial is not clear, but the decision most likely reflected the traditional attitude of society that nurses are "pure" and seeing a pregnant graduate would somehow distort that view. When a door closes, however, another opens. She was relieved and grateful that she had not been forced to take an earlier pregnancy leave, allowing her to graduate at the expected time and to begin earning money toward the support of her new family.

Recalling her early staff nurse years, on one hot summer day on 2-East with no air conditioning, she learned that patients paid $2.00 per day for a fan in their rooms, even though most could not afford the fee. Hazel Latondress, director of nurses, was often in the café at lunchtime where she could overhear staff nurse conversations. On one particularly hot day, administrator Bill Johnson was also present and overheard a conversation. Linda had been watching patients suffer with the heat, and she too was angry and hot. She vented her disbelief that fans were not provided in each patient room as part of the daily charge. Johnson said, "Maybe we can do something about that." The next day fans appeared in every room. Her unintentional advocacy paid off by enlightening an administrator who listened. Suffering patients at least could have the comfort of circulating air. She never gave her advocacy role another thought but was grateful that Johnson had overheard her words. Advocacy was inherent in her practice.

ANNA VAN'T ZELFDE STRYD '61

My first memory related to nurses' training involved the initial patient I was assigned as a "probie." She was extremely ill and when I started to care for her on 2 East, she tried to bite me. At that point, I wondered if I had made the right career decision. The incident occurred only six or eight weeks after I started school!

My favorite floor to work on was 2 East, despite being intimidated by the powerful presence and expertise of Dr. Littig. I spent about nine months of my training on that floor, many of them on the 11:00 P.M.–7:00 A.M. shift with other students who were in the same rotation. Sharon Schaller and I were usually scheduled together, and we had some memorable experiences. The elderly patients appreciated so much the care we gave them. I especially remember one 91-year-old, very tall man who crawled over his bed rails at midnight and came to the nurses' station where my roommate and I were charting. He proceeded to instruct us on how to touch our toes and insisted that we practice with him. We were fearful that he would fall and we would have to write an incident report.

My most unforgettable patient was a dear young mother with a wonderful husband and children. She contracted tetanus, I think through gardening, and we tried hard to provide her with the best care, knowing that any sound in the room or the act of moving her could trigger muscle spasms. What an uneasy feeling when she needed to be turned because she couldn't breathe and thus eliminate the fluid that was building up in her lungs. The morning that I was "specialing" her (as a junior student) she was scheduled to be turned, which we did, but then she quit breathing. Her heart stopped, and we couldn't clear her trach fast enough to successfully resuscitate her. Dr. Proos, resident at the time, worked long and hard, but saving her wasn't to be. Her husband was present, and I'll never forget his reaction. When there was nothing more we could do, he was devastated, as well as were all of the nurses who had cared for her. We realized that, in spite of wonderful and adequate nursing care, not all of our patients left the hospital able to move forward with their lives. We cared for all with the best tools we had available, but God has control over our final hours and days. I have thought of this patient, her husband, and the family frequently during the past thirty years and have wondered if there was anything more that we could have done for her.

Big errors were mistakes like throwing a sack of hair clippings, shaved off a patient before a craniotomy, down the incinerator instead of into a labeled bag and saved. The student who discarded the hair expected to be expelled from school, but she survived. Hair was always saved, just in case the patient wanted it for whatever reason, perhaps to make her own wig?

We often entertained ourselves at Truesdale Hall—the long halls made great bowling alleys. I have many dorm memories; a special one is of Dick Vander Molen being around to help us with all of our repairs. He was always willing to help the students if we had a problem; we really depended on him. I wonder how he ever got his "real work" done!

Throughout the years people have asked, "Why do you look so sober in your official graduation picture?" Our individual senior pictures were taken for a class composite. We loved to have a good time and weren't all that serious. The explanation is actually very simple. Mary B. Anderson, the director of nurses, would not allow a picture of us smiling. I don't remember the reason, but we couldn't smile and our hair had to be off our necks. In many of the pictures originating during Mary B.'s tenure, the students are not smiling and neither is she.

We were encouraged to treat our patients as individuals and not as a room number throughout our training. This mandate was sometimes difficult to remember when we had to "worry" about performing correctly in our instructor's eyes or when someone came down hard on us for committed errors. Most errors were far from life threatening and often could have been interpreted as another way of approaching a task. We had many nurturing supervisors, interns, and residents who helped to make our clinical experiences positive. We all had our bad days, but most of us can look back on our experiences and training as a positive experience that helped us mature and develop into the competent nurses for which the Bronson School of Nursing is known.

There were many good times, as well as sad times when a patient was unable to be "cured" and was sent home. Becoming a nurse was one of the best experiences of my life, and I learned much about life, death, and myself. These learning experiences have helped me to deal with many situations that I have encountered since graduation.

ELAINE K. MARSHALL FANSON '63

I have many memories of my three years at Bronson. Some of them are particularly happy and some are a little less so. Training was an intense and often stressful time of learning, working, and developing leadership skills. We, the student nurses, basically staffed the hospital in those days. Many times we were responsible for whole patient floors. We were also expected to work nights and attend classes during the day. I found that regimen to be extremely difficult.

Many of my fond memories are of life at Truesdale Hall. I am deeply saddened to learn that it has been demolished. My husband of 34 years picked me up for dates many, many times in that lobby. We were married two weeks after I graduated. I often go back in memory to our gatherings around the TV in the basement watching Elvis. How the girls would scream! I've always been nostalgic about Elvis because of those early-sixties' days at Bronson. I also remember how Dick would yell, "Man on the floor," when he would exit the elevator on our floor. How times have changed!

I was honored in my senior year, while I was working in the Outpatient Department, to have my picture appear in the *Bronson Bulletin.* I was holding a child and Mrs. Lord was standing beside me. I also recall some interesting events that occurred during my three-month stay at the State Hospital where I worked in female receiving. I enjoyed much of the time I spent working in OB and newborn nursery. Working in OR and on the surgical floor was enjoyable. Then it was graduation which was held at the large Kalamazoo United Methodist Church. It was a special day for all of us in the class of 1963.

> When I was six years old, I was ill with a kidney disease and spent some time in the hospital. I had to stay in bed, have shots, and take terrible-tasting medicine, but the nurses were all so nice to me and I was fascinated by what they did. As I grew up, my church put a good deal of emphasis on helping others in need. I attended a two-room school and my teacher for seventh and eighth grades convinced me that I might be capable of becoming a nurse.
>
> As a senior in high school, I spent half days in a co-op program, working and learning in the hospital. Thanks to the support of nurses and teachers, as well as my parents, I had the courage to apply to Bronson.
>
> ***Carol Peeks Gunneman '63***

JULIANNE DEBRUIN DEKORTE '63

My most memorable night on duty occurred when I was on Pediatric Service and assigned to work 11:00 P.M.–7:00 A.M. When I arrived at work my charge nurse told me that I was to "special" a little boy who had been burned in a barbecue fire. I walked to the room, not knowing what to expect. I opened the door, with no preparation to care for patients with burns, and was given a short report by a nurse who was anxious to leave. I never felt so alone in my whole life as I turned and looked at that little boy.

He was burned beyond recognition as a human being. His little mouth was open just enough to insert a suction catheter. At one point, he choked and stopped breathing. All night long I stayed in that closed room, with no break because it was busy on the floor. I was scared he would die, and I didn't know what I would do! I had to keep the room warm because of the exposed skin. It was necessary to wear a gown, gloves, mask, and hat for sterile technique. It was so hot and the air was filled with the smell of burned flesh.

All night long his mother, crying and watching me care for him, stood outside the glass door. There was little to do for him, except give him morphine and regulate the intravenous to the urine output every half-hour. I have never forgotten my feeling of sheer terror. We all knew he could not live—and I just prayed to God to let him make it through the night. He did—and in the morning, after I left, he expired in the ambulance while being transferred to the University of Michigan.

When I was back in the dorm I cried for hours, and it took weeks for me to get over the experience. If I had not been a senior, I do believe I would have quit school, for I remember believing that I truly did not have what it took to be a nurse and experience that kind of suffering. I never, however, had another night like that one again in training—and never since. As I look back on the amount of responsibility we were given as students, I am amazed! Yet we rose to every occasion without questioning. Those experiences formed character in many of us that would stand us through later adversities in life. I know I grew up a whole lot that night!

My Joys

- Getting my letter of acceptance when so few applicants were chosen from those who applied.
- Making it through the first semester when so many were cut.
- Earning my cap and first starched uniform with that name Miss J. DeBruin was a milestone.

- Finding out that I actually had what it took to give an injection to another human being.
- Being named as second in my class.

I took pride in being a Bronson School of Nursing graduate, knowing how hard I worked for my diploma and realizing what a great nursing education I received. I knew I could be hired anywhere and could handle any assignment because I was prepared. After I left work each day, I knew that I had served mankind; I had done a good job of making people more comfortable and meeting their health care needs.

Fears

My fears seemed to outweigh my joy, *e.g.*, being afraid I would be given a roommate who smoked—and then finding out that indeed did happen. We were allowed to switch after the first couple of days!

- Walking into that dorm room on the first day and seeing all those pins on the bulletin board and thinking, I'll never make it through all those months!
- Giving report to nurses who seemed to love to embarrass the students.
- Being in charge the first few times.
- Walking through the tunnel alone, only if the weather was blizzard conditions; otherwise, it was much preferable to run across the street no matter what the weather.
- Being "bone tired" from working 11:00 P.M.–7:00 A.M. and then having to attend classes and stay awake.
- Taking a body alone to the morgue on a gurney.
- Attending the required autopsies.
- Making rounds with a flashlight in the night to make sure the patients were still breathing.

We were required to spend one-week stints in the formula lab, nights in OR (alcoholing all the operating rooms down that dark hall), and the diet kitchen. We hated these weeks! If a "Code O" was called, all we did was grab the Emerson machine, stethoscope, and spyghmo. How does that compare with our ACLS[35] protocols of nowadays?

We worked extra shifts for $1.00 an hour. One time I needed some money so I worked for two months straight, without a day off, between student practice requirements and working for pay.

KAY COOK-DAVIDSON HANSON '64

I entered the School of Nursing in 1961. My enrollment at Bronson was a second choice; I was already accepted at WMU and planned to major in social work. Then, on a whim, I stopped at Bronson with a 4-H girlfriend. We located Mary B. Anderson's office, and I asked her for information on applying to BSON. The course of study offered a challenge; only applicants from the top one-third of high school graduating classes were accepted into the program. Daylong testing processes were held at both Western Michigan University and BSON. Even if accepted, one-third of the class would not make it through the difficult three-year training.

My mother was against my pursuing a nursing career. She said nurses had to work too hard for difficult, long hours. (She was correct for the most part.) Anyway I was allowed to apply and was tested, and lo and behold was accepted!

My future mother-in-law was an LPN at Bronson. She became friends with some of the senior graduating class of 1961 and thus was invited to attend graduation at the First United Methodist Church. She took me along after which my goal was certain—I would attend my own graduation in 1964! That was the power of positive thinking, and I do not remember ever wanting to quit BSON (as a dear roommate would choose to do). No one could have known less about the medical profession. I'd never heard of an enema, douche, and most other terms. I was just a happy, sheltered, only child, but one reason I wanted nursing as a career was my exposure to the Sue Barton nurse novels. True!

To get ready for nurses' training, we had a series of immunizations updated and added to. I hate shots, but had finally learned not to wail when receiving them. The typhoid shot gave me a fever and other symptoms of a nasty communicable disease (like chills, headache, nausea, and vomiting) but only for 24 hours.

The early sixties were a good time as I remember, with President Kennedy and family in the White House. We were still safe hitching rides to WMU for mixers, *etc.* Actually, hitching areas were available on the West Michigan Avenue campus. We were bused for classes to WMU, a process that encouraged closeness with classmates. Great new songs (I remember some), but familiar ones, were almost always sung—at least on our dormward trip. We learned a good deal that freshman year—how to relate to each other, our teachers, and our new life at BSON. I always lucked out with roommates and suitemates; we all still keep in touch. My first roommate left in the junior year—she did not like nursing, but it took a while for her to realize that it was an intolerable career for her.

We did have good times together, visiting each other's homes and enjoying BSON social life. Mixers (dances where WMU men were invited), were arranged and Bronson's sports activities were available to attend (Dick Vander Molen was active on all sports teams). We could walk to downtown movie theaters and to Chenery Auditorium for symphonies, *etc.* Many of us would go to the one TV set in the dorm Rec Room corner for viewing of Dr. Kildare, Ben Casey, *etc.*

Vividly I remember a lot of study and paper writing. Sometimes I prepared for exams in back stairwells. There was so much to know! We learned about the history of nursing from dear Mrs. Cripe—no notes, just underline in the textbook as she read. Here I longed for my exciting high school U.S. History teacher. (He brought history to life for me and I have always enjoyed it since, but I digress!)

I remember the rules about dorm life: hours to return at night (it varied a bit depending on your class), you must sign in and out for everything, no slacks, jeans, shorts allowed in the hospital (thus we walked around, not through, if we were so dressed). There must have been more rules, but I'll add only the "professional rules":

1. Address each other as Miss Cook, Miss Heneveld, *etc.*
2. Stand always when a doctor approached the work area.
3. Uniforms a specific length from the floor.
4. Hair off collar, hair pulled back and up.
5. No nail polish.
6. White clean and polished shoes.
7. No gum chewing or fingernail chewing (you would get the creeping crud, Miss Mason assured us).

Back to learning all those nursing skills, many of which I'd never heard of before BSON. We learned volumes in Nursing Arts lab—first how to wash our hands and the importance of it. I was destined to become an ICP (Infection Control Practitioner). My favorite pre-BSON books were *The Microbe Hunters* and *Rats, Lice and History* (Zinsser). The year I achieved Infection Control Nurse status (1981) was the first year we heard of AIDS, but that's another chapter!

We received the white uniform with the BSON emblem on the pocket as freshmen, then finally came capping. We were in! The great Bronson cap, harder than hell to fold just right, with that pesky button and pin in the back just so.

Soon we were giving baths, making beds, providing injections, and adding new skills every week. The poor patients: there were no neat, less-wrinkled fitted sheets; no rooms that were air conditioned except surgery and PAR[36]; no IVPB's[37] (at least not during my first two years) and so patients received more IM shots, like PCN,[38] streptomycin and lincomycin. Ouch!

We gave soapsuds enemas, and pre-surgical douches and helped doctors with rigid, metal-tube sigmoidoscopies. Laboring women were given enemas and their pubic hair was shaved. Even worse, husbands were not allowed in the delivery room.

Newborns were kept in noisy nurseries, noisy because, as a rule, you only took babies to mothers at set feeding times. Mothers stayed in the hospital four to five days following vaginal deliveries.

OB and surgery were junior-year services. We scrubbed hands and arms for operations, frequently to hold retractors with our bodies under some surgeon's armpit, but we did first scrub on many cases and therefore had to quickly learn general instruments as well as the surgeons' special instruments and preferences. I don't recall scrubbing for my future father-in-law [Dr. Curtis Hanson], but I recall a large back table loaded with every conceivable orthopedic instrument. We were assigned only partially by our OR instructor; other OR time was in the hands of OR management. We worked one week of nights and 3:00 to11:00 P.M. On nights we "alcoholed" the entire OR—each room, plus pulled supplies, scrubbed or set-up sterile [instrument tables] in each room, and covered them with sterile drapes to make turnover between cases more efficient. I remember that one of the RN's would upend IV poles, checking for that spot of blood. Sometimes a RN would sleep in the break room while students cleaned the OR.

I'll never forget how some doctors swore in surgery. We were not assigned to scrub with a few because they were so abusive. On off-shifts, however, there was no choice since the student and one RN were the only staff present, and the RNs always circulated, leaving the student to scrub. Once a classmate pulled a bovie[39] cord across the sterile field during a laminectomy and tossed drapes and instruments everywhere. I enjoyed my surgery rotation. I remember drawing pictures of instruments and memorizing doctors' preference and routines.

One of the biggest challenges was scrubbing during six T&A's (the doctor's private scrub nurse was on vacation). It was a rapidly done procedure with quick turn around. All went well, I guess. The surgeon never said a word to me—no thank you, no yelling, no nothing—he seemed strange.

I have many various thoughts; here are a few brief comments:

- The student choir, great fun.
- Talent shows each year given on the Rec Room stage.
- My classmate was asked to leave BSON due to blatant dating of a married doctor.
- Great black banding ceremonies were held in our Rec Room. Adding first a narrow black band to our cap meant attainment of junior status. The wider black band conferred senior or homestretch status
- Another important rule of student life was that we belong and attend Student Nurses Association meetings. We alternated meeting sites. I enjoyed our trips to the Borgess School of Nursing.
- I believe I became an adult at BSON. I've not regretted my decision to become a nurse.
- I had the sweetest elderly woman for a case study.

Senior students were next to God. They knew it all; at least I thought so until I arrived at senior status. Most learning did come easier as a senior, and I earned A grades for Clinical Leadership—imagine, shy little me. I was shy and much littler then.

Hell Week—first our turn as freshmen, then the reverse as seniors to the newest class. You haven't lived until you've eaten peanut butter from a bedpan. Being a slave to a senior for a week wasn't all bad. I remember ironing in the gathering room at the end of my floor when a group of seniors was there. They swore me to secrecy about a classmate dating a doctor. It worked out for Franny; she ended up marrying Dr. Dew.

I joined Kappa Chi Iota, the BSON sorority. We were a religious, service-oriented group. It was good to ground in such a group. First we met in the old church next to the dorm. We did have our own tiny chapel on the first floor of the dorm.

I have many memories of patients, especially the people who became my case studies. My Med-Surg case involved a 40-some year old man hospitalized for MI (myocardial infarction). People definitely stayed in the hospital for longer periods. My suitemate, Marilyn, also was following a man with an MI. The patients may even have been in the same ward. We came on the floor one morning and found that Marilyn's case study had died. The death was devastating. My Med-Surg case study featured a woman who had an abdominal hysterectomy. I saw her outside of the hospital months later, and her husband tried to give me money for taking care of her. We really developed close relationships.

When I first entered BSON we accessed the hospital either by a tunnel or by crossing Pine Street to enter near the then small ER. I was petrified of seeing some major trauma. Once I had rotated through ER as an older student, I could cope with just about any injury.

Major burns presented the most difficult cases. You were assigned to the private room and had constant dressing changes and other duties to perform while gowned in hair covering, gown, mask, and gloves. We had no Burn Unit or ICU. PAR was used for some major traumas until private duty nursing could be arranged.

My funniest doctor–nurse story occurred during a sigmoidoscopy in the treatment room on Hall 6. Big Dr. VanderVelde and an equally big senior surgical resident, a classmate, and I were in the tiny room with the patient. Dr. Van and the resident were using the old Gomco suction to clear the patient's bowel. Well, suddenly the top popped off the old, noisy Gomco. Feces flew everywhere. The procedure was terminated and the patient quickly restored to an upright sitting position and returned to his room. Luckily the patient was covered with a treatment blanket; remember them? My classmate and I laughed so much we both had to lie on the floor (outside the treatment room).

Surprisingly, as a senior I liked Peds. Having no siblings, I had a good deal to learn about sick children. Some good, young RNs worked on Peds. A small Preemie

Nursery was located on 3 where Peds was situated. An old RN ran the Preemie Nursery. From 3:00–11:00 P.M. and 11:00 P.M.–7:00 A.M., senior students were assigned to the nursery. One night, without warning, Dr. Birch (OB/GYN) brought a one pound infant to the door. He had the new father in tow. All I could do was place the baby in the tiny incubator and keep it warm. At the time, that size newborn was not long for this world. No pediatrician arrived. We had been taught to baptize babies under these conditions if the parents approved. The dad did so I baptized the little boy who remained alive through my shift. Almost everything has changed for the better. Our NICU nurses and doctors are terrific.

A word about the State Hospital Psych Rotation and all the old buildings there. It was a city unto itself with fire department, laundry, bakery (great bread), hospital, *etc.* We had the tour of at least all the female units. Great fun, with good instructors, and many new student friends. Other schools of nursing sent students there. We lived on the top floor of Linda Richards Building. We walked back and forth to the Receiving Hospital each day for three months. I played cards every night. After my stay at KSH, I had a week's vacation. Five of us (four Bronson seniors and one from Borgess) drove to Kentucky. Good fun.

By the time of graduation, we had all been transformed into well-prepared (my opinion, but not mine alone) young nurses. We all had jobs waiting for us, at Bronson if we wished. Graduation ceremony was wonderful, all that I'd dreamed of.

GAIL TAYLOR WILSON '64

I've always been grateful for my nursing education. Nothing has been more useful in everyday life; family, friends, neighbors, and even strangers have all benefited from my nursing/medical knowledge. I've come to realize that a nurse is forever a teacher and I continue to share what I know regularly.

We arrived on September 10, 1961, one hundred of us. Fifty would graduate. I still remember our arrival every year on that September day. I began and ended my career preparation with the same roommate and suitemates: Carol Gay, Jane Broker, and Barbara McKane.

My first patient, a 20-year old man with multiple fractures from an auto accident needed a complete bed bath. Oh my! It was before ICU or Critical Care units. Observing my one and only autopsy turned out to be a man I'd cared for many times; I didn't know he'd expired until that moment and have not been able to eat liver since that day. I also remember immunizing hundreds with the Salk polio vaccine and passing Levine tubes down one another in Nursing Arts lab, barfing on Miss Heneveld, our most proper instructor. I also worked Christmas Eve 3:00–11:00 P.M. and the following week specialing a comatose young woman in isolation on 2 East.

SARA GOLDSTEIN COLLISON '65

To be a nurse, a childhood fantasy? a Candystriper dream? a leap of faith? These were the questions I was asking as I entered my senior year of high school. My guidance counselor had cautioned me that science was my weakness and Bronson Methodist Hospital School of Nursing had the reputation of being a tough academic school, but also it had the distinction of being one of the finest three-year programs in the state!

As a new Christian, I found my life being challenged in so many ways. My greatest concern was to know God and find a life filled with love and service to Him. When I had the opportunity to visit BMH during Vocational Exploration Week, I realized that Bronson would provide the educational and spiritual opportunities that would help me to realize my life dream.

I will never forget our first night in the dorm. All of the students met in the little church next to Truesdale Hall for a Convocation service. I was feeling very lonely, overwhelmed, and apprehensive. God spoke to my heart, which brought such a peace and assurance that He would be with me to meet all of the challenges of the next three years.

Wonderful friends, support of excellent instructors, hard work, discipline, and dorm life second to none made those years rich and full. As a young adult, I faced life and death issues with our hospitalized patients. This indoctrination brought a new depth of faith and appreciation for life that is still my foundation. Serving God continues to be my passion. Bronson Methodist Hospital School of Nursing prepared me for this task. I will forever be grateful.

FRANCES BURKE KAKABEEKE '66

So many thoughts come to mind when I think of my years at Truesdale Hall. The excitement of moving in, meeting new lifelong friends, saying good-bye to parents who were to travel 300 miles back home. Only 18 years old and away from home for the first time, eating in the cafeteria was fun and the food tasted good for a while. Traveling by bus and often walking to and from classes at Western, we sang songs on the bus depending on the season. One night I took a free city bus to WMU to visit a friend from home and was planning to take the 9:30 P.M. bus back downtown, only to find out the bus was going back to the garage instead. The bus driver took pity on me, no money for a taxi and a 10 P.M. curfew, and took me, the lone passenger, to the door of 515 Pine Street!

I remember being anxious about my first clinical experience, possibly rectal temps and a backrub that included the buttocks, only to have the vital signs taken by other staff before I arrived! Whew! I admired the upper classmen who seemed confident and competent. Of course our class didn't appreciate "Hell Week" and bowing down to the seniors, giving backrubs, polishing shoes, and running errands for them. At the Friday night talent show each of us sat down at the piano and played "Chop Sticks." The seniors were pretty angry with us for showing such disrespect.

My clinical time was full of ups and downs, depending on the rotation, charge nurses, and instructors. One morning, after report on 2 East, when my patient reportedly had a "good night," I found him dead in his bed. As I reached for his pulse, all I could feel was my own, and it was bounding! I had a patient on 2 west, who was close to my age, with a family and even a dog like my own, who had terminal cancer. She became very dear to me since I had experienced the death of my own mother only two months before. We were never shielded from the realities of life. While in OB, I cared for a DNP/DNS (Do not publish, Do not show) baby. I was marked down for not discussing an unplanned pregnancy with the mother and asking how she was coping. At 19, I was not able to deal with these dramatic and sometimes tragic experiences in the lives of my patients.

I can remember cooling patients with tepid baths and giving 5cc syringes of paraldehyde to the confused elderly restrained in bed. The operating room was my favorite rotation because we scrubbed on many cases and learned the nurse's circulating role. The staff seemed to appreciate our presence (which wasn't always the case in other areas) and our instructor was well liked by the OR staff. Her great sense of humor supported us.

The years went by quickly; as seniors we became team leaders and mentors to the lower classmen. The hospital staff gave us their full confidence, and we seemed to mostly run the night shift. The house supervisor was our resource and we looked forward to sunrise. Dr. A.B. Hodgman would come in about 5:00 A.M., laughing and talkative to begin his rounds.

It was great to be close to town for shopping, movies, and restaurants within walking or hitchhiking distance to WMU. The intern and resident's families provided opportunities for babysitting and the COs (conscientious objectors), Amish and Mennonite orderlies, who lived in hospital-supplied housing, were always ready to party or hangout. Some had boats and took us water skiing on Gull Lake.

Probably one of the most memorable nights at the dorm was at the time the church next to the dorm was being demolished. A friend came screaming out of her room in pink babydoll pajamas and rollers in her hair yelling, "There are bats in my room!" We thought she was dreaming, but there truly were bats that flew into the hallway. We armed ourselves with coats, hoods, gloves, umbrellas, brooms, and a wastebasket of hot bleach water. We killed them by catching them in a corner with a broom, poking them with the point of the umbrella, and dropping them into the concoction in the wastebasket. When two more appeared, we called for help, and maintenance men from the hospital took care of them as we watched them duck and bob from the flying bats.

In June the seniors finished with six weeks of unassigned time. The week of graduation, seniors went around the hospital having uniforms signed and hanging uniforms and toilet paper from the dorm. A solemn graduation came next at the First United Methodist Church with a reception at Truesdale Hall, a pin and diploma, as well as a new job. Bronson hired all of its graduates who wanted to stay at the hospital. I graduated December 1966 in Mrs. Weber's office because, three months after my mother died, I left school for six months. I started employment on January 1, 1967, in the recovery room. It was New Year's Day, and no surgeries were performed so I was assigned to 2 West. It was interesting that on my first day of work, I was in charge of PAR without any type of orientation except that I had worked there as a student nurse a year before.

HELEN SHEPERD '66

Let me begin by saying that Bronson Methodist Hospital School of Nursing didn't prepare me with a well-known school name to flaunt here in Korea or any other place, (which seems to be all important at times,) but that omission is not as important to me as the real wealth of knowledge I received in classroom studies and through clinical practice. That clinical experience (known by students as WORK) was a good basis for clinical practice and teaching in the future. I remember being upset at times that the nursing school faculty wouldn't acknowledge that our "practice" was, in fact, hard WORK.

On my first day of clinical experience, I was on 2 East where we were assigned to take TPR's on two patients. I was excited and scared, too! Excited about beginning to practice and freaked out because the clinical practice was a foreign field for me. The one TPR went well, but the second one didn't. It was a rectal temperature, which was required on a elderly woman who couldn't hear well. As I remember, she told me to, "Take that damn thing out of there!" meaning that she wanted the thermometer out of her rectum RIGHT THEN. What a start, I thought. Well, that seemed like the time I should have stopped my nursing career, but I didn't.

Another incident that seems somewhat related occurred with a TB patient in isolation on 2 East. First thing in the morning was for breakfast to be served. As I dutifully delivered the tray and began to feed the patient, who was unable to feed himself, he repeatedly coughed and expectorated some very tenacious sputum, appearing not unlike the "runny" part of his soft cooked egg that was on his tray. As I remember, he hollered at me with some rather distasteful, foul words, telling me to feed him his egg, which I had been neglecting because I thought I might gag in the process. Perhaps this encounter was a good lesson for me, as I needed to go outside of my feelings of discomfort and meet the patient's needs, or perhaps the experience helped to move me along on the path of learning what empathy was when practiced.

Probably though, over time, the most important experiences were those that involved caring for cancer patients, especially a care-study patient who was 32, had two preschool children, and was a very pleasant woman. As a care-study patient, she was admitted for treatment of her leukemia and later she received palliative care. I saw her repeatedly and, was profoundly touched watching her go downhill with her advancing disease. Finally, as I returned to Ann Arbor for a weekend at home and visited her at the U of M Medical Center, where she died a few hours later, I was aware of a great sense of loss. I wondered what more I could have done to help her. It was a useful lesson in what we know as palliative care, accompanying an individual on the journey from physical life to death.

We experienced many instances in which cancer patients were cared for in our hospital but were often neglected emotionally because we were uncomfortable and didn't know what to say. (These were the days before Kubler-Ross' experiences in talking with, and supporting, people with end-of-life conditions.) It seemed we did well with the procedures and physical comfort issues, but were oftentimes at a loss in providing support to meet the rest of the patient's needs. Now those incidents provide fuel for the desire to give sensitive, supportive, skillful care to people with terminal illnesses.

The OB care-study experience was also memorable. When would "my" case come up? My name was written on the blackboard on the OB floor along with a few others. After days of wondering, I finally went to bed half-dressed so that I would be ready when the call came. Then, one Sunday as I ate in the cafeteria, I was called. My patient's first labor hadn't been too long and this one, for her second baby, definitely wasn't long! As she expelled the enema she hollered, "It's coming!" as she sat on the bathroom toilet. Yikes, what should I do? Does that emergency button in the labor room really work? As I helped the patient back to the

I always wanted to be a nurse and I had a favorite great-aunt at BMH (Marie Wantz), so I guess she was the primary motive for me attending this school. Truesdale Hall, fifth floor, was home. I remember our many "study parties" (we'd cram all night for a test), as well as our popcorn feasts and pranks (the good ol' Saran Wrap on the toilets). We hated the length of our uniforms and would tape them up for clinic (if you hemmed them, they'd come back from laundry lengthened again).

We created our own specialty clinics on fifth floor involving weight-loss, hair cutting and coloring, matchmaking, psychoanalysis, and personality typing (after State Hospital). We sunbathed on the roof and, more than once, I fell asleep after working all night and woke up "burned to a crisp."

My many experiences at Bronson gave me the background to do a variety of tasks in my nursing career. I loved my days at Bronson and am thankful that I have such good memories.

Edythe Merrill Rivers '66

bed, I hit the button! Yes, it does work! Immediately, a thundering herd of nurses came running and helped my patient to deliver her baby in the delivery room. This delivery was beautiful, as were all of the other ones! The miracle of this birth as well as all of the others still astounds me.

Kappa Chi Iota was a significant influence in my life, especially Chaplain Richard Clark and his secretary, Dolores Guy. Through this group and, especially through these two people, I learned about gentleness, kindness, and compassion.

My brother told me I would never be able to give injections. So, when it came time to practice, the prospect was one of the major traumas of the three years' experience. Classmate Joan Stone was my first victim. When she looked back to see what happened, I was standing there holding a syringe with a needle bent into a right angle. I guess this injection was like many to follow. Just as I approached the skin I hesitated, and these dull needles bent (because, as you remember, they were sharpened and checked for burrs in Central Supply). Thank goodness, with more experience and later with disposable needles, the technique got better. Again, after this incident, I thought I should leave nursing school, but I remember deciding that, unless I was told to leave, I wouldn't! I wanted to be a good nurse and already I had invested too much in the training to simply quit.

Pediatrics was difficult and yet I enjoyed it, too. We had a number of burn victims and a number of deaths during that three-month period. With children around, however, some humorous experience always added some lightness to the day. Taking temperatures near lunchtime maybe wasn't such a good idea. As I returned to pick up thermometers, a healthy child's temperature alarmed me. It was 108 degrees! How could it be? He was alert and not hot. The telltale hole in his sweet potato on his tray was the evidence I needed to provide a solution to this case.

The experience that took the cake was related to practice in the premature nursery. Miss Fox was a nurse whom I feared. She appeared to know everything about babies. She seemed to own the nursery and had no use for nursing students who lacked confidence. That was me because I thought I might break one of those precious little preemies. (In particular I remember that Miss Fox used to rap on the nursery windows to get our attention when we were doing something of which she disapproved.) So, this short experience was not short enough to please me, but it certainly was not made better by showing up for my clinical experience when it was my "day off." How could I have gotten confused and done that damage to myself?

Then there was the time a surgeon, who shall remain nameless but who was well known for his cantankerousness, threw a Jackson retractor across the operating room. That was an eye-opener, too.

NELLIE SANTINGA '66

During an extracurricular activity (a fun party), where we were to come "dressed as a song," a nursing student from Africa, Ruth Brower, arrived dressed as Little Red Riding Hood, as I recall. She then told the Red Riding Hood story in the Swahili language. It enlarged our horizon, as well as entertained us.

I vividly remember the patient who was my surgical case study. He was a salesman with severe G.I. problems, which ended up being diagnosed with an aneurysm, confirmed by a sudden rupture. By spontaneous, efficient action on the part of nurses and doctors, his life was saved by emergency surgery. The man's life was so changed; he gave up his career and worked for Bronson in appreciation until his retirement.

At my first practice shot experience I couldn't stick a needle into a fellow student. Terrified at causing pain, I froze, finally inserted the needle partway, pulled it out and sat down crying. The supervising instructor was an old army nurse, noted for zero tolerance, which terrified me more. Next, the patient, to whom I had to give a gluteal injection, happened to be a young, handsome, muscular youth in his 20s, another reason to be terrified. It was an experience to dread. As I thrust the needle into the gluteal maximus, the needle bounced off the tensed muscle of the nervous young man and bent into a 45-degree angle. The instructor went after another needle and I relaxed as I took on the nurse's role of reassuring comforter, forgetting my fears, and gave the injection like a professional to a terrified patient.

MARY ANN FINK REBERT '66

In 1963 choices for female higher education were primarily "secretary, teacher, or nurse." The reasons I chose nursing were the likelihood of just three years of school instead of four, (my reasoning was wrong, nursing was 33 months vs. 32 months), and it guaranteed that I would always have a job (I was right). In the state of Michigan, the two best nursing programs were located at Henry Ford (Detroit) and Bronson (Kalamazoo). My first glimpse of Kalamazoo was high atop the hill at WMU's East Campus when I came 200 miles for an application interview.

Truesdale Hall was a dorm with four-room suites and a view! The $1,000 tuition included food and lodging. Those of us in room 416 checked our mailboxes twice a day and once attacked a bat on our floor. Rosie was our housekeeper. We sunbathed on the fifth-floor roof in April and held backyard barbecues. Remember kissing dates in the "fish bowl," waiting for the phone at the end of hallway to ring, and making popcorn? Activities included praying in the chapel, traveling the "tunnel," and watching "Dr. Kildare" and "Ben Casey" on basement-lounge TV. To our study groups we wore baby doll PJs and large plastic hair rollers with bangs Scotch-taped to our foreheads! We also participated in a Hootenanny Hoot talent show, KXI sorority, the BMH Choir singing, "Let There Be Peace on Earth," capping, and black-banding ceremonies. Senior uniforms were autographed and hung on the front roof after graduation.

My memories of people include Miss McPhail, Dick Vander Molen, Mrs. Z on ortho, Jackie Wylie in OR, plastic surgeons Stillwell & Newman (trampoline artist), Dr. Weadon (neuro), Drs. CCC (Cooper, Callander, Clement, surgeons), Dr. Birch (gyn), Carole Wilt, and Doug Sturgill!

Kalamazoo, known as the Mall City, offered us the State Theater, Bronson Park, Whistle Stop Restaurant, Side Door Coffee House, tug-o-war at Milham Park, tobogganing at Echo Valley, and cruising at Schwartz's Drive-In.

Bronson Methodist Hospital itself had the Wesley Hall elevator, the first "Intensive Care Unit" iron lung, the 999 page for autopsy, 000 page for code, the lobby chapel, circle electric beds, TB isolation rooms, Burn Unit nitroglycerine treatments, OB enemas, a formula/bottle sterilizing station, case-study patients, care plans, team leading, 11:00 P.M. –7:00 A.M. shifts, and "specialing" a critical patient.

At WMU we had student athletic tickets—Go Broncos!—"Roll Me Over in the Clover" on bus rides; hitching with no destination in mind; Beatles, Four Tops, and the Supremes records on the Union jukebox; and mixers. We attended a Read Fieldhouse concert with Peter, Paul, and Mary, ate at Bruno's Pizza, and talked of panty raids and Wesson oil parties. My roommate and I had our A&P cat's hide tanned and preserved as a momento.

Memories about the State Hospital included keys, corridors, de-lice baths, chipped beef on toast, beautician therapy, hydrotubs, electric shock treatment rooms, autism/Huntington's chorea, isolation wards, the Tower, and the fire pole.

We made some radical choices: piercing ears, dying hair, Rolling Stone music, Ripple wine. Keeping toilet paper off bedside stands, and keeping glass syringes sterile were memorable challenges.

My deepest sadness was being present at the removal of life support from a 32-year-old father of three who arrested in OR while undergoing minor surgery, and my greatest joy is the outpouring of gratitude from patients whose lives I have enhanced positively through my physical and emotional support.

Far from being a young girl who dreamed of becoming a nurse, I am a woman fulfilled by nursing—transformation provided by BMH. The Alma Mater ALWAYS makes me cry!

LYNNE GAMBLE RASEMAN '66

My choice to become a nurse stemmed from a love for people, a love of helping people, and a desire to give something "uniquely me" to even one person which would make my life worthwhile. I attended BMH partially because it was highly rated and close to home but mostly because I felt a three-year school offered more opportunity for direct patient care and interaction compared to four-year degree schools that seemed to emphasize administration and management preparation.

My greatest fears throughout the three years were those of flunking out academically, making three medication errors as grounds for dismissal, and never inserting a catheter without violating sterile technique (Mrs. Grubb was my instructor). Chemistry with Dr. Stenesh was also another challenge.

My greatest joys all involved dorm life: the lasting friendships formed, the common bonds we shared, struggling to learn, to accomplish, to survive, and to succeed.

Lessons about life, birth, pain, and dignity of death came from patients during their bed baths, back rubs, bed changings, turning of Stryker frames and circle beds, A.M. and P.M. care, PAR., L&D, ER, and ICU.[40] Case studies were a pain to write but were immensely rewarding in terms of complete patient care and interaction from admission to discharge.

Humorous and pleasurable experiences are too numerous to mention. They range from bats on the fourth floor of Truesdale and burning bras in the dryer to leaving a thermometer in a patient's mouth while going off to a two-hour class or searching the room for a patient's second slipper, forgetting he was an amputee. There was no greater pleasure than mail in your mailbox or the buzzer going off in your room signaling a phone call or a "male visitor." My greatest sense of pride was receiving my all-white cap and BMH pin on graduation day—no more long string of safety pins on the bulletin board or on my uniform. The saddest day was leaving my home and family of sisters at Truesdale Hall. Nothing and no one can replace them.

The three years I spent in training marked one of the freest, happiest, hardest, and most rewarding times of my life. Those years have helped form the basics of who I am and of who I have yet to become. The lessons learned from the people and the experiences are passing from me to my patients and to my children, hopefully to benefit future generations. What more could I ask or expect from education or myself? I am truly blessed.

PATRICIA KLEYNENBERG LINGLE '66

Some early memories of my first times "on the floor" with a patient were those of terror! A first procedure involved an enema using the stainless steel container, rubber siphon hose, and nozzle. Such a proper process. Where are the good old days?

My first experience giving an injection was also one of terror. As I was doing my mental quadrants in preparation, an instructor grabbed my hand and plunged the needle at the intended area. Unfortunately, it bent. The process was interrupted to re-prepare another syringe and medication. Those glass syringes were the finest! Remember the preparation of streptomycin—hot water for mixing the powder to melt the substance, and how thick it was?

Humor was our constant companion. One day during Hell Week, the locks on our hall doors were taped shut to prevent entry with a key, and the wind blew them closed. Of course, no master key would work—idea for using the tape. Well, how do you enter a fifth-floor room without a key? The Fire Department was called. It arrived in a large red truck with full regalia: rubber coats, helmets, boots, and their axes. Guess what the axe was for? Right, to chop a hole in the door. Where else could one have such an adventure.

At another time, the church next to the dorm was in the process of being demolished. The church's tower, (where I received my nursing cap in a solemn ceremony) was home to many bats. Usually no one would prop a fire door open, but somehow the fifth-floor door access to the roof was open to allow the sunbathers on the roof to come and go. That open door was an invitation to an adventuresome bat that flew relentlessly up and down the halls until he was dispatched by the smack of a broom. A small sign on the wall at the site signifying "genuine bat blood," hung in memoriam for weeks.

My motivations to become a nurse were never clear. It was a skill necessary for employment. It did not occur to me that the medical model and disease concept was an attitude. Exposure to sociology outside the model opened a new perspective for me, those self-empowerment concepts that have enhanced the healing arts and began a process of reformulation. What a burden it was to "make people well" back then. Was it me or the system? Sharing treatment and selfcare information as inpatient teaching but permitting choice seems more effective. Motivation to utilize my nursing background in another setting—social work—was an interesting process and a difficult mental transition. I could not do the either/or. Fortunately, my career was in a model of practice that made education and theory of both professions very valuable. Families in crisis have all kinds of needs!

I felt I did my duty after practicing nursing for several years, and with enough experience to embark on a new career path. I have taken the plunge into business. Selection of the business type was careful: healing and wellness, customer participation in consumer informational resources, minimal stress for all—were all criteria.

Education came to us in many forms. Nursing opened doors for me for 30-some years. The people and opportunities have always given me new lessons to learn, and may I never be done learning until my final breath! I think the intimacy that develops because of relationships with people is part of the healing. I feel discomfited when I hear of experiences in hospitals and health care settings that make it apparent patient-provider relationships have become very sterile. What a sadness; our process has robbed us of healing intimacies. Perhaps *less* was more—less pay, less technology, less stress, less isolation, and less specialization.

The most valuable lesson I have had on my journey is that I can learn from *absolutely everyone* I meet, and they can learn from me if we have the inclination to allow the process. With time one discovers it is not the destination but rather the journey that has become one's goal.

With gratitude I remember Bronson School of Nursing as it was—with caring people, a wealth of information, staff who were innovative, and a cooperative can-do attitude. Why would we want to be anywhere else to learn life's lessons?

Thank goodness there are pearls of wisdom that keep us remembering that giving comes back to us. Was it nursing that exemplified such a concept? I do know that special people always are present in each of our lives at times we need them, but we seldom realize their impact. I have recollections of Dick V. who could make nearly anything work again, who knew where everything was, and who knew how to find anyone. He and his kind ways, and his memories of all of us whom he helped tutor over the years made Bronson a special place. Dick's remembrances have helped bind us, and I think this historical collection process is a wonderful project.

JANE SNY HARTMAN '67

As a child entering sixth grade, I attended a summer church camp at Lake Louise. The camp nurse was from Bronson Methodist Hospital School of Nursing. I was so impressed that I decided I would be a nurse and go to Bronson. I never wavered in my decision, and did not apply to any other school. I have no idea who she was but am grateful to her in helping me make a decision that developed into a good career.

When I think of the lack of knowledge that I started with and what I have learned in 33 years, I feel as though our plain cap stands for that freshman stage of learning. As a freshman during my first time on a floor taking temperatures, I could not see the mercury to read the thermometer. I have learned.

What a wonderful group of girls bonded together in Kappa Chi Iota with a goal of Christian fellowship. I had the honor of serving as president. I have served in many capacities in other organizations but none presented the same kind of challenge. It moved me into a way of life, both personal and professional, in which I have tried to serve subsequently.

Whenever I applied for a position and wrote that I was a graduate of Bronson Methodist Hospital, people knew of it approvingly. Thanks to all who had a hand in helping me have the life I've had.

SANDRA LEA WYCOFF PROUTY '68

The experience of being away from home for the first time was in itself very memorable. I still remember unloading my belongings at the dock that day in 1965. Being able to visit with new friends at any time was great. I had always lived some distance from my friends at home. A very rewarding friendship was made that first year at Bronson, which still continues. In fact, that friend and roommate at the time introduced me to my husband of almost 29 years. She was also the nurse on duty in Bronson's delivery room when I gave birth to my second child.

I remember helping staff the hospital when a huge snowstorm hit, I believe, in 1967. As students, we were proud to do our share to help our patients and coworkers.

My rotation at the Kalamazoo State Hospital was rewarding because our group of students became a small family. We did spend a great deal of time playing card games. The games we learned to play with patients were part of their therapy and we continued to play them at the end of our workday. We were at the hospital over Christmas and we decorated and even had a tree.

I felt that the training I received at BMH prepared me to be a self-starter and an organized, logical thinker. When I think how frightened I was the first time I took a temperature and then, at the end of training, when I was an essential team member, the contrast amazes me. The staff at Bronson really encouraged us and assisted us in our training. They were always helpful.

> With fear and trembling I mixed up my first penicillin and streptomycin injection in front of the instructor on 3 East. Oh, that thick white stuff was so hard to work with. I also trembled as I injected that needle into the patient's hip and was so glad that she could not see my shaking hand!
>
> I forgot to give my patient his 1:00 P.M. med. Oh no, a med error! How I trembled as I went to see Mrs. Weber, the school's director. How relieved I felt as she smiled, welcomed me to the "feet of clay" club, and told me of her first med error which involved a narcotic.
>
> ***Kay L. Taylor '68***

It seemed that every disease we studied, somebody thought she had it. My friends were sure I had meningitis when I had a high fever at one point. They took me to the ER but the doctors couldn't find anything wrong. My rotation in the Operating Room was the scariest for me. I thought I would never set foot in an OR for the rest of my life. Guess where I have been for 24 years? (Jackie Wylie will surely laugh about that.)

Once I was confined to the dorm for breaking curfew. Several of us were involved so we made the best of it. Living in the dorm was a good experience. I remember hearing the hall phone ring and hoping the call would be for me.

I always wanted to be a nurse, but I don't know the reason. I had never wanted to do anything else in my life. I recall playing nurse as a child. No nurses were role models in my life. Putting on that starched student uniform and cap for the first time was so exciting. It was an event I had dreamed about and it became a reality.

Thank you for the opportunity to reminisce. I will never forget my experience as a nursing student at Bronson. My graduation ceremony was such a milestone in my life. I still have my original pin and I know my caps are stored somewhere.

CAROLYN TENNANT FARTHING '69

In 1965, the choices were secretary, teacher, or nurse. My mother was a nurse, so I chose nursing. Bronson was well regarded and a Methodist school, so it was a natural choice for me.

Mrs. Weber was a great influence. She seemed the perfect image. She was always professional but with a great sense of humor. Her door was always open to students, as was her secretary's office. I'll never forget her standing there, white uniform, cap, and great smile with a twinkle in her eye. Mrs. Weber seemed to me to be everything a nurse should be—professional, but human, knowledgeable, and compassionate.

The atmosphere of BMH was also a great influence on my life. The testing and shots required to enter, the uniform standard, the dedication of the instructors, the focus of dorm life, the eating in the hospital cafeteria, and the dorm's proximity to the hospital spoke volumes about the mission of the school. BMH School of Nursing was solely about the education of good nurses. We were held to high standards and had to work hard to achieve that goal. In some ways, I miss the uniform and cap that set us apart.

The State Hospital experience was also memorable. Living in the dorm, eating with the patients in a locked cafeteria, working in the wards, and assisting with shock treatments, coupled with those beautiful grounds, made it quite a summer.

The housemothers and Daisy, the switchboard operator, were also people that I never will forget. The lobby, receiving late minutes, saying goodnight to young men, as well as the female dorm experience are great memories. I still remember some of the patients that I cared for at BMH. We got to know them through repeated assignments and the patient studies that we completed. The students that I see now in the hospital don't have that benefit.

MARILYN BACKUS PATTERSON '69

I have always felt that the school was one of the best in the state and turned out top-notch nurses. Besides the excellent education I received, the camaraderie I felt toward my fellow students was one of the highlights of my training. As students, we were together 24 hours a day and shared everything. Many times we felt we weren't going to make it, but the support we gave each other made the difficult times more bearable. These experiences helped me become a more caring nurse.

One vivid memory of my training was caring for a woman who had gone to a "quack" for an abortion. Abortions were illegal then. She had not passed the fetus and came to the hospital having contractions. She called me in her labor room when she expelled the fetus. Two other students and I had to take the fetus to another room to weigh and measure him. He had some bruises on his head and chest but otherwise was a beautiful, tiny (12 ounce), perfectly formed fetus. He was too tiny to survive. He gasped a couple of times and then made no further efforts to breathe, but his heart beat for 45 minutes. It was so difficult to stand by and watch the life go out of the little being.

I was upset that someone would want to kill her baby, but one of the Labor and Delivery nurses reminded me that we were here to give the best care possible to all of our patients and not to judge them. That was a valuable lesson I learned that day and one that has stayed with me.

I recently received my BSN from Florida Atlantic University. Its philosophy is based on caring. This experience represents a continuation of the caring I learned at the BMH School of Nursing.

LINDA WIGENT BURR '63

I had always wanted to be a nurse beginning when I was about four years old. I remember playing army with the neighborhood kids. They were all boys one to three years older than I was, and they had me be the nurse, just to be rid of me, I think. I was always in the "back lines" and occasionally one of the boys would let me bandage his arm. My cousin was a nurse anesthetist in WWII. I never thought of being anything else; I'm working full-time right now and still like patient care and contact.

I was raised a Methodist and was influenced to apply to Bronson by our local minister, Reverend George Beacock. I was concerned about being accepted, as I was told there were many more applicants than spots. I didn't apply anywhere else, however.

After Graduation

I moved to Cleveland immediately after graduation. Sharon Witmer and I were going to work in the OR; it had 22 OR rooms and different teams for the different specialties. We were impressed. On the hospital tour, the personnel director said, "While we're here on this floor, we have a new area that we like to show prospective employees as we're always looking for nurses to work here. We call it Intensive Care." Sharon and I were hooked the day we first saw it. Today both of us still work in this setting.

I met my husband in Cleveland within two weeks of my arrival. He was a dental student. The Vietnam War was at full scale, so he enlisted in the navy. Following graduation his first assignment was at the Great Lakes Training Center and then was assigned to Chelsea Naval Hospital here in Boston. We've been here ever since except for one year in North Carolina (1987–1988).

I went back to school at Boston University (1979–81). Lorraine Wilson, a BMH graduate, was the co-author of one of my favorite texts (pathophysiology). I read and outlined the entire book as a challenge, and I passed the test for course credit. The theory and courses at Boston U. were great and meant so much more to me the second time around. I absorbed a lot of information but was also happy to have the diploma background and clinical experience.

My greatest joy in nursing has always been interacting with the patient. I like people, and I like to allay their fears, and help to make them comfortable in a strange and oftentimes frightening environment. I love my specialty as I enjoy the challenge of serving the critically ill patient and using the technical skills required to do my job.

THE SIXTIES IN A NUTSHELL

The faster pace of life is exemplified in this barrage of incomplete sentences from the Class of 1966 members Cheryl Delobel Conner, Donna Easton Meninga, and Marilyn Emery Luther:

the need to pass two days of intensive testing (including psychological evaluation)
to be admitted to BMH
getting your acceptance letter
moving into Truesdale Hall at 515 Pine St. on September 15, 1963
paying $1,000 for three years of training
meeting roommates and suitemates
your big sis who had decorated your bulletin board and left your string of safety pins
signifying the months of training ahead of you
having the first married student who was allowed to live
in her own apartment in the freshman class
Hell Week
Capping
your first TPR assignment
riding the bus to WMU for first semester classes and
the songs we sang during the ride
curfews of 10:30 on weeknights, midnight on weekends with one 1:30/month
signing in and out on the cards at the front desk
the perfect Mrs. Kingsley as an instructor
the unofficial school song, *I Go to BMH Oh Pity Me,*
there's not a man in this damn nunnery
being buzzed in your room to let you know someone was calling,
and running down to the phones at the end of the hall
peeking through the mailboxes on the first floor to check out
your (or someone else's) date
hoping for even some junk mail in your mailbox
watching Dr. Kildare on TV in the basement recreation room
while eating hot dogs sold by the student council
using reusable needles and checking for burrs
mixing penicillin

patients on the sun porch
watching the seniors come across from the hospital to the dorm
wearing their capes and wishing the capes hadn't been discontinued
starched uniforms that had been measured for appropriate length
(14 inches from the floor)
clinic shoes
reusable treatment trays from Central Supply
meal trays coming up on the dumbwaiters
oxygen tents
counting IV drops
using med cards and pouring meds from multiple dose bottles
counting narcotics at the end of every shift
12-week rotations on all shifts
2 West
no air conditioning in the hospital
circle beds
black banding
cars lined up outside the dorm at night with everyone spending
the last few minutes with that special boyfriend
no men allowed upstairs
Truesdale Lounge and fireplace room
Daisy Manley at the switchboard
3 East with Mrs. Z and her BM rounds
scrubbing in OR
team leading with Mrs. Grubb
unassigned time
3 months at KRPH
being in charge of the unit as a student
nights with Mrs. Cripe
frequent visits from the Fire Department for padded bras burning in the dryer
the taped, locked door on fifth floor that had to be axed open
sitting under the hair dryer in the basement beauty shop at the dorm
sunbathing on the fifth-floor deck
pecan rolls from the hospital bakery
the snack shop in the hospital lobby
walking to the local ice cream shops (Carousel and Mursch's)
the Rexall drug store on Burdick
the $1 movies at the State Theatre
shopping on the Kalamazoo Mall
working for pay
milk and Maalox every half hour
Harold, Casper, and Lyle
the hospital softball and basketball games
KXI
bats from the church next door

watching the intern activities across the street
Schwartz's drive-in
selecting a little sis
playing cards with the psych patients at KPH
the song, *Counting Flowers on the Wall*
mixers at WMU
hitchhiking back to the dorm from classes at WMU
the squeaky shoes of Dr. Stenesh in chemistry class
dissecting cats
leaving Wood Hall at WMU and hearing of President Kennedy's assassination
pharmacology class with Mrs. Damvelt Tuesday and Thursday nights
at 7 P.M. in the basement of Truesdale Hall
only skirts allowed in classrooms and the hospital
linen days when we got clean sheets and towels
bells ringing for "man on the floor"
refrigerators in floor kitchens in the dorm
cooking in popcorn poppers
medical externs from England and Scotland
climbing out onto the Truesdale roof
the lockdown after the Richard Speck killings in Chicago
the tunnel between the hospital and the dorm
the ER trophy case of objects removed from patients (and they weren't all fish hooks)
Linda Richards Hall at KSH
cornflakes, peanut butter toast, and Spam at KSH
special care nursery with Miss Fox and the formula room
the T&A ward on Pediatrics
sign-off books
A.M. and P.M. care
learning proper backrub techniques
rubber sheets and mercury thermometers
surgery and PAR on the fifth floor
the first ICU opening on the second floor by the Personnel Department
always being addressed as "Miss____"
making rounds with the doctors
Miss Downy on 3 East, 3:00–11:00 P.M.
Mrs. Rice, Mrs. Klop, and Frosty
Mrs. Meninga, Mrs. Adkins, and Mrs. Cardiff on OB
Mrs. Weber
the threat of being expelled if you made three med errors
med trays with syringe and needle inside a cotton ball to be
carried down to a patient's room for administration
covering bed pans
folding washcloths into hand mitts
no nail polish or jewelry allowed while on duty
living in fear of failure resulting in disappointment for self and family

and as a result missing out on some learning opportunities
hypodermoclysis
assignment books
working four out of five weekends as students
Public Health and outpatient clinics with Mrs. Lord
the Alma Mater
graduation at the First United Methodist Church on July 28, 1966—
the largest class ever at that time with 64 grads

We will never forget good old BMH—the great education we received, the fantastic friends we made, and all the priceless memories . . .

CHAPTER 7 NOTES

---

[1] *The Charlotte Leader*, N.C. 1988 July 6, and telephone interview with Diana Dwan Poole by Jackie Wylie, 2003 November 29.

[2] *Kalamazoo Gazette*, 1960 December 21, "Auxiliary pays pledge."

[3] *Kalamazoo Gazette*, 1963 February 14, "Nurses receive valentine gift."

[4] *Bronson Bulletin*, 1960 Autumn; 4. "Bronson Hospital clinics expanding in both numbers and attendance."

[5] *Kalamazoo Gazette*, 1960 December 28, "Rates up $2 at two hospitals."

[6] *Kalamazoo Gazette*, 1961 January 6, "Asks 'why' of hospital costs."

[7] *Kalamazoo Gazette,* 1960 December 28, *op.cit.*.

[8] *Kalamazoo Gazette*, 1961 June 11. "New head of hospital defends service costs."

[9] *Kalamazoo Gazette*, 1966 October 19, "Tide of Medicare patients swamping local hospitals.

[10] *Kalamazoo Gazette*, 1962 February 25, "Hike rate for private nursing."

[11] *Kalamazoo Gazette*, 1965 June 8, "Battle on nursing duty shaping up."

[12] *Bronson Bulletin*, 1961 Winter; 1. "William C. Perdew, D.D., 1900–1960."

[13] *Bronson Bulletin*, 1969 December; 2. "Mr. Finch discusses comprehensive health planning."

[14] *Bronson Bulletin*, 1960 Summer; 3. "Income and expenses of operating Bronson Methodist Hospital."

[15] *The Catalyst Extra*, undated, Announcing organizational changes effective 1966 October 17.

[16] The first orientation is referenced on page three of an unnamed first-time employee newspaper which included a contest with a $25 prize, "Name the No Name News." The in-house paper became

The Catalyst, August 1963. The winner of the contest was senior nursing student Linda Cutright, announced in the second edition.

[17] *Kalamazoo Gazette*, 1961 June 8, "Federal aid okayed for Bronson.

[18] *Kalamazoo Gazette*, 1960 March 16," Dr. Perdew lists plans: Details hospital expansion."

[19] *Bronson Bulletin*, 1964 Summer; 1. "Community puts expansion drive over the top."

[20] *Bronson Bulletin*, 1967 Summer, p.1 picture.

[21] *Kalamazoo Gazette*, 1965 August 26, "Bronson Hospital to get cobalt unit."

[22] *Kalamazoo Gazette*, 1965 October 24, "Planned for 1968: Bronson Hospital to build three-story youth wing."

[23] Kal*amazoo Gazette*, 1966 May 24, "Cedar Street relocation."

[24] *The Catalyst*, 1965 December, "PAR and ICU units, 1965."

[25] *Bronson Bulletin*, 1965 Fall; 2. "Bronson nurse finds invention two-time winner."

[26] Sigma Theta Tau, International Biennial Convention speaker. 2003 November, Toronto, Ontario.

[27] *Kalamazoo Gazette*, 1960 August 31, "Bronson to graduate 26 from school of nursing.

[28] *Kalamazoo Gazette*, 1960 August 7, "Expect 84 in freshman class."

[29] *Bronson Bulletin*, 1960 Summer; 2. "Four Bronson School of Nursing students receive special recognition."

[30] *Kalamazoo Gazette*, 1961 April 25, "Nursing school choruses to sing at Muskegon."

[31] *Kalamazoo Gazette*, 1960 August 8, "Group writes legislators: student nurses plead for full mental health funds."

[32] *The Catalyst*, 1966 December; 10. "Nursing the art of origami."

[33] *Kalamazoo Gazette*, 1961 January 22, "Creates circus menagerie: local nursing instructor masters Japanese paper folding art."

[34] Oral interview with Linda Van Dyke by Jackie Wylie, 2004 June 28.

[35] ACLS, advanced cardiac life support.

[36] PAR, the post anesthesia recovery unit.

[37] IVPB, intravenous piggy backs, a term for intravenous infusion bottles (later plastic bags) that were inserted into the main intravenous infusion line.

[38] PCN referred to penicillin.

[39] "Bovie" referred to a cauterizing machine named after its inventor.

[40] Initials for the Post Anesthesia Recovery, Labor and Delivery, Emergency Room and Intensive Care Units.

CHAPTER 8

A MEDICAL INDUSTRIAL COMPLEX, 1970s

"When does it get easier?" This Class of 1974 theme, from Marsha Lewis's perspective[1], depicted her three years of Bronson nursing school education and also seemed quite apropos for hospitals that were trying to adhere to rules for reimbursement of medical and hospital services. Maintaining financial integrity didn't seem to be easier for hospitals, even with more reliable payment from private insurance and government units. Still, millions of Americans "fell through the healthcare cracks." Was healthcare a privilege or a right? The government, insurance companies and businesses started to ask the question, why the high costs for service? Could Americans afford a national healthcare system that was built on a medical model? Although the answer obviously was, "No," what would take its place?

Education of advance practice nurses and physicians' assistants was intended to create mid-level providers who could bring less expensive medical services to the public, with physicians as gatekeepers. The incredible knowledge increase in specialty disease management simply focused allied health professionals on that service, returning chronically ill people to a level of self-care and functional ability, important work but not balanced with other health-oriented possibilities. Public health options such as health promotion, disease prevention and a safe environment received less attention and less funding.

Could this be turned around? Not without a transformation of healthcare services which would balance resources given to invasive technology, and toward health promotion and disease prevention. Health promotion meant that each person had to be responsible for maintenance of individual, family and community health. This shift did not happen because of the amount of attention given to curing disease and the inattention to lifestyle and safe environment.

Newspapers told the story. Nurses and other allied health professionals were recognized only for their ability to provide delegated medical care and decrease high costs. Nurses and their non-physician colleagues, *i.e.,* nutritionists–dieticians, pharmacists, social workers, occupational therapists, physical therapists, *etc.,* all were paid mainly by fitting into the medical, disease-oriented model. Those outside the medical system, such as chiropractors and holistic health practitioners, were only considered to be non-scientific nuisances until it became clear that medical care alone was not the answer to developing a national healthcare system. If people recognized the need to reform the costly system, their voices were not heard. Dramatic technology always seemed to win over lifestyle changes that were less valued.

NURSE STAFFING, A MONUMENTAL TASK

Bronson Hospital, called a monument to women before it was built, became a monumental nurse staffing challenge. A December 10, 1904, news story described the hospital-to-be-built as a monument to women, " . . . for their untiring efforts which have produced a result to be proud of."[2] The result was a significant amount of money! Women had directed their energy toward generating community interest and dollars that provided a major portion of the capital to build the hospital. They continued to take active volunteer roles within a charitable system of care over the decades, one way to control costs. Nursing students in hospital-based schools contributed to low labor costs in exchange for service learning, board and room, uniforms, and inexpensive tuition. Less service meant that tuition would rise and amenities would decrease.

Bronson nurses numbered in the hundreds by the seventies and were the source of budget concerns, not because they made so much money—it took so many of them to manage acute, intensive patient care. Numbers of School of Nursing graduates averaged 70 a year, with Bronson hiring as many as would stay to offset high turnover rates and expansion of services.

Staffing challenges were newsworthy within Bronson's in-house bulletin, which described a three-part system: scheduling work hours for nurses, a patient-care evaluation (Medicus), and quality monitoring. Arthur Littlefield, chief nurse administrator, defined the term nurse staffing as, " . . . a process of identifying the individual patient-care needs and placing the right nurse with the right credentials at the right time and in the right place to meet those needs."[3] When census was down, nurses were given a shift or part of a shift off. Most seemed glad for the relief and often had the ability to live without a portion of their pay. This system had helped to manage costs over several decades. Nursing was not the problem. Instead, many considered it to be an illness care, over-utilization issue.

Nurses were and are in 2004 the biggest group of professionals employed in hospitals. One small wage increase for several hundred nurses was monumental in dollars required, compared to other professional group raises. The nurse wage scale, however, was compressed so that expert nurses earned little more annually for their expertise than did starting novice nurses. Starting wages were acceptable, but the flat scale did not reward the expert competencies that come with advanced critical thinking skills and years of front-line experience.

While nurse-staffing costs were being scrutinized in-house, governments scrutinized costs that they believed related to utilization and the need to halt capital expansion, which drove over-utilization. Efforts were beginning to slow down the apparent runaway train created by the Hill–Burton Act, which provided federal funds that increased the number of hospitals and services—not bad at the time—but not balanced with health promotion and disease prevention services. Public health and promotion activities received a tiny fraction of the dollar compared to money spent on hospital growth, equipment, and physician services (very different from services that could have been given by nurses and other allied health professionals).

LACKING RECOGNITION FOR CONTRIBUTIONS

How visible were women and nursing practice in the 1970s healthcare news? The annual announcement of graduation ceremonies, numbers of graduates, and names of those with local residences were reported. What else was there to write about? The system seemed to be working, and nurses were doing well with a wage that, overall, they accepted but that didn't compare well to wages for positions of less or equal responsibility and risks. Staff nurse responsibilities were burdensome. Nurses were the original multitaskers, expected to accomplish amazing feats and manage 50 jobs at once, not an exaggeration! Most of the time they managed well, but they went home at the end of their shift ready to drop the "hot rock" on other nurses coming on duty. Little energy was left to offer peer support.

Nursing education responded to the increasingly complex practice environment by creating curricula to educate clinical nurse specialists (CNSs) for roles required to assist the growing number of chronically ill people.

CNSs utilized physician protocols and practiced nursing within the dominant medical culture with the inclusion of nursing's answer to healing with caring, heartfelt relationships. Patients' editorials thanked nurses for their care, kindness', and technological competence. Nurses made the *Kalamazoo Gazette* editorial page on a regular basis, a source of public recognition, and to them the visibility felt good.

The nurses' presence was obvious in patient-care units as integral front-line providers directing daily activities. Interrelationships with all departments and providers made nurses hard to miss. Not to acknowledge their incredible responsibilities, 24 hours a day, seven days a week, apparently are a way of letting sleeping giants sleep.

An external layer of insulation appeared to exempt nurses and other nonmedical professionals from cost concerns when considering models of care and decision-making processes that could have helped balance the out-of-control, high-cost, technological system. Several of the so-called "allied" health professionals provided self-care and self-health management solutions that were not reimbursed or part of the medical model. They were not measured or considered as one answer to quality, effective care with less burden of suffering and dollar cost to the public.

The feminine factor seemed to wane over 75 years. It was often missing or hidden under layers of the hospital administration and medical staff. More than 95 percent of the physicians were men who viewed the 95 percent of women nurses as little more than physician extenders delegated to follow medical orders, although nursing care always involved so much more.

What if nursing and all of the other allied health professions with unique philosophies and ways of healing had been recognized for their real worth? Think of what a collaboration of health promotion educators, such as nurses, nutritionists, social workers, clergy, *etc.,* could have done for cost-effective care in health promotion and disease prevention as well as intervention during illness? Citizens held their health in their own hands—lifestyle choices.

HEALTHCARE IN THE NEWS: CONTAINMENT OF MEDICAL COSTS

The payment system—government and private insurers—recognized only the dominant medical culture and illness care as designed by the medical model. When the public lost sight of its self-care responsibility, it lived with myths that lifestyle didn't matter and, when the individual became sick, medical culture could cure him or her. Acute illnesses became most manageable, but chronicity was raising its head with a population that was living longer. It was easy to give up self-care responsibility and fall into complacence with sedentary lifestyles, TV, fast foods and fast-paced living.

Medicare and Medicaid were blamed for fast-rising, out-of-control hospitalization. Their entitlements created a payment mechanism and a demand for an expensive, masculine-oriented system that logically used every piece of existing technology, without regard for caring relationships—a major factor in healing.

Bronson's administrative officers at the top four levels were: Administrator, Daniel N. Finch; Associate Administrator, Peter W. Froyd; Assistant Administrators, William A. Johnson and William E. Johnson; and Administrative Assistants, F. Ray McConnell, Kenneth W. Huckendubler, and James K. Stroebel.

Mr. Finch's duties included, ". . . direct responsibility for Nursing Education," and Mr. William A. Johnson's, ". . . administrative duties included Nursing Service."[4] Miss Virginia McPhail was no longer at Bronson, the only woman since the early matron/superintendent days to rank with top administrators. She left her Bronson employment in June 1970.

The *Kalamazoo Gazette* published Sylvia Porter's editorials five days in a row describing the cost of illness as a desperate national situation.[5,6,7,8,9] Borgess and Bronson administrators talked about how to, " . . . avoid any unnecessary duplication of services . . . with the ultimate objective of increasing overall services available in the Kalamazoo area."[10]

Professional Standards Review Organizations (PSROs) were regional groups of local physicians, created by Public Law 92-603 to review utilization of healthcare resources and facilities. Physicians were considered the most competent in assessing appropriate medical care, given the rule that professional organizations police themselves. Who could argue that? It's just hard to see your own shortfalls. Probably all professions could have benefited by taking a careful look at practices that no longer made sense. Evidenced-based practice was only beginning. The recognition of health and healthcare overall had a long way to grow as more than medical management of disorders. A public attitude that medicine could fix any health problem appeared to be one factor that diminished interest in healthy lifestyles. One hundred years earlier Florence Nightingale referenced a woman being " . . . cured of self-mismanagement."[11] Knowledge of Nightingale's nursing diagnosis may have been an answer to rising seventies costs. The first-half century found most Americans engaged in home care. Few had access to formally educated professionals, and there was an acceptance of disease and death as natural life events.

During the seventies speculation on how long a person could live or be kept alive fueled rising hospital costs in the name of research. Immortality must have sounded good to most Americans, and no cost was too great to stay on Earth. A part of the resulting cost problem was the number of people dying only after all possible medical support had been used in futile attempts to save people even when death was inevitable. Americans along with health care providers continued to ignore the need for changing their philosophical underpinnings of health, wellness, safe environment and illness care.

Public Law 93-641, the Federal Health Planning and Resources Development Act of 1974, created local Health Systems Agencies (HSAs) to control expansion and rising costs by requiring *certificates of need* to be submitted before hospitals and other healthcare agencies could build, remodel, or buy new equipment. The federal government dedicated $97 million to the HSAs for the purpose of eliminating wasteful duplication of services. A competitive marketplace could not work since no one had a choice of when and where to be sick, although hospitals were beginning to market to the public as well as to physicians. Both were considered to be customers.

Hospital officials explained that compliance with government regulations was a big part of the added costs. Thirty-six dollars a day had to be added to hospital room charges to meet all of the paperwork requirements. Exploding costs created a vicious cycle with everyone blaming someone else.

An article in the June 21, 1978, *Bronson Bulletin* blamed everybody, probably rightfully so. "Everybody orders more when it's an expense account meal." Payments for hospitalization were covered by insurance and government plans for 90 percent of all patients. Indirect payment contributed to the loss of insight concerning costs. Who was really paying? Many at Bronson tried to cover the gaps with donations to the Good Neighbor Fund. Some people were ineligible for services but were treated; their costs then were integrated into overall charity care management operational expenses.

Costs were generated in response to medical diagnostics and treatments, since physicians were the only group of professionals who received direct reimbursement for services. Cost-cutting efforts did not directly study the imbalance of high-tech and high-touch care or consider a shift in thought. Medical providers couldn't do what they didn't know, not being trained in the ways of health promotion and lifestyle impact. The public was not ready to see the need for an integrative, interdisciplinary approach to care. Glimmers of system changes received small monetary rewards of $10 to $100. An example was nurse Marilyn Boer '62, who received a $10 award for suggesting the use of heavy plastic bags to enclose items used in a strict isolation room, a safe environmental practice that would protect employees from cross contamination and ultimately save suffering and dollars.[12]

WHO COULD BE BLAMED FOR RISING COSTS?

Medicare and Medicaid were blamed for costs rising from $300 a day in the sixties to $1,300 in the late seventies. The elderly were blamed for running up the cost of medical bills, for not transferring to less expensive care in nursing homes or to family home care, as if they had control over these choices.

If it was the elders, it was also those tiny babies. Baby buses (ambulance services for pre-term births), baby ventilators, and regional neonatal teams came into being. Costs to keep pre-term infants alive came with a huge burden of suffering and monetary output of $100,000 to $235,000— the largest hospital bill seen in 75 years to cover expenses for a 20-month stay.[13] It wasn't unusual for a baby to spend its first year of life in the hospital, only to go home with one or more chronic illnesses. Why wasn't more attention given to prenatal care and the prevention of pre-term births, along with the technological developments? It was and still is hard to disagree with the philosophy that every baby is priceless; but priceless enough to give it a healthy start by delaying pregnancy, preventing unintended pregnancies and providing their mothers with early prenatal care when conceived?

In some cases lawyers were blamed for climbing costs. Invasive technology, rising expectations, and less direct patient–physician relationships brought lawsuits and soaring malpractice insurance rates. The public fell out of love with invasive, high-tech care. As John Naisbitt proposed ten years later in *Megatrends*, ". . . there must be a counterbalancing human response [to technology]—that is, high touch—or the technology is rejected.[14] Except for pockets of nurses breaking out of the medical model, especially in university settings, nurses employed in hospitals for the most part were not conscious of the impact they could make given another practice model. Nursing care in public health departments and in industrial settings focused more attention on wellness but certainly never had the budget or influence needed to overhaul the ailing system. No one was blameless. Too few Americans engaged in daily healthy lifestyle practices.

HOSPITAL EXPANSION CONTINUES

In 1969 the Michigan legislature authorized the city " . . . to establish a hospital finance authority [to] issue city revenue bonds in an unlimited amount to finance the construction of facilities for a nonprofit hospital located in the area."[15]

Borgess planned a $10 million expansion, while Bronson decided to add third, fourth, and fifth floors to the new Center Building.

The center building at Bronson emerged in the seventies to house new emergency, obstetrics, and pediatrics departments. Bronson wanted to provide birth to death services and its expertise was in these areas. The population was also aging. Older adults were the greatest consumers, wanting to live functional lives without having to adapt to the infirmities of old age that were previously inevitable if they lived long enough.

The Emergency Department expansion was initiated in 1971 with $6.5 million[16] from federal and individual contributions that included $300,000 from the Kalamazoo Foundation.[17] It became a Trauma and Emergency Center in 1972 with 24-hour medical staff, traumatologists, nurses and paramedics, and mobile trauma units[18]; the operating rooms were relocated to the main floor of the north building; and the cafeteria was relocated to and enlarged in the basement.

The first local open-heart surgery was performed at Borgess Medical Center in January of 1972,[19] and Bronson's Burn Unit opened in February, 1973, to provide acute and convalescent care with multiple rehabilitative services within a sterile environment.[20] The medical director was Frank Newman, MD, supported by 13 nurses and other personnel. The women of the Bronson Methodist Hospital Auxiliary gave $9,000 to pay for a new Hubbard Tank, "a must for the burn unit," so that patients would not be exposed to potential infection when being transported outside of the unit. The total-immersion water treatment helped debride burn wounds, allowing new growing tissue to emerge. Attention to burn prevention may have attributed to the low patient numbers and eventual phase out of the burn unit, an example of how education could decrease costs and suffering.

Bronson's Kidney Center opened in spring, 1973,[21] and offered expanded hemodialysis services for people with end stage renal disease, many waiting for kidney transplants. Director of kidney care since 1969, H. Curtis Benson, MD, was

". . . responsible for an integrated program of treatment and training for patients with chronic renal disease, utilizing the artificial kidney machine." Patricia McDonald, '61, was the head nurse.

NON-INVASIVE INTERVENTIONS AND ALTERNATIVES TO HOSPITALIZATION

Outpatient surgery took on new meaning—a way to gain revenue yet reduce suffering and bed utilization. Surgery took on a less invasive nature with a variety of scopes that could be inserted into patients' abdomens, joints and other places. The outcome was a small aperture instead of greater trauma from scalpel-made incisions that took longer to open, close, and heal. Revolutionary laparoscopic technology paved the way for modifying a full week's hospital stay to one to two days and shorter recovery times at home.

Mandatory hospital bed reductions and cost containment failed miserably, as did voluntary physician measures to control expansion and use of technology. Costs continued to soar as medical research offered more body repair and lifesaving measures that required clinical trials for continuing research to occur. Over time, reimbursement mechanisms were changed when it became evident that the system was a runaway train that no one was able to stop.

Kaiser Permanente's Health Maintenance Organization (HMO) on the West Coast appeared to have one answer: health promotion meant to encourage healthy lifestyles and selfcare responsibility. Physicians and health care agencies received a specified number of dollars a year per patient. If the person became ill and required hospitalization, expenses rose beyond the amount received for care, therefore putting pressure on the system to keep people well using the least numbers of medications and treatments and definitely staying out of the hospital.

Somehow both the public and professionals were able to overlook growing mental-health problems: the numbers of people living depressed lives, in states of neuroses or psychoses, and myriad disorders that took their toll on functional abilities in adults and children. Treatment consisted mainly of medication and behavior modification and moving out of structured environments within institutions, like the Kalamazoo Regional Psychiatric Hospital, and into the community but without adequate funding. Bronson never provided psychiatric mental-health services, although occasionally psychiatric patients were admitted for surgical services.

Complementary Alternative Modalities

Some nurses and physicians saw the benefit of new ways to face health, illness, and end-of-life care. The American Holistic Nurses Association offered professional support for nurses who believed healthy relationships were a healing source. And the National Institutes of Health began to consider research proposals in complementary alternative modalities, looking for new ways to create a healthier nation at less cost.

Patient Education

People needed to be informed about the impact of lifestyle and environment on overall health. Healthy lifestyle alternatives crept into consciousness, while the first educational programs at Bronson focused on expectant-parent classes and patient management of their diseases, in between doctor visits.

Private industry, such as the Upjohn Company, was recognizing the impact of the cost of healthcare and the need to educate their employees. Company executives began to encourage employees to participate in preventive health maintenance programs and to develop healthy lifestyles, in the effort to decrease the coast of providing medical care for illness and injury. They also monitored the employee population exposed to hazardous or toxic materials for related health changes. Employee health services, staffed primarily by nurses and assisted by allied healthcare professionals, administered these programs. Anna Stryd, corporate occupational health nurse, directed the education health promotion and disease prevention programs in her company.

Education became not only a soft marketing tool but an intervention for helping people live functional lives while managing three or four chronic diseases, such as diabetes, heart disease, and arthritis. People would have to take self-care responsibility if they were going to live healthier lives and have greater potential for dying with their boots on.

Support Groups Led by the Public

People living with chronic illness benefited by hearing others' stories. As women's breast cancer numbers increased, support groups were formalized and offered healing modalities never considered to be part of medical care. Coming together and sharing stories seemed to be healing in itself. In addition, the groups provided an opportunity to learn about all kinds of interventions, from mega-vitamin ingestion to out-of-comfort zone foods that increased longevity, *etc.* In later years research actually verified that people facing life-threatening illnesses lived healthier and longer lives when they participated in support groups.

Hospice Care

Hospice care came into being first in England. Freestanding agencies and hospice home-care support helped face mortality. Thought processes changed to family care and comfort during end-of-life, instead of medical care and invasive technology that added to patient and family misery as well as burdensome dollar costs.

In 1979 the hospice idea was localized when a group of 40 Kalamazoo-based volunteers organized a fundraiser to begin offering hospice services to the dying and to their families who chose such care when diagnostics and treatment only seemed to prolong the suffering at end of life. Bronson's Chaplain, David Davis, was one of the promoters. St. Luke's Episcopal Church was to act as the fiscal agent until the group obtained tax-exempt status.[22] End-of-life care was transformed.

AN ENVIRONMENTAL MODIFICATION IN NURSING CARE DELIVERY

Nurses became more accessible to patients and their families when nursing decided to decentralize the nursing stations and create small mini-stations and nurse-servers[23] on each hallway. Previously one nursing station was located at the hub of the square-cross arrangement and had served all four corridors. The move included installing cupboards by each patient's room with the patient's chart and frequently used supplies kept close to the bedside for nurse convenience. The arrangement was not so convenient for physicians who wanted to access all patient records at one central location. The move was intended to decrease miles that the nurses' walked each day and reduce physical fatigue. Florence Nightingale, over one hundred years before, had the same concern for nurses who spent far too much time running up and down stairs to procure supplies. She had a dumb waiter installed to save the nurses' steps.[24] Norma Young, nurse supervisor on Hall 8, was one who helped to sell the new Bronson system to nurses and physicians. Though the nurse-servers and mini-stations had their benefits, some nurses missed the opportunities for collaboration with their peers when they had gathered around one central workstation. Confidentiality also became a concern since the nurse-servers were not locked. Anyone could access records or supplies. The system was eventually discarded.

MEANWHILE, BACK AT THE SCHOOL OF NURSING

The School of Nursing flourished during the seventies with the blessing of funds connected to medical education pass-through dollars and the ever-increasing tuition that students paid. Time spent in theory and closely supervised practice increased. Hours of nursing practice were more selective and directly related to classroom learning. The stronger work-study model used in prior years gave way to a more traditional academic approach. Experiential learning had offered repetition of previously taught skills. Less time in practice meant less repetition and a "tighter" program of study, one of the expectations for maintaining accreditation with the National League for Nursing (NLN).

Students from families who met low-income criteria qualified for Basic Educational Opportunity Grants (BEOG). They could obtain this money because Bronson was accredited by a government-accepted accreditor, the NLN. The Heyl Scholarship program was an additional boon.

A Gift to Nursing Education—Heyl Scholarships

Dr. Frederick Heyl, research scientist, and Mrs. Elsie Heyl will be remembered for their gift to nursing that continues in perpetuity.[25] The Heyl family philosophical underpinnings were socialistic and taught a sense of community economics along with a strong sense of giving service and worth in all people. Heyl's beloved father worked in the woodcarving craft, not a well-to-do man, but rather one who loved life and balanced work with fun. His mother was of German roots, and she was more practical and serious in nature.

F.W. Heyl's pharmaceutical career began in his Uncle Otto's drugstore. As he grew out of his teens, he was given more work responsibilities and was exposed to philosophical lessons learned from watching what this drugstore owner did for his community. His uncle's philosophy of community caring stayed with him for a lifetime. It guided his research and social conscience toward benefits to individuals and, ultimately, their communities. Dr. and Mrs. Heyl willed their accumulated wealth for the betterment of others. Heyl wanted healthcare products to be readily available to families at a cost just slightly higher than the cost of production, an idea that he had learned from Professor Ely at Yale.

> Delivering prescriptions to the upper floors of wretched tenement houses . . . made me remember unforgettably the filthiness against

> which some of the honest, God-fearing mothers struggled to rear their babies and . . . fought a losing fight against the vermin.[26]
>
> The drug store and its life have never left me.[27]

Dr. Heyl began his Upjohn career in 1913. "He brought with him to Upjohn an already developed sense of the purposefulness of the drugstore with its practical applications of remedies, time-tested for human benefit."[28] He was hired by S. Rudolph Light, MD, to begin a quality control program that would meet the regulations of the Federal Pure Food and Drug Act of 1906, the first drug law in the United States. His research came later.

F.W. Heyl tried to answer the question he saw as important about public and private domain—how could he best support the common folks and bring healthcare supplies and drugs to people who labored for small wages? He found his answer by giving the community a mechanism to support the education of its sons and daughters who chose to major in biological or physical science. A fortune amassed from drug patent royalties turned into endowments to Kalamazoo College, Yale University, the Bronson Methodist Hospital School of Nursing and, later, the WMU Bronson School of Nursing. Not only did individual students receive full scholarships but indirect expenses were also figured into his caring for students and their chosen schools, giving the three schools major boosts each year.[29]

"I am motivated by a desire to establish a fund consisting of the bulk of my estate, the net income from which shall be employed in promoting the education of young men and young women in the field of the exact sciences and in the field of nursing."[30] The combined teachings of his socialist father and his practical uncle, plus his own synthesis of ideas related to community need, set Dr. Heyl's direction. One quote of his is similar to the caring concerns of Florence Nightingale as well. "So far as the gospels are concerned, I decided that everybody who reads is entitled to his own interpretation." Florence and Frederick believed in natural laws that were subject to the interpretation of the men who built their specific religions using some, but not all, of God's laws. Natural laws also came from God and had to be learned in order to bring the best world to all of the people. Tolerance was part of their natures. "Unity of faith" crossed all religions, and encouraged the "evolution of human consciousness."[31]

Heyl continued his New Haven education at Yale University, which was located next door to the public high school, Hillhouse High, from which he graduated. Similar to the sons of nineteenth-century immigrants, his goal was to attend an eastern preparatory school. Heyl was proud that he and his classmates from the local high school could pass Yale's comprehensive examinations, be admitted, and graduate. He earned his first degree in 1904, with a major in chemistry, and a PhD in 1908.[32] Despite his fear of failure, Heyl had found the study of chemistry both "easy and interesting."

Dr. Heyl knew that children were dependent on financial resources, often a limiting factor in their educational choices. W. L. Orwin believed this factor was the reason Heyl limited the scholarship program to the Kalamazoo Public Schools (KPS)—central city children were less likely to have the resources found in the suburbs.[33]

The Heyls Impact on Bronson School of Nursing

While working at Upjohn, Dr. Heyl served as a Kalamazoo College faculty member. He held the college in high esteem and decided to focus his time, attention and future finances to help keep the college in excellent financial condition. Heyl's patent royalties, from early Upjohn Company patents, created the wealth for this community gift for graduates of the Kalamazoo Public School system, first Central High School and then extended to Loy Norrix High School when the second school was built.

The scholarship trust was created by Frederick W. Heyl, PhD and his wife Elsie L. Heyl. When setting up his legacy for future students, Heyl's words provided a glimpse of his sense of Kalamazoo's human capital, "We want to appreciate these hard working and well-endowed students and encourage them to develop their talents. This is an investment. This plan is an invitation to hard work".[34]

> It is believed that Bronson Methodist Hospital School of Nursing was chosen primarily because Mrs. Heyl has undergone two serious operations at Bronson, and was eager to reward the hospital for the compassionate care she had received. The nursing school scholarships are named for her. It is our understanding that she herself had an interest in nursing as a profession.[35]

Most likely the compassionate care received was within the hands of Bronson students and graduates who, before 1970, provided the majority of patient care at the hospital. Bronson women set the stage for the receipt of this prestigious gift.

The First Heyl Scholars

The Heyl Foundation made news in the July 1971 *Bronson Bulletin*, although only four Bronson students were recipients as of 1975.[36] By 1979, 12 Bronson students were receiving annual benefits.[37]

Lesley LaRoy was one of the rare nursing students who had not spent her early years dreaming about becoming a nurse. Career options had not been explored, and she assumed that she would become a teacher. She never considered nursing until her senior year at Kalamazoo Central High School when her physics teacher, Neil Norcross, mentioned the possibility of a Heyl scholarship to Bronson School of Nursing. He told her it was a new scholarship, and there was a good chance that she could qualify. She knew the value of a scholarship and figured that she would have to work part time while attending college, which was accepted by her.

Her parents were thrilled when the scholarship was awarded! Her father was a carpenter and her mother worked in a fabric store. Although the family was not poor, it did not have much discretionary income. The thrill may also have come from the recognition of their intelligent daughter's ability to succeed in a professional career.

Lesley worked "for pay" on off-hours at Bronson for spending money only. She never had to worry about tuition, only later becoming conscious of students who were not as fortunate as she. Until looking back, years later, when she was preparing her own children for college did she fully appreciate the value of the scholarship.

Use of Heyl "Indirect Dollars"

As dollars collected for indirect expenses grew throughout the seventies and early 1980s, a major remodeling of Truesdale Hall was completed, courtesy of Heyl's continuing gift.

- Truesdale Hall was put on a maintenance plan that Heyl dollars helped support throughout the remainder of its lifetime.
- Renovation of the Nursing Arts Laboratory gave students the opportunity to practice skills in an educational environment beyond the dreams of most Michigan nursing schools. We were proud! Jackie Wylie, in her director role throughout the eighties visited many schools. Few had learning laboratories that compared to Bronson's.
- Students and faculty/staff input helped insure the purchase of useful educational tools that were readily procured with the benefit of the Heyl funds.
- For 20 years, Bronson used these funds primarily for remodeling and maintaining the Nursing Arts Laboratory, and state-of-the-art educational

media and equipment, as well as environmental improvements in the student living quarters and classrooms of Truesdale Hall.

Heyl's Philosophy Opened the Door for Wylie

When I became the director of the school, one of my first self-care lessons for the school was to learn about its financing. Diploma schools were fading, closing across the nation in response to changing health-care economics and the funding of nursing and medical education. Kenneth Taft, Bronson's finance director, helped me learn about the school's resources, including the Heyl endowment.

Dr. Heyl wanted to help students who had the will and intellect to succeed. I wondered how I might connect scholarships with intelligent students who had less than stellar high school grade point averages (GPAs) that did not reflect their intellect or ability to succeed had they been given support rarely afforded students with fewer financial resources.

It was easy for me to see that intelligent students, who came from less well-endowed families or from different family cultures than did their peers, often struggled to succeed in the biological and physical sciences. Licensed practical nurses (LPNs), for example, were returning to nursing school to earn a diploma and the right to sit for the national licensure examination to become registered nurses. Not only was this group usually from the first family generation educated beyond high school, they came from families with the least resources to give, often socially and financially.

Though the LPNs high school GPAs were not always stellar, I decided to encourage them to apply for Heyl Scholarships and advocated for them. The chair of the Heyl Nomination Committee accepted my argument. I was a member of the nomination advisory group that recommended nominees in ranked order. At first the advisory group to the Heyl board frowned on my encouragement of applicants with less than stellar GPAs, but eventually members ranked Bronson candidates as last to receive the prestigious awards. The number of applicants applying to nursing school was always low compared to those applying to Kalamazoo College. It was natural that the Heyl high school advisors favored college degrees. It felt as if they did little to recruit for the non-degree granting School of Nursing. When LPNs applied to Bronson and we learned of their previous graduation from the KPS system, we informed them of the possibility of obtaining the Heyl Scholarship. Chronologically they were not young women but often they were young in terms of their educational development.

Finding Heyl recipients may have been viewed as self-serving since the school received indirect expense reimbursement based on the numbers of scholars. It's true that the extra funds enriched the education of every student. Everyone was a winner, including the addition of nurses with more education and the community for increased diversity in graduates. I never faltered in advocacy for the LPNs. It was the right thing to do, and I overlooked the resulting glares and frowns. So much money was being made as interest during the eighties that it was hard for the Heyl advisory group to deny the few Bronson applicants. Even though they were ranked low, in the end they were given this incredible benefit, which I'm grateful for to this day. I knew students' success did not depend solely on finances. But one of the stressors for Bronson's rigorous, full-time program was alleviated.

Bronson nursing students, the School of Nursing, and the hospital benefited from the Elsie L. Heyl Scholarship in Nursing, all during the early 1970s through the 1998 closure of the school. The yearly gifts financed direct and indirect costs of nursing students who met the academic qualifications as graduates of the Kalamazoo public high schools and who applied for the scholarship. When the Bronson Methodist Hospital school closed in 1998, I believed the Heyl money should transfer to the WMU Bronson School of Nursing and encouraged the director of the school to explore the possibility. I had lobbied for it as closure of the hospital school came closer to a reality in the 1990s, and I continued to lobby after I retired from the school in 1995.

In the year 2000, Heyl's philosophy again came into play when Western Michigan University's Bronson School of Nursing was able to make a legal case for their Kalamazoo Public School nursing student applicants to be eligible for a Heyl Scholarship. Kalamazoo College President Jimmy Jones and the Heyl Board did not recognize the "new" Bronson School of Nursing as the legal heir and predecessor to the Heyl program. A court case ensued and the judge, in his ruling favoring WMU, considered Dr. Heyl's philosophy, and told the administrators and lawyers involved in the case that, in the long run, they would remember the ruling in favor of nursing student applicants as a good decision.

With gratitude in our hearts, Dr. Heyl will be remembered for his incredible caring for nursing students and nursing education at Bronson School of Nursing regardless of administrative affiliation.

STUDENTS' STORIES

Seventies' students shared their frustrations and found stress release and fun within the context of humor. Humor was a source of strength while coping with nursing school demands—often expressed through exaggeration, all with elements of truth.

Marsha Lewis '74

It all started August 29, 1971. We arrived in Kalamazoo with bulging bags, boxes, and frightened hearts. We had the first night service, singing "500 Miles". At one o'clock in the morning, however, we were awakened to the famous first-night raid with clanging, crashing, turning on of lights, getting thrown into the shower. "I thought nurses were gentle, MOM."

The next day came. "Hey, where's the bus to campus? I missed it? Walk?" "It's only 2 ¼ miles," says a helpful senior as she drives away in her car. But thank goodness for big sisters! All they are trying to do is help, saying, "It'll get better, it will get better! But you wonder why they keep shaking their heads and laughing as they walk back to their rooms.

We attended Western Michigan University and Bronson classes, but the seniors were right. It did get better—Jim Price and his anatomy class, that is—it got a whole lot better! Sociology and Dr. Horton put a big dent in our minds, sex in India? Getting introduced to psychology—Mallot style—was a real experience in behavior modification. Remember your new friend? A white, fuzzy rat with a weird looking tail? Yuck! "What if he? Well, you know . . . " Reassured that he will, "Wash your hands!" Knowing that things could only get better. They had to; nothing could be as bad as the first semester!

Second semester we were hit with Microbiology. Oh, those three-hour labs, and then another three-hour lab in physiology. "See the frog jump? Why did the frog jump?" We didn't care why the frog jumped. Why weren't things getting easier?

January to April was a long stretch, but it passed. And it's time for black banding. We were juniors, WOW! At last things were going to get easier! Everything is going to fit into its place.

To the Orthopedic Nurses

Canes and crutches
Wheelchairs, too.
Stryker beds and
What have you?
Consultations
Some folks have
Operation.
Shave 'em here
And paint 'em there.
Can I sit up
In a Chair?
Carry bed pans
Change a sheet.
Cover someone's
Freezing feet.

You need a drink?
No, you can't smoke.
When I come back
I'll bring a coke.
Turn me over,
Crank me down
(I need time
To just sit down).
Start an I.V.
Or transfusion
Orthopedics
Is confusion.
Checks the charts
And answer light!
Am I tired?
You're darned right!

Ruth Rambodt
Room 341
Catalyst, 1970 June

Our first junior service was on 2 East, a medical patient unit. It's a real challenge: bedpans, blood pressures, passing medications and more bed pans and care studies and systematic assessments and bedpans and bedpans, bedpans, BEDPANS! I was up to my elbows in it. "MOM?" Then summer came, and sunshine and suntan oil, and the Truesdale sun deck—wall to wall roasting, burning bodies.

The next service was OB. Ah, all of the little babies. My first delivery—a boy! Seven pounds, six ounces. What a miracle, what a wonderful work of God. I just loved babies—until I wandered into the nursery. "Gosh, look at all of those babies! I have to feed them? And diaper them? And diaper, and diaper and. . . What an aim that kid's got!" Diaper faster!

On surgical service, PAR and Hall 6, terror strikes. Mrs. Rice and her reputation for eating students. "Does she really eat us?" Who is Edna? And what's this CS cart anyway? Forget it, what's PAR? I think I'll go to 3 East and Mary Mason. Look at all of those broken bones, and all of those casts, and fractured hips—a 90-year-old hip fracture? I think she's falling. Oh no! What if she falls? Thank goodness for help from Mrs. Z and Mike, or 3 East could have been another disaster.

In the OR, remember, "You scrub and I'll circulate." "No, you scrub and I'll circulate." I couldn't get the gloves on the doctor . . . hold your hands still please! These retractors are so big, and they're holding back so much flesh, human flesh. But it's still not easier.

Oh, wait, I'm forgetting our great halfway party at Bimbo's and Bowser's. Who can forget that? Remember Mrs. Wylie, our guest of honor, dancing? And Mary Mason, singing and sharing with us her wisdom and antics. It was a great party.

Hey, it's April 5, 1973, and black banding again, the wide ones! We were seniors! Wow! We made it! Far-r-r-r out! And, it was our first senior service, Pediatrics. And size-three pajamas, and IVs that snap shut, and those hateful medications. There was always something to do, and the parents were helpful, when they went home, that is. Tots were the most fun, but then it was back to diapers again.

The Burn Unit was indescribable, but the staff was kind to lend us the floor when we fainted.

Next came ICU! We all loved Ellie dearly, but we could never catch up to her. We all thought that she was trying out for track. Remember MCL1 Lead II? They all looked the same to me. ER was a mass of confusion, and HDU—wasn't that a bloodmobile? After five weeks of respirators, pulmonary edema and questions, questions, and more questions, a vacation was due. So, it was off to the clinics. They were fun, unless you were blessed with the OB Clinic. Then, once more, we vowed never to have any of those cute little babies.

On to psychiatric nursing and Joyce at State Hospital, plus "Hi honey!" Remember the Women's Unit staff and the Men's Unit staff? What about popcorn and movies, volleyball, and playing cards, cards and more cards? Best of all was our fantastic guide and friend, Joyce, "I can appreciate that." And we knew that she did understand.

Last, but by no means least, was team leading. Days and those long classes and book reports, and magazines, magazines, magazines. Then Tuesday night out . . . up on the floor for over four hours (if you were fast) and not even getting paid! And Mrs. Grubb, our instructor and the familiar, "Got a minute?" And wishing you didn't. And the even more familiar, "You *will* look that up." And bedpans, bedpans, bedpans, if you were so lucky to have a 2 East assignment. Nights were something unbelievable with the crashing of bodies to the floor, and the crashing of bedpans, the footsteps unrecognized. The three o'clock break was hysterical. Laughter, eating, and all of those juicy, obscene jokes that kept us going.

Our senior banquet and only one week to graduation! Our last party and maybe our last night to raise hell. Maybe our last week to complain that it never got easier during those hard three years, but it was a good three years—full of the best friends that we ever knew, full of loving, caring and sometimes overbearing teachers. And all of the help from Truesdale staff, Mrs. Dexter, Mrs. Maxam and Mrs. Manley.

Mostly we remember all of the good times, the best times! Remember Milham Park and winning the tug of war, and going to Mursch's, and our friendly bathroom talks? We were proud of our accomplishments and proud to have each other for friends who had made our lives "the happiest yet."

Anne Therese Hughes Schrider '78

> So what have you learned Dorothy?
>
> That the next time I go looking for my heart's desire, I won't go looking any further than my own backyard. Because if it isn't there, I never really lost it to begin with.
>
> —***Frank L. Baum***

It has been an interesting exercise for me to relive the feelings I experienced while attending Bronson. One of my personal "patterns" in decision making is to jump in, sometimes finding the waters distasteful, before I do any real thinking about why I choose a particular course. The times I have thought *first* stand out because they are so rare. The decision to attend nursing school, and Bronson in particular, was made without forethought . . . I was always going to be a nurse . . . I was always going to attend a diploma program. My mom did . . . so I did.

Once I began school at Bronson, I was continually plagued with doubt and unhappiness. I wanted to quit. I felt disconnected. I could do the work and succeed, but I felt deeply that doing so was not my path to personal and professional fulfillment. My parents, especially my dad, and my friends counseled me to stay. Mary Curtis used to say, "Don't look at the whole three years, just focus on one service at a time." So I did. And one day the training was completed.

There were positives, of course. One of the most indelible impressions was learning sterile technique. I assimilated the experience eagerly. It's still second nature to me and perhaps I'm comforted by the absolute principle inherent in the process.

Items were either sterile or they weren't—there was no in between. The code of ethics and related behaviors were clear. I always liked that certainty.

The other aspect of nursing I always liked, even as a student, was the art. Gentleness and a calm demeanor were soothing to patients and to coworkers. Compassion was the key to healing. I intuited that truism—but had no way to codify it, substantiate it, and justify my pride in it. After graduation, I spent 17 years in many acute care settings looking for my niche. I tried to reassure myself during those unhappy times in school with the thought: "Nursing is so vast, if you can't find something you like within the nursing field, you'll never find it elsewhere either." I don't believe that assessment now, but it made me feel better at the time. I did find many jobs that brought me satisfaction and pride in my work. One of my supervisors once said to a physician, "Anne is a very reliable nurse." My favorite compliment, though, came from a dying patient who said, after I had started his IV, "You are so gentle."

Even so, I began to believe that my greatest fear in nursing school was valid, and that fear was that I had made a big mistake. What I should have studied was astrophysics or some other subject that I never thought of at age 17 and that no one else thought to suggest. Then a curious turn of events filled in the center of the pattern. I entered graduate school. The bane of nursing education for most students was for me the saving grace, that is, studying the theorists: Jean Watson, Martha Rogers, and Florence Nightingale. They articulated what I valued about nursing. The writings of these nursing theorists lit the fire of pride in my path. Set in the context of these women's writings, my career choice looked different, and it finally made sense.

My nursing career is taking a new shape; I will be graduating from Michigan State University in spring, 1998, with a MSN degree and major in a family nurse practitioner role. The role in advanced practice leads some away from *nursing*, but for me nursing is the foundation, the center. Nursing *is* the "Philosophy and Science of Caring" (Watson, 1985). What I valued was there all along, I had just never noticed.

Ann Dimitroff '79

In 1976, as a new group of 73 student nurses[38] entered Truesdale Hall to begin the studies that would dominate their lives for three years, graduation seemed like a foreign word. Most of us, however, did graduate on March 15 and are pursuing our careers in different specialties, different hospitals, and different lifestyles, but with one common factor. We had all survived our years at Bronson Methodist Hospital School of Nursing and that feat was an unforgettable accomplishment, although I am sure some of us will try to forget a few details.

Freshman year was seemingly designed to weed out the weak from the strong. Our first shock was seeing our dorm rooms. For many of us, it appeared as if we would be required to eat, sleep, and study in a walk-in closet, not to mention having to live with a stranger. With four girls in a suite, it was also quite a puzzle figuring out how we could plug in four blow dryers and four curling irons in an outlet made for two.

After the shock of moving in, it was time to face the classes. The first year most of our classes were at Western where we were dropped off from our buses and left to wander aimlessly in an effort to find our classrooms. We learned the body inside and out at Western, but it was at Bronson that we learned the practicalities of nursing.

Our freshman nursing class had a month to prepare for the big step—actually working in the hospital for two hours a day. In nursing lab we had a chance to practice our skills on each other. We didn't really know our classmates until we had given them a bed bath and mouth care, put TED hose on their extremities, and administered both a sub-Q and IM injection.

When we did make it up to the floor in our fluorescent white caps and uniforms (which we ironed for two hours the night before), our duties seemed overwhelming. We were expected to do such intricate nursing tasks as giving a bath, taking a temperature and blood pressure, and making the bed. The mere sight of an attending physician would send a flock of students into the bathroom to clean the tubs or even hide in the dirty utility rooms testing already tested urine samples. A request from the doctor to get an item such as a stitch set would send the student hurrying out the door and triumphantly returning with the item—30 minutes later.

Freshman year finally was finished, and as we entered our junior year with only a few casualties, reality shock began to set in. The emphasis now was placed on a full eight-hour working day, three days a week. What do we do all day? We soon found out, as we rotated through Medical-Surgical Nursing, Orthopedics, OR, and Mental Health, that the bare minimum was all we could handle. Everything we did was a "Learning Experience" essential to our careers. We found out that the ones most essential to our careers were the ones no one else wanted to do.

Dorm life was dwindling to an all time low. We were now required to live with five people in a suite made for four. The hot pots were boiling away with such delicacies as macaroni and cheese, chicken noodle soup, and gallons of coffee. We supplemented our diets with cafeteria food only when absolutely necessary. The high point of the year was the extension of male visiting hours from 8:00 P.M. to 10:00 P.M. At 10:01 P.M., the receptionist would begin calling for any males not crossed off the sign-in list.

We were kept busy in our classes learning every major and minor disease process known to man and writing numerous care plans to apply this knowledge. Working on the floor offered such new challenges as passing medications and starting IVs. When a doctor asked a question, sometimes we even knew the answer without asking three other people first.

As we entered our senior year, we thought we knew everything until we started our new services. Advanced Med-Surg introduced us to a world full of machinery and wires, cardiac monitors, and arterial blood gases—a world surely we weren't ready for as we crossed the threshold into ICU. With our hands in a cold sweat, we clutched our EKG interpretation handout.

Professional development was our introduction into the realities of being a staff nurse. I don't think anyone of us can forget how crushed we felt when a doctor called up to the floor with orders and, when he found out he was talking to a student, asked if he could talk to a "real nurse." I guess that is the definition of RN.

Obstetrics showed us the beginning of life from a baby's first cry, and Pediatrics gave us more experience with kids, and they were still crying. Motherhood came early for most of us as we struggled to mix formula, change diapers, and chase three-year-olds up and down the halls for eight hours. Of course, we could always relax by coming back home to the dorm. Since cooking was now considered a hazard to our safety, most of us lived on a diet of carryout foods.

Looking back on the three years that have passed, we can never repeat our student nurse years but we can use our experiences, the good times and the bad, to go on and make our dreams become a reality. As we graduate wearing our new white uniforms, we will have to leave old friends and go on to new jobs and new hospitals, but all of us will have the memories of these years at Bronson Methodist Hospital to help us attain our goals. Wherever we end up, we have been prepared to be an asset to the nursing profession.

Sandra Quick Richards '71

Sandra Quick's parents in Detroit saved her letters during her freshman year. Excerpts[39] from them follow:

September 3, 1968

Dear Mom and Dad,

I got up at 6:30 A.M. today, surprise, surprise! There are so many things to see and explore. Beth and I decided to go for an early walk, and found a Catholic Church, although it is a distance away, I shouldn't have any problem getting to mass since we have no classes on Saturday or Sunday. I also found out that buses to Detroit are $5.15 one way.

I hope there is a place at Western to sit and study other than in the student union hall where, one of the juniors said to sit if you want a date. How are we supposed to study with a couple hundred cute, adorable guys in the same room!

Sept. 6, 1968 . . . Thank heaven it's Friday. I feel like I have been here a month. The homework and the classes are rough. My psycho class is the worst. We are on a 100 percent mastery, which means we must get everything right or we do it over. We have a quiz every day as soon as we walk in the door on the assignment we have read the night before. The two make-up quizzes have six different questions and, if you don't get all six right, you fail the class. Today I had my first make-up quiz along with about 200 other students.

Sept. 16, 1968 . . . Well, congratulate me. I went through a week of psych without having to take the make-up exam.

The kids on the west side can't open their windows because of the dust and noise [from construction of] both the interns' residence (across the street) and the pediatric wing (next door). When we go for meals we have to watch out for barricades, caterpillars, chains and manholes. Fun!

The food isn't getting any better. If it wasn't for my tremendous appetite, I would not try their new concoctions. I am always hungry.

On weekends, it gets rather quiet and lonely here. Please send me the following records from my room, if you know someone coming this direction: "Man of La Mancha", "Sound of Music", "West Side Story", "The King and I", Tijuana Brass albums, "Carousel", "Dr. Zhivago".

Oct. 1, 1968 . . . I'm sorry I haven't written in a while, but I have been too busy studying. It's been rough and I can't seem to make the grades no matter how much I try. I came pretty close to not passing my test. To make matters worse, someone has taken two skulls from the anatomy lab. If they are not returned by tomorrow morning, we all have to do a 5,000-word research paper on the skull. Our classes are mixed so someone not in Bronson could have taken the skulls for the heck of it, or then again— Halloween is coming up.

Oct. 17, 1968 . . . The juniors were playing jump rope in the hall using a couple of belts and restraints tied together. You never know what to expect next around here.

My mid semester grades were satisfactory. The only one that was bad was Sociology. I might understand it if this guy was in the younger, weird generation, but he is approaching 50. He has been teaching nurses at Bronson for 13 years, and every year Mrs. Weber gets the same complaints about him, but no other teacher will take the course.

From now on we are supposed to use the morgue entrance because construction is extending to the ER exit. Next we'll be using the front door. I was in the hospital library yesterday, and they are smashing the tunnel to pieces. Every time that big "boom" hit the cement, the building trembled.

We made pizza for lunch, somehow it turned out to be edible, I wonder how?

Oct. 26, 1968 . . . I wanted to come home last weekend but we had to bake something for our bake sale. I ended up making cupcakes. They look all right but the frosting leaves something to be desired.

Nov. 15, 1968 . . . In just 11 more days I will be home! We just had a big exam on the nervous system today in Anatomy. That was the best test Mrs. Rutherford gave us, but it was soooo long that I couldn't finish.

Last Wednesday I actually went out . . . with a couple of girls. One of the girls, Judy, is going into the Army. We went to her house [girlfriend Beth's] for dinner. It was nice to be in a home and the food was very good.

We dissected the cats' internal organs this week. Some of them had tape and thread worms in the stomach and intestines. In one cat, the stomach was full of hairballs and a mouse. Our cat was just pregnant.

No, we didn't get a chance to vote here. The faculty doesn't want any more fuss because the Students for a Democratic Society wanted to have a "sit out," but it was voted down.

Dec. 3, 1968 . . . Just before we left for vacation another student came down with the Hong Kong flu and lost 20 pounds over vacation. Mrs. Weber was admitted to the hospital last night because of dehydration.

When we walked into psycho lab Monday morning, 7:30 A.M., there was a rack of rat cages that had been left in the room since last Tuesday. About 30 of the rats were dead of starvation. The 10 that were alive were eating the dead. They were not the rats our class was using, but what a horrible sight.

Jan. 8, 1969 . . .There are 73 freshman left. One dropped out and the other nine failed Biochemistry. The classes this semester are a pain. Micro is going to be bad because there is so much to learn. Physiology lectures are dull. Right now in nursing, we are studying Pharmacology. The text is like reading an encyclopedia. Next week we start working in the hospital one morning a week for 2-1/2 hours. I am apprehensive about the hospital . . . I keep asking myself, "What am I doing here?"

Jan. 12, 1969 . . . My classes are getting harder, but it's the teachers that are driving me up the wall. Judy, my suite mate with the artificial leg, is having increasing difficulty with wearing the prosthesis and floor duty. She is advised to drop out until the skin irritation improves. I think she is hurting more than she shows, but she feels that God is doing this for a reason.

Feb. 3, 1969 . . .One day last week the heat and hot water were shut off—the coldest day too. Everything went wrong. I just about ignited the Micro lab today. I'm glad we learn by mistakes. I have learned a lot since September.

My junior year will only cost $360 for the whole year. Attended the District Student Nurses meeting at Nazareth College last night where the speaker was an industrial nurse.

Feb. 20, 1969 . . . From 3 to 5 P.M. we worked on a stupid lab experiment in Physiology and still can't figure out the damn thing. I caught a stupid cold again because last weekend this room had no heat. I went to bed. Three freshman, Geri, Kathy and Debbie are engaged to be married.

I was just thinking that it has been two months since I came home. No wonder I hate this place, the food tastes awful, and my nerves are a wreck. Last Saturday I took a job babysitting three boys. I wanted to get out of here so bad that I would do about anything. Friday I am going to see Bill Cosby. I hope he cheers my spirits.

One day last week the construction people dug into the water pipes, and we were without water for most of the day. Watched some slides on Vietnam presented by the Army recruiter. I never could have imagined how bad some of those mine, mortar, shrapnel and gun shell wounds can get.

Feb. 28, 1969 . . . This week has been great. I actually passed a test with a good "B." I worked on the floor both yesterday and today. I had the same patient and, by today, I knew the routine. The instructor left me on my own to irrigate the Levine tube, suction, and regulate the IV. We were rushed because my patient had to go to X-ray. I came back from class and my instructor had returned my care plan and evaluation. She actually complemented me. For Mrs. Forsythe that is a real accommodation and, in about two minutes, everyone on the floor knew that she had something nice to say.

Well, this week we learned how to give injections. We had to pair up and give each other injections with sterile water. They really hurt. I was the first to give an injection because I knew if I waited and watched too many others, I would get really shook up. I almost fainted anyway due to lack of sleep, tension, and exam just prior and the fruit cocktail for lunch. I'm all right now.

Mar. 28, 1969 . . . We have a big math test on April 7th. On that day the seniors graduate and we are expected to attend. I am in the choir so I pretty much should go. The next morning we have a Physiology test. If one more test is declared, I think I will stay here over Easter especially since it is going to snow anyway.

Say a prayer for President Eisenhower. He will be remembered along with FDR and Jefferson as one of our great presidents.

June 15, 1969 . . . Sue, Lin, and I have gone over to the Holiday Inn a number of times swimming. It is nice of the establishment to let us use the pool. When the nursing students are there, it seems to draw more attention and many people come out of their room to swim, lounge around or just talk to the students.

Love,
Your Daughter

Ruth C. Jorgensen Kneebone '71

I always wanted to be a nurse. Two of my great aunts were Bronson graduates: Gladys C. Jorgensen, Class of 1930, and Violet C. Comstock, Class of 1933. I admired them and wanted to be like them. All of our middle names are Christine.

> The Bronson instructors and atmosphere were most responsible for my development as a nurse professional when our focus was patient care. We were to look neat and be intelligent, caring nurses. Our profession needs more of us.
>
> ***Mary Conte Swander '70***

I applied to just one school, Bronson, and it was a great place. We had a taste of college at Western and then plunged into nursing. I still kept my ties with Western for a "social life."

Truesdale was a place to relax and study, a home away from home. On special occasions we would go down to the basement and watch a program on TV. It was usually something like the Miss America Pageant or a movie. We could all be critical of the contestants and root for our favorites. We would cry together over sad or touching movies or laugh over a comedy or two. "The Tunnel" was always great in bad weather, the early morning hours, or after the late night shift. Truesdale was always our safe place.

I had the luxury of a private suite on the fifth floor at the end of the hall. Lynn McPhall was my suite mate for one year. The next two years Mary Luckett was my suite mate. I worked for a year after graduation on Hall 8, the medical/surgical floor. A pediatric resident, Dr. David Burke, encouraged me to move to Denver and work at Children's Hospital if I wanted to be a pediatric nurse. I moved, got married and currently work in the NICU at Swedish Medical center in Englewood, Colorado, a suburb of Denver. Over the years Bronson has changed, but it will never be forgotten.

> The "wig lady," birthed by Sue and her roommates with the use of a wig head, broom and bathrobe, was set in a trashcan. She would ride the elevator in Truesdale Hall for hours.
>
> We liked to hit the alarm button on the first floor and have Daisy Manley, the switchboard operator and front door gatekeeper, come to see what the problem was.
>
> ***Suzanne Rosteck Morgan '74***

Santa in the Hospital

"Twas the night before Christmas
        when all through the wards
Everyone was rushing like thundering hordes.
Nurses in white and nurses aides, too
Ran hither and thither with so much to do.

The children were nestled in tents and cribs
Ten babies were bawling with toys 'neath their ribs
The Supervisor was off and making her rounds
When all of a sudden there arose such a clatter
Patients spring from their beds to see what was the matter.

A bevy of nurses all fresh and full-bloom
Were scurrying off to one patient's room.
I know what you're thinking
        but you're not right, you know
It was jolly St. Nicholas all covered with snow.

They put him to bed, he was frost-bit, you see
Poor Santa had a temperature of one hundred and three.

More rapid than eagles those nurses did fly,
Poor Santa got penicillin in his right thigh.

He whistled and shouted and called them some names . . .
Now Dash you, No Cancer, no Virus and Toxin
On TV, on Doctor, on Intern and Blitzed.
To the top of the clinic to the top of the hall
Dash away, dash away, dash away all.

So up to the Director, those nurses they flew
To get Santa a posture-pedic mattress all new.
And after a nap, Santa jumped from his bed
"Where's my meal?" he thundered
and his face turned bright red.

The Head Nurse came dashing right down the hall
"Why Santa, you're ill, the doctor I'll call."
The doctor said, "Santa, go straight back to bed.
If you go out tonight, by tomorrow you'll be dead."

His eyes how they twinkled, his dimples how merry
His cheeks were like roses, his nose like a berry.
"Just give me an aspirin and a hooker or two
And then I'll be off, I have plenty to do."
When the doctor had gone and the nurses had too
Old Santa put on his red flannels and boots.
He spoke not a word but went straight to his work
And filled all the stockings then turned with a jerk

And laying his finger aside of his nose
And giving a nod up the elevator he arose.
He sprang to the roof to his team gave a whistle
And away they all flew like the down of a thistle.

And I heard him exclaim as he drove out of sight,
"I sure fooled those nurses at the hospital, tonight."

Alice Hynes
Catalyst, 1966, 1973 December

Lynette Thompson Guyer '75

My first impressions of the School of Nursing are vivid. The reputation of being one of the best nursing schools in the nation was well known to me as a high school student. I was anxious to take the tests on the WMU campus and hear that I had passed them and was accepted into the program.

The school traditions of introducing the freshman students to their environment were greatly appreciated. Writing to my roommate in the summer before school started was a nice way to get acquainted. Having a Big Sister who could help you learn the ropes of the hospital cafeteria, direct you to the stores to buy your Clinic nursing shoes and white support nylons, and showering you with items to help your dorm room look "homey" was wonderful.

Mrs. Dunn was a great supporter in her quiet way as we took to the medical floor with sick, elderly patients to care for. She gave us time to gain confidence in ourselves and to spread our wings, being there to answer questions.

I remember trying to get off the floor in time to catch the bus for classes at WMU. The schedule was also tight to get home in time for a cafeteria supper after a late session in the Microbiology lab. It was a fast-paced, almost three-mile walk home.

I fondly remember our capping ceremony with reciting the oath, lighting the candles, and receiving our white New Testaments. The patch pockets on our uniforms were big enough for the book in one, leaving the other pocket for the all-important

> Before I started nursing school in 1974, I worked as an aide in a small rural hospital. The only anesthesia provider was a female nurse anesthetist. I was able to go back to surgery and see her work a couple of times. I thought, "Wow, what a cool job she has." So I decided to go to nursing school and on to nurse anesthesia school. It was the best decision I ever made.
>
> ***Deb Ringler Sponseller '77***
>
> During first year clinical practice, while taking a patient's temp, he decided to bite down on my finger at the same time. I told the instructor who thought the episode was an April Fool's joke (April 1, 1975). The scenario ended with a tetanus booster shot.
>
> ***Petronella Verhoog '77***

four-color pen and bandage scissors. No stethoscopes around our necks in the early seventies, though!

Pam Anderson Kusebuski '76

I will never forget that first night at Bronson. The rooms welcomed us with the little extras our "Big Sis" had provided. There was no need to lock doors; we were in such a friendly place! I had just dozed off, thinking this arrangement might not be too bad, when I thought I heard a stampede of horses coming down the hall. Then we received the "real welcome" from the "Big Sis" —Vaseline on the toilets, rice and crackers in the bed, toilet paper all over. It sure did bring my roommate and suite mates together. We planned next year's "fun" as we cleaned up!

The most memorable lesson I learned was from Mrs. Zolp, "Never assume anything!" It has been my saving grace! Thanks, Mrs. Zolp.

Leslie Fogelsong Gosling '77

So many wonderful memories come to mind such as dressing up for Halloween and trick or treating the children on Peds. They enjoyed getting candy, and we had fun coming up with a costume from what little we could scrape together at the last minute.

Another time, my suite mate and I decided to go to the hospital cafeteria for a midnight snack. Somehow we got locked in the hospital stairwell. Luckily someone came along to free us. To this day, I always check doorknobs to see if they are unlocked before I let the door close.

Linda S. Doctor '78

My first day of clinical nursing convinced me I would never graduate from BMH. Bedmaking was a serious and complicated process for me. Hospitals did not have fitted sheets and I had to learn how to fold military corners. I carefully made the bed. The corners were meticulous. There were no wrinkles. I confidently waited while Mrs. Gren inspected my work. My hopes were dashed as she slowly rolled the head of the bed up and the sheets, which were on upside down, fell to the middle of the bed! With a straight face she lectured on the proper way to make the bed so the patients can lie on sheets instead of a bare mattress. I knew I would NEVER make it.

Although my time at BMH was short in comparison to the rest of my life, it had a major impact on me. BMH gave me a skill I can market anywhere. Those two little initials – RN – have seen me through many job changes. I am grateful for the opportunities I have had because of my education at BMH. A hallmark skill I learned is organization. I am also grateful to Sondra Crow, who taught me team leading. Even though that concept is called something else now, I use it every day. BMH also gave me the best friend of my heart, Susan Bond Rubey. Our long-distance friendship has lasted for 23 years.

So eventually I did learn to make a bed (Thank you, Mrs. Gren!), and I feel my life has been blessed by attending BMH. I hate to see the program close, but the legacy it left in my life makes it easier to accept. Thank you, BMH!

Joni Sass Jones '79

Probably one of the most vivid memories I still have of Truesdale Hall is of "Miss Daisy" sitting behind the reception desk and making sure we weren't committing some type of rules infraction. She was adamant that "no men" would cross the line outside of the reception area, thereby having access to the dorm rooms upstairs. Not even fathers were spared her wrath should they innocently attempt to cross the line while carrying their daughter's luggage, *etc.* (We were safe only between 10:00 A.M.–5:00 P.M. on Sundays. After that, forget it!)

I also still smile when I remember Miss Mason and her deference to the physicians at Bronson. When any of the orthopedists walked down the hall, she would tell her group of students to "flatten up against the wall," to make sure the physician was in no way impeded in advancing to his destination.

Mostly, I remember the high degree of professionalism among faculty and staff. They were role models for all of the students—models of caring and commitment—whom I will never forget.

Your Dorm Helper

For three years I have seen you
Now it is time to move along.
You have made graduation,
Life's compensations now you seek.

Though, I am going to miss you.
I know you one and all.
Some I know better, but success I wish for all.
Your names you will be changing except for one.
He will give his to another.
I just hope your life is fun.
Remember, try, smile, do your best.
It all makes for happiness.

Daisy Manley
Truesdale Hall Receptionist,
Catalyst, 1976 April

CHAPTER 8 NOTES

---

[1] Copied from the 1974 Class History written by Marsha Lewis.

[2] *Kalamazoo Gazette*, 1904 December 10; 4. "Monument to women, will be the new hospital."

[3] *Catalyst*, 1979 September; 2. "Nurse staffing monumental task."

[4] *Catalyst*, 1974 September; 7–11. "Our administrative officers."

[5] *Kalamazoo Gazette*, 1970 January 26, "Hospital costs are staggering."

[6] *Kalamazoo Gazette*, 1970 January 27, "Medical care: our non system."

[7] *Kalamazoo Gazette*, 1970 January 28, "Hospitals try to hold costs."

[8] *Kalamazoo Gazette*, 1970 January 29, "Overhaul needed for health care."

[9] *Kalamazoo Gazette*, 1970 January 30, "Reviving home medical care."

---

[10] *Kalamazoo Gazette*, 1971 May 25, "Hospitals here join in planning, objectives: more service less cost."

[11]Dossey, Barbara M., *Florence Nightingale: mystic, visionary, healer.* Springhouse, PA: Springhouse, 2000. p.95.

[12] *Catalyst*, 1973 February; 8.

[13] *Kalamazoo Gazette,* 1976 July 28, "A quarter-million dollar baby, 20-month old tot finally able to leave hospital."

[14] Naisbitt, John, *Megatrends: ten new directions transforming our lives*. New York: Warner Books, 1982. p.35.

[15] *Kalamazoo Gazette*, 1974 May 14, "City action backs hospital expansion."

[16] *Kalamazoo Gazette*, 1971 November 19, "Bronson Hospital plans $6.5 million expansion."

[17] *Kalamazoo Gazette*, 1971 December 4, "Kalamazoo Foundation grants."

[18] *Kalamazoo Gazette*, 1972 January 26, "Bronson Hospital trauma-emergency center given approval by trustees, services to be expanded."

[19] *Kalamazoo Gazette*, 1972 January 12, "Open-heart surgery performed."

[20] *Kalamazoo Gazette*, 1973 October 25, "Bronson Hospital's burn center."

[21] *Kalamazoo Gazette*, 1973 March 15, "Bronson kidney center schedules open house."

[22] *Kalamazoo Gazette*, 1979 July 11, "Hospice group seeks money."

[23] Nurse-servers were cupboards next to the patient's room.

[24] Dossey, Barbara M., *op.cit., p. 89.*

[25]Orwin, W.L., 1980, "An invitation to hard work," 1980, Kalamazoo, F.W. & Elsie L. Heyl Science Scholarship Fund.

[26] *Ibid*, p. 14.

[27] *Ibid,* p. 5.

[28] *Ibid*, p. 6

[29] WMU Bronson School of Nursing qualifying students received direct scholarship funding. The School of Nursing did not receive indirect dollars that had benefited the greater good of all students.

[30] Orwin W.L., Appendix B, Excerpts from the Frederick W. Heyl Will, p. 33.

[31] Calabria, M.D., and McCrae, J. ed. *Suggestions for thought by Florence Nightingale: selections and commentaries,* Philadelphia: University of Pennsylvania Press, 1994. p.30.

[32]Orwin, W.L., *op.cit.* p.5

[33] *Ibid.*

---

[34] *Ibid, preface.*

[35] *Ibid,* p. 11.

[36] The first Heyl recipients were two 1973 graduates, Sarah Bahlke and Virginia Liebrandt, and two 1974 graduates, Lesley LaRoy and Patricia Schipper.

[37] Orwin, W. L., *op.cit.* p.1.

[38] Ann Dimitroff's story, published in the *Catalyst,* 1979 May, came from her.

[39] Richards, Sandra. "After twenty years of nursing, my mother presented me with all of the letters I wrote home when I was in nursing school. I lived in Detroit and did not get home often, and in those times there was no E-mail, so I wrote frequently to Mom, about anything and everything."

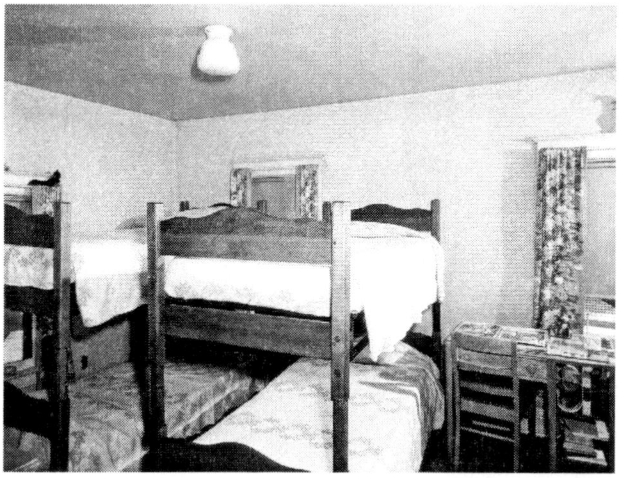

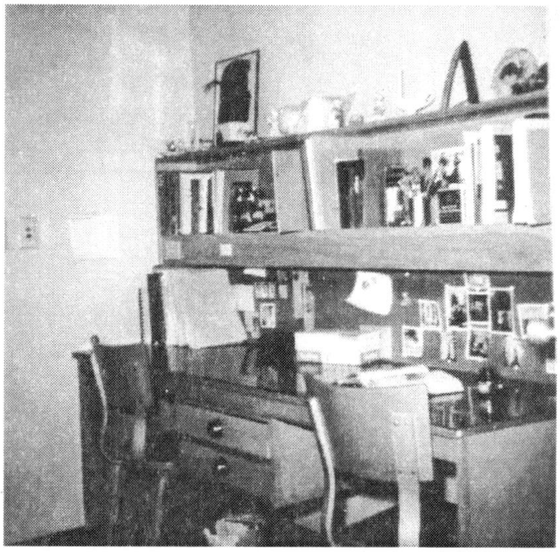

127. (above) An overcrowded dorm room, 1955. Designed for two beds, it had four, and was used for both sleep and study. 128. A typical Truesdale room (right) housed two students, 1960. As shown, this room is atypically clean.

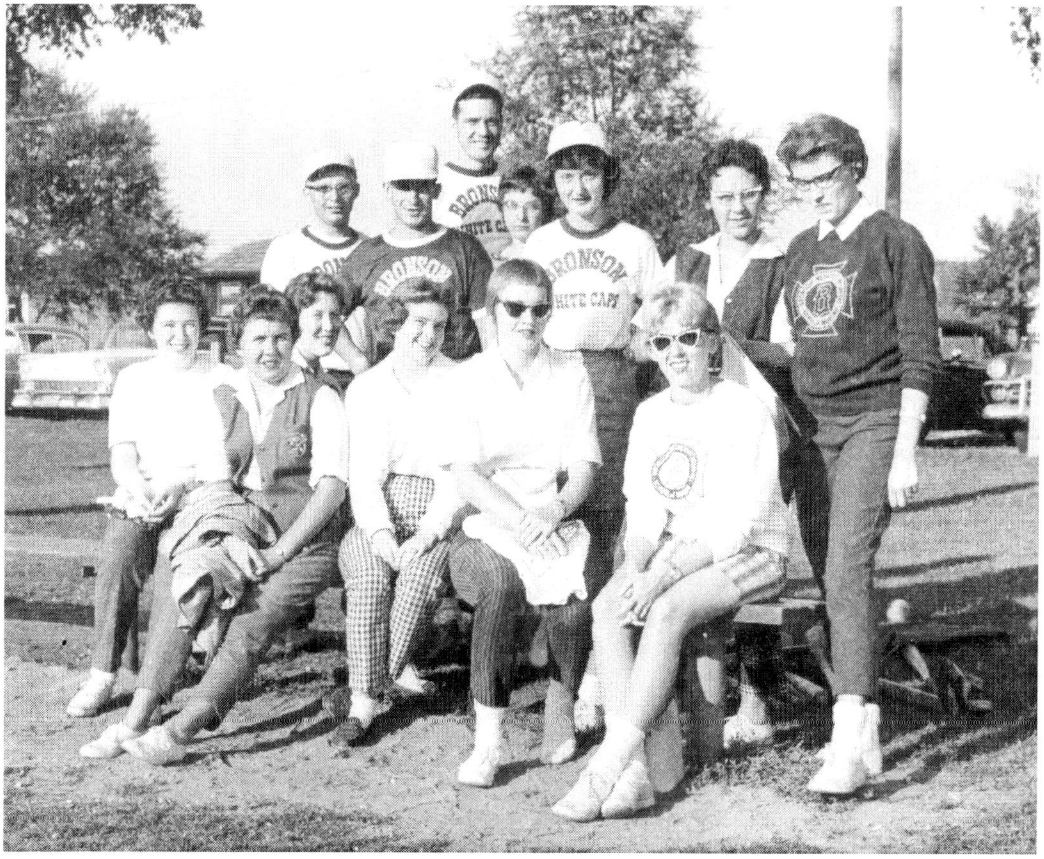

129. Students took an active part in the Bronson softball team, formed in 1960 (left to right) Joyce Hiatt, Gail Samborn, Maribeth Esch, Mary Winegar, Carolyn Lewis, Vernice Sherman; (standing) Dean Troyer, Jake Miller, Dick Vander Molen, Jolene Bowman, Phyllis Hollister, Sharon Schaller, Janet Krickhahn.

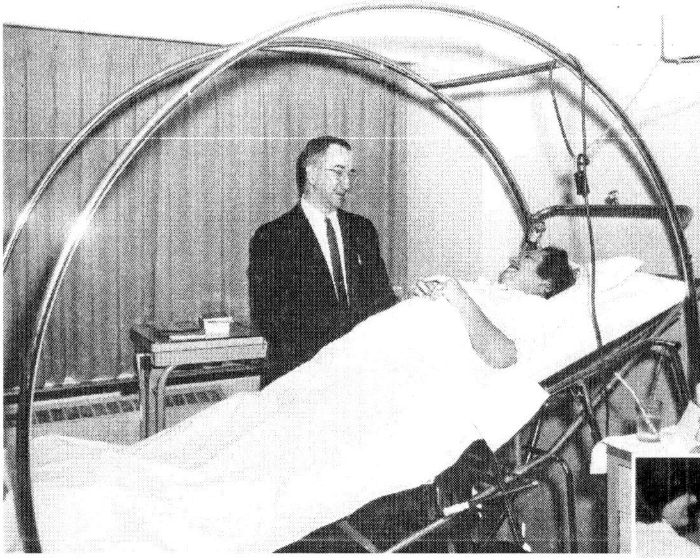

130. (left) Chaplain Robert Trenery counsels a patient in a CircoElectric® bed invented by Dr. Homer Stryker. It was used for patients unable to turn over, usually following back surgery. A "mattress" was placed on top of the patient, screwed in place, and the bed electrically turned in a circle so the patient was face down, relieving the pressure on her back.

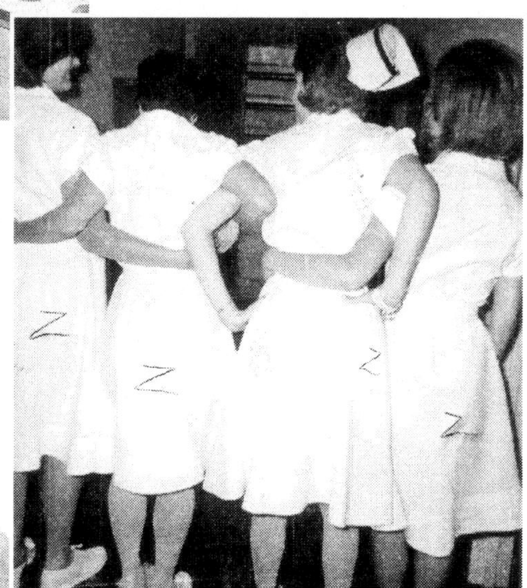

131. (right) Senior Autograph Day, 1967. Mrs. Z (Zeimelis) leaves her mark on these suitemates. (left to right) Sharon Hovarter, Beverly Prince, Ruth Schermer, and Sharon Ide. The last day of school seniors visited throughout the hospital to have staff autograph their uniforms as nursing school momentos.

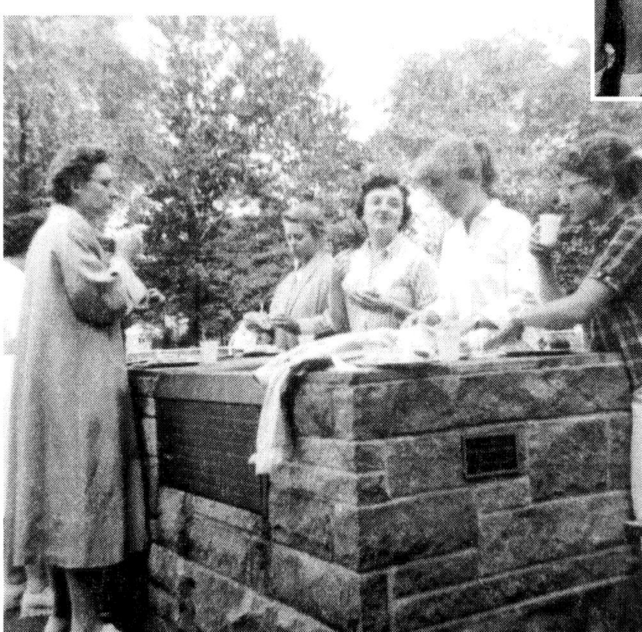

132. Students and instructors enjoyed a picnic at the back of Truesdale Hall, ca 1960. (left to right) Instructors Elizabeth Heneveld, Lois Wilkinson, and students Elaine Bartels, Dixie Ladd, and Mary Jo Rosa.

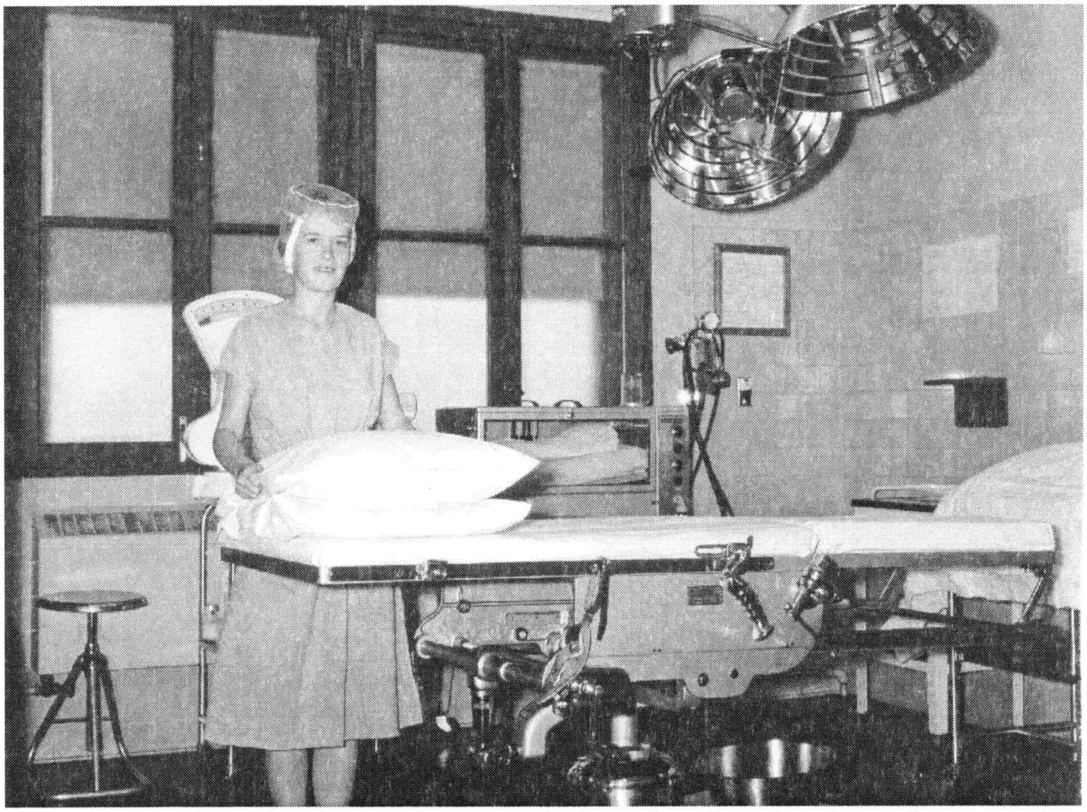

133. Esther Wyman in a modern delivery room, early 1960s.

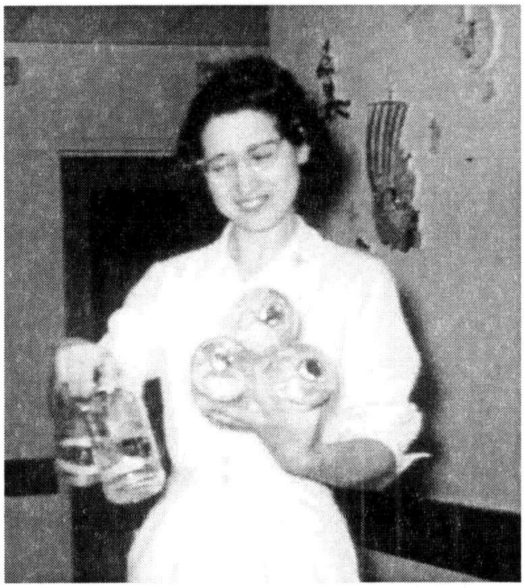

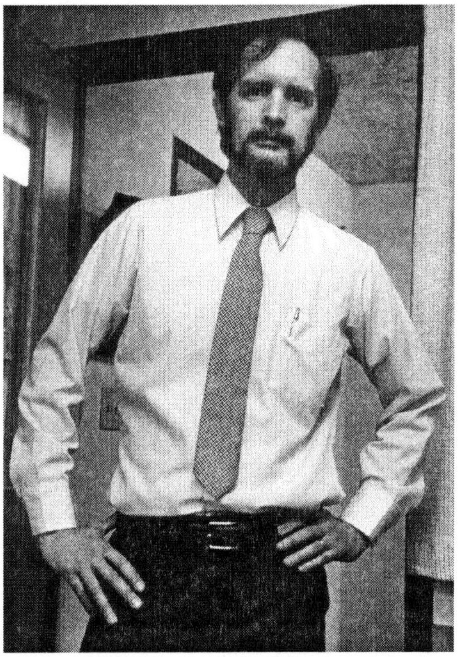

134. Marilyn Moored has her hands full with IV bottles, ca 1960. 135. Larry Wolf, hospital photographer, ca 1960, played a large part in documenting events mentioned in this book.

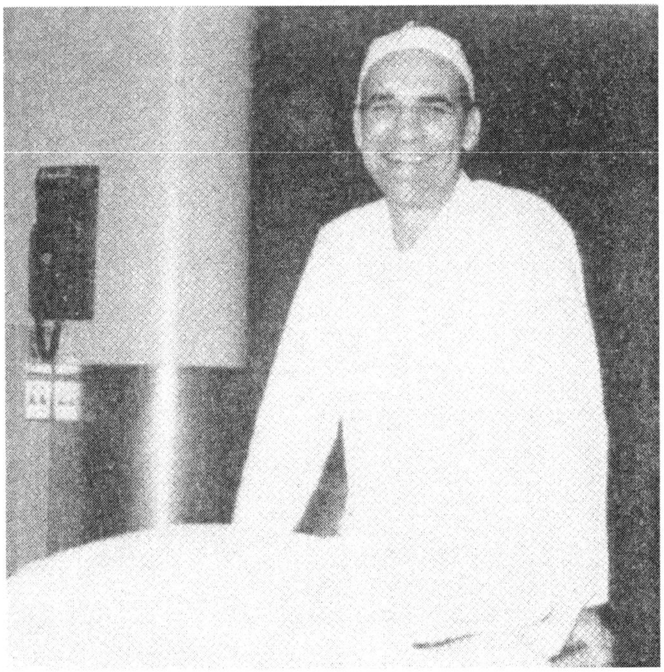

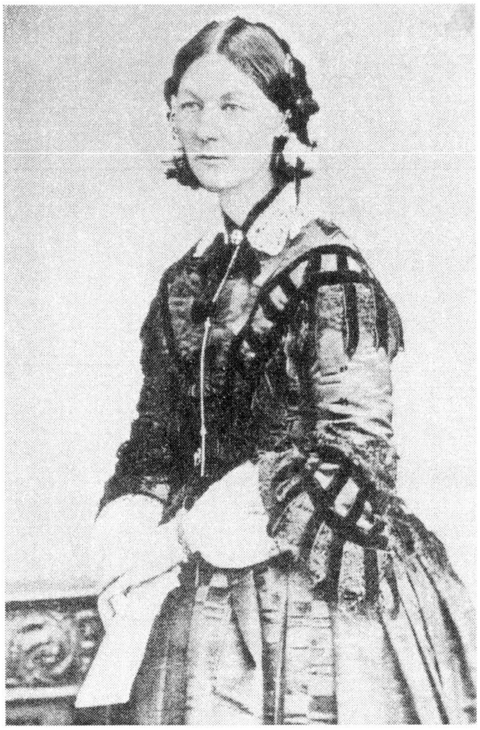

136. (above) Lyle Nottingham, surgery orderly, 1961.
137. (right) Florence Nightingale, 1856.

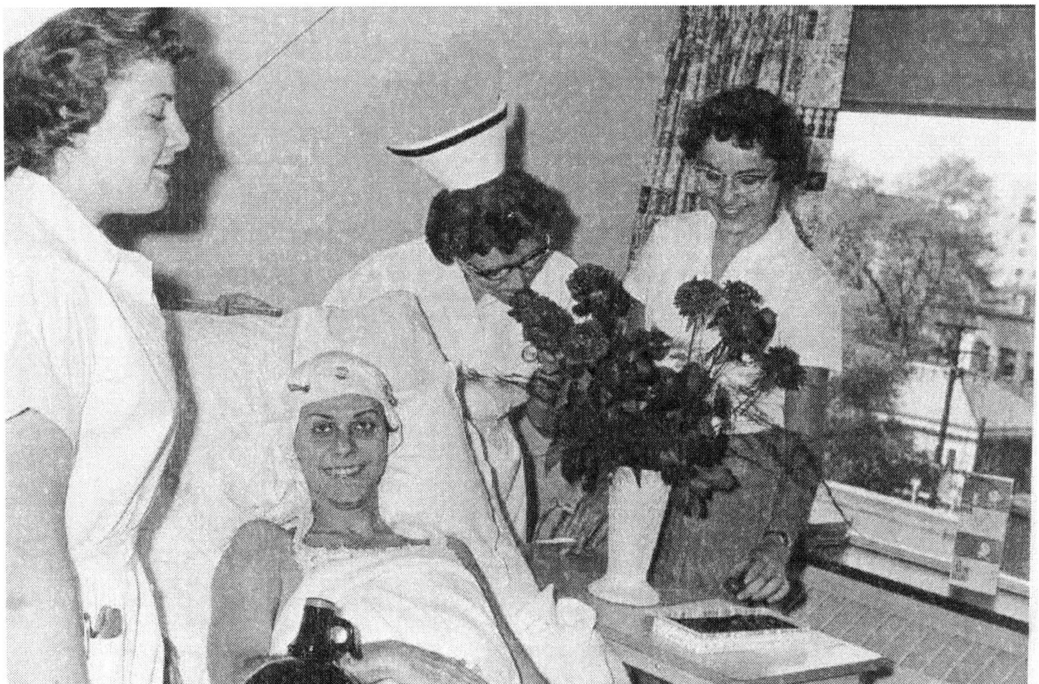

138. (left to right) Janice Baum, Janet Krickhahn, and Anna van't Zelfde provided comedy and comfort to Sharon Schaller who was hospitalized during her senior year.

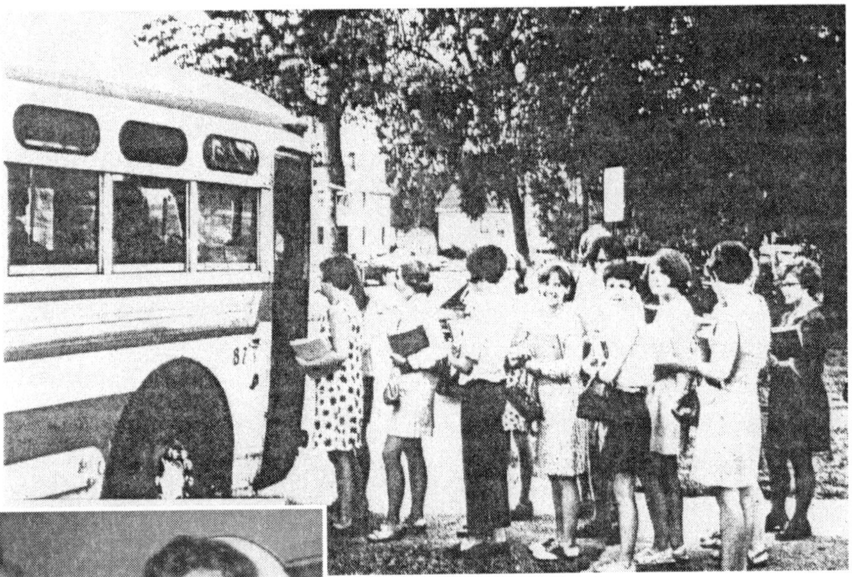

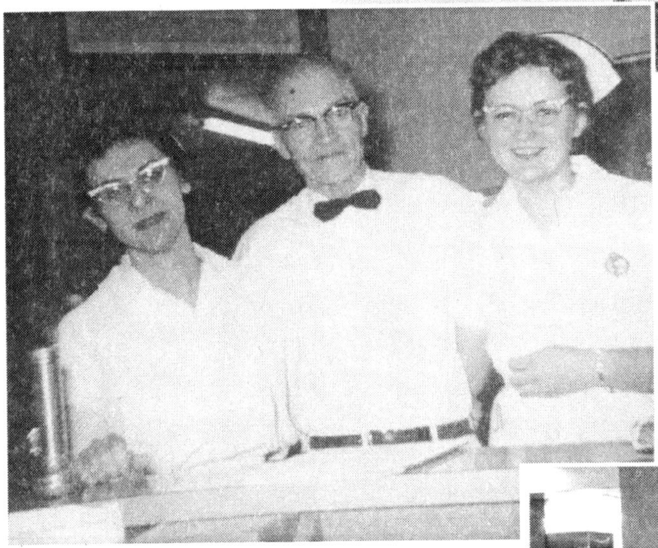

139. Waiting to board the bus to WMU.

140. Sharon Schaller, Virgil Sanford, and Charlotte Ward on night duty, 1960. Virg was everyone's friend, especially student nurses, as one of the few regular male attendants always willing to help on the night shift.

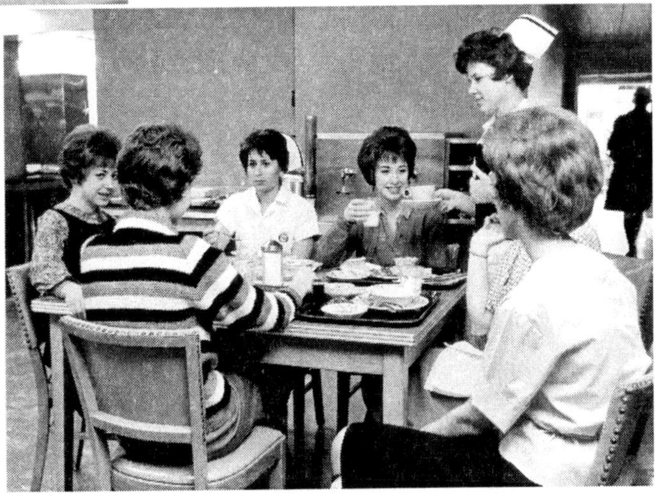

141. Gaille Lutz, in uniform facing the camera, chats after lunch in the hospital cafeteria, 1963.

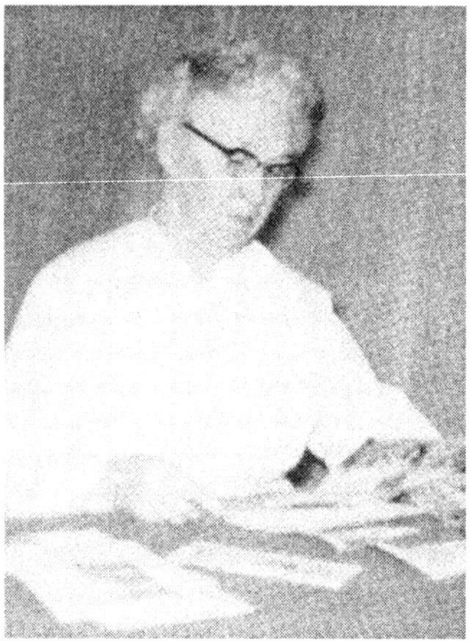

142. Esther VanBallegooyen ("Mrs. Van"), hospital hostess, greeted vistors, conducted hospital tours, and spent many hours as a Grey Lady. She was also the chairman of the White Cross Guild Nurses Group, which provided gifts to students and hosted new student receptions and graduate breakfasts.

143. (below) This 10-story hospital building, looking north from Cedar Street, was completed in 1966. The two round floors comprised its intensive care unit.

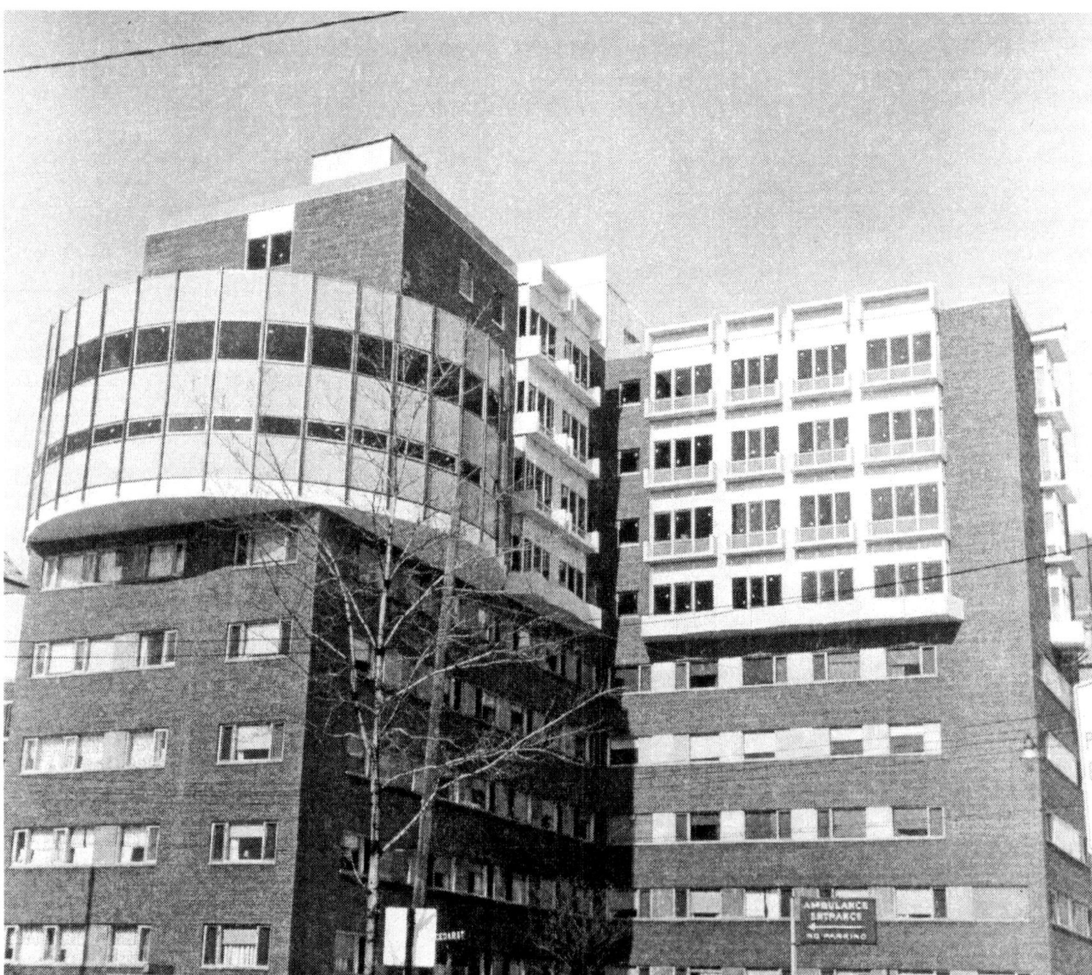

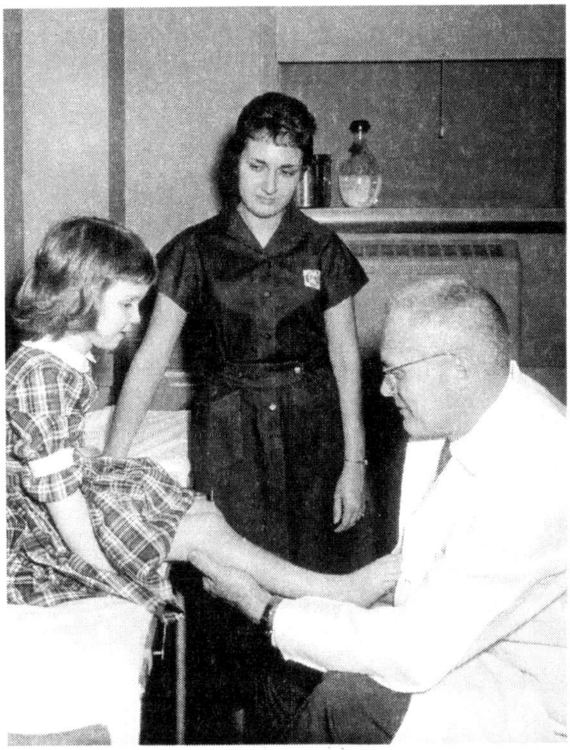

144. Outpatient clinics were an important part of student training, 1962. Nancy Bumstead, in her blue outpatient uniform, assists Dr. Russell Cashen in examination of a patient during Orthopedic Clinic.

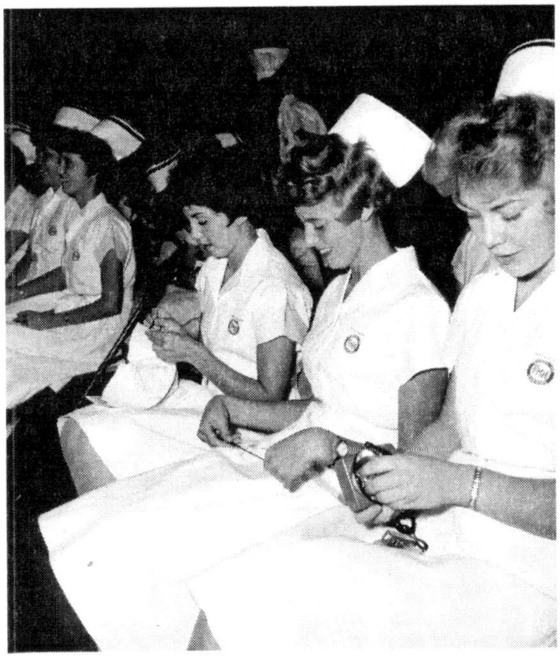

145. During Black Banding, junior students put on their narrow bands (right to left) Unidentified, Jeanne Teusink, Judy Baldwin, 1963.

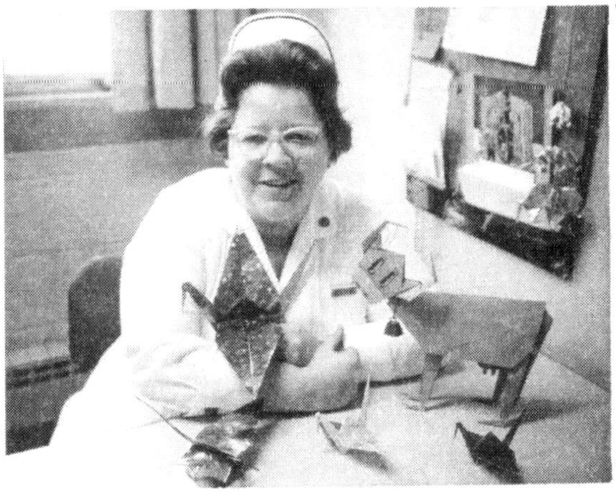

146. (above) Instructor Mary L. Mason, 1966. Her interest in origami figures arose while stationed in Japan as an Army nurse during the 1950s.

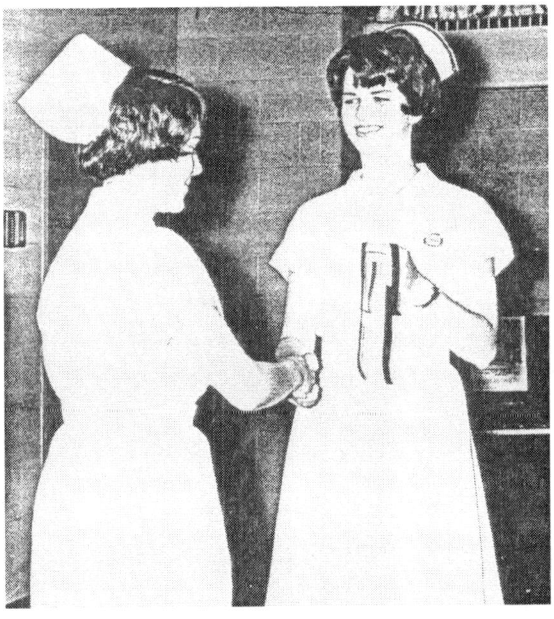

147. Senior Marilyn Backus presented Jacquelyn Page '72 her junior band during Black Banding, June 1968.

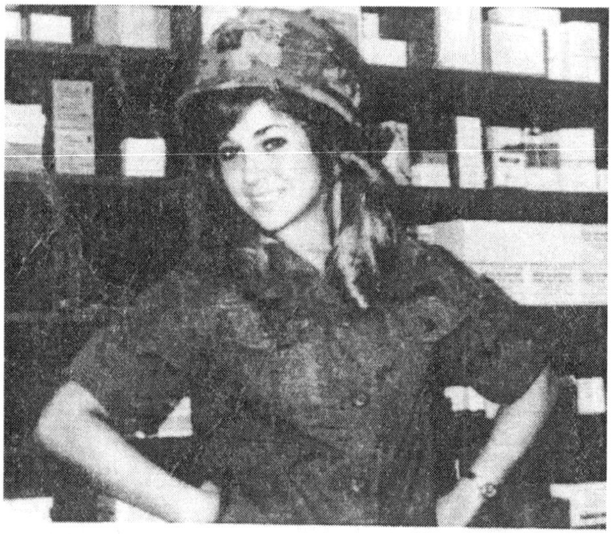

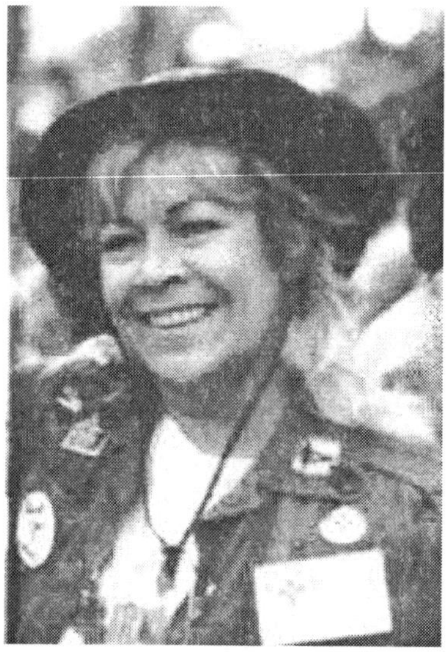

148. (left) Serving as an Army nurse in Vietnam, Captain Diana Dwan ran to the pharmacy during a Red Alert (incoming mortars) for penicillin, January 27, 1970 (her 24th birthday). The Pharmacy Tech told her, "Happy Birthday, Captain," and took this picture. 149. (right) Years later she was back in Washington, D.C.

150. (left to right, below) Representing the Education Department at Western Michigan University, Russell Seibert sits with Sarah Bahlke and Kalamazoo College President George Rainsford in Truesdale Hall. Sarah was one of the first Heyl scholars attending Bronson Methodist Hospital School of Nursing, early 1970s.

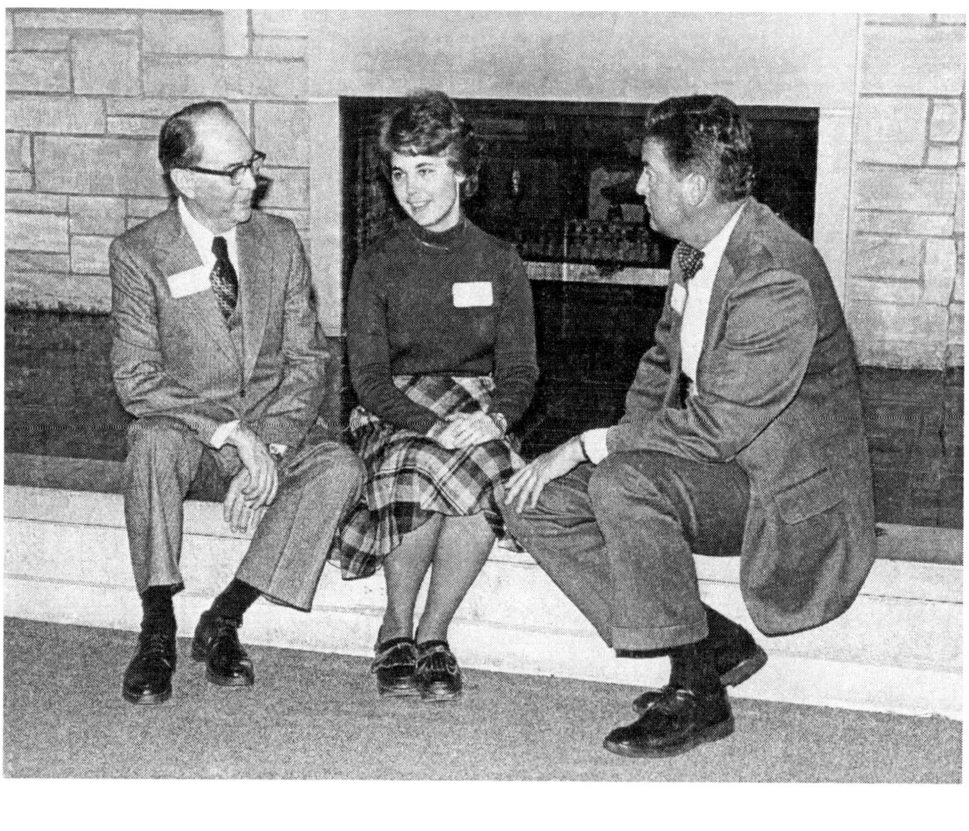

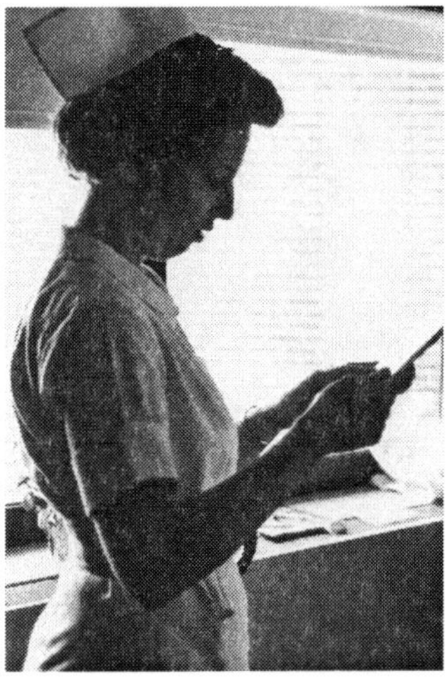

151. (left) Student Crista Yeiter reviews a patient record, 1972.

152. (right) In the recovery room, Head Nurse Mary Keeler cares for a patient, 1975.

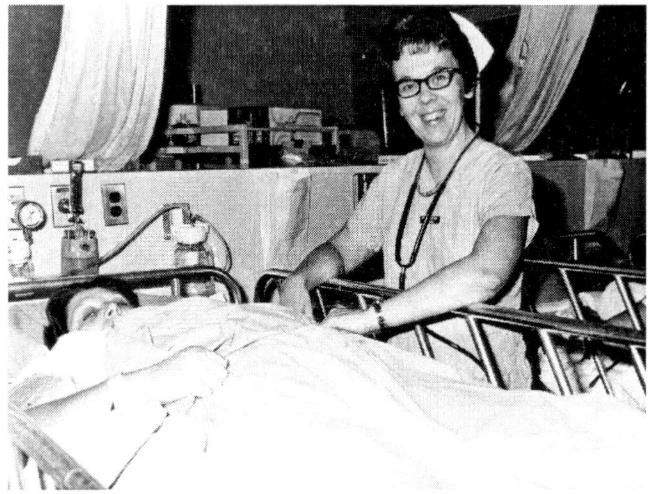

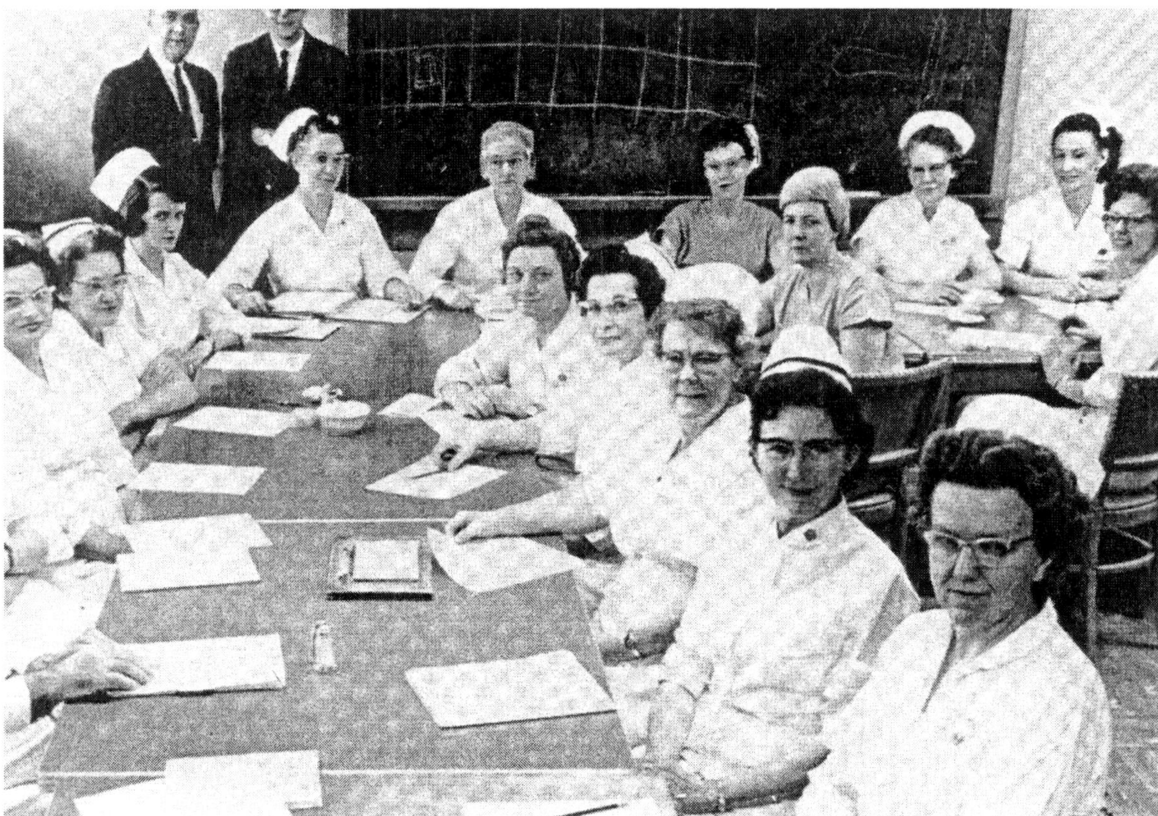

153. (Seated, clockwise from left) Ila Kain, Carrie Floyd, Marilyn Woodruff, Mabel Meyle, Maude Southon, Virginia Chamberlin, Estelle Theis, Hazel Latondress, Patricia McDonald, Donna Tosco, Unidentified, Mary Jane Bushhouse, Thelma Groat, Edna Lord, and Dorothy Meninga at a meeting of instructors and head nurses, ca 1970. (Standing, left to right) Stu Westbury, Jack Schwem.

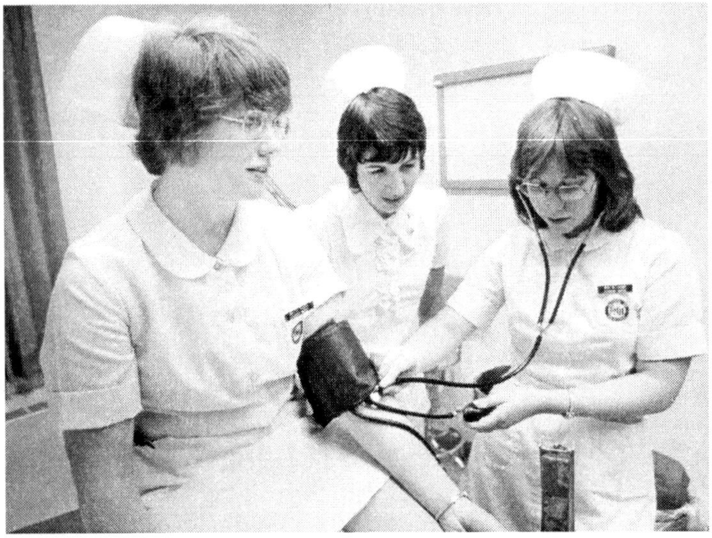

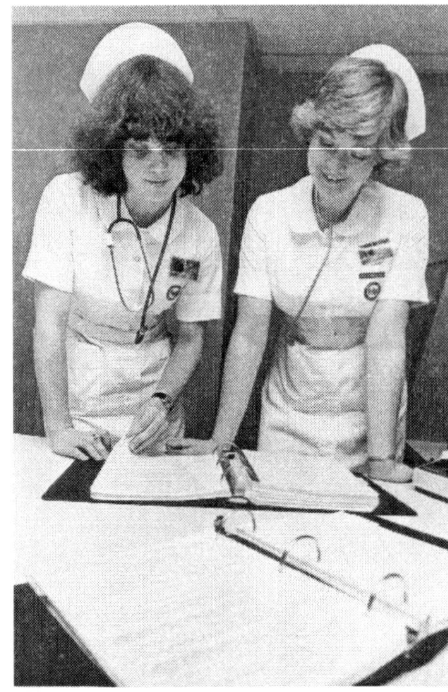

Clockwise from top,
154. Jackie Wylie (center) instructs students Shirley Tucker and Mary Ludwa in blood pressure measurement, 1975.
155. Freshmen Nancy Birge and Julie Stennett use the Hall 8 reference library, 1979.
156. Graduation ceremony with Big Bird, 1981.
157. (left to right, back) Shelly Kandt, Deb Madison, (front) Sue Rosteck and Jane Mayberry with Wig Lady of elevator prank frame.

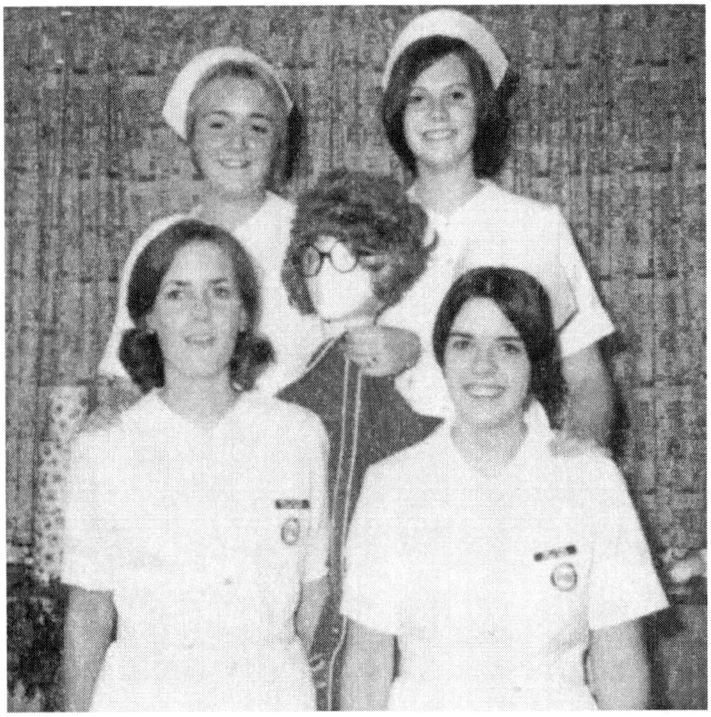

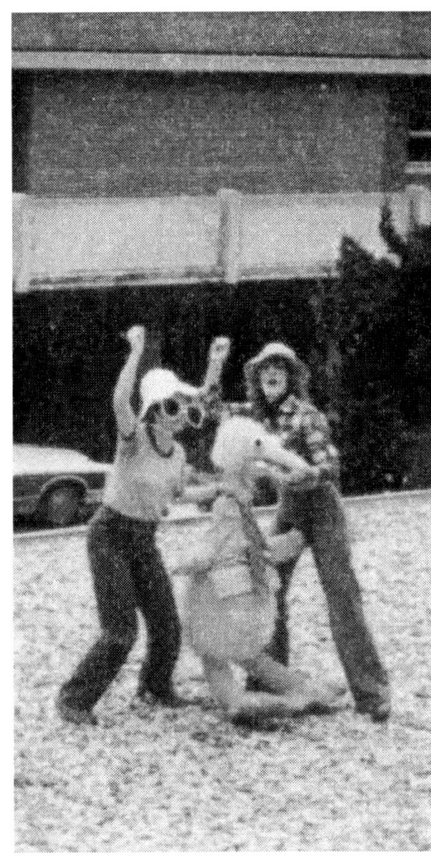

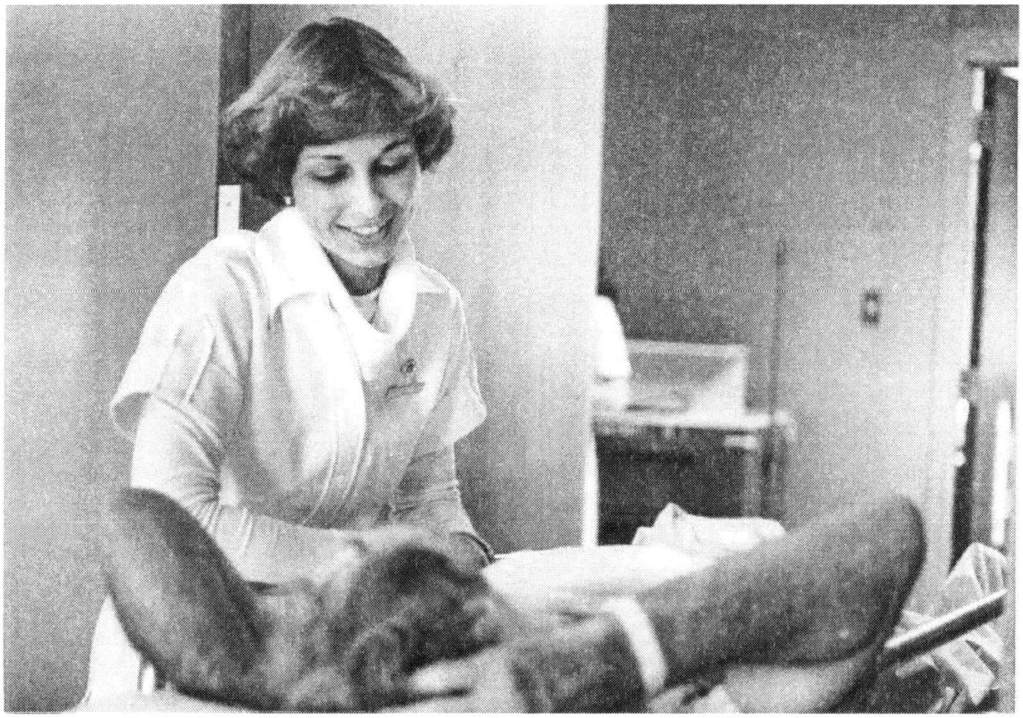

158. (above) Betsy Hoogewind comforts a patient, late 1970s.
159. (below) Photographed from the southeast Truesdale Hall, is the new addition to the Bronson Methodist Hospital complex, 1978.

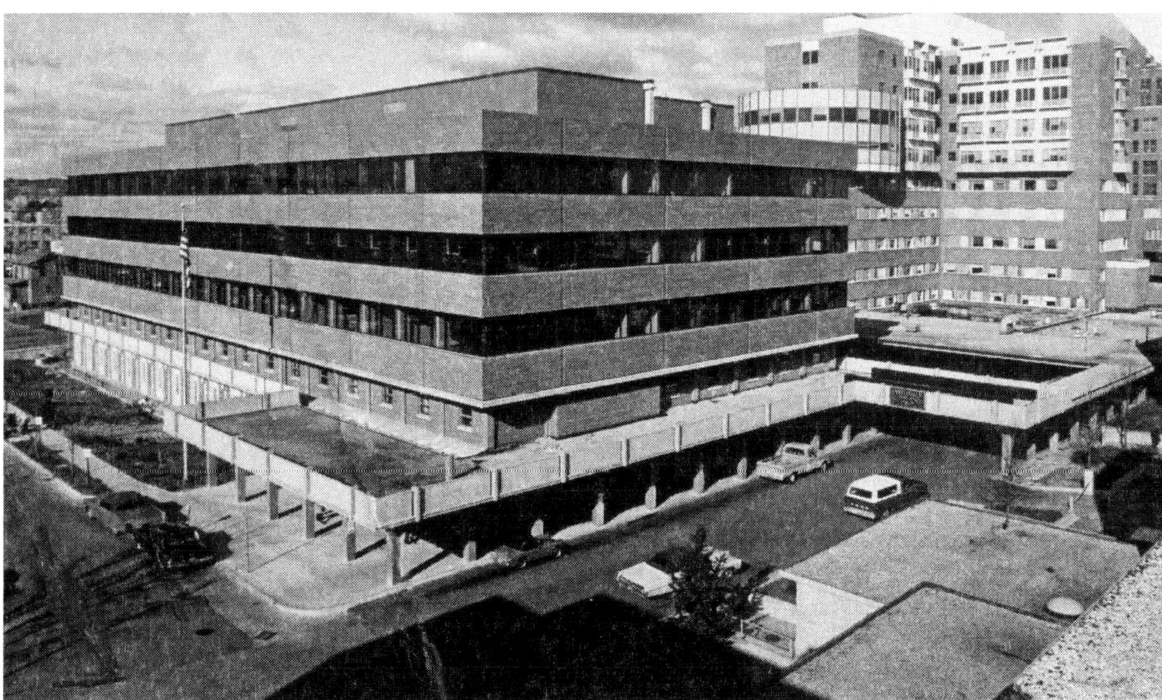

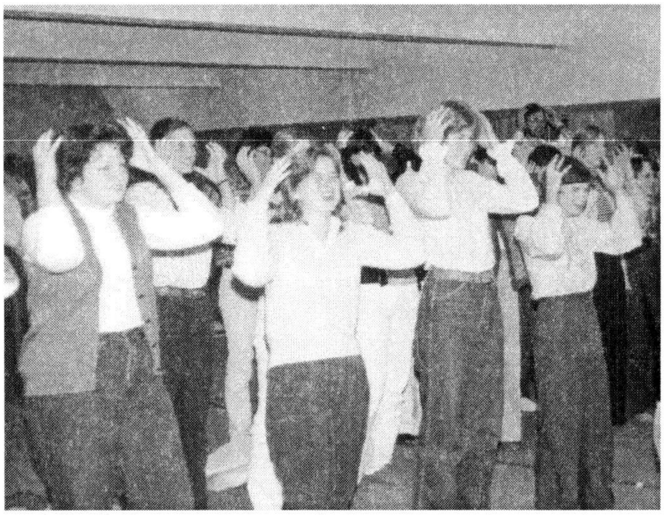

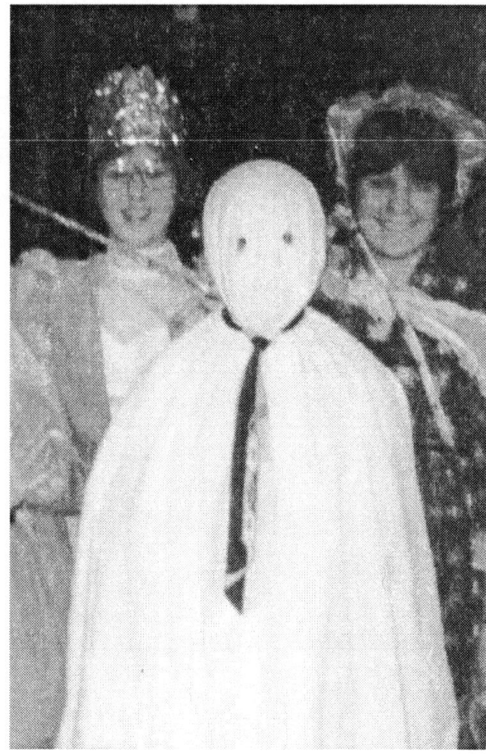

Clockwise from top,
160. Doin' the Motion during freshmen orientation, 1979.
161. Halloween on the children's ward, 1979.
162. Truesdale Hall (center) with Harding School (lower left) and hospital complex (lower right), 1979.

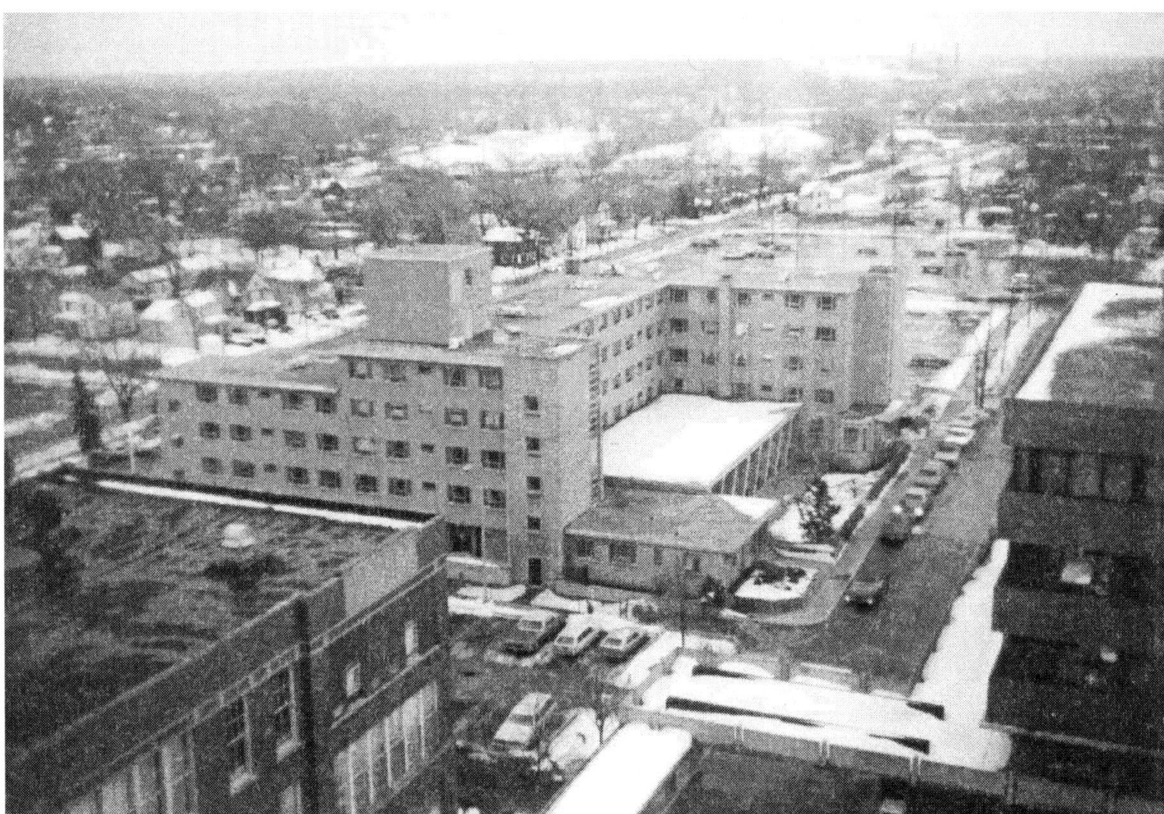

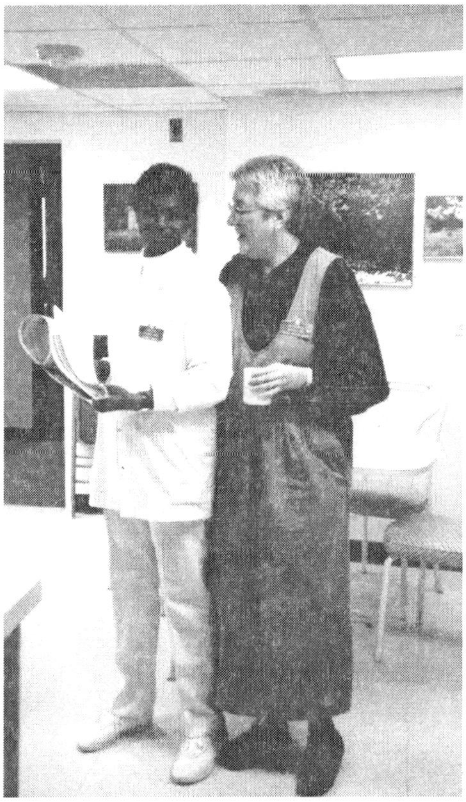

163. (left) Instructors Helen Truss and Barb Groh taking a break in the kitchen at Truesdale Hall, ca 1970s.

164. Three generations of furniture occupied the lounge of Truesdale Hall over its lifetime. Furnishings of the 1970s are shown below.

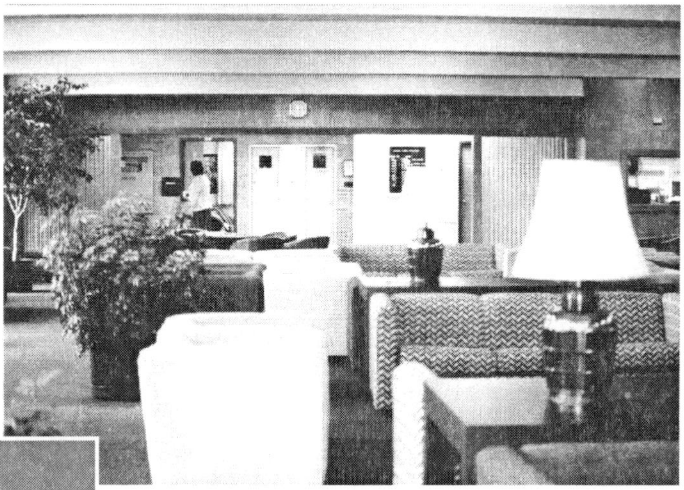

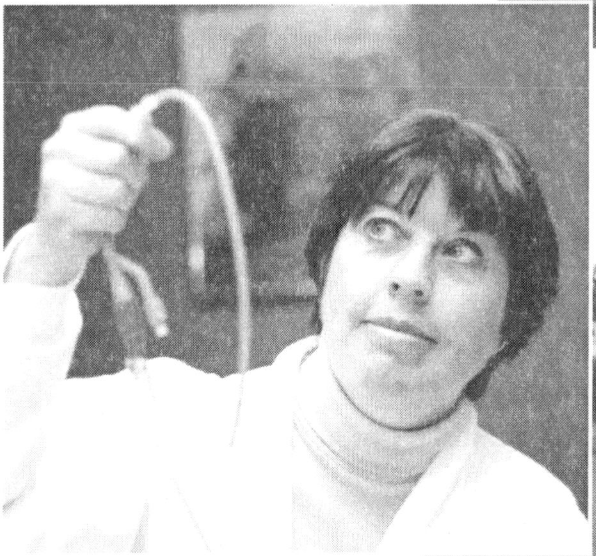

165. (left) Ann Orr carefully observes a Foley catheter after its removal.

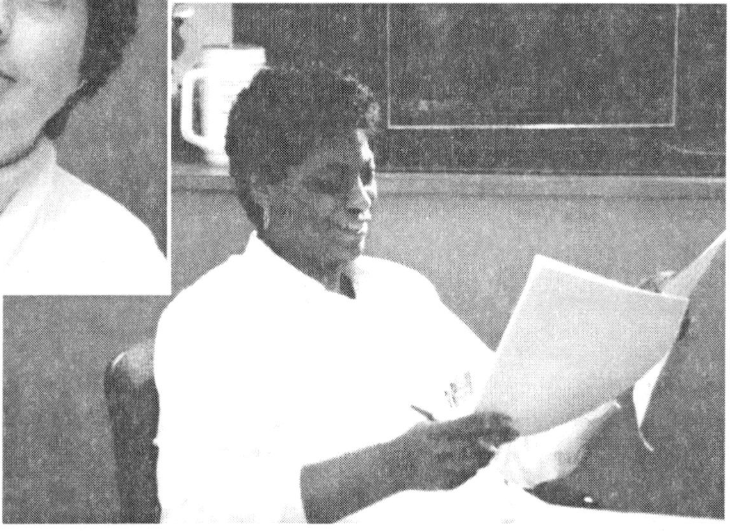

166. (right) Instructor Helen Truss reviews coursework at her desk.

Section III.

LEARNERS

CHAPTER 9

HIGH TECH-HIGH TOUCH: SELF CARE IN NURSING EDUCATION, 1980s

> On May 13, 1980, a tornado hit downtown Kalamazoo. We heard the alarms on the third floor of Truesdale and went to sit out in the hall where we heard something and felt a pressure change (all the doors banged even though they were closed). Then we learned that there really had been a tornado. During the afternoon we hung around the hospital to help as much as we could. That evening we wandered around downtown surveying all the damage.
>
> ***Deb Retsema and Gail Eberly '81***

A few figurative tornados also hit the hospital, medical system, and nursing during the eighties, a wake-up call. Accelerated changes in care delivery were on their way, in a dichotomous setting of medical-specialty expansion and a need for cost control in delivery of care. Would the dominant medical model support an increase in shared decision-making with other clinicians, administrators and consumers? Bigger patient roles toward self-care and self-health management didn't seem to fit yet. Financially insolvent small hospitals were closing their doors unless

> During the tornado we all hid in the tunnel between Truesdale and the hospital and sang hymns and prayed. Afterward I worked in the ER for eight hours as a phlebotomist.
> ***Patti Dell '82***

they could find larger systems that would include them. Could a win-win position be achieved?

In 1982, the hospital became a subsidiary of a parent company called Bronson Healthcare Group (BHG). The intent of BHG was " . . . to support the hospital by offering alternative healthcare services and new sources of capital and revenues."[1] Changes occurred in the face of government attempts to control costs and yet continue expansion—a redirection of services.

Daniel Finch, who retired on July 1, 1985, spoke in favor of expansion with arguments that competition was good and duplication of services could have a positive effect on cost control. In line with this thinking, Tom Langer, whose experience was in industry, was hired in 1985 as the vice president for marketing. Russell Kneen took Finch's place as chairman of the Bronson Healthcare Group. His past experience was finance in his early career as a CPA. He made it clear that expansion of services would be outside of the acute care hospital, with fewer beds and the need " . . . to conceive of ideas to keep patients out of the hospital."[2] The glitch—"out of the hospital"—meant healthcare consumers would continue to receive high-tech, diagnostic, outpatient services and interventions aimed at curing disease but would not necessarily be hospitalized. Health promotion and self-care just could not pay the bills.

Al L. Dixon was hired as Vice President of Enterprise Activities for BHG when the hospital had 453 beds, reduced from 464. The subsidiaries included 41-bed Bronson Vicksburg Hospital, designated the hospital's neurological center for patients who needed rehabilitation to gain functionality; Bronson Medical Center, the physicians' office building that had been part of the hospital for years; as well as Bronson Management Services Corporation, Bronson Health Foundation, Bronson Outpatient Surgery, Bronson Builders and Design, CareFlite, Inc., and Bronson

Clinical Investigational Unit in partnership with the Upjohn Company. Kneen said that the establishment of a health maintenance organization was in the making.[3, 4] "In January [1986] Bronson Healthcare Group Inc., holding company for Bronson Methodist Hospital, and IBA Health and Life Assurance Company joined forces to create the IBA Health Care Plan."[5]

Patric E. Ludwig was in line to become the next BHG president in March 1986; he replaced Russell Kneen in September 1988. Arthur Littlefield continued as Chief Nurse Executive.

COSTS AND COOPERATION

The First Health Development Corporation, created in December 1987 to promote cooperation between Bronson Methodist Hospital and Borgess Medical Center, began by hiring an independent consulting firm with a projected cost of $100,000 " . . . to study the best ways for the hospitals to face the uncertain future."[6]

Hospital reimbursements continued to decline amidst the creation of new health-care entities. "Kalamazoo, with average daily hospital charges of $1,139, ranks second highest in Michigan only to Ann Arbor, according to the Southwest Michigan Coordinating Council."[7] Bronson reduced patient room prices from $299 to $275 for a semi-private.

Kalamazoo's hospitals considered a merger plan in view of the costs of care in the fall of 1988, as part of their First Health Development Corporation led by Russell Kneen and Timothy Stack, Chief Executive Officer at Borgess Medical Center. "The real winners in this proposal are the patients in southwest Michigan,"[8] said Robert Kittredge, Vice Chair of the Bronson board.

Bronson and Borgess nurses, not to be left out, met at three rallies in October 1988, to voice their concerns about the possible hospital merger and what it would mean to nursing in the Kalamazoo area. The Southwestern Chapter Michigan Nurses Association (previously known as the Kalamazoo District Nurses Association), led the task force for this move. Nurses voiced their need to be heard in creating excellent care and drawing nurses into "magnet" hospitals.[9]

The nurses need not have worried about the hospitals' merger. This revolutionary idea did not get off the ground, although a joint effort would occur later with the development of the West Michigan Cancer Center.

DRGS BLAMED FOR HOSPITAL DOWN-SIZING AND THE NEW DIRECTION

One of the greatest forces that impacted hospital revenue was the federal government's prospective payment system, Diagnosis-Related Groups (DRGs), effective January 1, 1984. No longer would reimbursement be based on the reported cost of care for Medicare patients. Insurance companies followed the new system of assigning fixed payments to medical diagnosis classifications. The hospital could theoretically make a small gain if the care provided cost less than its reimbursement. Standardized care according to evidence-based practice made good sense, except there wasn't much evidence. Physicians and hospitals practiced in ways customary for regions, often not evidence-based. For example, hysterectomy was the treatment of choice for women's uterine problems in some regions while, in other areas, given the same patient demographics, care management was medical with similar outcome, at much less cost. Standards of care had been derived from what was customary in a region, not what research demonstrated as the most effective treatment for best patient outcomes.

The prospective payment system was phased in over four years to lessen potential negative impacts to hospitals and allow time for adaptation from what was usual or customary toward evidence-based practice.[10] The cuts were felt and forced administrators to look for other sources of revenue if they were going to conduct business as usual.

One outcome, based on acuity measures, was a limit on the time patients could stay in the hospital. No longer were people hospitalized for "observation." Patients were more acutely ill, and care more demanding and complex. The 24-hour preparation time to complete the homework for student assigned patients often disappeared because of early patient discharge. Students had to quickly learn the details for a new patient who had just arrived. Every day was a challenge of new information to learn and new experiences to absorb.

NURSING EDUCATION'S ANSWERS TO CHANGES

The BMH School of Nursing was rewarded for producing graduates who could manage complex medical technology as well as patient education. Health intervention toward self-care, control and self-health management became important and fit with the trend toward informed consumers within a competitive hospital environment. We were doing things right under the new model, but were we doing the right thing to meet long-term healthcare needs of the community? Dual roles of medicine and nursing were becoming visible and gave hope to nurses for increased recognition of their expertise.

Borgess Nurses and Their Five-and-a-Half-Week Strike

Two months after the tornado hit Kalamazoo, on July 14, 1980, the Borgess nurses struck! Tired of having no voice in their working conditions, they had voted earlier to become part of the Michigan Nurses Association's (MNA) bargaining unit. Represented as a collective, with all MNA nurses supporting them, they believed when negotiations broke down, that the strike was best for their patients in the long run. They took the risk and struck so their voices could be heard. It wasn't just about wages but about staffing patterns, mandatory overtime, and a sense of being second-class citizens within the hospital system. It was a time of discomfort for nurses, and Jackie Wylie marveled at the courage of her sisters for their bravery. Patient care wouldn't improve if nurses kept still and didn't step up to the plate. Nurses striking was an unheard of action in Kalamazoo, yet the Kalamazoo nurses voted to walk out and risk the censorship of those who would view and accuse them of being deserters for abandoning their patients.

Borgess prepared for the strike, decreasing patient census from 473 often-filled patient beds to less than half that number, with nurse-managers back in staff nurse roles. Bronson, with 453 beds, could manage the increase in patient census with some quick adjustments in scheduling elective surgical cases, which allowed for patients in emergency situations to receive immediate hospitalization. Bronson geared up for an increase in census and broke many records for the numbers of patients cared for that year.

> We continued to give patients the best care possible despite what, for some, meant long hours, missed breaks and meals, and missed time with families. Patients also recognized the situation and were cooperative and "patient". . . remarks such as, "Nurses were responsive to my needs, and everyone seemed willing to go the extra mile," were part of an in-house publication thanking all employees for their extra effort.[11]

All Kalamazoo nurses won increased wages with the strike. The loss was a developing adversarial situation for Borgess nurse administrators, managers and the staff nurses who seemed to be on separate sides. The role nurses played in decision-making and delivery of care, as well as the voices of other so-called "allied" health professions, didn't seem to change. As if there was no way to change the relational dynamics, nurses felt oppressed and often took on a victim mentality. The system had to change, but how could it be turned into a more caring, curing and cost-effective model? Consumers, providers and payers required a higher level of consciousness and a shift in thinking. The medical community could not be faulted for what needed to be a local community and national effort. Years away still, it would take transformation toward an integrated healthcare delivery system, not medical services alone, to build a new system of health with internal rewards—recognition for lifestyle changes and determinants of health, which are:

- lifestyle,
- socio-economic status (access to education and meaningful work, *etc.*),
- safe living environment,
- healthy genetic pool and,
- last on the list of health determinants, the healthcare system itself.[12]

Slowly nurses were returning to universities for nursing degrees or degrees in fields related to the evolving healthcare system: degrees in business, management, finance and administration on one end of the continuum and nurse midwifery, nurse practitioners, health education and holistic health practice on the other. A doctor of philosophy degree in nursing was an expectation for professors in nursing programs affiliated with upper-division colleges and universities. Bronson nurse–managers formed a nursing research committee with the "goal . . . to facilitate nursing . . . and other non-physician personnel [involvement in] research at the hospital."[13] The committee was interdisciplinary, with the Microbiology Department, Health Science Library, and Pharmacy staff represented. John MacDougall, nurse staffing director, a nurse with graduate-level preparation, chaired the committee.

> While physicians have traditionally dominated national medical research, today's trend is toward more involvement in research by nurses and other non-physician medical personnel. In the field of nursing, specifically, this growing trend includes incorporating research values and activities into the practice of nursing as a means of establishing a scientific basis for nursing practice.[14]

Although this effort was laudable, resources were not available to achieve its goals. There was one faculty member with the expertise to facilitate nursing research and no doctoral-prepared nurses who practiced full-time at the hospital. Secondly, the committee had no funding resources except for the possibility of applying for research awards from professional nursing organizations. Nevertheless, efforts were made to ask research questions and to recognize the art and science of nursing, even though a critical mass of doctoral and graduate-prepared nurses did not exist.

First Clinical Nurse Specialist Emerges at Bronson

Bill Selinsky, Class of 1975, was a nontraditional student. Men in nursing were few in number. Selinsky had been in the army medical corps. Later he became a nontraditional RN, in a sense, because he immediately continued his education after army tenure, earning a Bachelor of Science degree in health studies from Western Michigan University and a Master of Science degree in nursing, with an adult medical-surgical care focus, from Wayne State University. In 1980 he became the first clinical nurse specialist (CNS) at Bronson, with two more CNSs hired by the next year, *i.e.,* Judy Halpern, who specialized in the care of trauma and emergency patients, and Peg Malnight in neonatology. Clinical nurse specialists were graduate-level prepared, with advanced training and clinical practice in their specialty fields. "We are trained to synthesize data . . . make nursing diagnoses which are clinical judgments. Then . . . communicate these to the rest of the healthcare team. What we develop are comprehensive, long-range, future-oriented patient-care plans." [15] Hope developed that this type of attention would improve recovery and decrease length-of-stay. Little evidence existed on which to base their practice, which needed medical allies since, ultimately, physicians, controlled hospital admissions, treatment choices and discharge. Nurses were not perceived as income producers. They were numerous and viewed as expensive labor.

DID ANYONE HEAR THE NURSE LEADERS SPEAK?

Staff nurses appeared to be their own worst enemies at times. Threatened by the American Nurses Association resolution (June 1978) that professional nursing should require a baccalaureate degree, with a major in nursing as the entry-level degree, by 1985, nurses with associate degrees and diplomas resisted. Threatened administrators in community colleges and hospitals, who gave the impression that the status quo was just fine, supported them. Wasn't the system working for everyone? Why change it? Wouldn't increases in the nurses' education level just increase the cost of care? Probably so without a paradigm shift in how the business of healthcare was managed.

> In May, 1979, a Legislative Task Force was organized . . . to keep all hospital nursing personnel informed about pending legislation such as the "1985 Proposal" which may influence professional status. . . . The goal of the Legislative Task Force is not to take a stand on any of the issues, but to provide practicing nurses with information on existing and pending legislation, educational trends, and other issues relevant to the nursing profession.[16]

The Legislative Task Force had to do more than disseminate information. Most nurses were too threatened about the possibility of changes in nurse practice licensure, although they were assured of being grandfathered into the professional status with the licensure they currently held and would not be required to return to school. Only new graduates would be affected and appropriately assimilated into the system. The ANA resolution, in the hands of people choosing the status quo, pitted nurses against nurses. Nurses needed to learn that a win-win could happen if they would accept their educational diversity and value the expertise they offered as a unified whole.

If only the nursing career ladder could have been viewed as an educational asset with accessibility, advancement, and greater professionalism. Nursing was one of the few professions that offered a career ladder type of mobility. Women and men who could not imagine a four-year course of study, and who had no idea of attending college, found themselves in nurse aide or patient-care technician positions that opened their eyes to the world of caring for others. Some very bright, first generation, college-bound students emerged! It wasn't easy, but what a wonderful path a want-to-be nurse could follow. She or he could start at a nurse aide or patient-care technician level, learned from RNs the most basic functional needs of patients and nursing home residents, and get a taste of the meaning of supporting people during illness and end-of-life before enrolling in courses to become a licensed practical nurse. Once past its licensing examination, "want-to-bes" could then enroll in an LPN to RN ladder program. It's not easy to pull yourself up by your own bootstraps. Nurses and hospital administrators provided some support through scholarships,[17] but failed to recognize the emotional support needed to accompany the investment of time, energy, and dollars spent bringing employees' dreams to fruition—dreams of entry into the nursing profession. Administrators, too, dreamed of adding a more-skilled employee who already was loyal to the institution. Paradoxically, nursing leaders in southwest Michigan continued their search for nurses and employers of nurses who would stand with them to bring graduate nursing education to the region.

Logic for increasing nurse education levels had something to do with the fact that most entry-level professional degrees allow students the opportunity and benefit of development over six years and matriculation from graduate programs.

A Nursing Graduate Program Questionnaire

The Council of Nurse Educators and Service Administrators in Southwest Michigan appointed a steering committee early in 1979 to explore the possibility of creating a graduate-level nursing program which would lead to a Master of Science in Nursing degree. The program would be based at Western Michigan University (WMU). The committee included representatives from Bronson's School of Nursing,

Kalamazoo Valley Community College, Nazareth College, Bronson Methodist Hospital, and Borgess Medical Center as well as nurse administrators from local healthcare agencies:

> A questionnaire has been written [by Phyllis Nicolaou, RN EdD] and will be sent this spring [1979] to RNs and health service agencies employing RNs in the southwest Michigan health service area. The purpose of the questionnaire is to determine local support for the WMU program. Nurses and agencies need to demonstrate their interest. Presently there is no graduate nursing program in southwest Michigan. This deficit creates a serious shortage of nurses with advanced education and may limit some nursing services that will be vital to future patient care in our community.[18, 19]

One Voice

"A perspective on nursing: building bridges to the future," was the May 1985 *Catalyst* article[20] that voiced the professional direction supported by Bronson nurse educators. Judy Stewart,[21] EdD, MSN, RN, associate director, offered insights about the changing environment and nursing:

> What is happening to nursing at Bronson? What part are we playing in these changing times? Are we practicing nursing with as much style and productivity as we can muster? When I say "we" I mean all of the nurses employed at Bronson—ALL of us; for we know that it takes all of us to get the job done.
>
> Michigan Nurses Week's focus on *Bridges to the Future* provides an excellent opportunity to ask and answer these questions. We want to be involved in shaping that future and the bridges to it. We must be involved in order to see that professional nursing practice at Bronson continues to contribute in a maximally productive, cost-effective way.
>
> Nursing practice at Bronson is changing. The staffing ratio has dropped and nurses are questioning the quality of care that is delivered at Bronson. The reactions to the staffing situation are

understandable, however, I am suggesting that we build the skill or utilize the skilled nurses already in place to take a pro-active stance. The following are pro-active responses that are options for Bronson nurses:

1. Determine the cost of nursing care at Bronson. Fit this into the DRG payment framework. Determine if we are income producing. What ways can we reduce the costs at Bronson? What incentives are there for profit sharing? If we increase our productivity, can we share in the profits? Do all nurses have to meet the same production standards or could we contract for numbers of clients served? Are we utilizing a staffing system that provides incentives for improving delivery of care outcomes? Until we have a handle on the cost of nursing care and its relationship to the organization's income, we will not be able to redefine nursing practice at Bronson with the adjusted staffing patterns.

2. Redefine nursing practice at Bronson. Identify those problems that result in lowering quality care. Identify high cost, low outcome activities. For example, are bed baths and linen change essential daily? Take charge of shaping nursing practice so that outcome objectives are met in a profitable way.

3. Improve our relationship with the medical staff and Board of Trustees. Because we make up one-third of the employees at Bronson and because our services are essential, we are visible and strong. We cannot, however, get our job done without strong collaborative relationships with the medical community and without resource support from the Board of Trustees. Strategies for strengthening this aspect of nursing practice should be developed.

4. Develop and move on risk strategies. Realize that there is discovery in failure! You win every time you learn and gain data to improve the system. One project in five may be immediately useful to nursing practice and the organization. We must venture forth with resources, innovation and creative thinking. The rules of the past no longer apply. The future is ours to shape, and we must restructure. "Front line" nurses must be involved in the planning of innovative changes so that

> their ideas are realized. Seek information. Ask questions. Together we can build an exciting future.

> Bronson has a long history of taking good care of employees. This is based on the principle that productivity is a result of the way people are treated. The framework for taking care of Bronson nurses in the future must be one in which nurses take charge of their professional nursing practice and assume an assertive role in contributing to productivity at Bronson. Let's celebrate Michigan Nurses Week by participating in the making of that bridge to the future rather than letting it happen to us!

Collective Nursing Support

What would Florence Nightingale have said about Stewart's words and her plea for all nurses to collectively support nursing services? Be pro-active, and propose changes without compromising standards of nursing care. Nightingale would have approved! The Legislative Task Force had to do more than disseminate information.

Nurses honor Nightingale each year during the annual May Nurses Week celebration in holistic nursing circles around the world that light candles in remembrance of a nurse leader and genius, born May 12, 1820. She set standards and assertively aligned with influential people who could help nurses realize their potential. Nurses of the 1980s needed to follow her lead.

Nursing Advancement Week held November 16-21, 1987, was an event cosponsored by Bronson's Human Resources Department and its nurse recruiter, Gail Durant, RN, BS and its School of Nursing administrator, Crystal Richman, RN, BSN The newspaper advertisement said, "Nurses from across Michigan are coming to share experiences, discuss the future of the profession, and explore new areas of specialization." Uplifting events that week were intended to recruit nurses and nursing students.[22] Nurses needed to hear their voices and believe in their healing powers.

Loving Patients Back to Health

William Selinsky '75, Bronson's first Clinical Nurse Specialist, wrote these words[23] about his mentors:

> Mutuality and relationship with a nursing technician is a story of extraordinary influences. To describe Roberta Ferguson would take a great deal of effort[24] [and] a gifted writer to choose just the right words . . . a sensitive poet to paint a picture in words of Roberta's love for humanity, kindness and sense of duty . . . a talented comedian to relay Roberta's affability and sense of humor . . . and much more space than is allowed here.
>
> However, all of the right words and the sensitivity and humor can be rolled into one six-letter word, "Fergey." To those who know her, just the mention of her name brings a smile to their faces, a momentary pause and then a statement that borders on the refrain, "You can't get any better than Fergey."
>
> Fergey has worked on Hall 6 as a nursing technician for several years. Her experience in the nursing department and orthopedics spanned 23 years. During that time, Fergey loved more patients back to health, helped more student nurses and became friends with more staff members than most people around here can recall. "Fergey's the only one I know who has her former patients take her out to lunch all the time," said Annie Higgins, a nursing technician and good friend of Fergey's for many years.
>
> Mirzda Zeimelis, RN, Fergey's friend and supervisor for 17 years, remembers a story that is typical. "Fergey would always befriend the little old patient from a nursing home who had no friends or family. She would take his/her few worn and tattered clothes home with her to wash and mend. If they were beyond repair or fell apart in the washing machine, Fergey would make new ones. Always above and beyond the call of duty: that's Fergey."

Was it possible that gifts of caring from a nursing technician [later called, patient-care technicians] brought healing presence? Not only was it possible, it was obvious.

AUXILIARY CONTINUES GIVING

By the 1980s the Auxiliary was managing a lucrative gift shop at Bronson with all proceeds donated back to capital campaigns and other projects that needed funding. Auxiliary gifts were wonderful—not only in dollars but in wanting to give community input. They recognized that community members valued hospital services and chose to support them. Administrator requests most likely influenced Auxiliary decisions.

Julie VanderNoot was hired into the business office in 1985 to assist the Auxiliary as the gift shop manager at a time when outpatient pharmacies often connected with gift shops. This next step occurred in January, 1987, with the Auxiliary removed from managing the gift shop service and losing its privilege of saying for what the generated revenue would be used. Logical though the change may have seemed, to some it was a sad day for the Auxiliary. The gift shop had been its major source of fundraising throughout the seventies and eighties. It was also a sad day for Bronson which lost this interesting community connection and the infusion of thousands of dollars each year by very caring and dedicated volunteers. It was a sign of the times.

Volunteers have worked in the gift shop since its transfer to the Pharmacy Department. Dutch Market, originally held in 1963, and a bazaar became the Auxiliary's major focus, with fundraising events taking the form of book and jewelry sales on the hospital grounds.

The Bronson Methodist Hospital Auxiliary led the volunteer efforts of the four volunteer divisions, with 300 members contributing services. The Bronson Red Cross Division added 125 workers, and 50 people were members of the Bronson Service Volunteer Division, while 30 teenagers worked as Health Care Volunteens during the summer. Maria Collins, the volunteer coordinator, said that an average of 40 volunteers gave service every day.[25]

Their contributions were more than the time spent in direct service. They made up a team of loyal community good will ambassadors. The Auxiliary celebrated its fiftieth anniversary in 1985 with 236 members.[26]

EXPANSION AND REMODELING

On the southeast corner of John and Lovell streets, a courtyard and new lobby, with seating for 64, welcomed the public by appearing more hotel-like and as a safe place to pick up and drop off people who often needed wheel chair assistance.[27] A security department helped manage logistics.

A place of strong healing is the translation for the name of the sculpture, *"Locus Curae Validae,"* funded by community donations and dedicated April 27, 1983. Kurt Newman, a Kalamazoo sculptor, created this piece to grace the main entrance at the Bronson Lovell and John street's corner. The Reverend David McShane's dedication speech explained the connection between the bronze piece and the symbolic, " . . . promise of wholeness to the wounded and the ailing. This place is here to heal."[28]

SOFT MARKETING OF CARING

Part of a series of TV ads to be aired on stations throughout southwest Michigan and northern Indiana appeared on the cover of the September 1982, *Catalyst.* They highlighted the warmth and caring of Bronson and its people:

> 'Tis the human touch in this world that counts
> The touch of your hand in mine
> Which means far more to the fainting heart
> Than shelter, and bread and wine
>
> For shelter is gone when the night is o'er
> And bread lasts only a day
> But the touch of the hand and the sound of
> The voice, sing on in the soul always.

Bronson and Borgess found some ways to join ranks toward cost reductions and less duplication but, for the most part, emerging marketing made Kalamazoo medical services seem like a major hospital competition for patients and the newest technology. The *Gazette* referred to the "B and B" saga as a second story of "*War and Peace*."[29]

Certainly the *Kalamazoo Gazette* was a winner in the number of full-page ads that touted the services offered by both hospitals. The sidebar (page 424) is an example of Bronson's message to the staff and the public. Its slogan became, "We're with you all the way," intended to let the public know that Bronson offered birth to end of life medical services. "While advertising by hospitals was once heavily criticized, it has become a valuable informational tool which aids and equips the consumer to make appropriate healthcare decisions," said Dick McDonald, president, McDonald Davis and Associates.[30] Why? McDonald said that declining censuses, soaring healthcare costs, and an over-abundance of services made advertising necessary.

Patients became more involved, not in responsible lifestyle changes, but in choosing a hospital, specialty medicine and invasive technology to manage chronic illnesses that limited their daily functional ability, and as "better informed healthcare consumers [who could] become primary decision makers in their care."[31]

Looking for new markets often brought problems to light that in the past had been unmentionable. Bronson ran a quarter page advertisement on May 20, 1987, "Impotence Can Tear People Apart!" The public was invited to hear physician Mark A. Lucas "conduct the discussion, covering symptoms of impotence, testing, and treatments."[32] Anonymity would be respected.

But what about informed self-care, self-health managers? Advertising was first about healthier hospitals, not about healthier families, though there seemed to be some movement toward a healthy America 2000.

For a smile
Or for a teardrop
For the way
You are today
In a time when things are
going wrong
In a time when it's okay
We know it's never easy
When a loved one is away
We're here to help you
understand
"We're with you all the
way,"
We're with you . . .
BMH *Catalyst*,
1985 July-August

Jackie Wylie's favorite patient-care unit provided a healing environment that epitomized the slogan, "We're with you all the way." Hall 4 exuded comfort, first with its warm staff attitude that welcomed families and friends at any time of day or night. It was common to see families snuggled in all corners of the large living room area when arriving on the unit at 6:30 A.M. A kitchen was available for families to bring special foods to sharc with their hospitalized family member and a scream room behind two doors if grieving needed release.

The Kalamazoo Hospitality House opened to care for families of critically ill patients at Bronson and Borgess hospitals. Sponsored by the Kalamazoo Junior League, the house opened on South Street with lodging free of charge.[33]

Caring Committee and Employee Well-being

Meeting for the second year, the 1980 Caring Committee's goal was to improve relationships and job satisfaction among staff. Edith Leppke, RN, MA, Bronson home care coordinator and a School of Nursing instructor during the seventies, was its first chair. Randy Ailes from the Medical Social Work Department succeeded her in 1980. Sponsored events included a motivational seminar, presented by Karen Kaiser Clark, called "Growing Together," the committee's theme.[34]

"Choose Health" became the 1983 theme offering a "series of health and wellness programs" for personnel. Lorraine Schneidenbach, School of Nursing instructor, who chaired the committee, said, "There is so much expertise within the hospital in so many health-related areas. We are encouraging personnel to take advantage of this expertise to lead a more healthy lifestyle."[35] Health was hard to sell and didn't come out of a pill bottle. Even in the School of Nursing, health promotion was harder to sell than disease management for patients. Helping other people to change their lifestyles was easier than changing oneself.

"Stress is always a direct response to a stressor, and it is necessary to first identify the stressor before being able to effectively cope with it."[36] Gloria Meert, RN, MA, nurse-patient/relations coordinator, directly counseled nurses and other personnel seeking assistance. She provided educational sessions to enhance interpersonal skills through the identification and management of stress. Introduced self-awareness techniques helped employees recognize their preferred styles of communication and discover how they might change with exposure to activities such as assertiveness training. Group sessions offered listening and empathizing opportunities, again to raise consciousness levels. Was the service successful? There were benefits, but the underlying causes of nurse stressors often related to the system itself and required long-term efforts to address needed system changes. The process wasn't going to be easy and Meert was often frustrated that her proposals to administration did not fit its traditional way of operating.

Meanwhile, construction of a $2.2 million center began in 1983 on the old Sears and Roebuck department store at 150 East Crosstown, which included sufficient parking space for easy entry and egress.[37] The original plan was to build an "11,200 square-foot structure . . . on land owned by the hospital at Dutton and Jasper streets, south of the hospital. . . ."[38]

HISTORICAL CHANGES

Layoffs

Layoffs came to the 2,845-member work force in January, 1985, the first time in the hospital's 85-year history! Based on seniority within job classifications across several departments, 260 employees got the word that they were no longer needed, including 23 RNs and 37 LPNs. Blame for the layoffs included the new prospective payment system, increased emphasis on outpatient services, shorter length-of-stay, and less hospitalization benefits offered in industrial Michigan and the nation which ultimately decreased the in-house patient census.[39] For the first time in eight decades, nursing students weren't assured of a job upon graduation. Employees "let go" had the benefit of outplacement counseling.

Employee opinion surveys in 1986 were used to address morale. The outcome was the establishment of a Response Committee and Action Commitment Teams (ACTs) of 8–12 employee volunteers. One result was the hiring of 251 employees; 87 were nursing personnel.[40]

Bronson was the fourth largest Kalamazoo employer in 1988, with 2,825 employees, just 20 short of where the organization was in 1985 after the layoffs.[41]

Shortening Patient Lengths-of-stay

Free-standing Ambulatory Surgery Center

As a cost containment measure for patients having minor surgery, outpatient surgery expanded and fewer patients were admitted to BMH. Patients were discharged "sicker and quicker." Most patients liked the quicker part, but could their families and friends be informed in their postoperative treatment to recognize impending complications? Discharge instructions were meant to meet an educational need for patients and their families who went home immediately after a brief stay in the recovery room. Not all patients had family for support, however. Their anxieties were evident, as were those of staff, when taxis were called for transportation home. Social workers helped make postoperative care arrangements to ensure patient safety.

Short-stay Options for Birthing

Choices provided parents (without delivery or birthing complications for either mom or baby) the opportunity to go home within 24, 36, or 48 hours at reduced prices, whereas patients in the past had stayed four to five days. The new time frames fit the growing Family-Centered Maternity Care Program's response to patient requests according to Crista Hull, RN '74, assistant vice president of perinatal services. Reduced length-of-stay meant advantageous available bed space and cost reductions to patients and/or their insurance carrier and to the hospital. Nurses called families' homes after patient discharge to assess the convalescent's condition and make recommendations for further care if deemed necessary.[42]

Development of Trauma-emergency Specialties

The work of the seventies paid off. "In 1981 the State of Michigan designated Bronson as the region's trauma center,"[43] a short-lived glory because the state designation system soon was discontinued due to lack of funds. To gain that status Bronson had opened several services in the preceding decade: a burn center in 1970, pediatric intensive care in 1972, nurse education in 1978, and continuing education programs in 1979 for pre-hospital trauma personnel such as paramedics, as well as provided sponsorship for the first annual day-long seminar for Michigan trauma professionals.

A trauma-emergency nursing course offered another advanced education resource in 1981. That was followed by a second program in 1983, "The Nurse As Part of the Trauma Team."

Express Care was the cost-effective answer for treating minor emergencies that would ordinarily be treated in the physician's office, if the patient had a primary-care physician and if the emergency occurred during daytime hours.

The expansion of trauma services continued in 1985 with the region's first aero-medical transport service (the Bronson helicopter) and an inpatient unit dedicated to trauma patients. Two years later a full-time medical director supervised Bronson's trauma services, and the state granted approval for the building of the largest trauma and emergency center in southwest Michigan.[44] Quicker entry into trauma services was an argument for long-term cost savings because fewer patients would develop complications, which would decrease overall hospital days. "When moments count most, CareFlite will help ensure quicker access . . . to specialized care," said Russell Kneen, Bronson Healthcare Group president.[45] CareFlite, Inc., complemented the expanding trauma services, bringing critically ill or injured people to Bronson from rural southwest Michigan and northern Indiana. One of the first flight nurses was Wendy Finsterwald '76, though flight nursing was never integrated into the School of Nursing curriculum. Medical drama won again over the cost-effective measures of accident prevention and a focus on self-care and self-health management. Self-care models apparently didn't impact the bottom line positively.

A new $3.5 million trauma center with 15,000 square feet opened in 1989. In 1987 the hospital had projected a census of 38,000 patients by 1989, so more room was needed. Nurse Director Sally Berglin said that the center was, " . . . designed to complement Bronson's role as regional trauma, burn, pediatric critical care and perinatal centers."[46]

Finding Quality of Life While Living with Chronic Disease

Rheumatology Coordinator Joyce Cutler, RN, praised team efforts in caring for people with arthritis and the support that patients gave each other through being together in one unit, learning exercises and joint protection skills. Team members included nurses, a social worker, a physical therapist and physician.[47]

Diabetes education at Bronson, " . . . provided access to a nurse specialist, a clinical pharmacist, a therapeutic dietician [and] social worker [who offered] private consultations, counseling and group discussions."[48]

Hemodialysis Unit

Patient inclusion and self-care became part of the teamwork evoked during patient-care conferences in the successful treatment of end-stage renal disease that required a well-informed patient and family, dietician, social worker, nurse and physician who knew their clients well. Treatments two to three times weekly in the hemodialysis unit provided relational and monitoring opportunities. The dietician was necessary since daily water and food intake made a tremendous difference in the success of the patient's control of toxic body waste not easily eliminated with kidney failure. One of the goals was to normalize life and find quality according to the patient's perspective.[49] After five years in the oldest part of the hospital (Wesley Hall), a new ten-station unit, projected to cost $507,000, was constructed in the Bronson Crosstown Center.[50]

Gerontology Center

The Gerontology Center opened in 1987 to help manage the care of older adults who were living with three to four chronic health problems and were thus more apt to be hospitalized for longer lengths of stay. The center focused on how to best maintain functionality. It provided, " . . . five main services: GoldenCare Plus, a counseling and benefits program [started in 1984]; a Community Division offering self-health management clinics [started by the BMH School of Nursing]; an Inservice Division [to improve care during hospitalization]; Geriatric Services [with Dr. Lee Russcher and] . . . a Research Division [under Dr. Russcher's supervision]."

The manager of the center was Rosalind Proos, RN, who shared responsibility for the development and coordination of the service with Dr. Russcher.[51] Proos had been a faculty member in the School of Nursing prior to this appointment. It was a natural process for the School of Nursing to turn over its self-health management clinics for development within the center.

An advertisement in the *Kalamazoo Gazette,* September 9, 1987, offered, "Bronson's Homecoming Program for Seniors," to decrease hospital days. "After you leave Bronson, we don't just send best wishes, we send a nurse." The service was provided in partnership with the Visiting Nurse Association of Southwest Michigan.

Purchase agreements for three nursing homes in the spring of 1987 were considered a way to move people who needed longer recovery periods into less expensive settings: Brookhaven Care Facility on Olmstead Road with 50 beds; Plainwell's Bridgewood Manor, 124 beds; and, Arboridge Manor, 93 beds in Galesburg.[52] Eventually Arboridge became a separate corporation within the Bronson family of companies, Brookhaven was sold to the Kalamazoo Probation Enhancement Center, and the purchase of Bridgewood Manor never materialized.

An $18.9 million upscale retirement village was planned north of Maple Hill Mall to be a part of Bronson Properties Corporation of BHG. At its ground-breaking in April 1988, Russell Kneen said, "We want people to be able to live independent lives with a sense of security. Fifty jobs would be created by the project." [53] Its name was Bronson Place.

Open Heart Surgery

It was deemed necessary for Bronson to expand the cardiology service that it began in 1956 since 43 percent of Bronson patients had cardiac disease as one of their medical diagnoses.[54] As a tertiary care center, Bronson needed to respond to diagnostic results of cardiac patients with the ability to perform open-heart surgery, which was becoming commonplace. Bronson was able to gain approval for what had become a standard, specialty practice.

Hyperbaric Chamber

Treatment of carbon monoxide poisoning and some infections required pressurized oxygen for effective results. A chamber to support this approach was another technological addition, costing $150 per treatment.[55] The Great Lakes Institute of Hyperbaric and Diving Medicine was established a year later under the direction of physicians Dircks and Grambau, who had first directed the addition of the West Michigan Hyperbaric Unit at Bronson.[56]

Radiation Therapy

Approval was given by the Southwest Michigan Health Coordinating Council for "Bronson's request to spend $2.7 million on the [therapeutic] center and a linear accelerator. . . ."[57] Treatment of cancers continuously improved with new radiation technology. The *Catalyst* reported that an application had been filed with the Health Systems agency to purchase a Magnetic Resonance Imagery (MRI). MRI was considered to be the "greatest breakthrough since the discovery of the X-ray." It was projected to be operational by 1985 and would be housed in a facility separate from Bronson and Borgess.[58]

Women's Health

A breast screening clinic opened and more women learned to do their own exams, a great example of self-health management based on outcomes. Women found 75 percent of the variations from normal breast tissue on self-examination. Access to early detection saved lives from breast cancer, a leading cause of death in women, and readily available mammograms could detect lumps too small to be palpated by the woman.[59] Post-mastectomy support groups proved to be a service that saved women's lives. Those who participated in support groups survived longer than those who did not.

Pain Control

Patient-controlled analgesia (PCA), piloted at Bronson in 1986, was an incredibly powerful message of what was yet to come. Hospitalized patients were able to push a button to deliver a small dose of pain medication delivered from a computerized intravenous pump. Patients managed their own pain effectively and actually used less medication when they controlled its release. Recovery was even quicker.[60]

HEALTH EDUCATION AS A LONG-TERM, INEXPENSIVE INTERVENTION

Construction began on the Donald S. and Genevieve U. Gilmore Center for Health Education in 1981 and was completed in 1983. Built south of and adjacent to Truesdale Hall, with a tunnel extension from the hospital, it took a swatch out of the original recreation room. Tom Jenkins, director of educational services, noted that seven hundred students from diverse disciplines were mentored annually at Bronson. In addition to student practice, continuing education programming kept clinical staff updated with current practice.[61,62, 63]

The Bronson Institute for Health Education formalized, "continuing education services for physicians, nurses and other healthcare professionals [and was] housed in the Bronson Gilmore Center for Health Education."[64]

The Health Sciences Library at Bronson played a role in that education. It had been open to the public for years but was used mostly by health professionals. "We're in the business of information," said Jeanne Hartenstein, Director.[65] A *Gazette* article made it clear that an informed public was within Bronson's service goals and, with computers and connection to the National Library of Medicine and other databases, information was available. A public focus became more apparent in 1987 with a library extension called Health Answers that invited the public to stop in or call. "We help people become intelligent, informed patients," said Hartenstein.[66]

> "Your system can benefit from ours," was the slogan used at the time, "*Health Science,"* a new [*Kalamazoo Gazette*] . . . quarterly publication . . . full of tips for disease prevention, nutrition, fitness and other topics," was introduced by Bronson, " . . . Kalamazoo's leader in health education and information." [67]

Client-substitutes

A growing trend in nursing education was the use of client-substitutes. They were local families and friends who partnered with first-year students for practice and demonstration of how to complete basic health assessments and use communication skills fundamental to a broadened perspective of nursing care.

Search for client-substitutes led beyond the acute-care setting and promoted the development of several practice opportunities. Director Jackie Wylie and School of Nursing faculty had the vision and enthusiasm to support the development of diverse nursing practice opportunities. They made efforts to balance learning about clients in acute-care medical settings with caring for clients who were managing self-care or chronic health issues in the wider community,

Self-Health Management Clinics

The BMH School of Nursing's Curriculum Committee was responsive to Russell Kneen's words—creative practices were required to meet the changing healthcare needs of the community. One solution was the establishment of community clinics for family access to healthcare professionals on the Western Michigan University campus; a second was self-health management clinics for older adults at several Kalamazoo congregate meal sites. Both services were offered free of charge as a way to engage Bronson students and faculty with functional families and adults in the community and, in a way, meet a soft marketing goal of the hospital. The public had this opportunity to meet Bronson nurses and students. Would this influence their choice if or when they faced hospitalization? Patients often went to the hospital of their physician's choice, although newspaper ads encouraged their readers to become involved in that choice.

Barb Groh, instructor, designed and managed "portable" self-health management clinics that were transported to older adult residences, senior centers, and congregate meal sites.

The Self-Health Management (SHM) Clinics emerged from several trends. At the time, healthcare was mostly defined as medical acute care and hospital-driven. Winds of change, however, were blowing with concerns about rising costs, increasing technology, and complexity, as well as with an expanding aging population. Faculty recognized the need for nursing practice grounded in whole-person perspectives, with physical and social assessment skills in addition to traditional nursing competencies.

Community Involvement

The School of Nursing was known for "breaking out" in the eighties, piloting programs that encouraged nursing students to explore aspects of their own self-care before delving into the health of the community with its soft-marketing connections to Bronson if and when hospitalization was needed. The new word was partnerships between patients and healthcare providers.

This movement toward whole-person caring and enhanced assessment was demonstrated in many ways. One of the most obvious was the school's shift from caps and capes to nursing bags. Navy canvas bags, embroidered with BSoN, became part of the school uniform. Bronson students were well equipped with basic assessment tools including stethoscopes, sphygmomanometers, otoscopes, scales and Bates' *Physical Assessment* (textbook and video tapes).

Holistic health was a concept gaining acceptance among consumers. The school applied the term to mean attention to the whole person. Many faculty hours planned students' chances to learn holistic approaches to nursing care.

The Bronson curriculum introduced, "Family in the Community," a senior level course. Wellness and holistic-care concepts led to self-care promotion as a way for students to practice patient teaching. Wellness fairs were the venue for service delivery, first with educational posters, mini-sessions and handouts to the school's own students, then with those at elementary and high schools, and at places where elderly or disabled people gathered, beginning in the hospital's own "hood" at Skyrise Apartments, west of John Street on the corner of Burdick and Walnut streets. This urban housing facility was subsidized for disabled and elderly residents and gave nursing students and faculty access to clients living with chronic health problems at a location convenient to students who lived at Truesdale Hall.

These community-involvement roots took hold, as the Medicare system moved from cost-based reimbursement to DRG driven, capped arrangements for payment of services. As a result, senior citizens became more interested in self-care and health management. These older adults were willing patients and became School of Nursing clients in the process. At an advocacy event for elders, standing-room-only seniors wanted to know how to talk to their doctors and secure the treatment they needed with the resources they had. This progression led to a partnering between Senior Services, Inc. (SSI) Friendship Centers (congregate meal sites) and the BMH School of Nursing to provide Self-Health Management Clinics.

Ann Thoms, director of SSI Friendship Centers, offered a place for the SHM Clinics to operate prior to and after meals were served. Bronson faculty members Mary Mason, Sondra Crow and Barb Groh created a place in the school's curriculum so that, during a second-level, medical-surgical course, students could select two of three placements: at the nursing home, in surgery and/or with a SHM Clinic. It took some time for faculty and students to be reassured that all learning experiences didn't need to be the same and that course objectives could be met in a variety of ways. The ease with which students selected between the three choices reflected the diversity of learning, practice, and population preferences among the students.

These SHM Clinics grew to be very popular with the older adults. By the mid 1980s the SHM Clinics had a client base of about 2,500. Clinics were held weekly, bi-weekly or monthly for two to three hours at twelve sites. Two to four students and RN faculty carried files of client records, as well as assessment and teaching equipment to them. Clients participated in SHM Clinics at the Mount Zion Baptist Church, Comstock Senior Center, Milham Meadows, and Washington Square and Evergreen North Senior Services meal sites, as well as at the Rickman House on Burdick Street, Skyrise Apartments, Crossroads Mall, and Bronson Methodist

Hospital's lobby. Services offered included the monitoring of health indicators, consulting and coaching about best ways to manage chronicity, and identifying resources available. The nurses kept client records and also provided clients with tools for their own record keeping, as well as provided support for assertive discussion with their other providers.

Clients and students learned vigorously from each other. A sit-on scale was used for clients who couldn't stand to be weighed. One of these clients was a wonderful 260+-pound woman who came weekly to be weighed and have her BP checked. Each week she wondered why her weight did not go down since she ate like a bird—only one potato chip at a time.

Clients helped students discover that nutrition teachings at the Rickman House needed to focus on—not low sodium or low cholesterol—but balanced, dumpster diets. Students found out from a 70-year-old woman who had life-long diabetes about re-using disposable needles because, "you don't want to waste them after only one time." She was able to demonstrate stellar aseptic technique by pulling her skirt over her knee to prove her thigh injection sites were every bit as healthy as the nurse's choice of injection sites. The very next week a nursing research report was unearthed that described the re-using of disposable needles with correct technique as safe and effective!

Students and their clients came to value the time to meet and focus on communication, consultation and caring about health concerns. Hundreds of hard-of-hearing clients helped novice students to speak up, maintain eye contact, and start with open-ended questions in managing their assessment interviews. Queues of waiting clients assisted students in conducting focused, time-managed interviews and assessments. Perspectives about aging, resourcing, chronicity, reality-based health management, and humor grounded the nursing practice of those who participated in the clinics.

The SHM Clinics eventually acquired two part-time RNs to manage and maintain them. In the late eighties, responsibility for the clinics transferred to Bronson's Golden CarePlus and Older Adult Service Line. Over the years, several spin-offs based on SHM principles and values occurred: Foot Care Clinics; participation with Yesterday's Youth in Today's World, a Self-Health Management Community Access TV series; and functional health assessments in the Kalamazoo Probation Enhancement Program (K-PEP). The K-PEP clinics continue in 2005, managed by United Nursing Service RNs at sites in Kalamazoo, Battle Creek, Benton Harbor, and Muskegon.

Thanks came in multiple forms including stories like these. One client who shared her nightmare fear about vivid red blood, scissors and a pig, came a week later thanking the nurse and student for helping her remember to schedule her annual cardiac check-up for her pig-heart valve replacement. Well after the end of a clinic, the nurse and student waited for a caseworker to see an elderly gentleman who was just, "going to end it with his WWI revolver." A thank you note from him two weeks later informed them that he was alive and well.

AGING

As I sit with 26 years behind me,
I look to you.
Your skin is quite wrinkled,
will I soon be too?
Your hands are arthritic,
your legs just won't hold...
Tell me, will I be that way
when I finally grow old?
Your activity is limited
but your medicines are not.
Do you think I'll be that bad?
Oh God, I hope not!

Then I talk and I listen
to things that you say,
And your experiences lessen
my fears in a way.
You laugh and remember
how things used to be
You accept what life offers
and like me for me!
I discover your shell
is fastly decaying,
But the inside's alive if I hear
what you're "saying."

As I walk to the car
at the end of the day,
I turn the ignition
in the usual way.
I glance at the building that
shelters the old
And lock away all the words
that you told.
And when I'm fifty
I hope I remember you,
And all the bouts
of life you survived through.
As the years go by, many things
I'll engage in,
But the final step will be
of a natural aging.

Kathy Shinn '83
February 23, 1982

Older adult care became a curriculum focus, with Lorraine Schneidenbach and Phyllis Curtis teaching students about aging as a developmental process and experientially with the "Aging Game".

FAMILY NURSING CENTER AT WMU

The Family Housing Nursing Center (FHNC) developed as a senior-level clinical experience to enhance the pediatric course at Bronson's School of Nursing. The downward trend of pediatric admissions to hospitals, coupled with an awareness of unmet needs of children in the community, prompted its development. Another important impetus was a desire by the faculty to practice from a nursing, rather than a medical, model. FHNC began at Western Michigan University in 1985, through the hands-on efforts of BMH School of Nursing faculty Carol Van Antwerp and Anna Mae Spaniolo, and offered nursing students the opportunity to gain some understanding of cultural differences and skill building in cultural competency.

In June, 1985, VanAntwerp and Spaniolo contacted the nurse educator at the WMU Health Center to propose a nursing clinic in the WMU Campus Apartments for families. Among other reasons for the proposal, nursing students at BMH School of Nursing needed experience with nurse-managed ambulatory care for families with children. Additionally, at that time, no organized healthcare services existed for the children in the Campus Apartments where the largest concentration of students with children was located. According to a survey done by WMU Campus Apartment staff in February, 1985, 142 children age 5 and under, 66 U.S. citizens, 44 Malaysian, 23 Middle Eastern, and 9 Nigerian lived in these apartments. Faculty believed that the international families would especially benefit from such a nursing clinic because of the barriers such as language, transportation, insurance, and unfamiliarity with local healthcare services. All these factors limited access to care.

Representatives from the University Health Center, Campus Apartment Office, Office of International Student Services, and BMH School of Nursing formed a Steering Committee which met that summer to develop a cooperative pilot project for a nursing clinic. Bronson Methodist Hospital and its School of Nursing, as well as the three WMU offices, provided administrative support.

The Steering Committee met periodically throughout the year to assess and evaluate the project. It promoted the development of protocols for referrals and acquisition of teaching materials from drug companies and hospital sources. Bronson pediatric faculty wrote articles for the *Campus Apartment Newsletter* that focused on health concerns, *i.e.,* preventing frostbite, promoting school readiness, managing bee stings, and so forth. The FHNC opened on September 10, 1985, and was open every Tuesday afternoon except during holiday and student breaks. The Steering Committee enthusiastically agreed to support continuation of the project through 1986–87.

WMU developed and marketed a brochure, which outlined hours of operation, address, phone number, and a description of the free services. This brochure stated:

> This is a nursing service provided by the BMH School of Nursing to help families with children meet their own health needs and goals, based on the belief that families are responsible for controlling their own care. The service is open to WMU student families and offers:
>
> - W.I.C. recertification assessments
> - Denver Developmental screening for children up to 6 years of age
> - Monitoring of children's height, weight, and head circumference
> - Vision and hearing screening
> - Blood pressure check
> - Ear exams and follow-up for suspected ear infections
> - Guidance on a variety of issues parents may wish to discuss, including nutritional needs of the infant and toddler, healthcare options in the Kalamazoo area, managing minor health care problems such as the common cold, discipline, and toilet training

- No appointments necessary.

During one academic year, the services of three pediatricians were paid for by WMU; the physicians would rotate one morning a week to see sick and well children. The addition of the pediatricians allowed the nurses to offer immunizations through a relationship with the county health department. The pediatricians were under-utilized, however, and their contract was not renewed the following year. Nurses continued to give immunizations as well as the services described.

The FHNC enriched the experiences of students and was rewarding to the faculty who developed the service, Anna Mae Spaniolo and Carol Van Antwerp. They treasured the time spent with Steering Committee members Christine Zimmer, RN, Jolene Jackson, Bob Sprick and Janey Lutzka. The BMH School of Nursing faculty were gratified by the experiences students had and appreciated the opportunities to learn from the clients who utilized the service. The Nursing Center closed in 1991, following the untimely death of Spaniolo and Van Antwerp's resignation from the School of Nursing. Van Antwerp left Kalamazoo upon acceptance into a post-Master's program at Emory University in Atlanta, Georgia. In December, 1991, she completed requirements to become a pediatric nurse practitioner. Appendix B includes examples of their publications and honors bestowed upon these two innovative nurses who were distinguished members of the faculty.

Pediatric Nursing Teaching Projects

Education had always been an important pediatric nursing intervention that Van Antwerp and Spaniolo instructed students to pursue. Students were expected to demonstrate their competency teaching children, having only practiced with adults in past courses. A good teaching project connected the patient with a helpful lesson. Lori Vining, '84, designed a children's coloring book, *Tami Turtle Goes to Bronson*

Methodist Hospital. It included a maze meant to help a child find his or her way around the hospital. It used characters depicting patients, nurses, physicians, and several of the departments that a child might visit as part of his or her hospital experience. Well children often were provided with friendly tours of the hospital to reduce anxiety should future hospitalization be needed. The coloring book was also distributed at the Bronson Young People's Health Fair, an annual event in Bronson Park.[68]

BMH SCHOOL OF NURSING RESPONDS TO CHANGE

Nontraditional students[69] became commonplace in the eighties, so much so that they shaped a new tradition. For years students had been admitted once a year in the fall. To wait a year, if one was ready to start school, seemed a waste of time and resources for the students and their future employers. It was time to respond to students with diverse lifestyles and needs. Why not pilot an admission process and flexible curriculum structure within the confines of development progression? Faculty adapted courses to respond and students were successful.

By the eighties the computer age reached Bronson and nursing moved into computerized record keeping. The School of Nursing became the first department to obtain word processors, given the support of Harriet Perdue, Administrative Assistant to Mr. Finch, and a newly employed, computer-literate, business education major, Linda Ickes. Next came Linda Thede, a graduate-prepared nurse with a passion for the integration of computers into nursing. With funding available, a small computer lab was built under Thede's direction.

The Nursing Arts Laboratory was extensively remodeled to include state-of-the-art equipment. Hospital supplies were readily available from the hospital's Central Supply, while educational models and teaching aids were selected by faculty and ordered directly through the hospital's Purchasing Department. The new laboratory was dedicated with rhyme written by faculty member Anne Orr in honor of her colleague, Dorothy Patow Dunn '48, who made learning fundamentals of Nursing Arts a warm and caring experience in itself.

Tribute to D. Dunn's Courage During the Remodeling of the Nursing Arts Laboratory

There once was a lady
 named Dunn
Who ran a lab that was lots of fun
But one day it was gone
And then came the dawn
When poor Dottie was on the run!

Upstairs and downstairs
 and hither and yon
She hustled and bustled
 and pushed bravely on
Such grief finding beds!
She had, it's been said
Barely time to go to the john!

JCIC and BCIU and Wesley Hall
 and Harding, too
And to far parts unknown
With barely a groan
Dorothy daily got a new view.

But at last she no more does roam
 And so comes the end
 of this poem
The lab is complete
And that's no small feat!
So we say, "Dottie,
 happy new home."

Anne Orr
BMH School of Nursing

JAN DeVRIES WALCOTT '80

My greatest joy came after I completed nursing school. It was the feeling of accomplishment that followed graduation. I knew that I could become clinically proficient at procedures like starting an IV, inserting a catheter or nasogastric (NG) tube or changing a dressing. I remember starting my first IV on a patient on Hall 7—a butterfly-heparin lock for a gentleman having a cardiac catheterization. I got into his vein on the first poke and flushed and taped it in place as if I'd done a million of the procedures. My critical care instructor was quite intuitive because, as soon as we sedately left the room, she showed her true feelings by giving me a big bear hug! Better yet, I knew how to look at each patient as an individual and give him or her care by establishing a relationship first through dialogue, maybe laughing or crying but always by listening!

Becoming part of another community for three years was a very broadening experience for me. Kalamazoo was the first town I learned to navigate on my own! I remember how thrilled I was after living in Kalamazoo for awhile when someone asked me for directions, and I could correctly direct the person to where he or she was headed.

After years of existence as an only child, the atmosphere of Truesdale Hall was truly exhilarating. Socialization! Cooking wasn't allowed in our dorm rooms. For a treat, my roommate and I grilled burgers on a hibachi in the back courtyard for supper one night. A Truesdale "official" knocked at our door and accused us of using the barbecue indoors—at least that time we were not guilty.

When a physiology test was postponed after the big blizzard of 1977, we went traying (using cafeteria trays instead of sleds) down the hill outside of Truesdale Hall. We walked down the middle of Crosstown Parkway to the Jewel store to purchase and enjoy non-cafeteria food during the time we were "snowed-in."

After having had chili for supper the night before, I taped two kidney beans to my Med-Surg renal unit test and drew a diagram of the ureters, bladder, *etc.,* for extra credit. I earned no extra credit for my effort, but Lorraine Schneidenbach's subsequent students heard this story for years to come.

I appreciated the mentoring of Bronson faculty at the time and still do. Students were encouraged (or downright nagged) to continue their education. It has been important for me to keep current in my specialty area whether completing my bachelor's degree or maintaining certification in my area of practice. At Bronson's School of Nursing, I learned that a nurse's education is never over.

I believe our class was the first not to have every new graduate hired who wanted a job at Bronson. The age of DRGs was upon us!

[Walcott continued her education to receive a master's degree in gerontology. After passing her board exam, she became a west Michigan geriatric nurse practitioner (GNP) in 2000. More recent comments about her practice[70] indicated that her practice was:]

> . . . going well. I need to increase my productivity but there's no pressure . . . yet. (Oh yes, there is my own internal pressure to diagnose fast and right.) The patients are marvelous and I have experienced no resistance when folks are scheduled to see me rather than the doc. This was a most pleasure surprise! Friends who worked in long-term care had more difficulty with patients accepting them during visits instead of the doctor. The learning curve is steep but I'm getting there.

I purchased and read *From Silence to Voice*. I found to my horror that when patients thanked me for my thoroughness or for suggesting an effective intervention, I tended to reply self-deprecatingly, "Oh it was nothing," or "It was no big deal." After reading the book, I have trained myself to reply, "That's what nurses do." A small thing, but every little bit helps! [Walcott's confidence gain is visible in her 2004 story:]

> Hopefully, this story will make you smile the next time you feel physician rage: Last Friday a woman who lives in the retirement community where my partner and I see patients came in to see me rather sheepishly. She said the facility's Christmas brunch/buffet was Sunday and the tray on her twelve-year-old walker was broken; no tray meant no way to carry plates from the buffet to her table. For a seasoned GNP this was a one-phone-call finagle. It took about six minutes before a van from the durable medical equipment provider was dispatched with a loaner (which we later found would be permanent since Medicare coverage applied, given the age of her original walker). My patient was so grateful she went on and on as she left saying, "I'm sure glad I saw you today instead of the doctor. He never would have been able to manage this so fast" . . . as the aforementioned physician stood in the doorway of his adjacent exam room! Reimbursement for the office visit, non-existent; the look on his face, priceless!

CAROLYN VESTAL '82: A HEYL SCHOLAR STORY

Carolyn Vestal was a 1962 Loy Norrix High School graduate who was tired of being poor. "I was determined to make something of myself!" Nursing education, though coming 20 years post-high school, was a natural choice. At 19, she was called home from Chicago to be at her mom's bedside. Earlier she had been her mother's caregiver during a three-month terminal illness. When her mom died, she made all of the funeral arrangements, as her father was not the one who managed the family affairs. Her mother had been the home manager and the one who paid the bills.

Though estranged from her father, she had promised her mother that she would care for him. She kept the promise, and when he became ill, cared for him 24 hours a day until his death in 1978, making the best of a challenging relationship. A small inheritance allowed her to consider the possibility of pursuing a program of study and she chose nursing. Her husband supported her decision.

Carolyn's previous paid experience had included 16 years as a dental assistant with on-the-job training at Henry Ford Hospital in the oral surgery department, a preadmissions and scheduling clerk position at Borgess Medical Center, and a deputy sheriff job with Kalamazoo County that was definitely not her "cup of tea." Also, Carolyn had accumulated science credits from Kalamazoo Valley Community College. A Bronson graduate and faculty member, Marilyn Luther, influenced her to attend Bronson. Luther, Vestal, and their husbands were friends, connected by previous employment.

So, in 1979, she applied to nursing school. The BMH School of Nursing's admissions' staff had informed Vestal of scholarship possibilities and encouraged her to follow through and apply.

She became the recipient of a Heyl Scholarship. Not only was it, "a nice surprise" but a wonderful gift. Along with her small inheritance the scholarship gave her the privilege of focusing on her education without the stress of financial need. She remembered attending a Heyl function at Kalamazoo College with other Heyl scholars. The event included dinner and a scientific lecturer whose talk was "indecipherable":

> I was with the blue blazer folks and felt out of place until I met another Bronson candidate, Kelly Walton, and her parents who were about my age. We bonded immediately and that relationship gave me the courage to make it through the evening and continue on.

Carolyn was considered a "nontraditional" student since she had been in the work force for 20 years before applying to Bronson. Through the eighties, nontraditional students became traditional as people began to choose second careers more frequently. She remarked, "It was all a blessing from God. All I had to do was show up and do the work."

KELLY ROWEKAMP '83

Choosing a nursing career no longer meant putting aside past passions. Kelly Jo Rowekamp, a high school softball athlete, was a "two-way winner," meeting the challenges of both nursing school and a softball tournament. In her second year at Bronson, she led her team by pitching the winning National Senior Division Championship game of the Miss America Softball Organization in Tampa, Florida! Rowekamp was a Heyl Scholar. She said, "My summer hands-on experience in the float pool[71] was the best learning experience of all. My participation in the operating room has given me a new goal. I'd like to become a surgical specialist."[72]

CHERYL LYNN HILLA '83

I have life-changing memories from Bronson's School of Nursing since I was challenged in every area of my life. I am thankful for the lessons I learned.

My greatest fear in nursing school was the fear of failure. After my first semester, I decided that I would quit because I could never be smart enough to be a nurse. This was not a result of my grades . . . I was doing excellent academically. But it was my lack of self-confidence that left me with a constant fear of failure.

Before I left for Christmas break, I went to see Mrs. Gren (one of the Nursing 101 instructors). I shared with her my concerns, my feelings of inadequacy, and fears of failure. She listened intently. I told her I had decided to quit. I will never forget her response. She looked me straight in the eye and said, "Cheryl, you are one of my best students. I'm not concerned if you leave nursing school. I know that whatever you do, you'll be the very best at it. That is the kind of person you are!" Her words changed the course of my life. I want to thank Mrs. Gren for the positive affirmation I received. It has been a precious gift to me. I returned to nursing school and graduated.

I learned many lessons throughout my years at Bronson. The greatest lesson I learned was that I could do hard things. I now teach this to my three children.

PATRICIA FLANDERS '83

I was an older nontraditional student, who had already been a part of the work force, when I transferred to Bronson in 1982. I put high expectations upon myself, and because of this requirement, I got frustrated and was ready to drop out. My fiancé (now husband) and I talked about my decision to quit. I had a good job working in Bronson's General Surgery Department as a scrub technician. Why was I putting myself through all this stress? I called to report my absence from clinical practice on a Friday. Atypically, Lorraine Schneidenbach, my clinical instructor, called me back and I told her I was going to quit the program. She asked me to come in and I reluctantly agreed. I had made my decision, and I was going to stick to it. Lorraine, Phyllis Curtis, and I talked for two hours and we all became emotional. At the end of our conversation, I decided to stay in the program. These two women cared enough about me to help "save me" from making a very wrong decision. I have thanked them over and over in my mind and heart. I don't know how many others these two excellent nurses and educators saved from making this mistake. I do know that without their caring intervention, a dream would not have become a reality. And with that, I want to again thank Lorraine and Phyllis—Thanks!!

> Nursing is something I had always wanted to do. I remember my mom coming home from work and talking about the people she took care of, and this career sounded exciting to me as a small girl. She also attended Bronson . . . which is why I chose to go there, even though I grew up on the east side of the state. I'm not sure if she's aware of the impact that choice made in my life.
>
> My friends from Bronson are friends for life. The closeness we all shared was something unique, that I'm not sure exists now that Truesdale Hall is gone and students graduate at different times.
>
> Our class came at the end of an era, I believe, when nursing was changing in many ways . . . and Bronson certainly prepared us for that contingency. I feel my education was one of the best you can have in nursing.
>
> ***Patti Harner '83***

Now I am an educator also. I have had the opportunity to do the same with a few of my students. I like to relate my own story to them, and I have been able to convince them not to lose hope and quit.

MARIE STOLINE '84

My nursing career began with an anonymous telephone call. "Hello, Bronson School of Nursing? I'm calling to inquire about the age limit for your nursing program." "Well, let me check . . . I think you have to be at least 17." "Is there an UPPER age limit?" I asked. "I've never heard of one. Shall I send you an application?" Given that I was soon to be 41 years old, her response made my heart beat fast! It was the first of many times I experienced a rush of excitement at Bronson.

I had already graduated from the University of Iowa with a degree in sociology. Then we had nearly finished raising our family of four, when my husband and I moved to Kalamazoo where he took a job. I worked part time as a receptionist at Pleasant Pediatrics and was actively involved in volunteer activities in the community, but I just couldn't let go of my childhood dream of becoming a nurse.

Younger people may be surprised to learn that marriage used to disqualify one from attending nursing school. Student nurses were required to be single and were usually female. Later I learned that professional nurses' roots were in religious orders and military service, initiating this tradition of "dedicated singleness."

Once officially registered in the BMH School of Nursing, I was able to take microbiology at Western Michigan University. We were introduced to high quality microscopes and allowed to see real live microbes in the lab—another rush of adrenaline. When we could see the beauty and orderliness of such tiny life forms, it was further evidence of the great mysteries of creation. This "show" was better than any production on the Discovery Channel!

> My daughter, Brianne, arrived months before her due date, a preemie weighing 391 grams (14 ounces), who required hospitalization for 15 months. When she was able to go home it was with a tracheotomy and a need for extra oxygen related to her premature lung develop-ment. Brianne was the smallest survivor in the history of the Methodist Medical Center in Dallas where she was born in 1996.
>
> I'm grateful for my nursing background that allowed me to care for Brianne at home.
>
> ***Sharon Beals Cox '85***

I recall another moment of high emotion on my first day, taking care of a real patient. Oh, how afraid I was that I would do something stupid! The day before, we had each been assigned one person, and given complete background information on his or her condition, medications, and treatments. So we had plenty of time to study up on what we would need to know . . . or at least, that was the plan. We arrived with caps pinned in place, shoes polished snowy white, no fingernail polish, no perfume, and a sense of enormous responsibility on our shoulders. As a supposedly "mature" student, I was still not exempt from feeling very aware of my limitations and my concern that everything be perfect.

Our instructors were very supportive—they wanted us to succeed. They patiently answered questions, redirected our awkward efforts to deliver bedside care, and kept us keenly aware of the high standards of our vocation. We cherished every bit of the wisdom and experience they shared with us during our clinical rotations. I vividly remember how one instructor picked up a soiled sheet that had an unusual stain, still fresh and damp. She sniffed it, then brought it to us to do likewise. "Never forget that odor," she advised. "It can only be caused by a specific disease process, and we will learn more about that in an upcoming lecture." We were taught to make complete use of all our senses and every opportunity in the assessment of a patient's condition. There can be no substitute for this experiential learning process.

Just as this was a time of transformation in my life, it was a time of transition in the nursing profession. I had previously visualized myself functioning as something like a well-trained stewardess, making patients comfortable, carrying out the doctors' orders, keeping rooms tidy. I soon learned that these tasks were only a small part of my duties. Over and over, I heard the mandate:

> You must be each patient's final advocate. You must know anatomy, physiology, microbiology, pharmacology, medication management, ethics and treatments so well that—should an inappropriate order be given—you can intercede on behalf of the patient who cannot speak for him or herself.

Did that mean that we should ever question a doctor's order? "Absolutely! You are equally responsible for the well-being of those in your care. You must be knowledgeable and skilled to be part of today's healthcare team." In the work that I currently do, as a geriatric care manager, I am often a patient's final advocate. How glad I am to have that early introduction to my responsibilities.

I vividly recall an episode in surgery. I was scrubbed sufficiently to be free of infectious contaminants but had assumed that I would only be observing the procedures. Midway in the operation, the surgeon said, "I'd like the student nurse to step up here close to the table, please." I did as requested, and then—quite unexpectedly—he carefully took my gloved hand and slowly maneuvered it into the incision. "Feel that throbbing at the tip of your finger?" he asked. I nodded my silent, "Yes." "That's the patient's heart. This gives you a better sense of the anatomy than you can get from studying it in books." I was absolutely overwhelmed with the enormous impact of that moment—to be so closely involved with the life processes of a human being, to be part of a team that was changing my life for the better, to be learning how to help others in the future. I was close to tears of pure joy.

As I drove home that day, I reflected on others my age who were busying themselves by playing cards or watching TV, and I was immensely grateful that Bronson's School of Nursing did not have an upper age limit for admissions. I am still grateful all these years later. Nursing has been the keystone for a life filled with satisfying service.

MARGARET ROSE HAMBLIN MITCHELL '85

What I treasure most about attending Bronson was the kindness, patience, and willingness of the instructors to go the extra mile helping me to succeed and graduate. The years I spent at Bronson were difficult because I was being forced to grow up in a new way for which I had not been prepared. The hours I spent in the offices of Mrs. Schneidenbach, Mrs. Passero, Mrs. Curtis, Mrs. Zolp, and Mrs. Wylie, to name a few, must have been frustrating as well as exhausting for them. All of these women were very much a blessing to me.

Others I did not mention for their support to increase my chance for success will not be forgotten. That includes the day I drove 17 miles in snow up to my bumpers to the State Hospital only to find clinical practice cancelled but the instructor, Rosemarie Nedeau-Cayo, waiting for me. School had been cancelled while on my way, and just a couple of miles away in Truesdale Hall, my classmates snuggled warmly in their beds. It was nice to have the instructors' undivided attention for the day. Then there was Linda Thede. How I appreciated her matter-of-fact manner in setting me straight when I needed it.

Anne Orr, Bea Gren (I spent a lot of time seeking advice from both of them), Dorothy Dunn, Barb Groh, Marilyn Luther, Mrs. Damvelt, Mary Mason, Roz Proos, Karen Lachstadter—how blessed I am for having known you all including those I didn't mention. I am very thankful for the unselfishness of these people.

NANCY GEORGE '89

> I was a licensed practical nurse (LPN) working at Bronson when I applied to school, and I am thankful to Bronson School of Nursing because the instructors and staff looked out for the well-being of all the students. My fear level was less because of them.
>
> Bronson School of Nursing taught me that there are still caring people who are willing to take time with students, even with an older student like me.
>
> Thanks for everything.
>
> ***Gracie Harris '87***

While in the Peace Corps in Kenya I had an opportunity to work with an UNESCO researcher on a reading project for hospitalized children. While volunteering, I thought it would be interesting to work as a nurse midwife. I spoke with as many nurses as I could and they all enjoyed their jobs. I applied to three nursing schools from overseas. Two of the schools had a year's waiting period. Bronson didn't.

What I learned from nursing school was a) I didn't want to be a nurse–midwife, b) nursing education taught nurses to meet the needs of their clients, while the educational process remained rigid and often didn't meet the needs of the students, and c) nursing is ultimately a flexible profession that opens many doors.

Many of the nursing instructors and administrators influenced my values and how I wanted to practice. Those who positively influenced me helped me think beyond the here and now in meeting my own needs and the needs of my clients. Those who negatively affected me helped me see how I didn't want to practice or act. Overall, nursing has opened doors for me and let me explore new horizons.

SUSAN KAY AMMON ROBINSON '81

My mother was a Bronson graduate and from the time I was five, my determination was to be just like her. I made my decision to go to Bronson while in junior high. Living in Battle Creek, it seemed ideal geographically as well as academically. I was already convinced then that the diploma route would afford me the clinical experience necessary. From that point on, I never seriously considered a different school. By high school, I was planning each year's class schedule around the pre-reqs listed in my BMH handbook. My junior year brought the exciting news that I had been accepted into Bronson's nursing program. I took it rather nonchalantly, it simply had never occurred to me that I wouldn't be going to Bronson.

When I arrived at Truesdale Hall in the fall of 1978, my "big sister" had already prepared my room. I was completely mystified about the purpose of the tiny paper nursing cap and the paper clips attached to it. Little did I realize then how encouraging it would be to see those paper clips accumulate on the "months gone by" side.

The first few weeks were a blur of new faces, new terminology, and the mysteries of Nursing Arts Lab. I was overwhelmed at the number of different verbs that described urination and awed that my suite mate knew what an enema was.

During this time I briefly worried that I had made an error in my career choice. For all my careful preparation for nursing school, I had never obtained any practical experience such as volunteering in a hospital or nursing home. I found myself nervous about going into the hospital environment and interacting with real patients. Still, I found that I enjoyed the patients once clinical practice began. As intimidating as Tuesday nights were going up to the floor in a lab coat to pour over the chart and learn about the patient assigned before Wednesday morning, then making up med cards, starting the week's nursing care plan, and meeting the patient the next day and putting a face to the medical history never failed to put the humanity of nursing back into the clinical experience for me.

It was in my 20 weeks of med-surg and later advanced med-surg that I began to find myself professionally. As I worked in a general ICU 16 years later I could still hear the lessons that Lorraine, Phyllis, Ellie, and Felicia taught me. I especially recall Felicia teaching us in the Pediatric Acute Care Unit (PACU) to be vigilant in our assessment of unconscious patients. Because they were most vulnerable, they required our protection more than anything else. I always think about that admonition when I'm caring for an unstable neuro patient. When I can't account for an elevated intracranial pressure (ICP), I've learned to search carefully for a source of discomfort that my patient is unable to report.

> The solid nursing education that I received at Bronson School of Nursing gave me a confident and positive feeling about my career as an RN.
> ***Cindy Tokarz '81***
>
> [Cindy was a LPN who furthered her career opportunities by moving beyond the dependent practice, LPN level.]

As time went by, we sometimes found it stressful to be surrounded continually by other students who jointly ate, slept, and breathed nursing, as we shared the same studies, environment, and instructors. And yet, we had support and camaraderie because of our common experiences. You could wander down the halls of Truesdale at almost any hour and find someone's door open, the room's occupant willing to talk.

During the flurry of activity in the final weeks before graduation, it occurred to me that very soon I would be on my own, professionally and domestically. It was strange to think that I would no longer be living with the other students who had been part of my daily life for nearly three years. And it was frightening to think that very soon I would be turned loose, on my own, with no instructor to back me up. How could they send us out there before we knew everything? Well, I still haven't learned everything, but Bronson's School of Nursing gave me a good start. My staff-nurse orientation on Hall 6 taught me that wisdom. I went through orientation with a KVCC and a Nazareth grad and was on my own weeks before either of them. We had noticed in clinical how our shoes showed many more signs of wear than those of students from the other two schools. Yes, clinical experience was the backbone of Bronson's program, and I've never regretted going the diploma route.

Thanks, BMH, for preparing us for the real world. Even though many of us couldn't wait to leave, we now look back fondly on our days with you.

PATTI DELL TIBBLE '82

I entered nursing because, since I was a little girl I'd never thought of doing anything but helping people get well. I was excited and nervous at age 19 to move away from home (200 miles), but Jackie Wylie wrote me the nicest letter of encouragement and support. I admire and respect her dearly for the love she could give to a scared little girl, when she obviously had other tremendous responsibilities to handle.

The mentoring from other RNs made such an impression on me—Mrs. Gren, Mrs. Carr, and Mrs. Leonard were incredibly kind to me as I questioned and challenged everything (my "D" personality!). The love of nursing was so evident in every instructor—they truly were admired by all of us. I wish we'd been grown up enough to tell them of our esteem at the time! My other fondest memories are of the wonderful "sisters" I met while in Truesdale. Natalie Ferris and Marshe Scott became as close as family. Michele Parker saw to it that we had fun, and Laura and Rachel had the best stories to keep us laughing. Bronson, for example, had just installed new flame-orange carpeting, and we student nurses helped move patients' belongings to the new floor. One of us on duty needed to give Maalox to a patient, didn't check the lid, and shook the liquid all over that brand new carpet, christening it on the first day!

My freshman year, I was taking care of a patient with a traumatic injury who was in all kinds of traction, casts, *etc.,* and I had him as my "primary" patient for a long time. We talked so much getting to know each other that I kept forgetting to carry out all of my nursing care tasks, and the instructor wondered whether I was cut out for nursing—or was I just working on my "M.R.S." degree.

During one terrible snowstorm Natalie Ferris and I worked 18 hours straight in the baby nursery due to all the "call-ins."

I vividly remember trying to make a bed the first day, with Instructor Marilyn Luther observing my progress. I couldn't for the life of me understand why the sheets had to be so tight, and why the hospital couldn't obtain fitted sheets with elastic corners, why, why, why—poor Mrs. Luther. I feel sorry for her now, having to explain the logic of our routine so many times. Remember trying to start an enema, but forgetting to take off the end cap? Remember changing the stripes on our caps as we advanced—yes, even in the 1980s.

I spent nearly ten years in mental health nursing. When placed in a layoff position, I had the opportunity to move into OR nursing; both were my "loves" in nursing school. One of my best feelings about nursing school was of great pride, not only for going to the best diploma school in Michigan, but in our excellent experiences—long, 10-week clinicals in every area! Even today, when I tell people I had 10 weeks of clinical practice in the OR, they gasp. Now it's one or two days of observation in most schools!

I recall being quite hurt for being voted "biggest parting-pooper," but now I am proud to say I don't have the regrets others may have. It was fun learning to be grown up in that protected but unparented environment. Daisy was adamant about those doors staying locked after10:00 P.M. Another dear lady, Mrs. Dexter, was our housemother. She was kind and helpful and obtained all kinds of items for us—safety pins, stamps—just like a mom. Hugs, too.

MICHELE PARKER SANCHEZ '82

Memories at Bronson always bring a smile to my face. In my first year, I brought a kitten back to Truesdale Hall and got away with it for a week, but then Mrs. Dexter called my mom and told her that either my cat or I had to go. So, after much thought and a survey of the girls in my hall, we decided that one of the girls would take the cat home to her farm.

One of the funniest things happened when we were at WMU in Phoebe Rutherford's class. I was very, very tired, and happened to doze off. She was talking about cervical cancer and I woke up with a start, raised my hand, and asked, "Is that only in women?" The whole class of two hundred plus people laughed and I didn't know why.

The years at Truesdale making great friends were some of the most memorable. I had always wanted to be a nurse and have never regretted becoming one. I take great pride in my profession—to help people!

ALICIA WANK PASSOW '81

I was in my OB rotation and caring for a laboring mother who grabbed my uniform dress by the collar and screamed, "Get this kid out of me! NOW!!" The act and the comment would not have been so alarming except that I was pulled off balance and fell into her bed during her crazed moment. After the contraction, I was released to standing position. While shifting my uniform back in place I heard a meek voice from the bed saying, "I am so sorry." I dismissed the situation, only to have my college boyfriend repeat the story to me, as he heard it while attending church a few weeks later. During her labor, she had no recollection of what I looked like, but she was appreciative of the comprehensive care provided. I learned from that experience that people don't always remember who we are, but they do remember what we do for them. I was glad to leave a positive, lasting impression that the woman could take home with her.

Nursing and my feelings toward the profession have certainly had their ups and downs, but I will forever embrace this profession for all I have learned from it and all it has given back to me. I was sad to read that Bronson Methodist Hospital School of Nursing closed its doors, but it outlived many diploma schools. Thank you to all . . . who are keeping the Alumni Association intact. I was the president of the BSN program for California State University for a couple of years and I know how labor intensive the work of the association can be. Your efforts do not go unnoticed.

DEB RETSEMA LAUGHLIN and GAIL EBERLY MERCER '81

When we arrived at school "big" sisters had decorated bulletin boards for each incoming freshman. My board had a paper clip for each month of nursing school and caps at the month when we were due to earn them, and the narrow and wide black bands to be utilized later. We were welcomed in the evening by senior skit night and an after-dark raid. We had wisely locked our doors, but some of the freshmen were scared.

Memories of WMU included riding the "special" bus to class. All the girls would exit the bus and parade to class, and we felt like spectacles. Often we would walk home to avoid taking the bus. Plus, there was the good old "rat lab."

Clinical practice included big writing projects—case studies that included a care plan with all of the rationale for the nursing interventions stipulated for the patient. During our OB rotation we followed a mom-to-be from labor to discharge. We eagerly anticipated the call, and arrived at the Labor and Delivery Unit as quickly as we could. We cared for the mom during her labor and assisted at her delivery as well as with follow-up care. Retsema's case-study baby was born with spina bifida.

Fun times included popcorn parties. Deb Laughlin would make popcorn and a bunch of us would gather around to eat and talk. Trips to the High Wheeler for ice cream, great costumes at Halloween, secret Santas at Christmas, the half-way through training party, and the Senior Banquet were all part of our social itinerary.

During our second year of nursing school, Amy Hull spearheaded the beginning of Nurses Christian Fellowship, to meet weekly for Bible study. We focused on topics related to the spiritual care of our patients as well as for ourselves. We even sponsored a musical group to perform in Truesdale Hall, and the event was well attended. Ginny Mange was the faculty member who assisted.

Just before graduation a group called Kook and the Gang came out with a song called "Celebrate," which became our theme song. We danced on the roof to it, sang it, cranked up the sound, and just generally enjoyed the upbeat music. We made signs with a big CELEBRATE to announce graduation. It was a wonderful song to graduate with.

MICHAEL PHILLIPS '89

Michael Phillips wrote a letter, dated January 11, 1993, to Bronson's School of Nursing requesting support for a nursing school in India. A syllabus and nursing diagnoses accepted at the Fifth National Conference on Nursing Diagnoses were included in the envelope. Apparently Phillips had taken this list of nursing diagnoses and accompanying care plan examples with him on a visit to north central India in November, 1992, as a member of a work project team invited to Clara Swain Hospital in Bareilly. Phillips said, "I believe it is the only Methodist managed hospital complex in the country."

As one of three staff RNs on the visiting team, Phillips spent most of his time with the hospital staff and nursing students at the Mary V. Gordon School of Nursing on the hospital campus.

The purpose of Phillips' 1993 letter, with an accompanying prospectus for the Mary V. Gordon School of Nursing and Midwifery, was to open dialogue with Bronson's School of Nursing. In the letter, he said that he would inquire if the program director or any nursing colleagues would be interested in corresponding with Mrs. Rosie Bisht, the Indian school's principal:

> Although the school and hospital are located in a city of close to one million people, they are actually quite isolated. Material resources are scarce. Phone and fax lines are often inoperable. Electricity is intermittent and there is the frequent droning of gas-powered generators. At night the lighting is dim and the acrid scent of dung-fueled cooking fires fills the air. Outside the city are few roads and for one hundred miles in any direction are bleak and remote villages, farmland, and jungle. The nursing and medical staff are hard working and very dedicated, and the people they serve are generally very poor and do not seek attentions until they

> are gravely ill. I believe that any contact between the Bronson and Gordon schools would provide a tremendous morale boost there.

Regretfully, this relationship never materialized due to lack of follow-through on the part of Bronson's School of Nursing administration and staff. Maybe someday connecting with the Western Michigan University, Bronson School of Nursing can rectify this regret.

BMH SCHOOL OF NURSING'S EXPECTED OUTCOME—GRADUATION!

Dr. Julie Hover '63 served as chairperson for the Department of Nursing, Edgewood College (Madison, Wisconsin). She spoke on "Nursing in the World of Tomorrow," at Bronson's 76th annual commencement on April 23, 1980, in the First United Methodist Church. Her topic called for advanced nursing education that was needed to meet the care needs of future citizens. Dr. Shirley Bach, medical ethicist at Western Michigan University, gave the 1987 graduation address, "In Celebration of Human Care."

Kathy Shinn '83 reflected on student life as she came closer to graduation:

OUR LIFE

The chains are all broken,
the handcuffs removed.
No longer our "know how"
do we have to prove.

The days of instructors
and papers are through.
It's time for a vacation
that's long overdue.
We'll say our final farewell
and last goodbye.
And on graduation day
we may even cry,

But we'll always look back
on our stresses and strife
After three years at Bronson,
we've earned to live "our life."
Kathy Shinn, SN
March 22, 1982

Graduation numbers reported in *Catalyst* over the years verified that there were lower attrition rates in 1987 than in previous years, with a decade average near 70. More than half the graduates in 1982 began their professional careers at Bronson, but by 1985 graduates were concerned as to whether they would find employment when hospitals were laying off staff.

CHAPTER 9 NOTES

---

[1] *Kalamazoo Gazette*, 1985 June 20, "Reflecting, Finch says competition good."

[2] *Kalamazoo Gazette*, 1985 July 4, "Healthcare chairman sees bright future."

[3] *Kalamazoo Gazette*, 1985 July 4, "Kneen, Hospitals to survive despite gloomy forecasts."

[4] *Bronson News and Information,* 1985 October 29, "Bronson Healthcare Group names vice president for enterprise activities."

[5] *Kalamazoo Gazette*, 1986 October 2, "Kalamazoo-based health plan is growing."

[6] *Kalamazoo Gazette*, 1987 December 23, "10 from area to oversee hospital's partnership."

[7] *Kalamazoo Gazette*, 1987 May 29, "Hospital costs here 2nd highest in state."

[8] *Kalamazoo Gazette*, 1988 September 8, "Hospital merger draws applause."

[9] *Kalamazoo Gazette,* 1988 October 14, "Nurses seek a voice as hospitals discuss unity."

[10] *Catalyst*, 1983 December; 1–3. "DRGs: new payment classification system to impact healthcare at Bronson."

[11] *Catalyst*, 1980 September; 1. Elliot, P., "Thank you everyone—you did a great job!"

[12] Office of Disease Prevention and Health Promotion, Department of Health and Human Services, *Healthy People 2010.* http://www.health.gov/healthypeople

[13] *Catalyst*, 1984 December, "Nursing research at Bronson: guiding the delivery of quality patient care."

[14] *Ibid.*

---

[15] *Catalyst*, 1981 May, "Clinical specialists: providing long-range patient care."

[16] *Catalyst*, 1980, April; 4. "Legislative task force keeping BMH nurses informed."

[17] *Catalyst*, 1981 February; 7. "Nursing scholarships."

[18] *Catalyst*, 1980 April, "Nursing graduate program questionnaire."

[19] Nurse leaders believed that a local public baccalaureate education was needed more desperately than a graduate level program. However, the Nazareth College president had the support of the local president's council voting against initiating baccalaureate-level nursing education at Western Michigan University as unfair competition. Nazareth was dependent on the RN–BSN program for revenue. Only when Nazareth College closed was another program considered.

[20] *Catalyst*, 1985 May, "Perspective . . . nursing: building bridges to the future."

[21] Judy Stewart married and her name changed to Judy Hoelscher.

[22] *Kalamazoo Gazette*, 1987 November 12, "Nursing advancement week: where is nursing going? where can it take you?" (an advertisement)

[23] William Selinsky a 1975 Bronson graduate died at a young age in California, during open-heart surgery to replace his mitral valve. Selinsky became Bronson's first Medical-Surgical Clinical Nurse Specialist in 1980. His story reminds us of all the nursing aides (later called nursing technicians and later still patient-care technicians), whose warmth and caring came directly from their heart and love of their underpaid and undervalued services.

[24] *Catalyst*, 1981 August; 10. "Above and beyond the call of duty: that's Fergey."

[25] *Catalyst*, 1981 April; 10. "Adding the human touch."

[26] *Kalamazoo Gazette*, 1985 September 12, "Bronson auxiliary observes 50th anniversary."

[27] *Kalamazoo Gazette*, 1982 April 5, "New entrance opens today at Bronson."

[28] *Catalyst*, 1983 May; 9. "Locus curae validae, strong place of healing."

[29] *Kalamazoo Gazette*, 1987 May 21, "B & B: a saga of competition and cooperation."

[30] *Catalyst*, 1985, July–August, "Bronson's marketing program: aimed toward excellence."

[31] *Ibid.*

[32] *Kalamazoo Gazette*, 1987 May 20, "Impotence can tear people apart," an advertisement.

[33] *Catalyst*, 1985 March, "The Kalamazoo hospitality house: reaching those in need."

[34] *Catalyst*, 1980 January; 12. "Caring committee begins second year; growing together 1980 theme."

[35] *Catalyst*, 1983 March; back cover. "Choose health."

[36] *Catalyst*, 1984 March; 4–5, "Programs available to promote well-being of Bronson employees."

[37] Catalyst, 1983 June; 5. "Construction begins for ambulatory surgery center."

[38] *Kalamazoo Gazette*, 1982 June 17, "Bronson outpatient surgery clinic gets conditional approval from the state."

[39] *Kalamazoo Gazette*, 1985 January 23, "Bronson reduces work force by laying off 260."

[40] *Catalyst,* 1986 November, "Employee opinions prompt ACTion."

[41] *Kalamazoo Gazette,* 1988 January 1, "Top 10 employers."

[42] *Catalyst*, 1984, "Special delivery package arrives at Bronson."

[43] *Healthlines*, 2(24):1989 November 13. "The Bronson trauma system."

[44] *Ibid.*

[45] *Kalamazoo Gazette*, 1984 October 12, "Bronson Healthcare plans helicopter ambulance service."

[46] *Kalamazoo Gazette*, 1987 October 8, "Bronson trauma center plan OK'd."

[47] *Catalyst*, 1983 June; 1–4. "Rheumatology care at Bronson: a team effort.

[48] *Kalamazoo Gazette*, 1986 August 8, "Diabetes unit receives $10,000 gift."

[49] *Catalyst*, 1980 September; 3–4. "Hemodialysis unit: emphasis on individual patient, self-care."

[50] *Kalamazoo Gazette*, 1986 May 29, "Bronson projects."

[51] *Kalamazoo Gazette*, 1987 January 21, "New Bronson gerontology unit to open."

[52] *Catalyst,* 1987 March/April, "Bronson buys three nursing homes."

[53] *Kalamazoo Gazette*, 1988 April 29, "Ground broken for Bronson's retirement center."

[54] *Bronson News and Information*, 1985 May 3, "Bronson seeks cardiac surgery program."

[55] *Kalamazoo Gazette*, 1986 March 20, "Pure, pressurized oxygen overcomes infections, poisons."

[56] *Kalamazoo Gazette*, 1987 April 9, "Bronson opens center for diving-related experiments and activities."

[57] *Kalamazoo Gazette*, 1987 May 26, "Radiation therapy center endorsed for Bronson."

[58] *Catalyst,* 1984 April, "MRI: A new breakthrough in medical imaging."

[59] *Bronson News and Information,* 1985 July 3, "Bronson conducts first Kalamazoo breast disease screening clinic."

[60] *Kalamazoo Gazette*, 1986 November 22, "Patient in pain can 'order' own morphine dosage."

[61] *Kalamazoo Gazette*, 1981 February 15, "Health education center to be built at Bronson Hospital."

[62] *Kalamazoo Gazette*, 1983 June 18, "Health center named after Gilmores."

[63] *Kalamazoo Gazette*, 1983 June 18, "Bronson to dedicate new education center."

[64] *Kalamazoo Gazette*, 1987 April 16, "Bronson opens health institute."

[65] *Kalamazoo Gazette*, 1986 March 6, "Medical answers found in this library."

[66] *Kalamazoo Gazette*, 1987 April 23, "New health library can field questions."

---

[67] *Kalamazoo Gazette,* 1987 November 11, "Some health tips from Bronson."

[68] *Catalyst*, 1984 April; 11. "Bronson School of Nursing student designs children's coloring book."

[69] Students who came to nursing school after working or pursuing a different career and not directly out of high school were considered non-traditional.

[70] Walcott, J. 2002, February 1, e-mail to J. Wylie sharing a recent nurse practitioner story.

[71] The float pool was a temporary solution for an understaffed patient-care unit, providing nurses and nurse technicians to fill in the gap. Students could work as nursing technicians and find hands-on experiences that supplemented their nursing education.

[72] *Catalyst*, 1981 November; 13. "A two-way winner."

CHAPTER 10

TRANSITIONAL DECADE FOR ONE HOSPITAL-BASED SCHOOL OF NURSING, 1990s

Student stories from the 1990s speak of an environment at once similar and different from earlier decades. In the midst of downsizing and closing, students were provided with individualized attention and contracts to meet their learning needs for socialization into the nursing profession.

REFLECTIONS

Denise Heath '90

I can't believe it has been over seven years since graduation from Bronson School of Nursing! My life has changed for the better since beginning the program in 1987. Our school is gone now but not forgotten. I remember the close feeling we had with the instructors and staff. I was not a traditional student; I was married and had a child. I made the destination, even though the road was tough at times.

I can credit Carma Williamson for steering me toward a nursing career. We had gone to high school together! I ran into her at Bronson while taking courses at KVCC and WMU in computer science and business. She had graduated from

Bronson's nursing program earlier and enjoyed working there. So what do I remember?

Early clinical mornings came with feeling so unsure of myself and thinking, "What am I doing here?" The day we all hated was "IV and Injection Day." We were guinea pigs for each other, testing our poking techniques. Even our instructor didn't escape our needles. Due to an uneven number of students my partner was instructor Brad Corbin. I was so glad to insert the needle into his vein on my first try.

My fellow students and I remember the day Jessie (my son) accompanied me to finals! Day care had closed that morning, and Jessie wanted to "talk" and play during the tests. Exams that day were in the hall for Jessie and me! I also remember writing, writing and more writing.

My husband followed my footsteps and became a nurse also. He works at "that other" hospital. I plan to teach aspiring new nurses-to-be. I have found my place.

Sharon Smotherman '91

When I first started school at Bronson, what I knew about nursing was what I had personally experienced, that nurses "made beds and gave shots." During my years of schooling, I learned that nursing skills included teaching, comforting, and lots of paper work. My greatest joy in school surfaced each time I learned something new and especially when I was able to teach one of my patients, for instance, how to prevent or control high blood pressure.

Truesdale Hall was my home for all three years, and I stayed in the same room for the last two years of school. When graduation came, the other seniors had already moved. I was able to stay in the hall until I was ready to move to Nashville, Tennessee, where I had accepted a position at Vanderbilt Medical Center.

Looking back at all the roles I have played, I wonder how I kept anything straight my senior year. I was a nurse extern, resident assistant, computer lab assistant, yearbook editor, president of the Nurses Christian Fellowship and I babysat in my spare time. I still am amazed that I managed to attend class. Bronson gave me an excellent start for my nursing career.

Deborah Voikin Berkenpas '91

I have many fond memories of Bronson. My roommate, Sara Seat Boyd, and I are still close friends, even though she moved to Florida. When we get together, we often talk about our days at Bronson. We laugh about how nervous we were before giving our first bath and how we practiced "hand washing" before the test.

"Let's drop out of Bronson and go to beauty school," we said when times were stressful. On particularly stressful days in my nursing practice now, I still think, "Why didn't I go to beauty school?" But the good days far outnumber the bad and on those days I am thankful I did not drop out. Nursing is a hard profession—but I have enjoyed the challenge.

Jerri Robinson '91

My motivation to become a nurse stemmed from the compassion I have toward people. I enjoy helping people in all phases of their lives—sickness, health, joy and sorrow. I truly believe God put me here to help those in need. I also feel my true calling is to work with the elderly. Seniors have so much knowledge and wisdom that they are willing to share, and I have learned so much from them.

My greatest joy was graduation. As I looked around the church auditorium, I could see the smiling faces of my children, mother and family. I had finally completed my goal—to become a REGISTERED NURSE! My father, who passed away in February, 1981, would have been proud of me. Being the first daughter to complete a formal, postsecondary education program made my mother happy.

My greatest fear in nursing school was starting an IV on Suzie Themins in front of the entire class. What was scary was the fact that she let me try three times!

Phyllis Curtis was the most memorable person who influenced my beliefs, values and career outcomes; and she accounts for the most memorable lesson I learned at Bronson School of Nursing, always to have another RN check insulin types and doses before giving an injection. I remember when she and her family gave my children and me Christmas ornaments for our Christmas tree. I was recently divorced, and our ornaments had been discarded accidentally. I had no idea how I was going to decorate the tree for the kids. During lunch, Phyllis sat at a table with students as she often did. She heard me discussing my problem and offered to give me decorations for my tree. Not only did Phyllis give the decorations, she gave each of my children and me a gift to put under our tree. I will never forget this gesture. Although we didn't have much that Christmas, we had a beautiful tree and four neatly wrapped gifts from the Curtis family. Thanks, Phyllis!

Andrea Meeder '92

Suzie Themins was an excellent clinical instructor. She taught us so much more than clinical skills. We were encouraged to seek out learning experiences, and she (as well as other School of Nursing staff) supported our enthusiasm and helped us move past our fears.

One lesson is that nursing school doesn't teach you everything. It provides an introduction to multiple aspects of nursing—and that exposure encourages later choices and decision-making toward life-long learning after graduation. Open communication between clinical instructors and students helped us to understand that you can never know everything, so just keep learning every day. Now when I precept students, I always remind them of these lessons.

Thanks, Bronson, for such excellent starting ground! Never once have I regretted my choice. I will put my education and experience up against anyone's, and I have always been proud of my diploma. As I go forward and collect more initials behind my name, I send my heartfelt thanks for all the lessons taught and encouragement provided by Bronson faculty and staff. Everyone was wonderful!

My latest endeavor has been to create a new business opportunity with a group of obstetric nurses—a legal consultant business. The process has been quite an education! Through it, I have learned to value, more than ever, teamwork and diversity.

Jon Towne '92

It's been over five years since I graduated from Bronson on a Friday and started orientation at South Haven Community Hospital in critical care nursing on the following Monday. Since then I've earned my CCRN[1] and am now the part-time patient-care supervisor. None of these milestones in my life have I regretted, and I appreciate the continuing daily challenge that my career provides.

Closing of the program leaves me with great sadness. When I last went to Bronson accompanying a patient on an ambulance run, I saw the hole in the ground that was formerly Truesdale Hall. It seemed strange to tear down a perfectly good building full of memories and make the area a parking lot. A certain sixties' song came to mind, but the reality of economics, change and the evolution of the health-care system, for better or for worse, apparently left little recourse.

My two years at Bronson are fading in memory, but they facilitated a needed transition for me from the remnants of a sixties mentality that careers were a decadent lifestyle to the reality of supporting a family. In a way my idealism was not sacrificed, since choosing nursing as a career was to provide service. I helped people in need. Going to the Bronson School of Nursing is something I will never regret or forget, no matter how many years I remain in nursing.

Amanda Speedy '93

My sister, Jill Barnum, graduated from Bronson in 1992 and was working with people. I had graduated from Kalamazoo College in 1986 with a Bachelor of Arts degree in Biology and was working in medical research. I liked what my sister was doing. Her work became my motivation for choosing nursing and breaking free from the isolation of medical research. I learned to interact and help others in difficult circumstances.

> My greatest fear was attending my first nursing class and meeting the teacher. My greatest joys involved living in the dorm and graduating.
>
> Susan Manifold was my most inspiring teacher. She was a new instructor at the school with a wealth of knowledge and ability to apply it.
>
> ***Kelli Smith Miller '94***

My science background made the book-learning part of nursing easy. The challenging part was the people that I worked with every day: patients, and healthcare teams, giving and taking reports, and with fellow staff with varying degrees of motivation. Nursing was excellent preparation for future family care and life experiences, such as birth and death. It was emotional learning versus an intellectual approach for me.

Once I graduated, I didn't practice nursing other than in a volunteer capacity at a migrant free clinic where I met my future husband. Even though I never earned a paycheck as a registered nurse, I never regretted the decision to attend nursing school. I learned everything that I needed there, but the work was too hard to do for the rest of my life. Nursing, I discovered, was a more difficult task than medical research. Now I analyze and write Pharmacia and Upjohn (currently Pfizer) research reports. The activity is pretty cut-and-dried with a model to follow, but I went back to that work which I found easy.

Mary Beth Sanders-Jones '96

From as far back as I can remember, whenever I was asked what I wanted to be when I grew up, the reply came naturally, "A nurse." Becoming a nurse was a long-held dream not realized until I was 35 years old.

My nursing school experience was very "nontraditional." I was married at age 19, and began a family shortly thereafter. When my first two children were toddlers, I enrolled at KVCC and began taking one prerequisite class per semester toward enrollment in a nursing curriculum. It took ten years to finish the non-nursing coursework. Once these courses were completed, I enrolled in the Bronson School of Nursing and continued to work part-time as an Employee Benefits Specialist in Human Resources at Bronson. Prior to that position I had worked in the School of Nursing as the administrative assistant to the director from 1983 to 1989. Knowing the school and staff helped firm up my desire to attend Bronson. The faculty and staff struck me as having a high level of commitment to achieve the goal of graduating successful nurses.

When the time finally came to enroll, I didn't have to think twice about which facility I would attend. Bronson was home to me. The support I received was phenomenal. Everyone from family, friends, coworkers, fellow students, and nursing school staff wanted me to succeed. I also received a scholarship through the Kalamazoo Foundation that provided generous financial support. It made my journey through nursing school less stressful than it might have been.

Attending school as an adult with a husband, three teenage children and a job was quite a challenge. I'll never forget my first clinical at Upjohn Nursing Home with Anne Orr. Even though I was supposedly a confidant, self-assured adult I was just as nervous as the 20-year-olds. I had so many questions, like how could I approach someone I didn't know to bathe him or her? What if the patients didn't like me? What if I made a mistake? Anne was just as patient and kind with me as she was with the younger students. After all, our learning objectives were the same, and I wanted to be successful.

I don't remember anything out of the ordinary during nursing school. Many of my classmates, however, viewed Bronson as a step toward achieving goals in higher education. They planned to continue their education immediately after nursing school: some would pursue a bachelor's degree, midwifery school, nurse anesthetist school and other options. Quite frankly, I couldn't understand why they weren't satisfied with being a registered nurse. I had wanted only that role for a long time and I was sure it would be all I needed—or so I thought.

That was seven years ago. A lot has changed since then. I began my nursing practice as a cardiac nurse at Bronson and held the position for 18 months. One year after graduation, I was offered a position as a case management nurse at a local health insurance company. Not wanting to lose my clinical skills, I held both positions simultaneously until I became pregnant with my fourth child. Reluctantly, I resigned my staff nurse position at Bronson to work full time as a case management nurse. I continue in this position today. A lot can be said for having weekends and holidays to spend with family, but at times I miss the hospital setting and actively taking care of patients. I've also changed my opinion about continuing education, and realize that I need to be constantly challenged to grow in my field. I have learned that I have significant leadership skills and a strong desire to help guide others to develop their best selves.

Beginning this fall, I have enrolled at Western Michigan University to pursue a Bachelor of Science degree with an emphasis in Interdisciplinary Health Studies. My three teenage children have all graduated from high school; two are enrolled in college and one is serving in the U.S. Army. My youngest started kindergarten today. I begin my first class at the "big university" on Thursday.

I am blessed to have had a friendship with Jackie Wylie throughout my nursing career. Jackie was my boss when I worked at the School of Nursing, was the director when I was a student there, and has been a mentor and friend since graduation. She has truly been an inspiration and has helped guide me along the path to becoming my best self.

Mark Witteveen '97

I remember walking through the doors of Truesdale. It was dark, not one person was around, and I was probably 30 minutes early. This was one of the biggest steps I had ever taken in my life.

After fulfilling prerequisites at KVCC, I went right to Bronson. As early as I could remember I wanted to be a nurse. Getting involved immediately by attending Student Council, I was voted class president. The best times shared at Bronson were with the friends I met. We all got along quite well. We would go to lunch and on breaks together, whether in the cafeteria or downtown on the mall. We would sign up for lab times to practice and sign-off skills. Mostly I remember a lot of laughter and smiles.

I can honestly say that during school I had no significant disappointments, but of course there were minor ones, such as my first NLN score.[2] I think the major disappointment came when my time at school ended. I had to say goodbye to very close friends. My greatest fear encountered was my first patient assignment at the nursing home, and I have never shaken so badly in my life. My voice quivered and cracked, and my hands tremored. I felt like jelly. What Bronson taught me was *CARING*—caring for the sick in spirit and body.

I want to thank Susan Manifold for all of her guidance. She was the Great Encourager throughout my schooling and helped me stay focused. I saw in her what I wanted to be. She was the ideal picture of a nurse. Fun, kind, and caring. I can honestly say that, because of her, I am a nurse today. Thank you, Susan.

BRONSON HOSPITAL'S NURSE EXTERN PROGRAM

The nurse extern program began in 1984,[3] bringing together the Department of Nursing, Educational Services and the School of Nursing. Its popularity increased when 1990s student requests for increased experiential learning matched Bronson's clinical nurse experts' knowledge and its recruitment need for quality novice nurses. Here was a practical approach to a modern-day problem—students supplemented their income and gained needed clinical expertise as they approached graduation. Their expertise then matched patient–employer expectations of their readiness to practice in demanding staff nurse roles. Work-study models had their place when the model was truly about "growing" clinical expertise and was not simply an apprentice-maintenance system.

> Students and staff recognize the growing complexity of nursing and the economic advantage an extern program can provide. . . . Nursing students seek healthcare employment to improve their technical and professional skills and to supplement their income. Nursing departments need well-prepared, new graduates as accelerating change drives the healthcare system in times of dwindling resources. . . . Numerous publications describe the need for clinical experiences and preceptors for professional socialization of new graduates beginning in staff nurse roles.[4]

The nurse extern program was further developed with integration into the School of Nursing curriculum in 1991 to provide a three-credit, experiential, work-study course that was an upgrade of the early student work-for-pay years. Learning contracts were individualized to respond to the student's level of development. The course, however, was squelched by the National League for Nursing Accreditation visitors who thought they saw shades of the past (students simply working for pay as inexpensive labor, not connected to their education). The visitors did not see the need for an elective course, with earned wages, that increased hours of students' protected practice. Course credit was omitted and the nurse extern program flourished in a work-study format separated from the curriculum. Neither learning nor accreditation was compromised.

> The School of Nursing acted in June 1990 to delete the extern program from the curriculum. The decision was based on the NLN recommendation. The 1989–90 Nurse Extern budget was $184,610 for 23,944 hours of work-study or 11.51 full-time equivalents and average salaries of $7.71 per hour.[5]

When the school closed in 1998, the nurse extern program was continued under the supervision of director, Linda Van Dyke '61, and Barbara Groh, instructor in Education Services.

BUILDING A *COMMON* NURSING LANGUAGE

Another move to facilitate nursing's unique role in healthcare was the development of standardized language research by nurse educators and local pockets of nurse service administrators and practitioners. It seemed important for nursing students to clearly understand that nursing care was more than an extension of medical interventions ordered by physicians. Nursing nomenclature was well integrated into the 1990's curriculum. Nursing students were expected to diagnose and treat human responses to actual or potential health problems.

> There is one scope of clinical nursing practice. The core, or essence, of that practice is the nursing diagnosis and treatment of human responses to health and illness. This core of clinical practice of nursing is dynamic, and evolves as patterns of human response amenable to nursing intervention are identified, nursing diagnoses [are] formulated and classified, nursing skills and patterns of interventions are made more explicit, and patient outcomes responsive to nursing intervention are evaluated. . . .[6]

Leading this movement was the North American Nursing Diagnosis Association (NANDA) which had grown out of a national conference held October 1–5, 1973, in St. Louis, Missouri, when 100 nurses came together to begin the work of classifying nursing diagnoses.[7] The director and some Bronson Hospital School of Nursing faculty had continued to participate in conferences throughout the eighties and nineties. Nursing diagnoses submitted by nurses for peer review described what nurses did that was separate from physician extender work. Some nursing diagnoses focused on wellness and accompanying health promotion interventions intended to maintain or increase spiritual, mental/emotional and physical abilities.

CLOSURE OF THE BMH SCHOOL OF NURSING

The hospital-based School of Nursing held its head high and met National League for Nursing accreditation standards throughout the 1990s budget paring for nursing education, when the school was caught in the hospital's process of changing its allocation of healthcare dollars.

Costs of nursing education gradually moved into academia and away from hospitals, as medical education dollars decreased with the decrease in student-practice education hours. State of Michigan finances replaced federal medical education dollars that were tied to hospital-based nursing education.

Budgeted hours for faculty and staff decreased. Some faculty welcomed the 1990 summer break with fewer courses to teach, while those who were major family breadwinners sought replacement work as staff nurse summer relief in the hospital and community. The good news was that work was always available for faculty who wanted or needed it. The break was a way to maintain and learn new clinical skills and, not least, to build relationships with nursing staff. Faculty agreed by consensus that summer cuts were the least disruptive to the School of Nursing curriculum, a way to retain the most expertise and not lay off any of the nurse educators.

Pediatric nursing expertise was lost when Anna Mae Spaniolo died March 12, 1991, and her nurse-educator team member[8] and friend, Carol Van Antwerp, resigned to enroll in the pediatric nurse practitioner program at Emory University's Nell Hodgson Woodruff School of Nursing in Georgia. Their replacements were pediatric staff nurse experts from Bronson Hospital, Sally Vliem and Elizabeth Phillips, who were new to nursing education. They became an excellent team to fill the huge hole in the pediatric curriculum, and later, in the late nineties, accepted faculty positions at the WMU Bronson School of Nursing

With school closure, Bronson nursing students lost a natural practice advantage with regard to the mentoring relationships among themselves, and with Bronson faculty and nursing staff. The school was well integrated into the hospital culture, even during the last 30 years when students were no longer counted into the daily patient-to-staff ratio. But in other ways, the students' acute-care clinical practice advantage became a disadvantage since graduates earned a hospital diploma with credits that were not always transferable to a college or university. A college degree was the credential graduates needed in order to advance their careers. As nurse professionals, the degree was also needed for the practice of nursing.

Diploma school educators' strength was the maintenance of stable educational systems and production of RNs, but they lacked the skills and time for nursing research and the development of best nursing practice. Few were educationally prepared beyond the graduate level. In order to advance the profession, doctoral-prepared nurses were essential for the conduct of research and inclusion of new nursing knowledge into daily clinical practice. The movement to the university was required for the collective good of healthcare, the students, and nursing practice. Diploma educators had been rewarded for hospital system maintenance, not for research and nursing innovation. Still, faculty within the School of Nursing were encouraged to design innovative practice opportunities for students. Faculty and students gained personal satisfaction and community recognition for bringing nursing services to people in their environments. Art Littlefield, chief nurse executive, supported School of Nursing community endeavors quietly.

Total graduates[9] since the program's 1904 beginning numbered 3,299, when the Bronson Methodist Hospital School of Nursing's ninety-fifth and last class matriculated on May 1, 1998. The school remained open until the following December to facilitatc program completion by a small number of remaining students, to compose the closure report for the Michigan State Board of Nursing, and to move official student transcripts to the WMU Registrar's office.

CLOSING BMH SCHOOL OF NURSING.

Leaves of
Old texts,
Outlines,
Care plans.
Brittle bones of this season.

Trapped in crannies of my soul.
Compost of re-design.
Fertilizer for caring.
Dry. Dark. Dust to dust.

Smoldering ash burns old ways
and smoke carries
School's soul home.

Phoenix rising to
Bless and be Blessed.

Barb Groh, 1998
BMH School of Nursing

All past student records were packed by Sandy Pritz and Kathy Stewart, school support staff, and transferred to WMU for future transcript release when requested by graduates. First-year instructors Suzanne Nahan, Sally Sutkowi and Anne Orr completed their teaching assignments in 1997. Remaining faculty included Rosemarie Nedeau-Cayo, Barbara Groh, John Hall, Helen Truss, Susan Manifold, Susan Vrobel, Teri Davis, Dianna Hargis, Susan Kay Clark, Wendy Kerstner, Elizabeth Phillips, and Sally Vliem. Phyllis Curtis was always willing to teach part time on a contractual basis during the last years.

NURSING ADMINISTRATORS' IMPACT, 1990s

Linda Van Dyke '61

Linda Van Dyke's nursing expertise and teaching skills led to a night clinical instructor role, first reporting to Hazel Latondress. Then a reorganization shifted her educational position into Education Services, led by Director Roberta Hunt.[10] Van Dyke subsequently became the Education Services director when Hunt accepted a position as director of the Bronson Clinical Investigational Unit.

Van Dyke accepted the position in Education Services the year Bronson laid off employees for the first time in its history. Discomfited, but knowing what had to be done, she took responsibility for decreasing the nurse educator hours, part of the hospital downsizing. With the cuts in nurse-education hours as well as clinical nurse specialist positions, nursing appeared to lose some of the empowerment gains made in the early eighties. Adaptation was a skill that Van Dyke had learned, and she adjusted to changing times, doing the best possible job with the resources given. She had a "take control" attitude and had a good relationship with her staff and nurse managers. She understood the cyclic nature of healthcare financing and was able to respond positively and proactively.

Later in the nineties downsizing continued to impact nursing. Art Littlefield had had the benefit of nurse special-project administrative assistants, *i.e.,* Sue Kovats-Bell '79 focused on nursing quality assurance, while Beverly Adams '67, managed policy and procedure interpretation. Van Dyke had watched when Roberta Hunt Utrecht followed Littlefield in the chief nurse executive role at a time when all nurse administrative assistants had already been eliminated. Consequently, it was a difficult time to advance nursing practice within the Bronson system, whether in an administrative or educational role. As cycles have their ups and downs, however, the tides changed in 1996 with Frank Sardone's leadership. Slowly the groundwork was laid for advanced nursing practice at Bronson, taking four years for clinical nurse specialists and other nursing support positions to be opened in 2000.

One of the highlights of Van Dyke's career was her role in the orientation of all staff for the move to the new millennium hospital in 2000. The organizational philosophy embraced by administration and staff led toward the creation of a healing environment and balanced culture for all who entered through its doors. The hospital became the new monument to Bronson women for the new millennium.

Before the elevators were operational, Van Dyke's education team walked the stairs, teaching volunteers the building layout and how to conduct public tours in preparation for the hospital's completion date! Betty and Dick Vander Molen were part of the group preparing for tour-guide status. During her interview, Van Dyke smiled with satisfaction, stating, "It was an amazing day and such a reward to see peoples' faces light up when they viewed the spacious environment, so open and receptive to all. They were awestruck!" The patient rooms were all private. They included sleeping sofas or chairs if it was important for a family member to stay for an extended period. Aware of the transformation, Van Dyke hoped that everyone who earned a paycheck at Bronson would never rest on his or her laurels but be constantly working to improve customer service. Striving for improvements in Bronson's caring services was not just for patients and families but for themselves as employees.

The Human Resources Department sponsored a fashion show to facilitate uniform and color decision-making. A dress code was introduced to facilitate customer recognition of staff positions. RNs wore white tops and forest green scrub pants; patient-care assistants wore all teal blue.

Van Dyke nostalgically watched the 2003 demolition of the main hospital North Tower where she had practiced nursing as a student, staff nurse, supervisor and nurse educator. Memories of patients and families in her care flooded her mind, and she saddened to think of the many people who would not remember the care they received in the old, medically archaic building now gone from view. The edifice was as unsuited for renovations as it was for downtown apartments. Having once said, "I'll retire from Bronson when 2-East is air conditioned," she recalled, thinking that such an innovation probably never would occur, but it did. Van Dyke stayed on for years after the 2-East area no longer housed patients, and saw the building leveled except for most of the ground floor, preserved, and remodeled for ancillary hospital services.

Van Dyke's 40-plus year career is expected to culminate when she retires at a time of her choosing. She entered Bronson as an employee in January, 1962, and is the Bronson graduate with the longest, uninterrupted Bronson career. When interviewed on June 28, 2004, she anticipated that her allegiance to Bronson would endure throughout the rest of her life. Besides her myriad work hours, her husband and his sisters were born there when the Labor and Delivery Unit was located in the original 1906 structure. Her three children were also born at Bronson. The Van Dyke family will not forget the hospital located in its multiple 20th-century structures.

Arthur Littlefield

Art Littlefield, former vice president of nursing and patient-care services, with 20 years of service as a gentle and caring nurse at Bronson, died March 20, 1998, a month before the last class graduated. He was remembered at a special Bronson memorial service and continues to be remembered by those who benefited from his open leadership and supportive mentoring style. His leadership was manifested in a quiet presence: empowering, nonjudgmental with a hint of humor, and always open and supportive of all the School of Nursing innovations for practice in the community.

Littlefield was never a micro-manager. He supported students and faculty in their freedom to learn. The School of Nursing, as a department of the hospital in a late eighties reorganization, reported to a newly established department that focused on education and marketing. It was under the supervision of Tom Langer and Robert Doud, EdD. Doud's previous position included management of the Kalamazoo Valley Community College Nursing Program.

Rosemarie Nedeau-Cayo, the School's Last Director

A graduate of Borgess Hospital's School of Nursing in 1970 and Nazareth College's School of Nursing in 1975, Rosemarie Nedeau-Cayo[11] received her first nursing credential and baccalaureate degree within a five-year period. She earned a Master of Science degree in nursing in 1982 from Wayne State University, majoring in the promotion of mental health and the care of adults with mental illnesses.

Rosemarie Nedeau-Cayo was appointed director in August 1995, cognizant that closure of the School of Nursing would most likely happen within a few years. She was the unanimous pick of the faculty by consensus, a process facilitated by retiring director, Jackie Wylie. Faculty knew and trusted Nedeau-Cayo's reflective, open management style and believed that she was the best person to represent the school. They preferred the known to the unknown, and she had no enemies.

Nedeau-Cayo, in the new director role, and Barbara Groh, Nursing Education instructor, favored a plan to keep the school open, even if on a smaller scale, as a way to hedge the hospital's potential program loss. They wanted to prevent a Bronson nursing shortage by continuing to support staffing with a local product of their own making, a process that had worked so well for 90-plus years. They wrote a proposal to that effect, but the die had been cast, the doors to the school were closing, and monetary support went to the new, university-based, soon-to-be-named, WMU Bronson School of Nursing.

Some students had graduation requirements to meet following the last formalized graduation at the First United Methodist Church on May 1, 1998. By August, all but one student had met requirements. That exception successfully completed the last course by invitation at Grand Rapids Community College School of Nursing, with the credit transferred back to Bronson for conferring of the diploma.

Nedeau-Cayo and Groh were two of the last full-time faculty attached to Bronson. Both transferred to the hospital's Education Services Department, then directed by Linda Van Dyke '61. Nedeau-Cayo was invited to accept a project-writing role to establish a critical care-nurse intern program, envisioned earlier by Roberta Hunt and Van Dyke as a way to mentor novice nurses. Groh wrote the nursing education coordinator-liaison proposal that facilitated the WMU and other schools' clinical placement contracts for nursing student practice opportunities. Some schools of nursing that consistently use Bronson services are Kalamazoo Valley Community College, Kellogg Community College, Glen Oaks Community College and Western Michigan University. Groh also became responsible for managing students in nurse extern, work-study positions throughout the Bronson system. Numerous students benefited by the coaching skills offered by these nurse educators.

Closure of the school was formalized with a report written by Nedeau-Cayo to the Michigan State Board of Nursing in December 1998. Many Bronson administrators and nursing staff, in both education and service, who understood cyclical professional nursing shortages, met the issue of closure with cognitive dissonance, but the school closed with honor and respect. Program adaptations for individual students allowed all who had enrolled to have the opportunity to complete program requirements and take the State Board exam. The faculty had chosen well. Nedeau-Cayo was the right person to be the last director of the Bronson school.

Her transition into Bronson's Education Service Department provided an educational bridge for novice nurses requiring extensive post-graduate education to move toward expert nurse competencies in caring, clinical judgement and invasive technical skills. After designing the first critical care-nurse intern program, Nedeau-Cayo extended and managed two more nurse intern programs in building medical-surgical and peri-operative competencies.

Roberta Hunt, Vice President and Chief Nurse Executive

Roberta Hunt's Bronson career spanned 19 years[12] that included several promotions. Her goal was to advance the profession of nursing and its caring, cost-effective, non-invasive services that fit with Wylie's notions for creating a healthier professional nursing culture and work environment. Hunt and Wylie, two nurse educators, dreamed of a professional nursing practice model that would require a different staff mix—an increased percentage of baccalaureate and graduate-prepared nurses who could practice at a higher professional level in an interdisciplinary hospital. Such a transformation did not occur as envisioned, but each step built on the work of previous nurse leaders. The model would take a critical mass of nurses dedicated to change, who were willing to take the risk of returning to academia to learn more about nursing science and its possibilities for the enhancement of community health. Success would require influential administrators, physicians, and a paradigm shift, fondly called redesign, with new standards that were found in magnet hospitals.

Hunt's Early Career

Prior to Kalamazoo, a move prompted by her husband's career, Hunt earned her graduate degree in nursing from the University of California at San Francisco. She wanted a nursing education position and wanted to teach with Phyllis Nicolaou, RN, MSN, EdD, director of the Nazareth College nursing program. She liked Nazareth and would have taught a management course with Helen Truss if the salary had been close to her expectation. Just $11,000 for the academic year was not enough, an observation she shared directly with Phyllis. Having been paid more at the University of Connecticut, she took the opportunity to teach at the University of Michigan School of Nursing, then found her way into Bronson. Still, it wasn't easy adjusting to two weeks of vacation after an academic schedule and its generous time off during the summer months. Money played a part, and the salary differences at that time were so great between academia and acute care:

> When I started my nursing career, I was working as a medical-surgical nurse for $300 a month. We were salaried and didn't earn overtime pay but, when the patient census was low, we could go

> home early.[13] Staff nurses receive hourly wages in most hospitals today.

Hunt was hired in 1982 to teach in the University of Michigan baccalaureate completion program and to supervise the U of M students on Bronson's Hall 10. Donna Asma, medical-surgical vice president of nursing, commented, "If you ever decide to leave teaching and education, come to Bronson. We want to develop a program with the Michigan Nurses Association so that we can grant nursing continuing education units.[14] So would you think about it?" Hunt said she would, never believing she would follow through. She preferred nursing education, but the salary difference was a great incentive to change her career path into hospital acute care.

> I liked the people and the atmosphere at Bronson. That's what pulled me here, and the position was related to education for staff nurses and other hospital personnel. Hazel Latondress was the director of nursing when I arrived. Then Art Littlefield was promoted to administration. I remember Hazel saying, that to play ball with the boys [in administration], we needed a man and Art was it.

He had a business background that was required to bridge the gap between clinical nursing practice and the masculine business reality that drove most of the eighties hospital management teams in the Midwest region.

Tom Jenkins was the director of Educational Services when Hunt was hired. Barb Sipe '66, Linda VanDyke '61, and Dorothy Kavalhuna were the three educational supervisors. The education budget was healthy so programs were numerous. Nursing staff-to-patient ratios also allowed the nurses time for educational opportunities within their work schedules. Nurses delegated care in their absence, then reversed the process so that all nurses had the benefit of on-the-job continuing education.

Still, Wylie's heart and mind were excited by the possibilities of new Bronson nurse leaders. She never lost hope that transformative nursing practice would somehow emerge in a mutual partnership with medical practice. The process proved to be evolutionary, not a quick change. Cost containment focused on labor costs while advancing medical technology continued to build expensive diagnostics and interventions into the system, creating a "catch 22."

Several interviews with this chief nurse executive occurred over the period between 1997–2004. When Wylie asked the former Roberta Hunt, remarried as Roberta Utrecht, "How could nursing philosophy and science be woven into hospital acute-care nursing practice?" Hospital reimbursement was based on physician admissions and medical treatment. Nurses were often perceived to be only following medical orders, an extension of physicians' hands, and were paid for just that, rather than for their unique non-invasive skill set including 24-hour nursing presence. So much of nursing care was simply not visible or submersed into the medical model.[15]

Utrecht's philosophy of nursing practice had been strongly influenced by graduate school and being in the university setting. To perennial questions of how nursing roles played out in acute care, and how did you reconcile nursing practice differences, Utrecht replied:

> Staff development within an education department was somewhat like academia. I was still in education and took my time to learn what acute care was really all about. I remember some sessions that Nancy Figel, Lois Richmond, Jan Dax, and you and I had about the nursing philosophy at Bronson. You and I wanted to choose a nursing theorist for the Department of Nursing and Education to follow. We earned the names "Drifter and Dreamer" because the nursing patient-care directors and managers said that we had our heads in the clouds. What I found out was that, in acute care, one nursing theory doesn't cover the complexity of nursing practice. I think the self-care model[16] was part of the unwritten Bronson nursing model, and I think it still fits.

It would take an interdisciplinary model of health care, however, to move the system into the 21st century. How could hospital administrators, medicine, nursing and all of the health professions put their heads together to transform daily practice? The definitive answer to that question was and still is elusive.

The School of Nursing faculty followed its own version of a self-care model and self-health management to inform healthcare decisions. Still the traditional medical model was the dominant overlay of all care given in the hospital, with nursing practice more of a counterculture. A sense of unified nursing practice among the nursing departments and the school was missing. A shared nursing model that could be integrated into the medical–hospital structure would take time to develop.

When asked about NANDA, Utrecht said, "I think the School of Nursing faculty participation in NANDA and the MNA did influence nurses' practice here." Utrecht also became active and learned more about nursing languages to try to effectively articulate nursing practice at Bronson.

Balancing the Feminine and Masculine in Hospital Administration

More women were administrators by 1997, and a number of them had nursing backgrounds. It was a big change from when Utrecht first came when all the administrators were men. Clinical administrators were needed—physicians and nurses—to balance the business end of the spectrum.

Nursing administrators walked a fine line—supporting nursing staff and working to contain labor costs. They seemed more vulnerable than nurse educators who enjoyed a less volatile environment. Did Utrecht feel vulnerable?

> It depends on what day of the week you're talking to me and it's the middle of the week—I'm still all right. When I took the job as vice president in 1992, nursing at Bronson was compartmentalized. Nursing directors reported to different vice presidents. I was responsible for surgery, some medical-surgical units, and Bronson Vicksburg Hospital; Jon Dixon managed the Trauma and

> Emergency Department; and other VPs oversaw other areas of nursing. So nursing units didn't work closely together. We all had our silos in our own departments and managed and directed them according to our own styles and philosophy.

Flight from Bronson

Seven hundred employees, including RNs, left Bronson in 1995 when it offered them early retirements or lump sum payoffs for those not eligible for retirement. Bronson had almost 100 percent RN staff prior to this exodus. As an economic measure, the RN full-time equivalents (FTEs) were replaced with unlicensed trained personnel who, according to Utrecht, consultants said were numerous in the work force. The labor market, however, was not plush with well-trained, unlicensed direct caregivers, and Bronson had to fill a gap by quickly hiring people who needed extensive training. More time was needed than taken for a thoughtful replacement procedure. After a "weeding" process occurred, some of the unprepared, newly hired employees mutually agreed to resign because the work did not meet their expectations any better than their performance matched Bronson's need.

Right-sizing the Bronson Organization, a Downtime for Nursing

The buck stopped with the nurse executive. Before Frank Sardone assumed leadership in 1996, Utrecht was caught in an untenable position with the hospital's expectation that the quality of patient care could be increased with a change in nurse–patient ratio from 1:4 in medical-surgical units to 1:8 or 1:10. More unlicensed, patient-care assistants (PCAs) were recruited to fill the professional nurses gap.

Utrecht attended patient-care unit meetings when nursing staff invited her to listen to their perceptions about staffing. Some nurses appreciated PCAs and delegated care well. If the PCA was well trained, had a positive attitude and could do the job, the nurse and PCA teamed well. The nurses were also tired of frequent mandated changes in their practice. A staff nurse said to Utrecht,

> It seems like one part of the country tries something new so we do it—everyone gets on the bandwagon. We had team nursing years ago! We had primary-care nursing! And once again, we have something similar to team nursing. Are we going back to primary-care nursing again?

Utrecht could not answer her question. No one seemed able to articulate the best cost-effective patient-care staffing mix involving registered nurses and unlicensed personnel, although hospitals with magnet status appeared to be closer to the solution. Nursing did not have the answer and neither did the frequently hired consultants who did not experience the consequences of frequent changes in staffing patterns.

Actually, some of the patient units worked well with unlicensed staff. Critical care units had maintained 100 percent RN staff, and some units were returned to 100 percent RN staff instead of a RN mix with unlicensed staff. Conversations with colleagues at national meetings indicated that some parts of the country were returning to all RN and LPN staff. Southwest Michigan had few LPN's, however, since most had continued their education to become RNs, knowing that the acute care environment more often hired at the RN than LPN level.

Reflecting on her past, Utrecht said that she had practiced in a team nursing model, and it worked efficiently, with division of labor between RNs, LPNs, nurse aides and orderlies. Functional assignments meant that the work was divided based on functional areas of care with one nurse giving medications and another treatments, while aides helped with activities of daily living, as opposed to one nurse giving total care to one to four patients. Patients who were progressing well received little care from the RN, which appeared to be satisfactory then.

Nurses in the 1990s continued to learn the more complex technical skills that had to be mastered for clinical competence, feeding the need for more expert nurses with never-ending education. Patients expected RNs to be direct caregivers and voiced their complaints when they only saw nurses on occasional rounds and when medications were administered. Some patients said the nurse aide was nice and attentive, but he or she wasn't the same as having nursing care. The expectation was, "If I'm admitted to the hospital, I will have a nurse care for me," so patient and family education about PCA competence was essential, and the unlicensed staff had to prove themselves. It was an uphill battle because patients weren't sure they wanted less than professional help when they were acutely ill. When it was a positive experience, discharged patients said, "That's an O.K. system." If it wasn't a positive experience, they believed we needed an all RN staff. It was as if the patient was on one end and the nurse on the other—both feeling disenfranchised.

Utrecht mentioned that the re-engineering of healthcare had brought chaos and incredible challenges for the nursing staff. "Consultants and the re-engineering gurus maintained that, if the environment is not a state of chaos, you're not moving quickly enough." Utrecht, however, wanted to have a sense of what the outcomes would be:

> I like to know where I'm going and it's frustrating when you're working in a re-engineering mind frame where consultants say you don't need to take all this time. "Don't worry about the time. You'll get there—just trust that you'll get there." Well, where is there?

It took an accountable, supportive administrative team, well-engaged, with competent staff, to accept a discovery model where there was no failure, only recognition of what worked and what did not. Sardone continued to build the relationships that would eventually bring nursing into a more positive light. Best patient care depended on well thought-out practice and was essential to healthy outcomes for patients and the organization. Discovery learning required expert nurses within expert teams and resources for quick adaptation and physician support when patients' conditions changed. Utrecht continued:

> Speeding up change is so frustrating for me, for the staff nurses and their managers and also for physicians because clinicians are logical and organized in their approach to patient-care management. And now we must function in a complex, accelerated change environment without experience or predictable outcomes. Accelerating change is frustrating for all, not just nursing.

HOSPITAL SCHOOL OF NURSING CLOSURE IN SAFE WRAPS

One of the tasks that came with Susan Ulshafer's appointment to Human Resources was to support the phasing-out period leading to the School of Nursing closure. Robert Doud, vice president of the Bronson Institute for Health Education, shared administrative support for the school with her during a 1995 fall transitional period while Ulshafer learned the Bronson culture and established relationships with employees who would report to her. Doud shifted roles to vice president of Public Relations. The decision to close the school with the establishment of the WMU School of Nursing had already been made before Ulshafer arrived in Kalamazoo.

Impact on Nursing Education

The School of Nursing continued to teach the caring staff-nurse role and the scientific method via nursing process—how to explain and manage nursing practice. Most content and clinical practice were built on the bio-psycho-social sciences, framed into a nursing assessment of health patterns, nursing diagnosis, patient goal setting, interventions to reach goals, and evaluation to measure outcomes. It was an educational challenge to help novice nurses understand how nursing's system fit into hospital services. Critical thinking skills had always been essential. Sicker patients meant potential for more complications, which required expert judgment, often without time to reflect and consult. Knowledge of every disease was not essential, but knowing how to recognize patient condition changes, where to find resources, to respond quickly, and to be a partner in caring, to be a team player, and to be sensitive to the patient's and system's needs were all essential. Novice nurses and students had to be paired with expert nurses over extended orientation periods for safe caring practice.

Some students were alarmed at the challenges of clinical decision-making. They had come into nursing believing that all they had to do was follow the doctor's orders, as if that would protect them from having to think critically and from being accountable for patient-care outcomes. Students graduated to become novice nurses who were fearful of thinking and acting independently, and it was easy to understand why. No machine was able to replace human caring or clinical judgments, and blindly following medical orders never was an option. Critical thinking had always been essential. It seemed as if it might have been easier to go to medical school in order to have more authority in the system than nurses felt they had. Assessing, monitoring and mediating among patients, families, hospital administrators, and myriad professional clinicians and unlicensed staff required expert nurse negotiators. Later Ulshafer and Sardone helped build an inclusive team where the nurses' voices could be heard.

Bronson had designed an acute-care delivery model with the RN as the manager of care for a group of patients, including the supervision of unlicensed personnel, for which most RNs had not been educated. They had grown accustomed to peer support from other RNs who practiced close by in primary care—helping hands, hearts and minds for each other. Team nursing distanced the RN support for each other. If a nurse had asked a colleague, "I'm running behind. Could you check Ms. X's catheters and IV?" the nurse peer would know exactly all the parameters that needed to be checked. When the nurse asked a PCA, however, the PCA did not always know what parameters had to be monitored and measured—especially those PCAs who had minimal knowledge and little hospital experience.

Bronson nurses had been educated to provide total care for patients. Their practice behaviors had to change to include delegation and on-the-job training and support for PCAs. Hospital courses in delegation and risk management did not ease the transition from primary care to team care. Nurses worked to adapt to the changes. Those who were old enough to have experienced team nursing had less difficulty, but the younger graduates, who had only experienced nursing practice in a primary-care model, had the most difficult time. A few courses in supervision, delegation and risk management were not enough support in the complex, acute-care environment. Expert empowered staff nurses took time to grow. They had to believe in and "own" their practice.

Moving Toward a Professional Practice Model and Effective Use of Staff

The dilemma had several parts. It was not just the change in ratio of nurses to patients but also the ongoing relationship building and education for hospital staff nurses. Graduates prepared at the baccalaureate (BSN) and associate degree (ADN) and diploma levels often held similar positions with similar professional practice expectations once they passed the State Board exam to become licensed RNs. Nursing service administrators' and educators' arguments about similarities and differences in graduate performance had gone on for years. Increase in educational qualifications offered a strong argument. If nursing was practiced at a baccalaureate (BSN) professional rather than the associate degree (ADN) technical level, it could be assumed that nursing would have more to offer to the patient-care team. Advanced education, BSN, MSN and PhD degrees overall, meant more knowledge to back a complex care system. Later, a 2003 study demonstrated that " . . . surgical patients experienced lower mortality and failure-to-rescue rates," when hospitals employed " . . . higher proportions of nurses educated at the baccalaureate level or higher."[17]

While nurse researchers were demonstrating that educational levels did make a difference, nursing lagged behind other professions' educational expectations that the graduate master's degree is the appropriate entry level into practice. Why nursing could not educationally upgrade appeared to be a matter of economics and tradition. Professional status for nursing could not be won without advanced practice degrees to match its colleagues in the transforming interdisciplinary healthcare marketplace. Michigan RN licensure laws were not about to change. Movement toward a professional practice model sought by Utrecht was destined to be evolutionary, even with the support of chief executive officers like Sardone and Human Resources Vice President Ulshafer. Both used "magnet hospital" leadership styles that supported nursing in its development toward greater professional status.

Utrecht thought that nurses could stay closer to patients at their bedside if Bronson had a professional practice model. Advanced practice roles meant that nurses managed with a competency skill set more in tune with the complexity of patient care. "Those are the kinds of people that I would like to see manage a care team—to take care of patients in the hospital," Utrecht said. But unless incentives to stay in the fast-paced, demanding acute-care hospital were built into careers, nurses would leave. Recruitment and retention incentives were needed for young graduates. The average age of RNs in acute care settings was 43!

New graduates feared the demands placed on staff nurses in hospitals. They needed mentoring and building toward the autonomy often given to nurses practicing in outpatient clinics, community health or home health; and if they hired into an acute-care hospital setting as novice nurse graduates, they often stayed until their mastered technical skills blended with increased competence in critical thinking. Then they resigned for positions that offered more autonomy.

Nurses perceived their lack of authority in hospital nursing practice yet they accepted accountability for desired outcomes. Wylie had sensed this dichotomy early in her career and, as a result, had transferred into nursing education, "That was why I left the acute-care setting." How nurses could gain autonomy in their hospital practice setting was the question.

Magnet hospitals seemed to have the answer, with RN staffs that enjoyed a sense of authority and connectedness to the interdisciplinary hospital team. Nurses needed to step up to the plate, be conscious of forces that were intimidating, and name them to manage fears. Opportunities came and went, but getting into healthy, interdisciplinary practice models took a higher level of administrative support, nurse consciousness, values changes, education and time. An interdisciplinary course to facilitate the change and practitioners to back it up were few, so Utrecht laughingly suggested, "Let's put together a course—we'll do that in our spare time."

Bronson again hired advance practice nurses in 2001 when Katie Harrelson became the chief nurse executive. Utrecht said:

> I think a good use of clinical nurse specialists is offering their support to staff nurses learning how to best document patient education as the intervention that it is. Programs are being designed for specialty areas where we expect to use clinical nurse specialists.

Staff nurses and clinical nurse specialists may not have realized how all Bronsonites could win from everyone's support—the concept of mutuality coming into play. In return, the staff could reach out to mentor nursing students and novice graduates who enriched the system with their enthusiasm, new ideas and eagerness to become expert nurses.

Utrecht and Wylie, in the late nineties, reflected together on 20 years of Utrecht's tenure at Bronson, including establishment of the WMU School of Nursing. They agreed that the future needs of nursing students and graduates could better be met with more nurses advancing their education within the university. Risk awareness of alienating nurses with less than a BSN was with them always.

Often nurse mentors for students were from the ADN and diploma schools, loyal and expert in the care they provided, but not knowing how to gain satisfaction or how much more they could accomplish if they chose to advance their education and support system changes in which nurses could become equal partners. It took both an advanced education and clinical practice-setting expertise to affect that decision. Students paired one to one with expert caring nurse mentors produced amazing outcomes. Utrecht reiterated,

> I'm always trying to determine how best to engage nurses as mentors. They are so busy now. There's so much pressure to manage more patient care that they can hardly think of mentoring a student. So that condition is a big concern. How might nursing service and education work together so that students experience acute-care complexities and hospital case management? It's important for recruitment—it's important for students to have state-of-the-art mentors and know that they have the best role models.

SELF-MANAGEMENT OF THEIR OWN PROFESSION

Moving toward shared governance, the Nursing Council had been established in the early nineties by Art Littlefield. Its replacement in the late nineties, was the Nursing Advisory Committee led by Roberta Utrecht. The earlier Council had evolved into a policy and procedure committee whose members balked at continuing its deliberations, based on the cost/benefit of their time. How could nurses best address needed changes? A different approach was taken by the Advisory Committee to manage policy and procedural changes. Each nursing unit had its own unit council, some of which were effective, and some, not. The Nursing Advisory Committee's status was consistent with the revised hospital organizational structure. The advisory group included other caregivers, moving toward a collaborative, interdisciplinary practice.

Did the change from the Nursing Council to the Nurse Advisory Committee increase nurse power and influence? Did the nurses perceive themselves as having more power to better manage patient care? Utrecht reported in 1997:

> The new group that we pulled together, for instance, identified patient issues that needed to be addressed. We divided issues into internal and external customers with each group, focusing on how to work with each other and with the community-at-large. I think nurses now have more say on operations—how patient issues should be addressed. The ideas are still new. A survey will be administered to ascertain nurses' perceptions.

Advisory meetings were held once a month with dialogue about patient-care challenges and staffing issues; for example, nurses were concerned that patients were not able to identify and differentiate between the nurses and other caregivers. They suggested that clothing worn should clearly identify employees to patients because name badges did not seem to suffice. Patient vision was too often compromised when glasses were not in place and pain management clouded thinking. Advisory nurses surveyed their colleagues and, by consensus, concluded that nurses would wear white and dark green uniforms. Administration was pleased with this advice, and soon all hospital employees who had direct contact with patients were choosing clothing to represent their services to patients.

Another resolved issue was the long wait for patient placement on units. Families and patients complained that admissions were not managed in a way that was the best for the patient or for the physician. Work with employees who made patient bed assignments was in process. Customer service was a concern. Bronson had so many new employees that cultural expectations had been lost, and employees did not know how to help patients or each other. The Nursing Advisory Council recommended that intensive customer-service training was needed to rebuild caring as an institutional value that would recreate a friendly environment for patients, visitors and staff. Greater customer service soon became a hospital-wide initiative.

Nursing Advisory Council outcomes also included dialogue about mentoring and unanimous group support for the nurse extern program. Council members said the externs' attitudes demonstrated engagement in professional practice. The work-study employment was great for recruitment, often requiring a simple job status change and a modified, less costly orientation upon graduation. Council members wanted new students from the WMU School of Nursing and surrounding colleges and universities to experience nursing at Bronson since the on-site School of Nursing was scheduled to close in 1998. Utrecht reflected,

> We've been fortunate for all of the Bronson graduates who want to stay here. We won't have new Bronson graduates after 1998, and we will still need nurses! A positive learning experience is necessary to encourage students to become staff when they graduate. Next may be a nurse intern program. New graduates cannot be expected to carry a staff nurse load without having the extra experiences as externs and interns. With all of the changes in healthcare, there is no way you can take a new graduate, put him or her on a patient unit, and say, "Go to it."

The investment in student development insured a stable staff nurse supply, a process that had occurred naturally for the first 60 years between the parent BMH and its diploma School of Nursing. Staff nurse recognition or remuneration for the role in student development vacillated between remuneration and recognition only. Budget restrictions eliminated payment for the skill of mentoring students and engaging them in daily practice. Remuneration was perceived as a perk not required because mentoring was an expected professional obligation.

The challenge of mentoring while engaged in actual nursing practice was important to recognize. Clinical nursing judgment and other professional skill sets took attention and time to teach and learn. The Human Resources Department worked with management and staff on one of the nursing units to identify ways to recognize mentor work in the form of bonus points. Preceptors for externs could earn "x" number of points, or points could be earned for committee service. Mentoring or working an extra shift when staffing was short could earn points exchanged for a monetary bonus.

Enhanced nursing leadership was Utrecht's vision for nursing and a futuristic Bronson nursing practice:

> Nurse leaders are needed to take care of groups of patients, and whether we will stay with the model that we have now or go back to more of a primary-care model, with RNs and LPNs, I'm not sure. Nurses who can think critically are needed. Most patient-care decisions are best made by frontline staff nurses without deferring to their charge nurses or manager. I like to see them think through the situation, identify alternatives, and act upon their rationale, and say, "This is what I did," instead of asking for permission from their supervisor, *i.e.,* "Should I do this or should I do that?"

Professional practice models gave staff nurses not only accountability but the authority to act. Best clinical decision-making and risk management required expert nurses with extensive knowledge, not only of whole person responses to health and illness, but also how to advocate for patients, delegate to non-licensed staff and facilitate organizational changes toward a healthier environment for all. Nurses had to know that nursing administration and hospital administrators would value their decision-making rationale. They had to have confidence that what they did was the best nursing or medical intervention and that they would be supported in changing patients' plans of care when the plan was ineffective. Best practice required utilization of research and new knowledge within a safe, learning environment. Logical, rational nurse decision-making had to be valued, supported and understood by patients and the health-care team.

Utrecht acknowledged the challenge of changing to an interdisciplinary culture. She said,

> It's difficult right now [1997]. Everyone admits that this is probably one of the most difficult times that any of us has ever experienced in healthcare. But to be pro-active and not whiny is essential. Speak up and identify problems. Staff nurses have good ideas and I'd like them to take action.

Be part of the solution! Be mindful of desired outcomes and confident of what can be achieved in interdisciplinary practice. It was hard for many nurses to change after years of learning how to defer or work around authority to meet patients' needs. Authoritarian systems did not turn history around easily, even when a newer version of team gave support and shared authority to the nurses. Utrecht explained,

> I think that many nurses want to use their critical thinking skills more and be more direct and proactive in their management of patient care; they want that independence. So if we could build the acute-care setting, and change the environment to meet their caring practice needs, then I think we'd have very satisfied nurses.

Overall, the Nursing Advisory Council provided feedback. Decision-making was limited and required staff development to move to a shared governance model. Utrecht was no longer alone by the end of the nineties. Other nurse leaders were hired into administrative positions above the director level. Katie Harrelson was one of them. She would carry the council model toward shared governance with nursing practice principles utilized in magnet hospitals.

DEVELOPING A CRITICAL MASS TO CHANGE NURSING PRACTICE

The years 1995 to 1998 were a troubled time for Bronson nurses and employees who were upset by the 1995 staff exodus. The friction among departments and peers, and across departments rubbed everyone the wrong way. It was a time of disharmonious relationships, out of balance, with no common path toward mission unification.

A major part of the nursing challenge was the decrease in RN staff that had occurred beginning with the eighties layoffs and nineties hiring of unlicensed patient-care personnel. The professional skill mix of nursing had been reduced from 95 percent RN staff to 50–60 percent RN staff, depending on the unit, with unlicensed personnel intended to provide the same level of patient care. Responsibilities of RNs included:

- bedside clinical judgments,
- unit management,
- execution of most invasive technical skills and medication management as ordered by physicians,
- delegation and supervision of patient-care assistants who had been trained to perform selected, less-invasive technical skills,
- patient-care outcomes, regardless of who gave the care.

The pressure of managing patient care with the supervision of unlicensed personnel added stressors for the nurses who had been educated to practice within a primary patient-care model where the RN delivers total patient care. Patients seemed to be too sick and discharge planning too complicated to expect unlicensed personnel delegation. Many skills and services just could not be delegated. Frictions increased between units, even though there were attempts to bring the nurses together.

Utrecht as Chief Nurse Executive

Utrecht led a Nursing Council, and, in doing so, built a relationship for further development of shared governance. Nurse managers, however, could not seem to find the personal and economic resources to relieve the perceived pressure on nursing, lack of a professional critical mass, and recognition of the challenges they faced. The council allowed space to air hurt feelings and frustrations. Sometimes, for Utrecht, it felt as if anarchy was the rule. Utrecht and Harrelson knew that frustrations had to be managed if nursing practice was going to change. Nurses collectively had to take ownership of their practice, recognize their collective power, and become healthy partners in clinical practice decision-making with others.

Eldred as Senior VP

The nurses' level of consciousness needed a boost! Philosophical approaches to nursing care were unclear. A critical mass makes a difference! Utrecht's attempt to bring nursing together under one roof needed the right timing, nurturing, and empowering dialogue that came into being with support from Sardone, Susan Ulshafer, Mary Ann Eldred, Jo Ulrich, Jackie Wahl, Linda Van Dyke, Barb Groh and Katie Harrelson to name a few of the key players. Nurses had the opportunity to reframe their thinking, by bringing healing professional relationships to individualized nursing care for each patient and family served. All were catalysts needed for continued evolution toward becoming a nursing center for caring excellence. Nurses, other clinical staff and administrators behind the scenes who helped to achieve this result consciously or unconsciously are to be commended.

Still the nurses were often unhappy and struggled to regain their roots, forgetting why they had chosen nursing as their profession in the first place. They sometimes reverted back to victim roles, complaining about their plight of having no say, without offering a proactive plan or other proposal. They were unable to hear their own discontented voices or realize that the change needed was within their own hearts and minds. Complaints could only be fixed if they took the lead in describing the best kind of nursing practice and found ways to do it. It was a challenging time.

Support by Harrelson

Wounded nurses needed to emerge from a relatively comfortable victim role of blaming others and not taking control of their practice. They had to regain their professional identity by losing behaviors akin to pawns on the chessboard; they were out of touch with the power positions that influence the system and services to improve patient care. They needed to realize that the nursing knowledge they collectively owned would help patients, the healthcare team and the community; an awakening to their roles as equal players in the complex healthcare game was imminent. Katie Harrelson believed that the nurses could change themselves and change nursing practice in the process. A major cultural shift was needed. She believed she could help to make the shift happen and found herself in the role to do so when Utrecht chose to join her husband in retirement.

Harrelson understood the challenge. Her voiced vision for a professional practice model emerged, given a supportive administration. The history of caring nursing practices needed revitalization. Professional practice could only be gained by stepping up to the plate and taking the risk of being heard and acting on nursing values. She proved that she could do the job! She was recognized as the catalyst for changes that would occur in the new millennium. Closure of the hospital-based program gave way for movement toward nurse advancement and best practice outcomes for patients within a valued healing environment.

END OF A HOSPITAL-BASED NURSING EDUCATION ERA

Bronson employed Susan Ulshafer, Vice President in Human Resources, in August 1995. The School of Nursing was one of her responsibilities. Ulshafer was the last vice president before school closure. Nedeau-Cayo continued to be responsible for all school inquiries after the December, 1998, closing. Financial support shifted to the new baccalaureate program of the WMU School of Nursing, which graduated its first class in April 1999. Nedeau-Cayo was well supported by Ulshafer in planning a dignified path toward a school closure date, one that provided a win:win for students and faculty. Its components allowed

- successful completion of all commitments to students,
- faculty to gracefully apply and transfer to positions in and outside of Bronson,
- its last class to graduate just one year before WMU graduated its first.

The hospital's 98-year history was intertwined with the school, virtually existing as a unit since their inception. Loss of the School of Nursing would require a grieving process to honor thousands of nurses who had received their first nursing credential there. Numerous Bronson graduates were employed by the hospital and in the community. The Alumni Association of BMH School of Nursing was the glue keeping all living graduates throughout the U.S.A. and world in close contact through its newsletter and Kalamazoo-site brunches each year in the spring and fall.

Ulshafer understood the grief and loss that would accompany the school's closure and was instrumental in financing and planning a weekend commemorative event in May 1998 that was the frosting on the closure cake. The event was congruent with the graduation date of the last class and six months before December, 1998, when all students were officially graduated, records transferred to WMU, and the school's doors closed. She supported Nedeau-Cayo, the faculty, Bronson's newest graduates and the Alumni Association in this significant emotional event! She was the mistress of ceremonies as a fitting end to almost one hundred years of nursing education services. The ceremony will never be forgotten by those who participated and, to this day, hold school loyalty close to their hearts.

CHAPTER 10 NOTES

---

[1] CCRN represents certification in critical care nursing. Nurses must apply, have experience in critical care nursing, meet continuing education requirements, and pass an examination periodically.

[2] The National League for Nursing offered standardized exams focusing on areas of nursing specific to course content. Schools could purchase the exams and receive data comparing students in diploma, associate degree and baccalaureate programs. The exams offered the opportunity to improve the program and to counsel students about interpretation of exam outcomes.

[3] The original nurse extern program, as conceived by Christine Davis, Judy Stewart and Jacqueline Wylie, was established in 1984. Davis, then an Andrews University graduate student needed a class project, and Bronson School of Nursing faculty mentored her.

[4] Davis, C., Stewart, J. & Wylie, J. "Nurse externs–an economic way to strengthen your nursing staff." Unpublished manuscript, 1985.

[5] Quote from an in-house 1990 October 31 memorandum to the nursing directors from Linda Van Dyke and Jacqueline Wylie, "Recommendations for 1991-92 Nurse Extern Program."

[6] American Nurses Association. *The scope of nursing practice.* Kansas City, Missouri: ANA, 1987. p. 2.

[7] Gebbie, K.M. & Lavin, MA *Classification of nursing diagnoses, proceedings of the first national conference.* St. Louis: C.V. Mosby, 1975.

[8] Nursing instructors were paired to teach specific nursing courses, most often with 16 to 20 students enrolled per class.

[9] *Healthlines*, 1998 May 12–25, "Bronson's final nursing class graduates."

[10] Roberta Hunt changed her surname to Utrecht when she married in 1992.

[11] Frequent conversations with Rosemarie Nedeau-Cayo, from 1995 to 2004 provided stories related to the School's last days, closure and her transition to the Educational Services Department.

[12] Oral interview with Roberta Hunt Utrecht by Jackie Wylie, 1997 November 12.

[13] When census was low, it was not uncommon for nurses to go home early. Because they were paid hourly wages, they lost a portion of their wages. Nurses often welcomed the relief and did not object, and the nurses who needed a full day of pay worked. Overtime was paid to hourly workers. Staff nurses worried about remuneration if they were paid a salary that they would most often work 50 to 60 hour weeks, which many did.

[14] Twenty-five continuing education hours every two years became mandatory for nurses, regulated by the Michigan State Board of Nursing.

---

[15] Buresh, B. and Gordon, S. *From silence to voice, what nurses know and must communicate to the public*. Canadian Nurses Association and Cornell University Press, c2000.

[16] Orem, D. *Nursing concepts of practice*, 3rd ed., New York: McGraw-Hill, 1985.

[17] Aiken, L.H., Clarke, S.P., Cheung, R.B., Sloane, D.M. and Silber, J.H. "Educational levels of hospital nurses and surgical patient mortality." *JAMA,* 2003: 290(12); 1617.

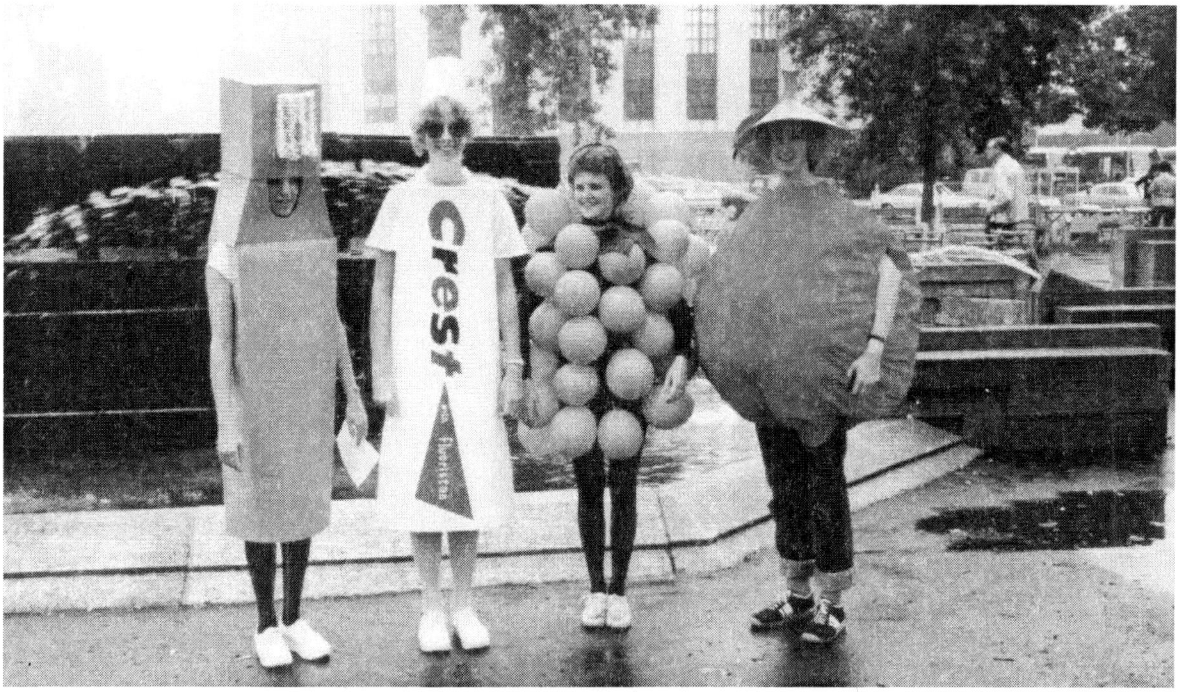

167. (top) Bronson Park Health Fair, 1980.

168. (bottom foreground) Instructors Brad Corbin and Barbara Potts confer with student Cheryl Howard (center), late 1980s.

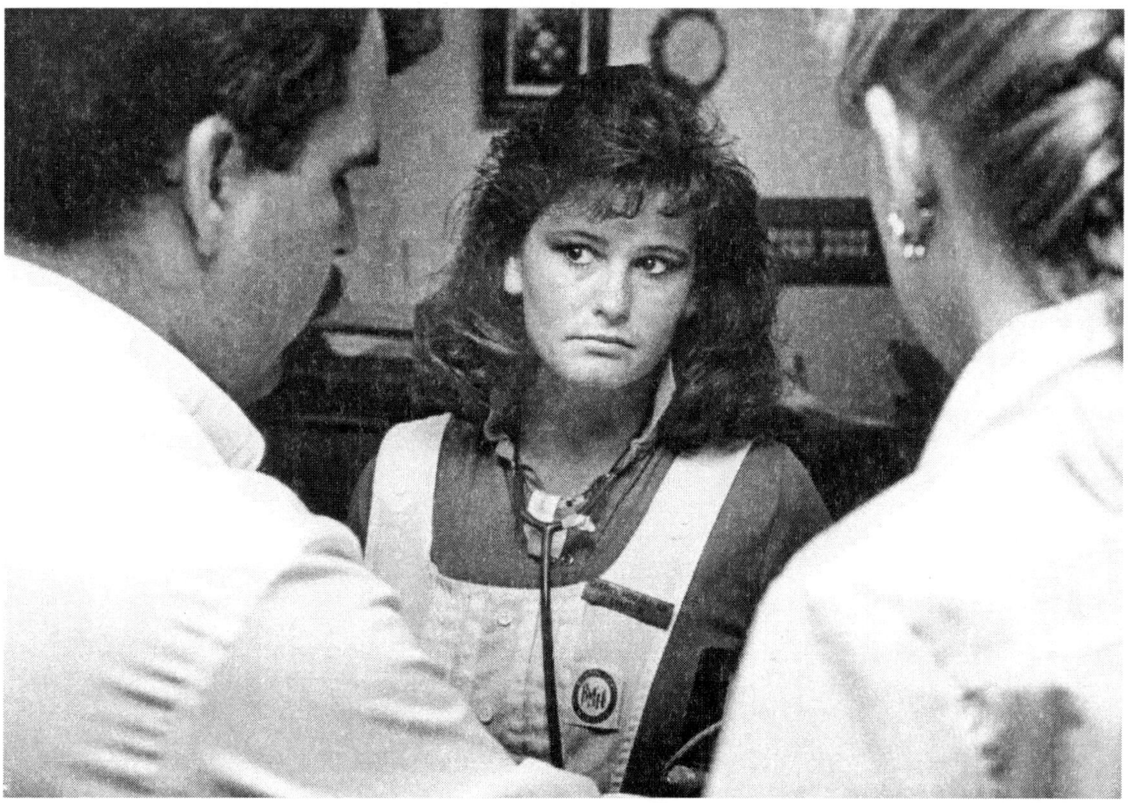

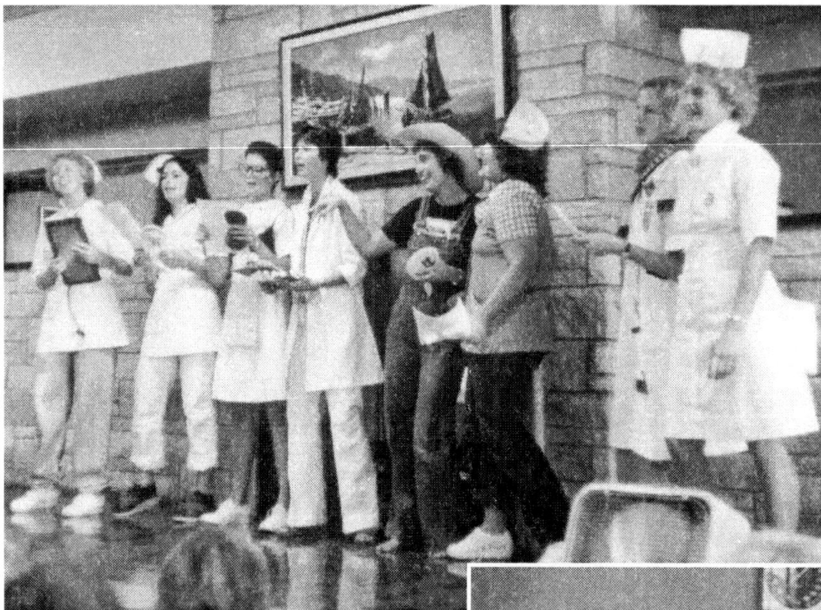

169. (left) Welcome Freshmen Skit, Truesdale Hall, 1980.

170. (below) Rebecca Lusso takes a patient's blood pressure, 1980.

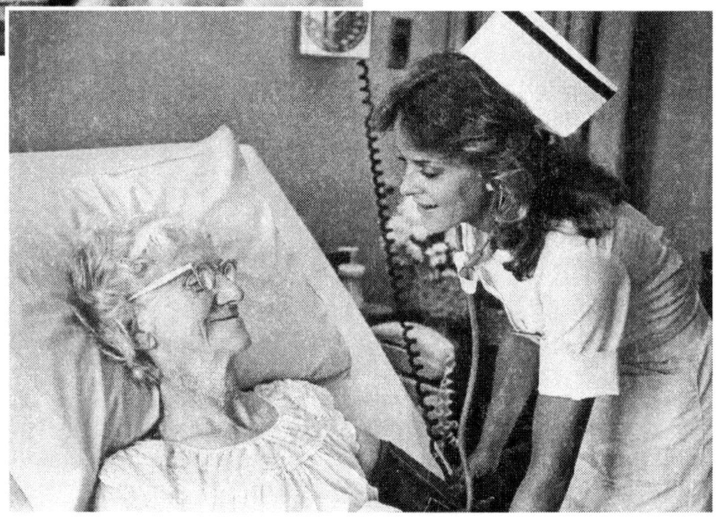

171. (below) Mary Lou Stewart, Bronson archivist, consults with Jeanne Hartenstein, Bronson Methodist Hospital librarian 1980s.

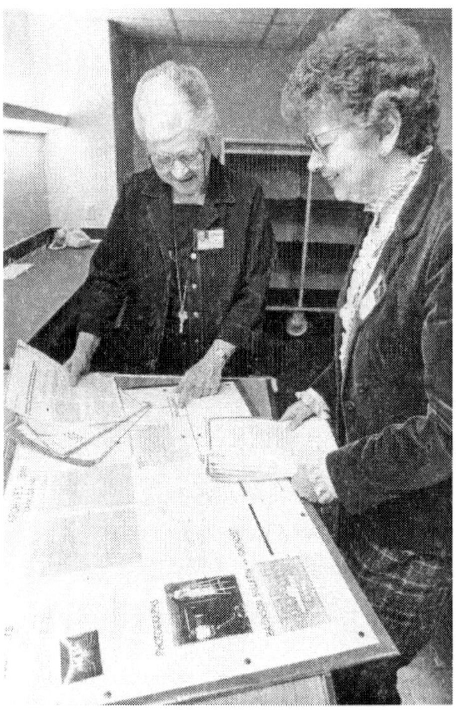

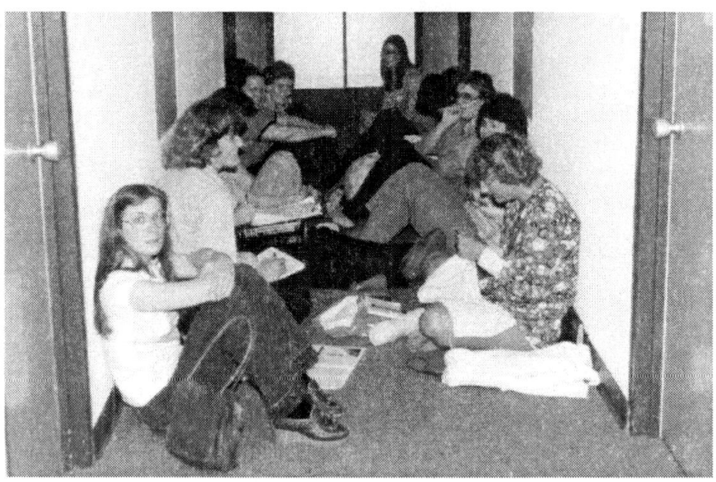

172. (right) Corridor safety shown during the 1980 tornado.

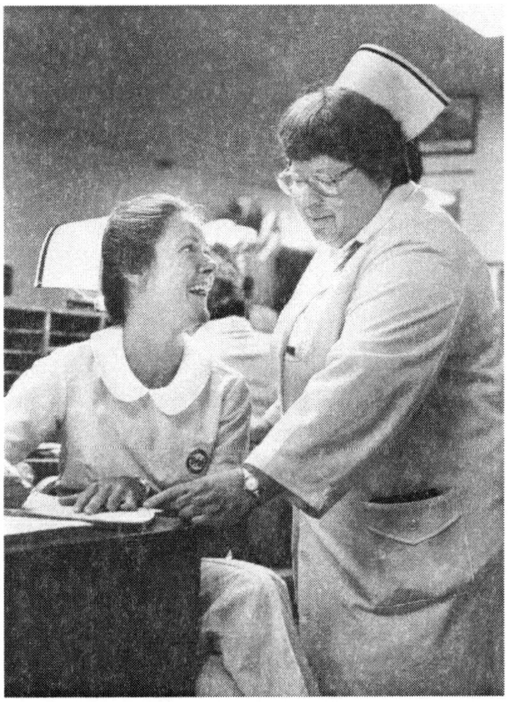

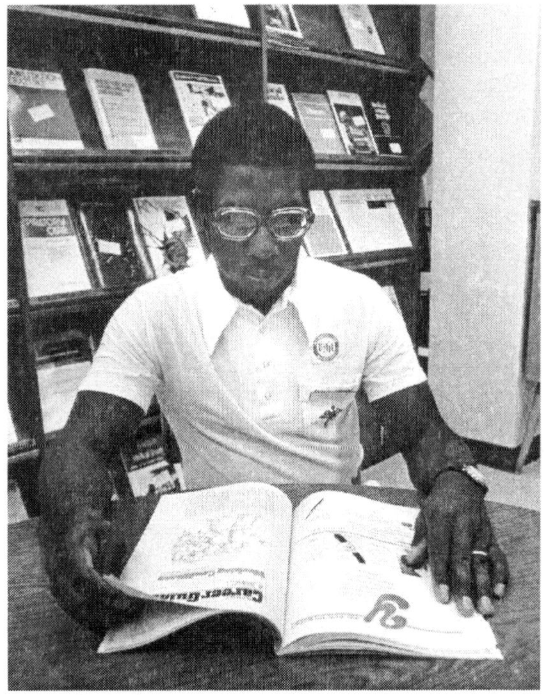

173. (above left) Student Joan Ratliff receives instruction from Mary Lou Mason, early 1980s.
174. (above right) Leonzo Hudson, Jr., studies in the library, 1980.

175. (below) Laura Karsonovich checks the vital signs of an Oncology Unit patient, 1985.

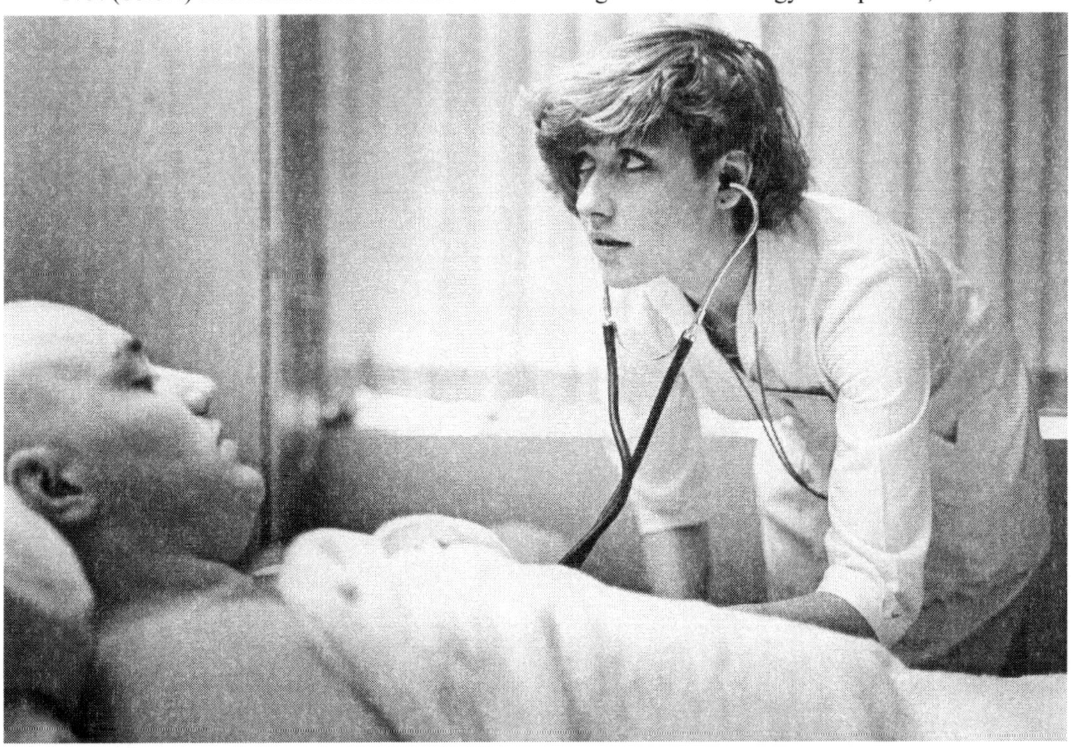

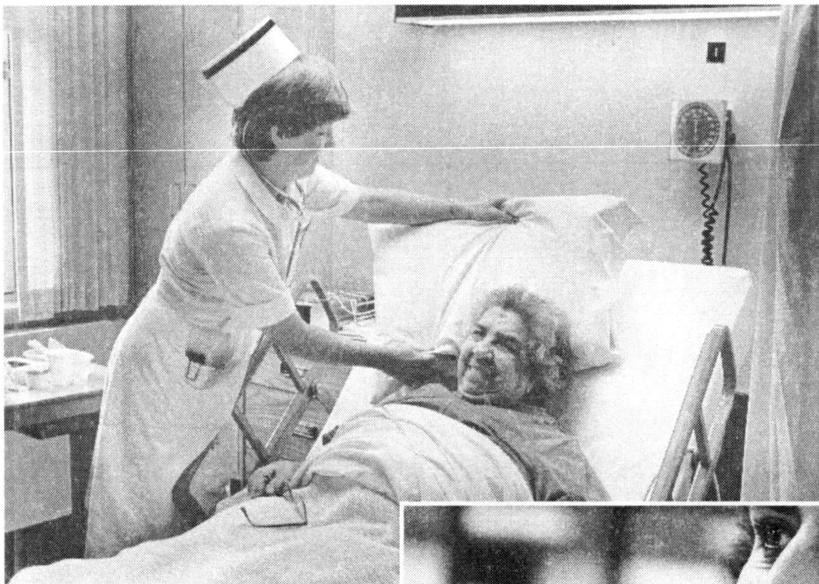

176. (left) Sandra Rohwetter adjusts the comfort pillow for her patient Georgia Wier, ca 1981.

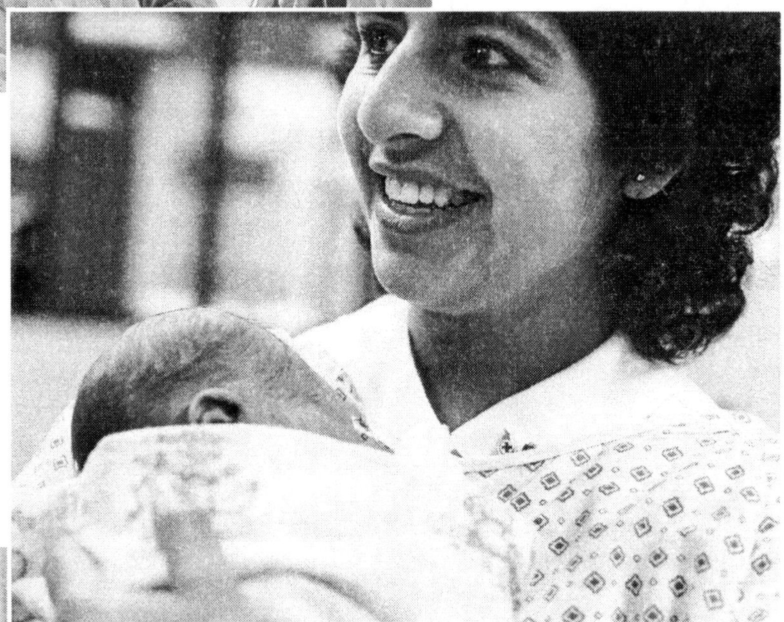

177. (right) Amal Mansour holds a newborn, ca 1984.

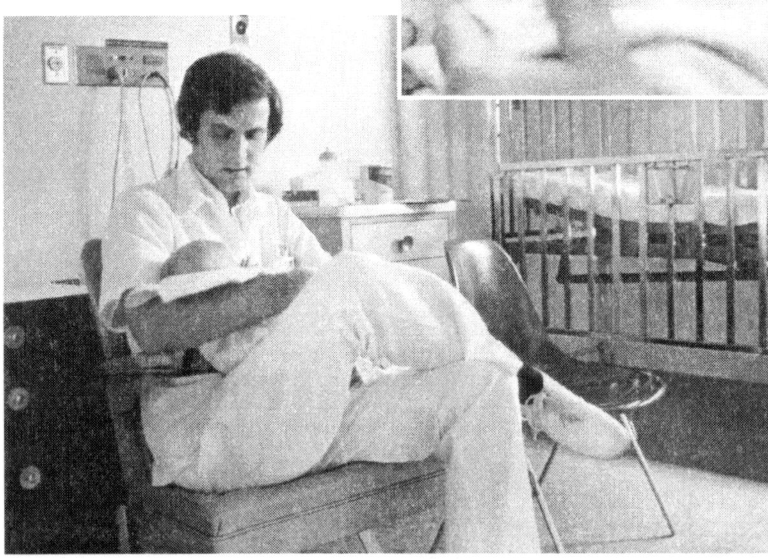

178. (left) Steven Rice cares for a pediatric patient, 1981.

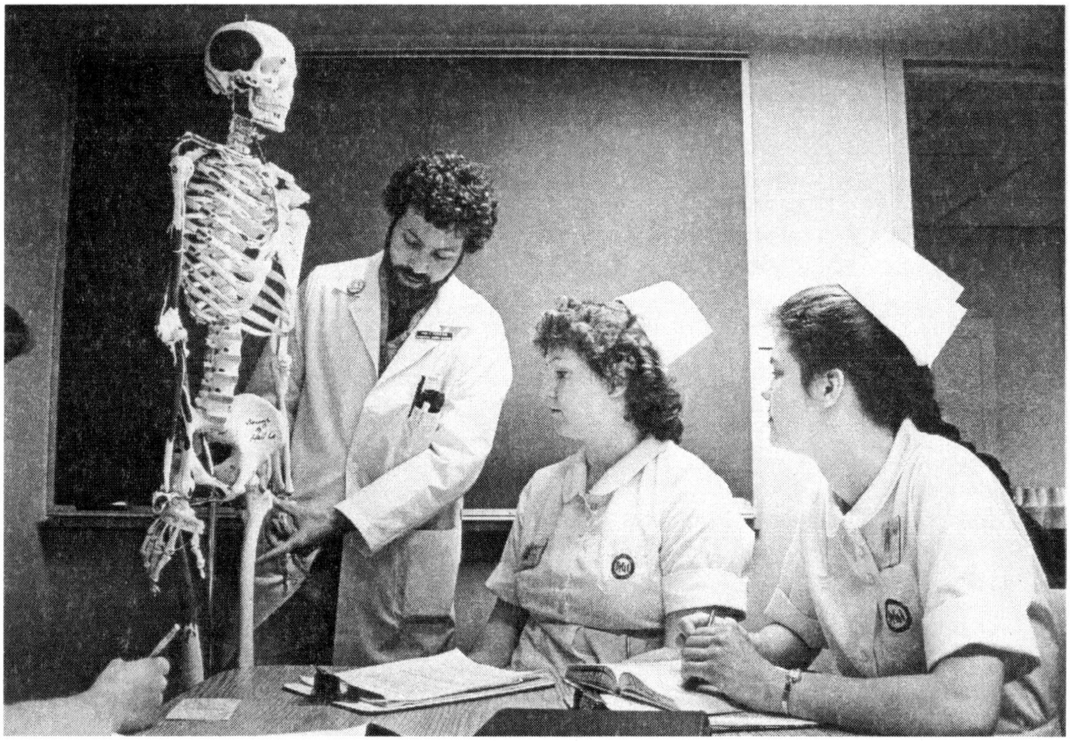

179. (above) Students Jina McIlvenny and Teresa Olsen receive an anatomy lesson from an Orthopedic Surgery resident, 1983.

180. (bottom left) Helen Weber, Director of the School of Nursing, 1970s
181. (bottom right) Marie Stoline giving foot care to a geriatric patient, 1984.

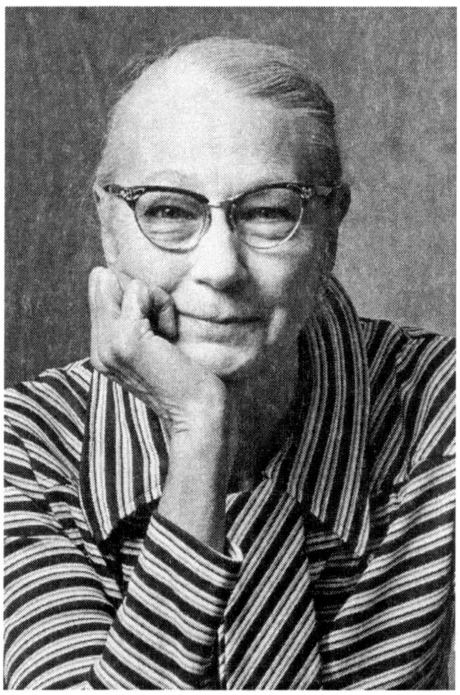

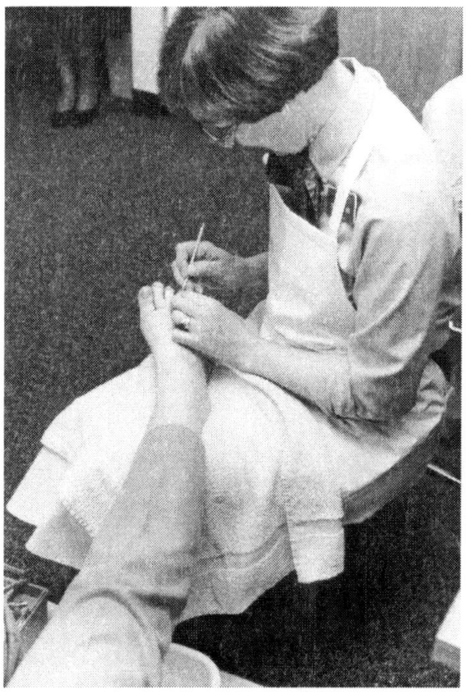

182. (right) Lori Rolph shows concern for a critical patient, late 1980s.

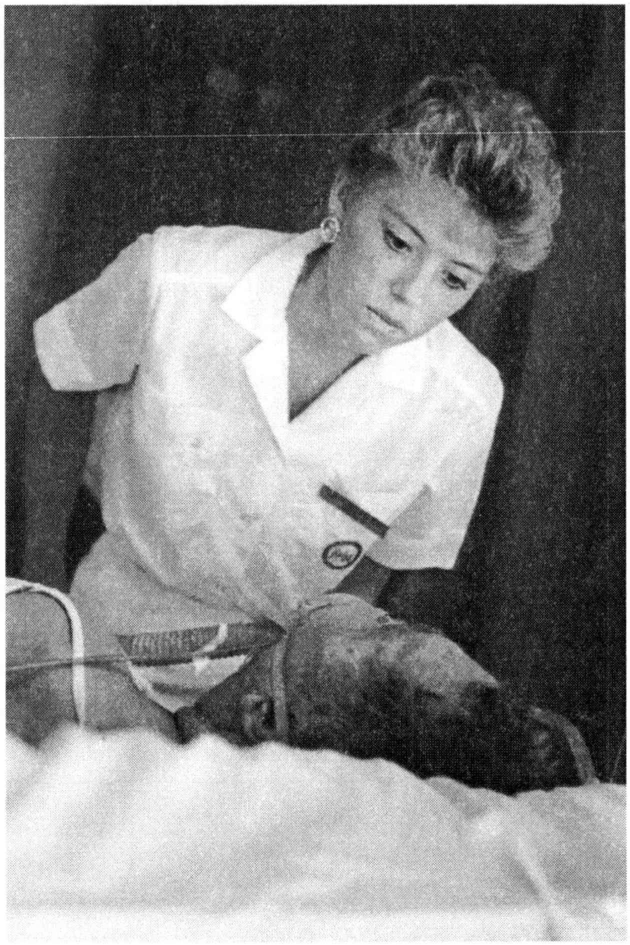

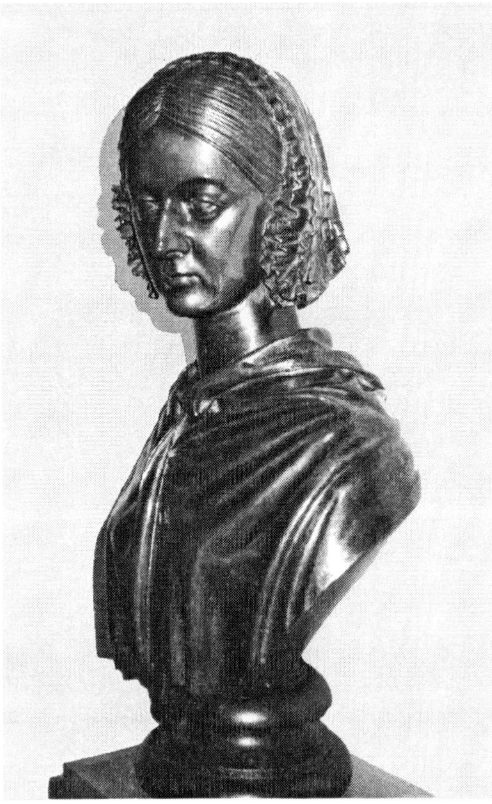

183. (above) Florence Nightingale bust located in her namesake museum, London.

184. (below) CareFlite nurses Michelle Weese and Jim LaForge, late 1980s.

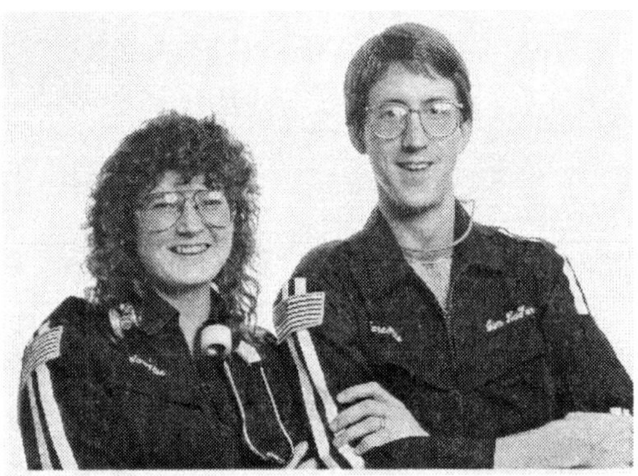

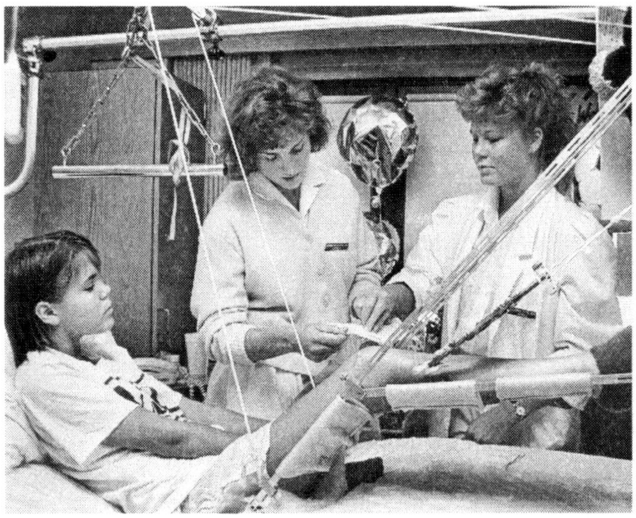

185. (above) Duana Webster and Susan Vite with patient on Orthopedic Ward, ca late 1980s.

186. (right) Jackie Wylie, Director of the School of Nursing, 1980s.

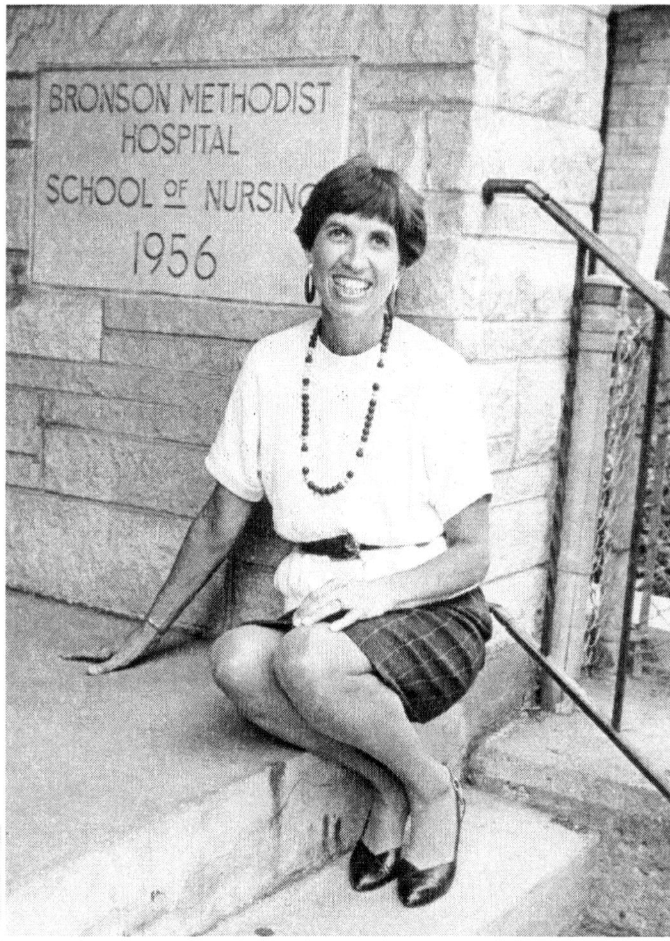

187. (below) Bronson Methodist Hospital looking southeast from the corner of Lovell and John Streets. The building facing John Street is the entrance to Wesley Hall and, directly behind it, is the Center Building.

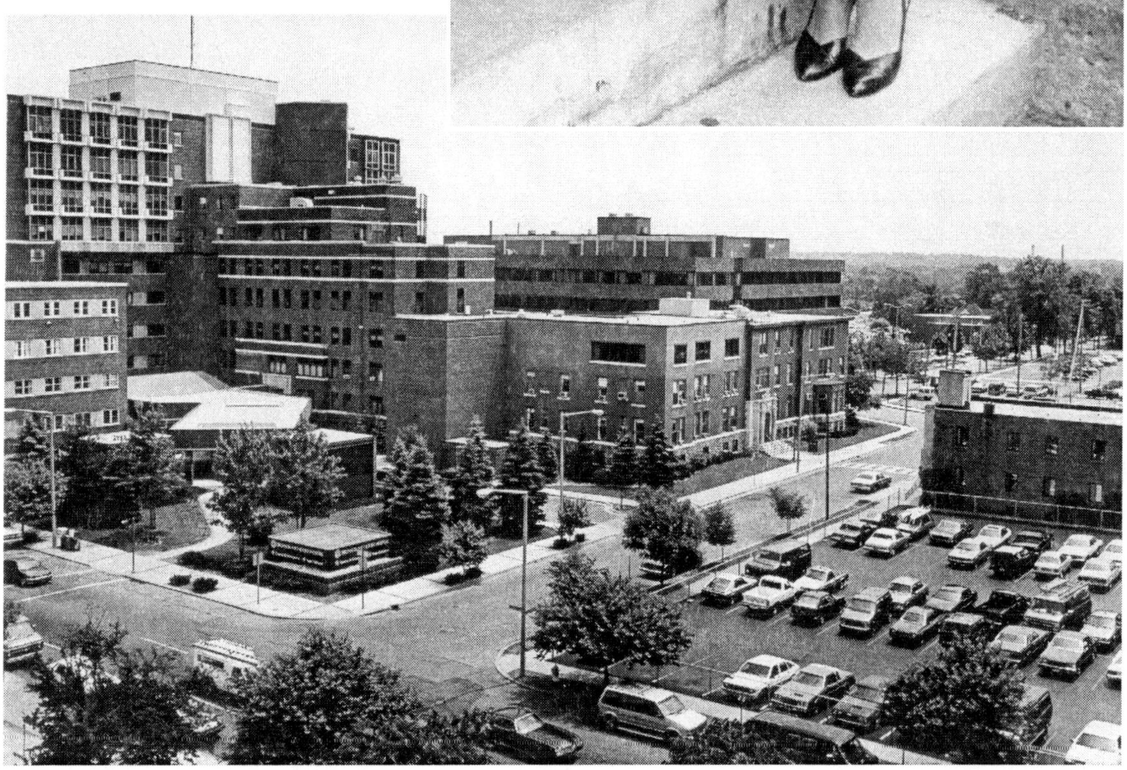

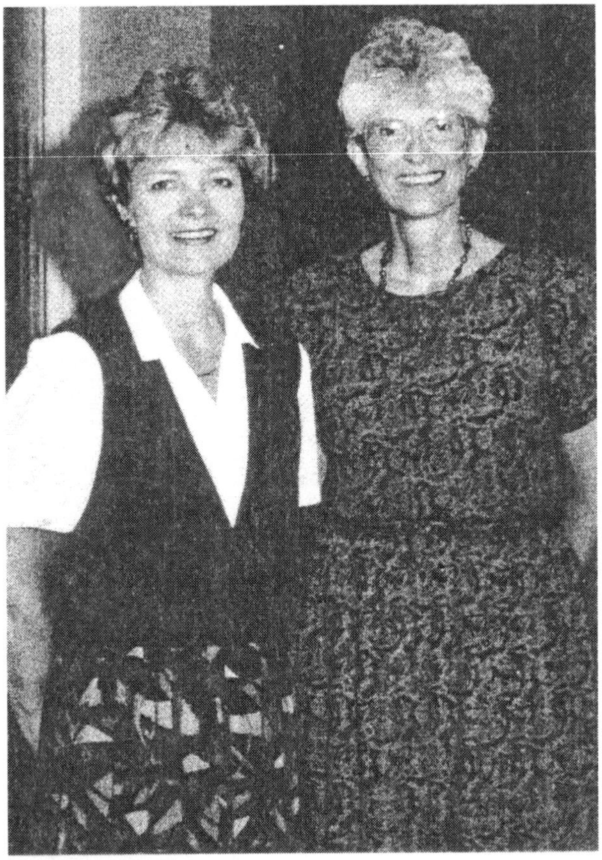

188-189. (left and near below) Carol Van Antwerp and Anna Mae Spaniolo developed this nursing center in Western Michigan University's married student housing center.

190-191. (below) Cultural competence is the focus for these unidentified nursing students with youngsters from international student families

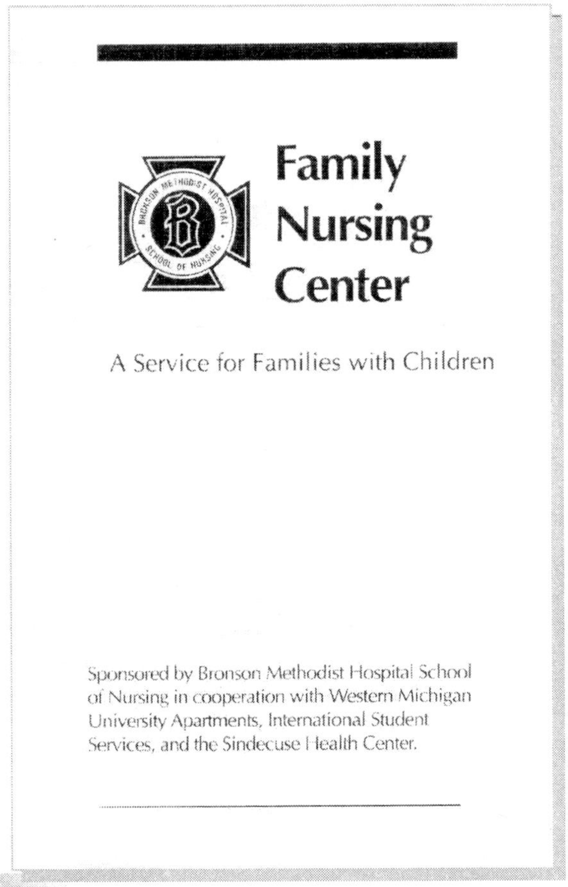

Family Nursing Center

A Service for Families with Children

Sponsored by Bronson Methodist Hospital School of Nursing in cooperation with Western Michigan University Apartments, International Student Services, and the Sindecuse Health Center.

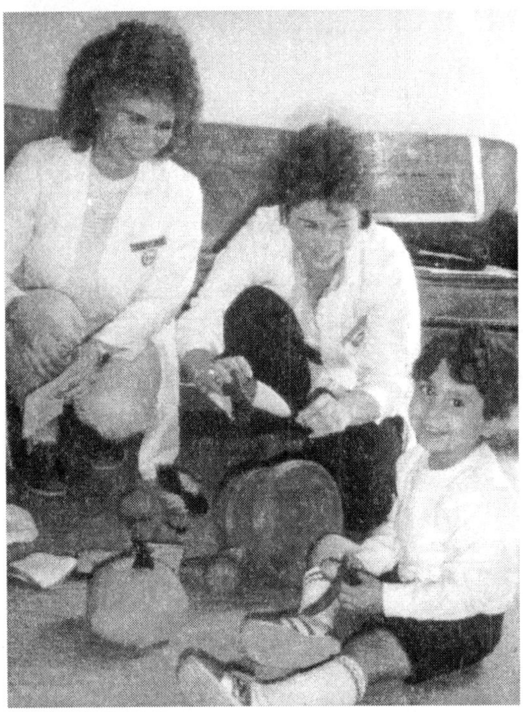

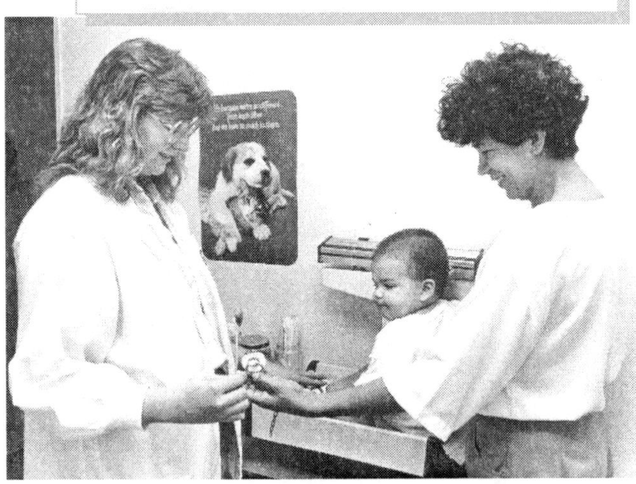

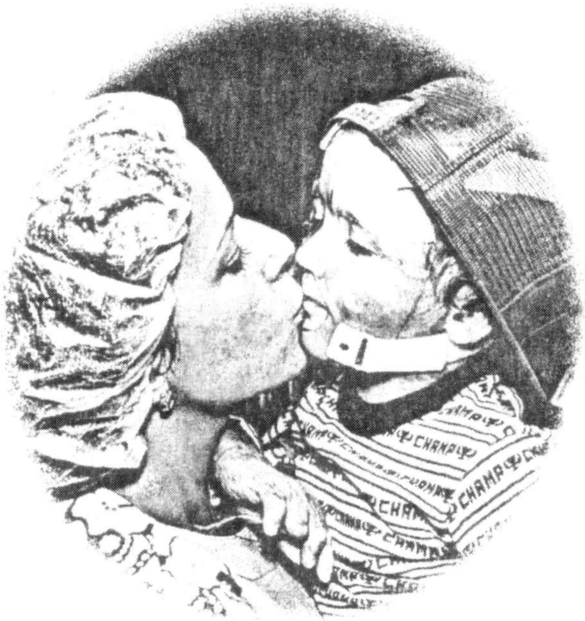

192. Nurse kisses child with burns in photo from the *Catalyst* cover, March 1983.

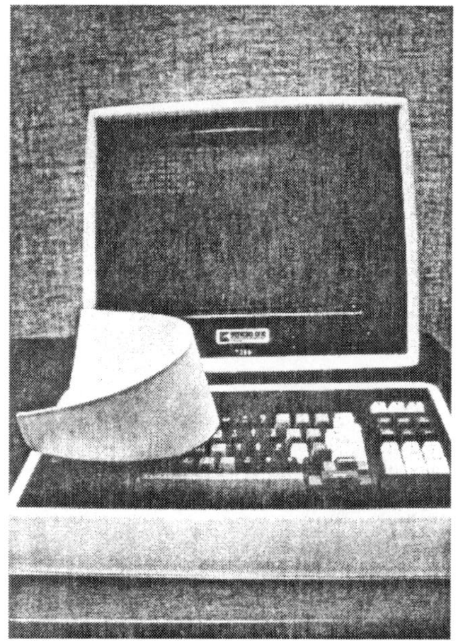

193. Computers come to Bronson, 1980s.

194. (below) Elizabeth Thirtle works with an orthopedic patient, late 1980s.

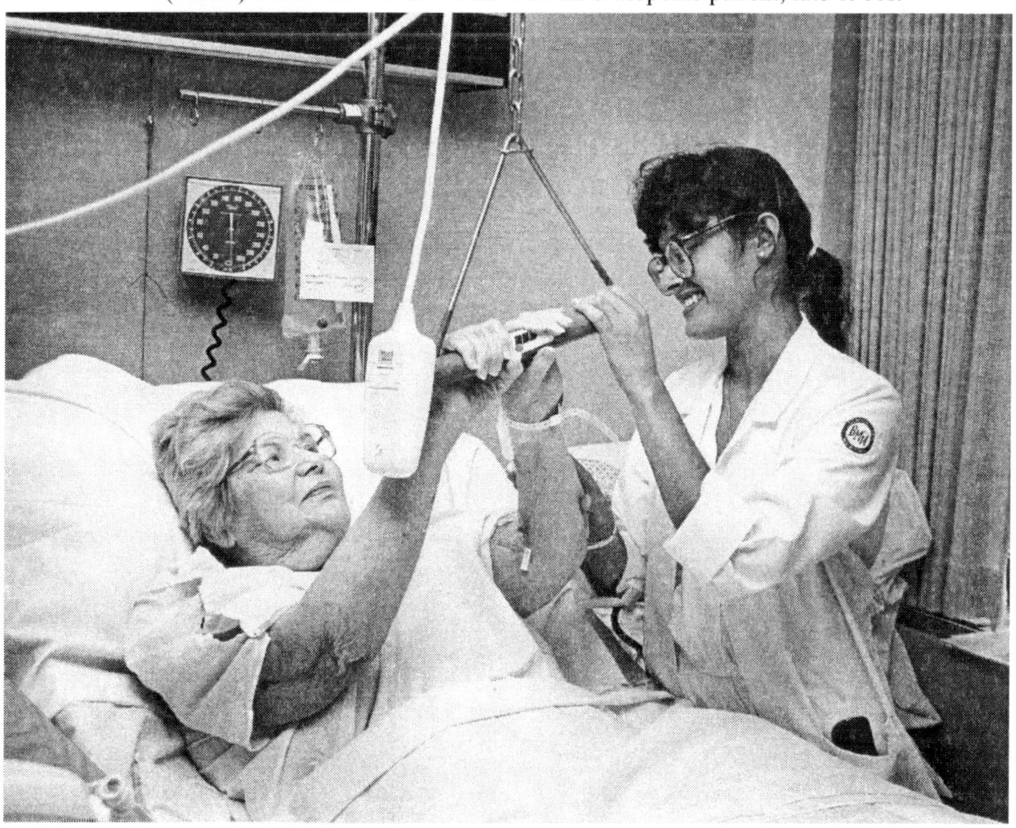

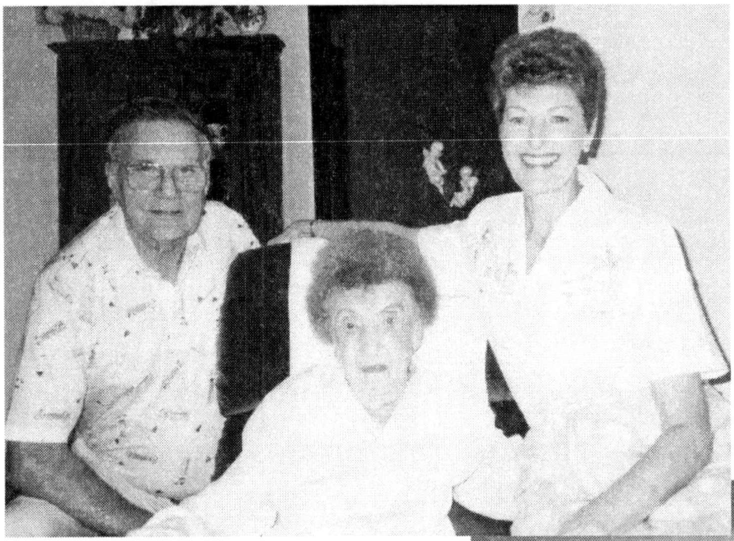

195. (left) Dick and Betty Vander Molen with Jean Lemmer Vander Molen, a 1922 graduate, on her 100th birthday, late 1990s.

196. (below) Instructor Phyllis Curtis, 1980s.

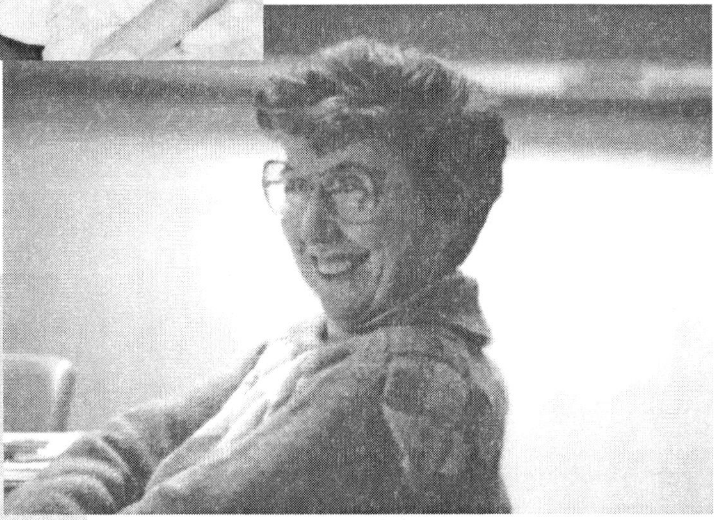

197. (below) Nursing student Aaron Keefe leads a seminar for his peers, early 1990s.

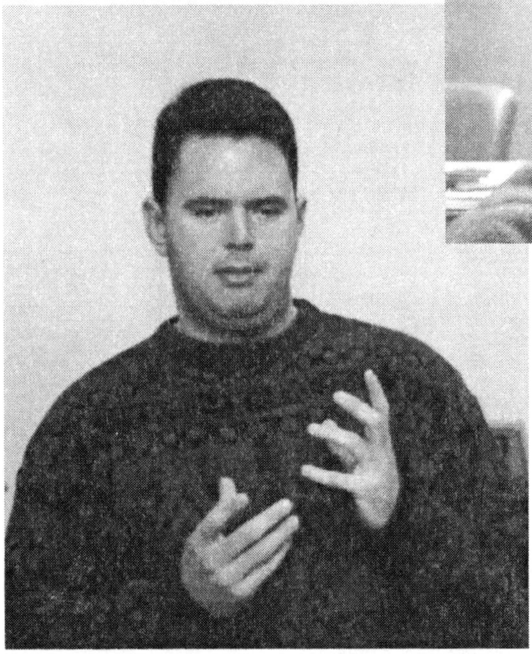

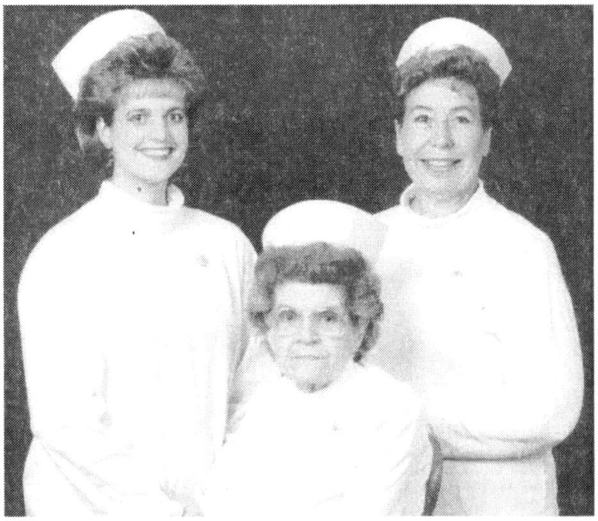

198. (right) Three generations of Bronson School of Nursing graduates: Tracy French, Class of '96, Ruthanna Luttenbacker French, Class of '39, and Linda Meints French, Class of '69.

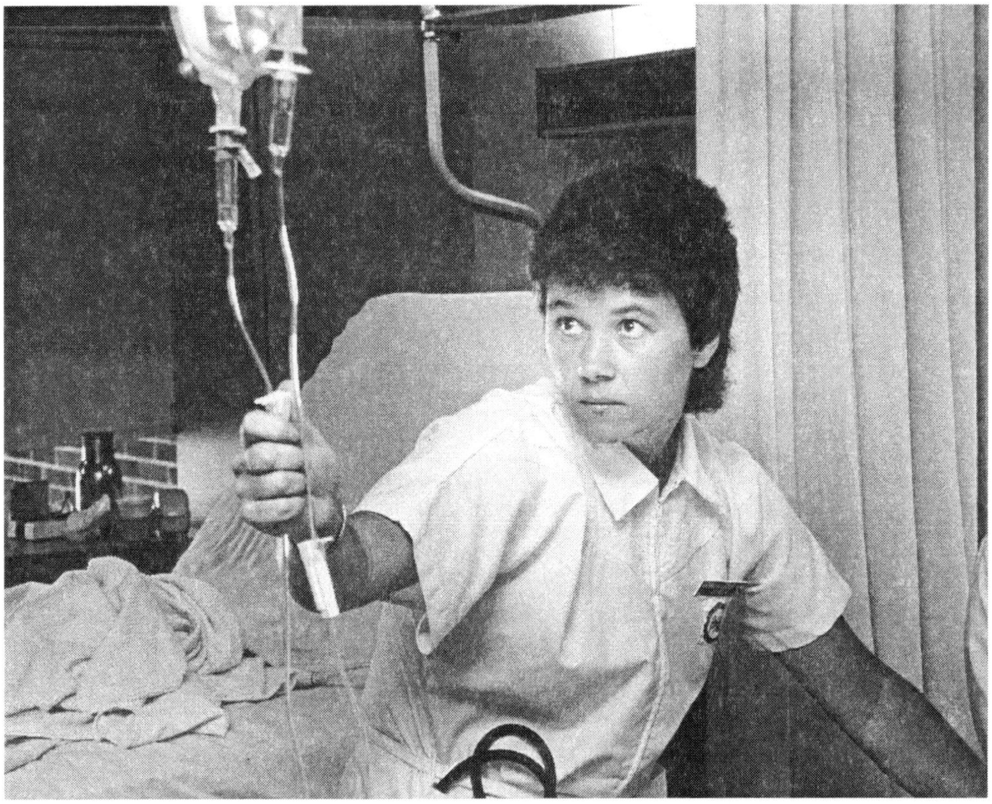

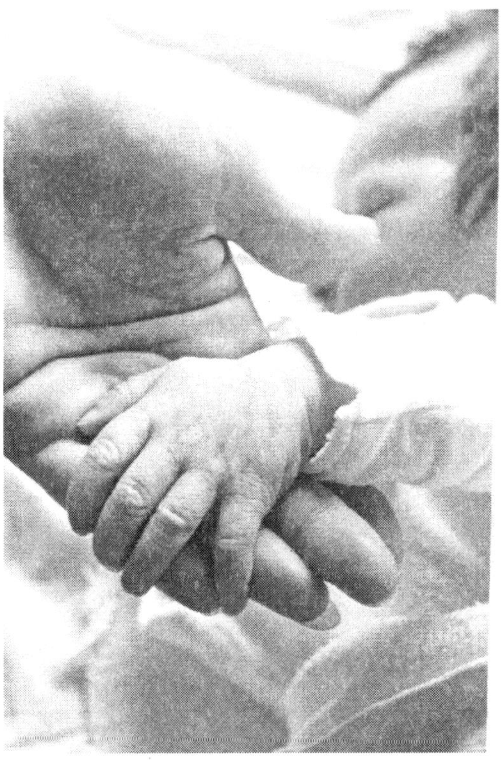

199. (above) Barbara LeDuc adjusts the flow of intravenous feeding, early 1990s.

200. (left) Newborn care.

201. (below) This Bronson logo first appeared in the 1978 *Catalyst* (September).

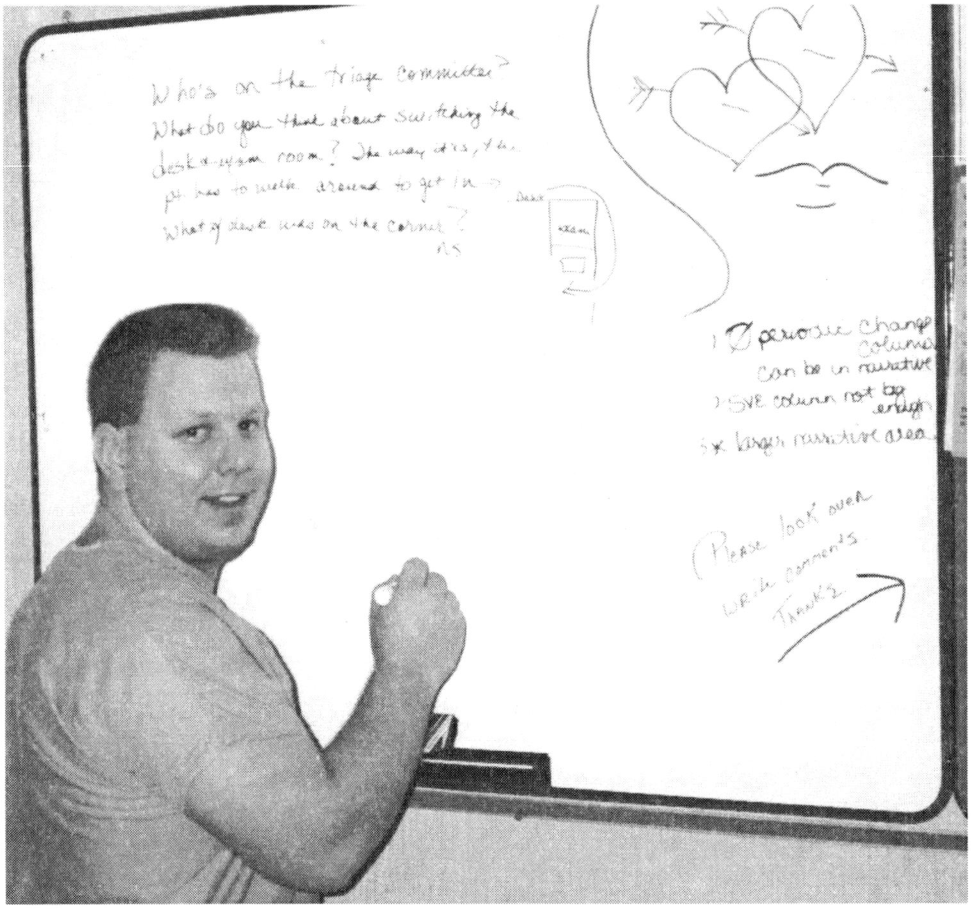
Who's on the triage committee?
Please look over
write comments
Thanks

202 (above) Jim Switzer leads a problem-solving group of fellow nursing students, 1993.

203. (below) Camaraderie at a Christmas brunch for alumni, early 1990s: (left to right) Carol Lawrence, unidentified, Marilyn Ely, Cherie Delger, Wanda Boekhout, Betty Kaub.

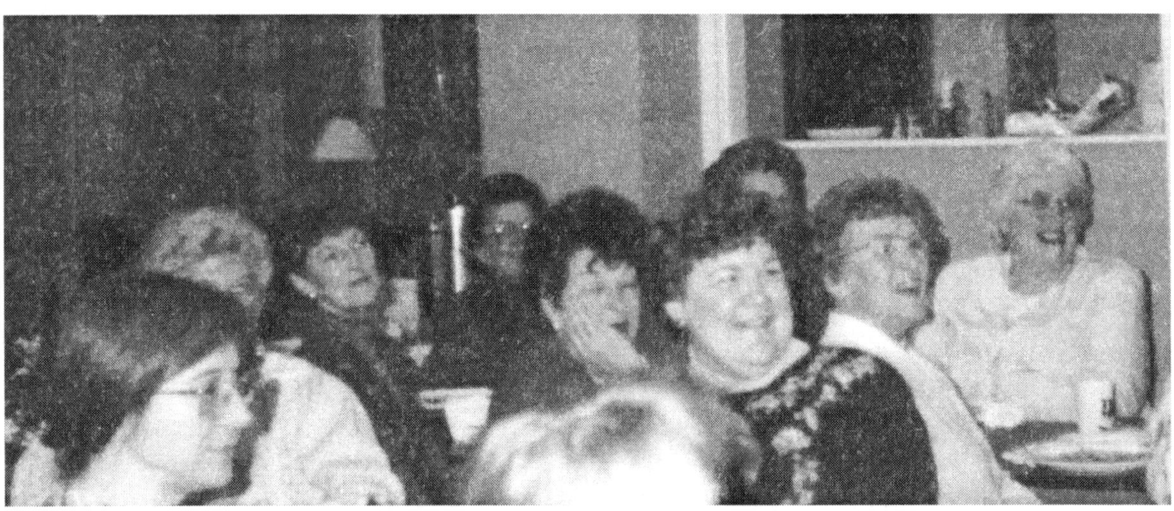

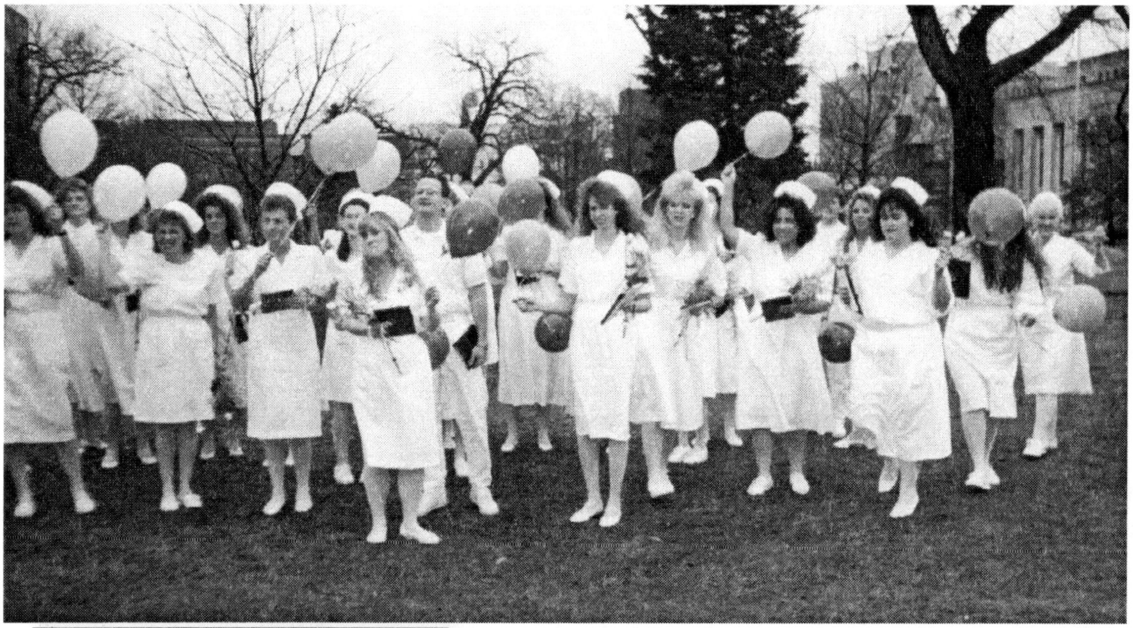

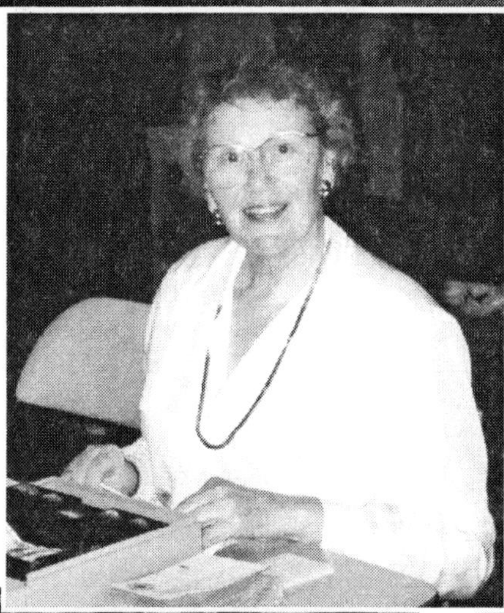

204. (above) At Bronson Park, graduates released colorful balloons after their ceremony. March 1991.

205. (left) Wanda Boekhout and 206. (bottom left) Marie McLeieer work at the Holiday Bazaar, 1996.

207. (below) Amy Beebe, Class of 1994, gives a class presentation.

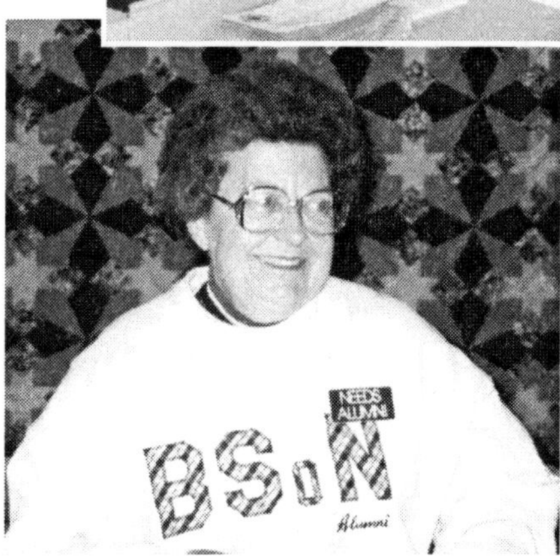

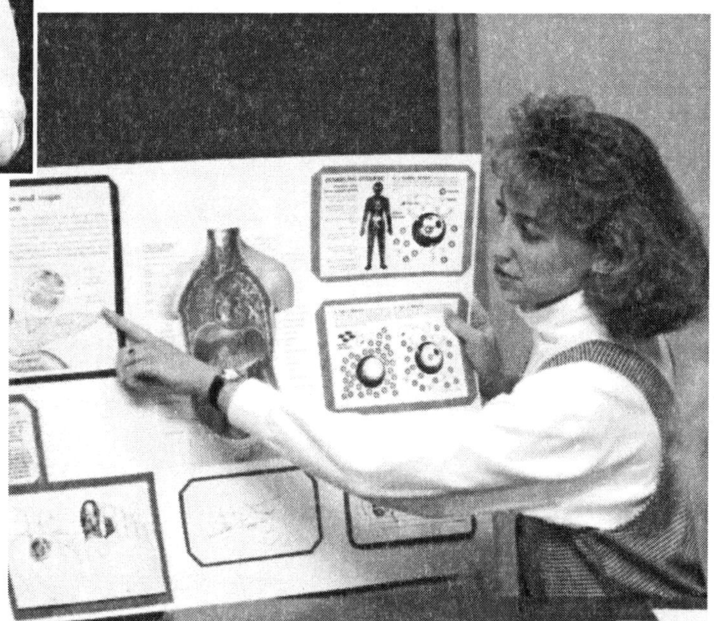

208. (left) Doug Bell gives a nephrology presentation, ca 1993-94.

209. (below) Scott Stockinger hangs out in a dorm room, early 1990s.

210. (right) Katherine Sirlin takes a break at the nursing station, ca 1993-94.

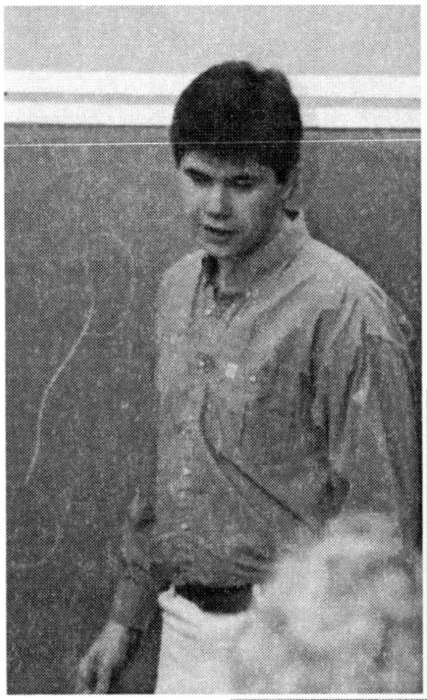

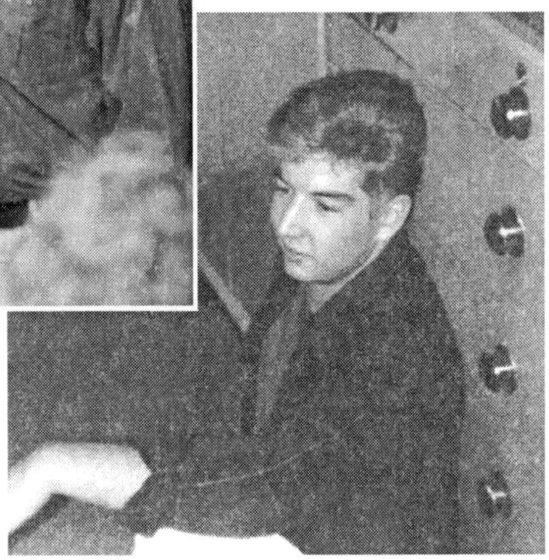

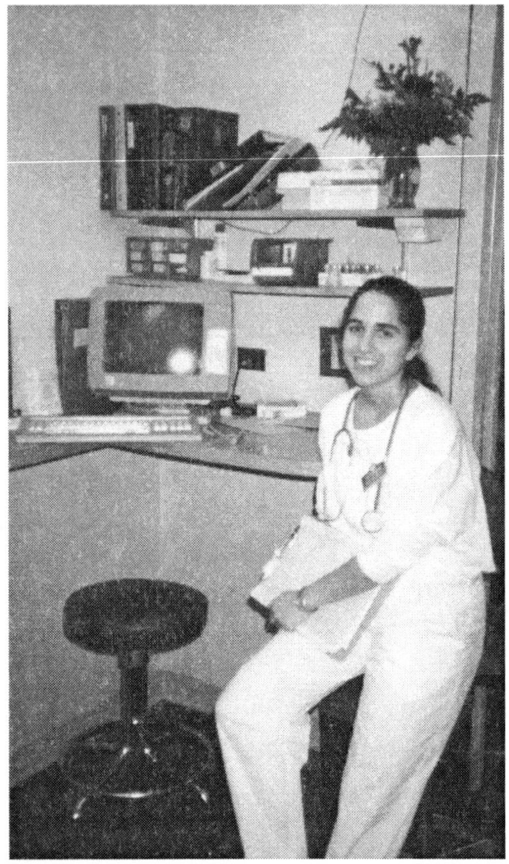

211. (below) Nursing 100 class, September 1993. Back row: Lynnae Brovant, Michelle Battie, Kelli Smith, Mary Good, Lisa Aldrich, Gail Wagoner, Karla Goodman, Lisa Blissick, Melissa Hakes, Jennifer Dull, Julie Dolan, Jennifer Moored, Wendy Cook. Second row: Jennifer Lutri, Leslie Cooley, Monica Mikowski, Dawn Barnard, Katherine Sirlin, Julie Vanbuskirk. Third row: Kim Bickley, Aimee Amos, Amy Beebe, Anne Thomas, Doug Bell, Robin Ray, Mark Vazana, Aaron Keefe. Fourth row: Janet Gillette, Kari Piell, Lynnette Burleson, Tricia Opicka. Not pictured: Cecelia Aaron, Trina Gomez, Polly Pelong.

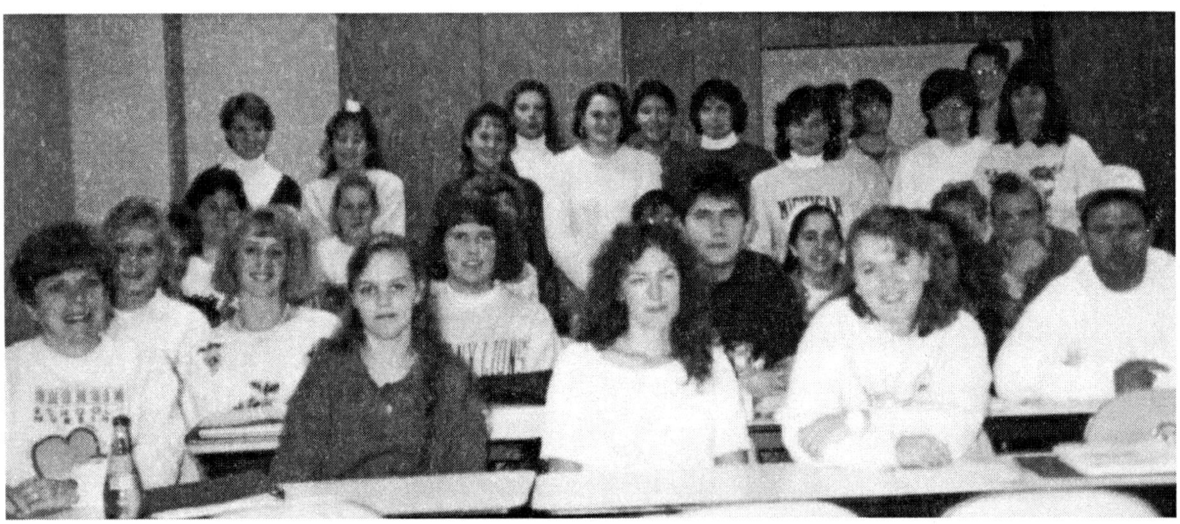

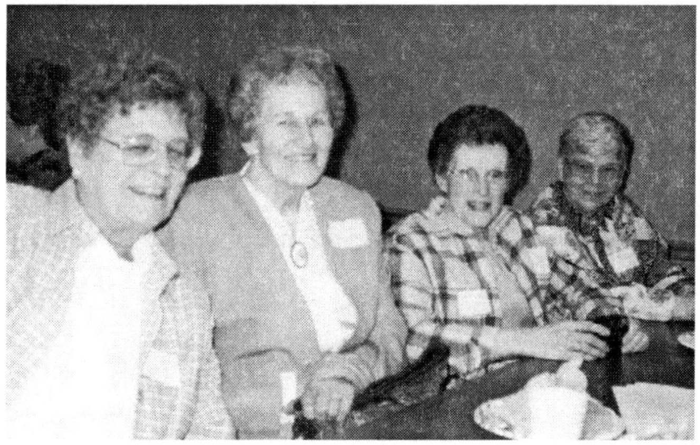

212. (above, left to right) 1949 classmates Ruth Matteson, Marilyn Cardiff, Florence Manning, and Betty Dunn enjoy their time together at spring brunch, 1997.

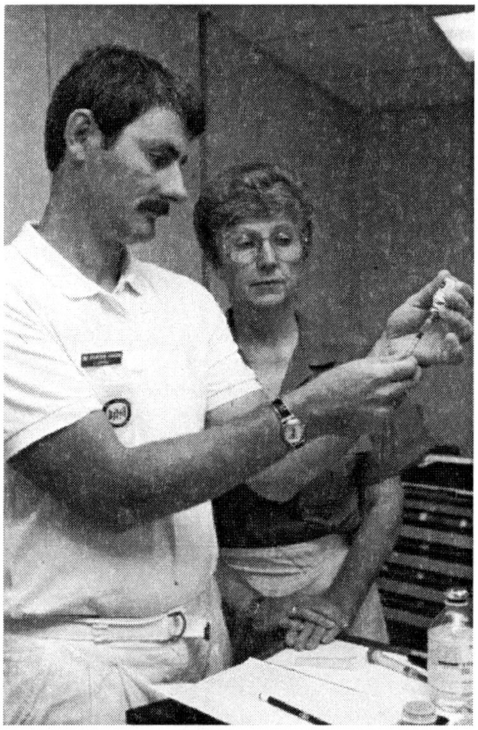

213. (above) Phyllis Curtis observes Mike Koehler demonstrating proper injection technique.

214. (right) Checking for their mail in Truesdale lobby are (left to right) Stephanie Pollum, Janet Bestervelt, Christine Dorey, and Mike Rodgers, 1993-94.

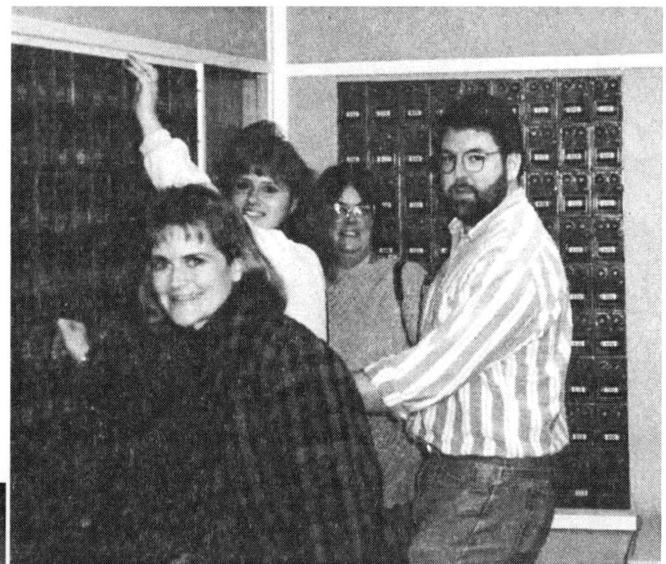

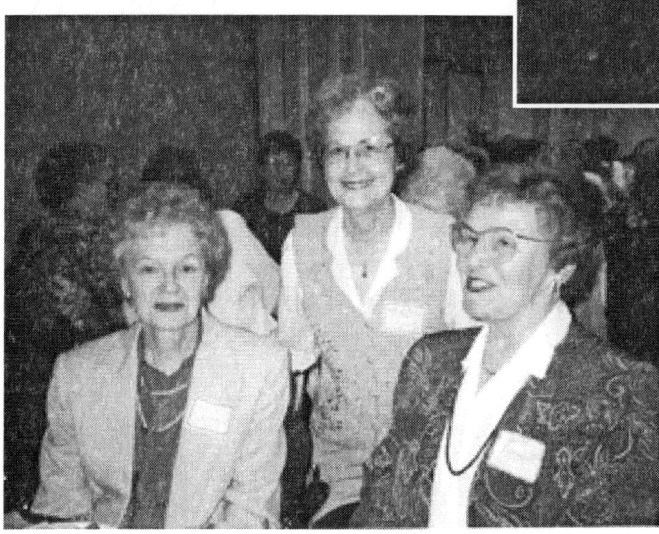

215. (left to right) Lois Vermeulen, Gertrude Sparks, and Wanda Boekhout, Class of 1947 reminisce during spring brunch, April 1997.

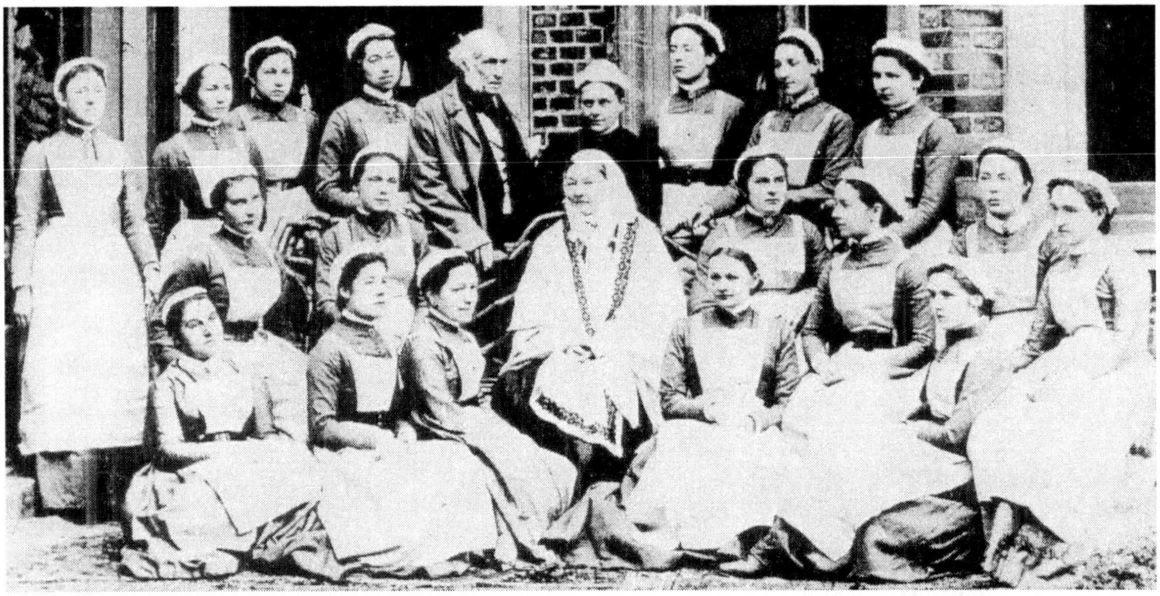

216. (above) Students and staff of the British clinic, Clayton House, that F.N. reorganized in London, 1886.

217. Embley Hall, Nightingale family residence, is now a school, 1990s.

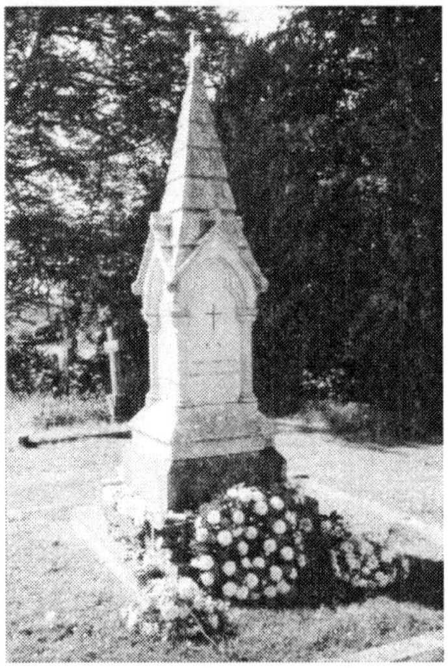

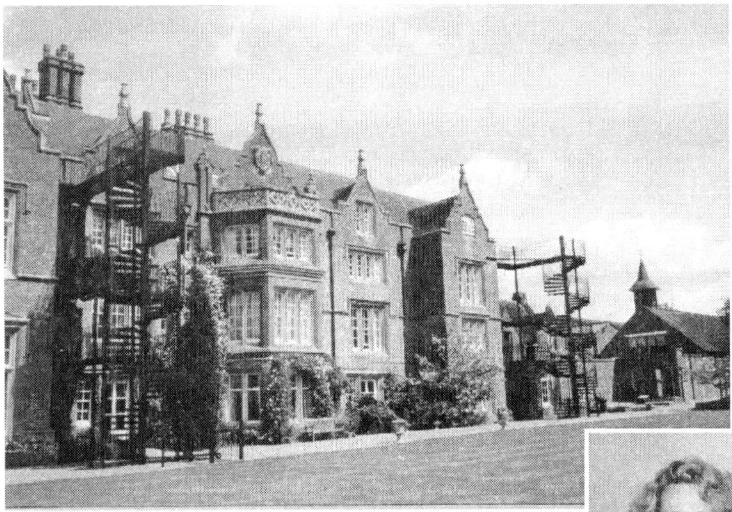

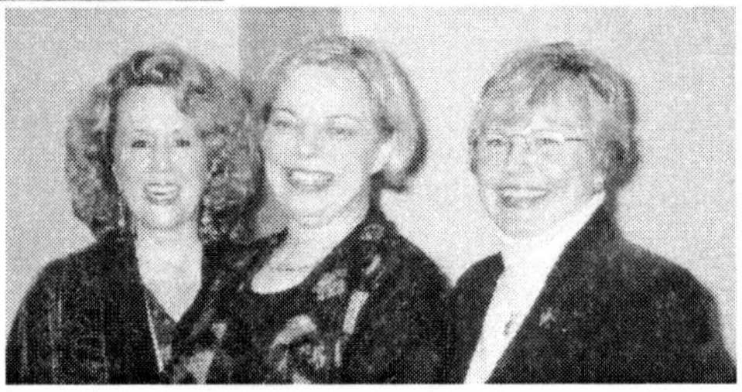

218. (above) Contemporary Nightingale scholars: Barbara Dossey, Diva-Marie Beck, Louise Selanders at ΣΘΤ International Biennial Convention, November 2003.

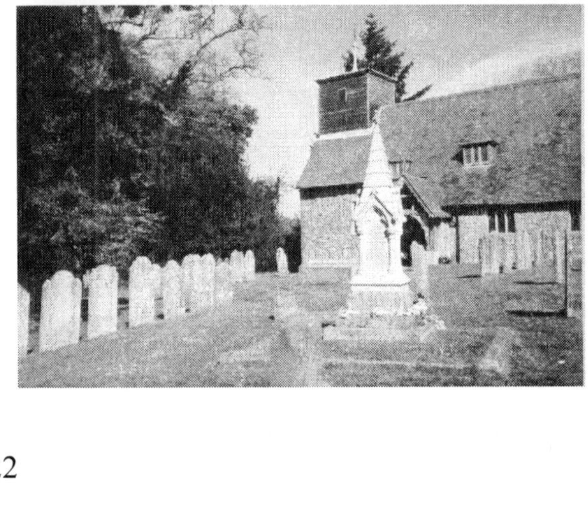

219-220. (left and right above) St. Margaret's churchyard with F.N.'s grave marker, 2003.

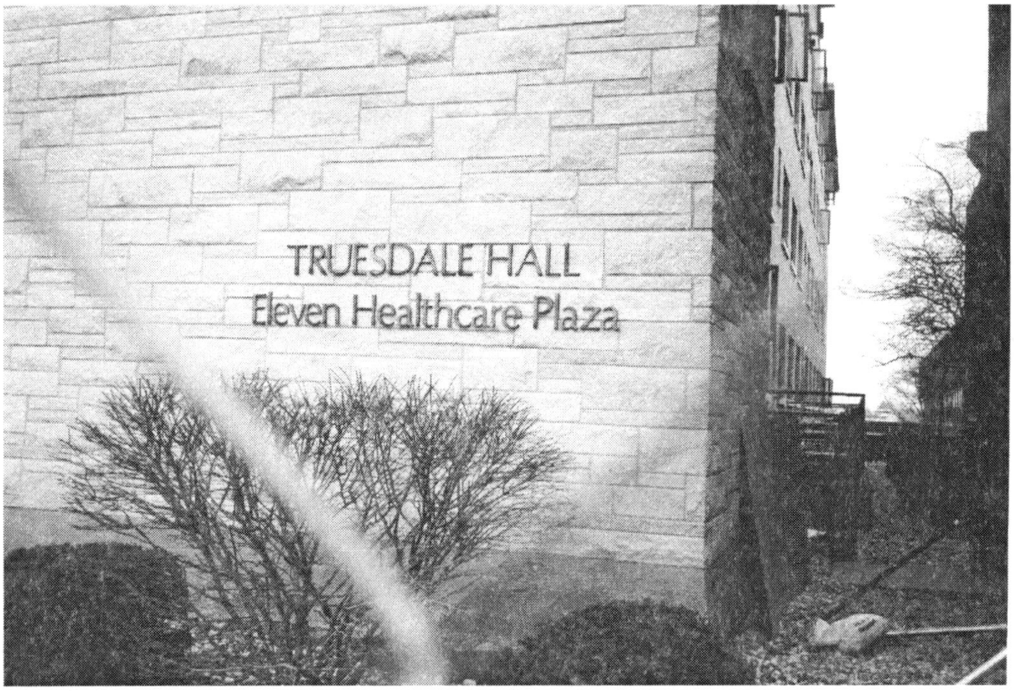

221 and 222. Days before demolition and the alumni's last brunch, 1997.

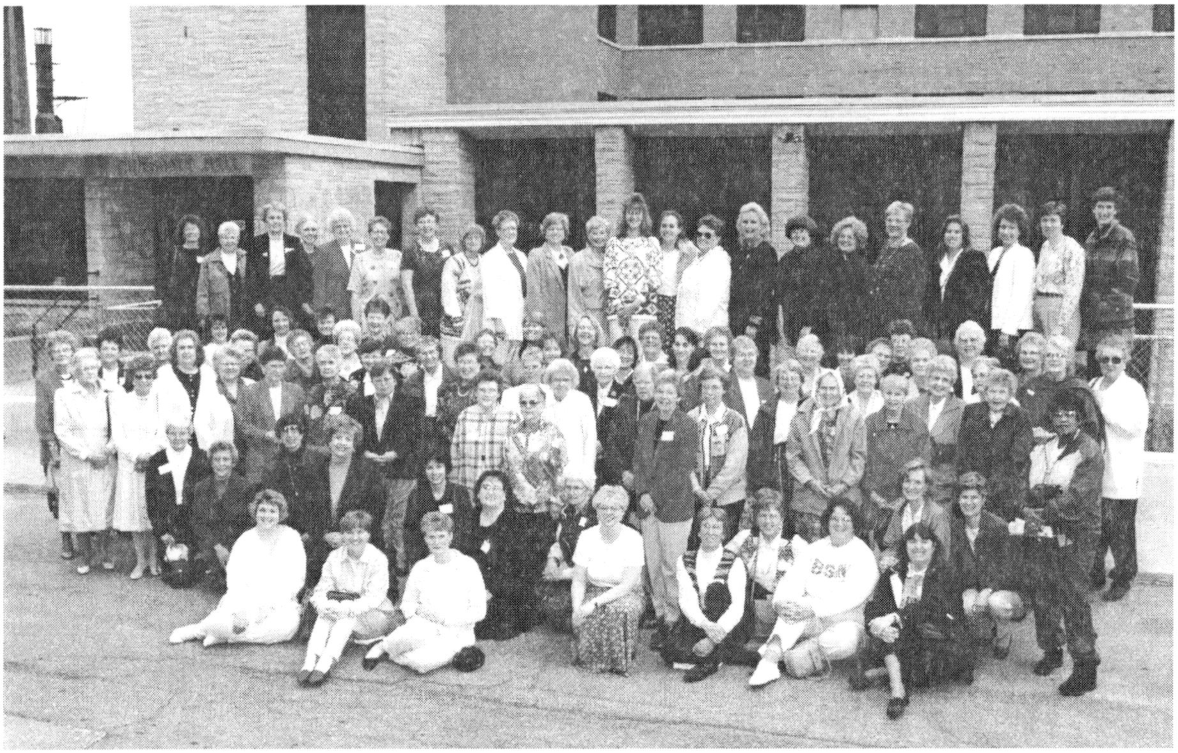

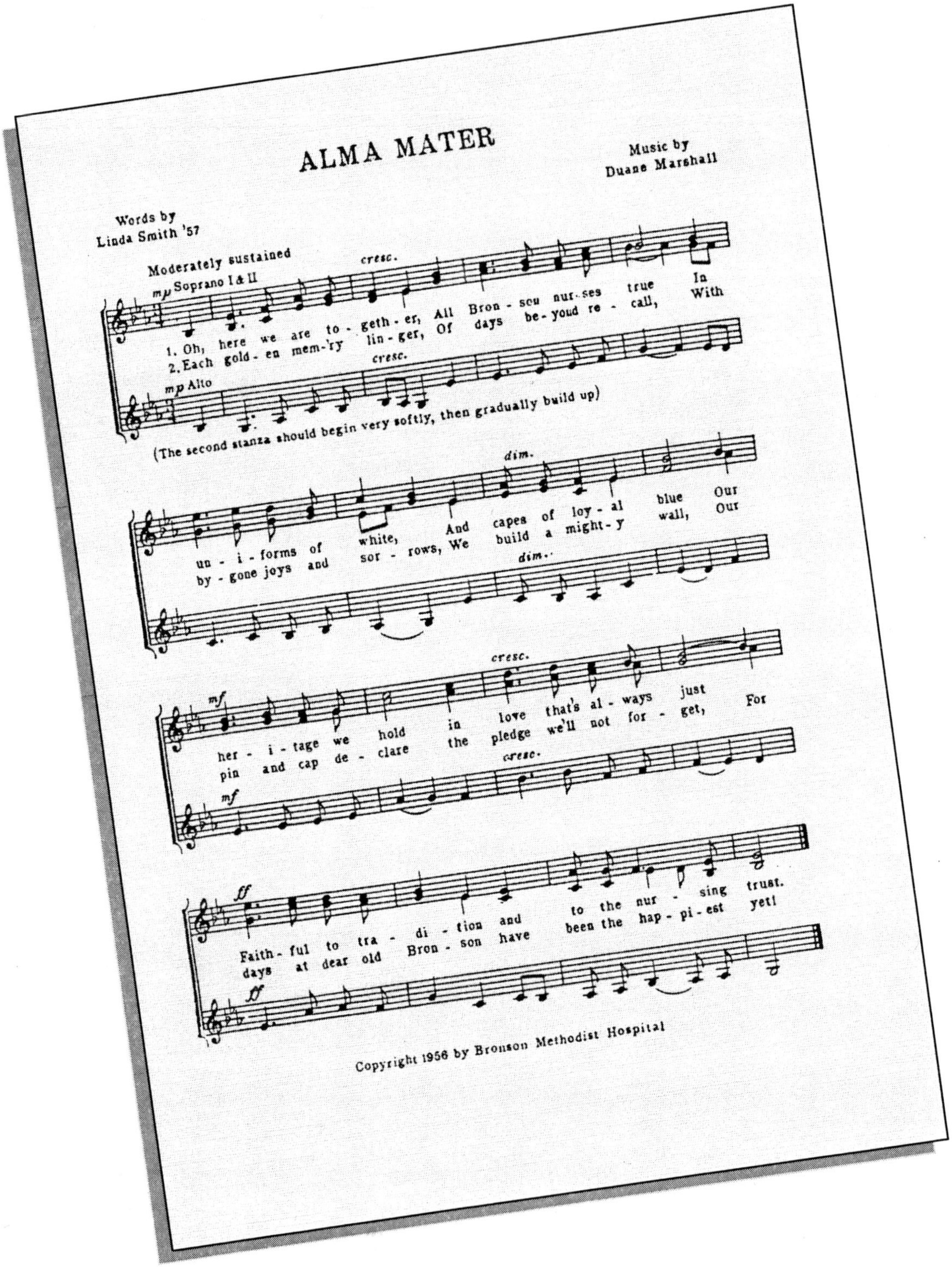
ALMA MATER
Music by
Duane Marshall
Words by
Linda Smith '57
Moderately sustained
cresc.
mp Soprano I & II
1. Oh, here we are to - geth - er, All Bron - son nur - ses true In
2. Each gold - en mem-'ry lin - ger, Of days be - yond re - call, With
mp Alto
(The second stanza should begin very softly, then gradually build up)
dim.
un - i - forms of white, And capes of loy - al blue Our
by - gone joys and sor - rows, We build a might - y wall, Our
mf
her - i - tage we hold in love that's al - ways just For
pin and cap de - clare the pledge we'll not for - get,
ff
Faith - ful to tra - di - tion and to the nur - sing trust.
days at dear old Bron - son have been the hap - pi - est yet!
Copyright 1956 by Bronson Methodist Hospital

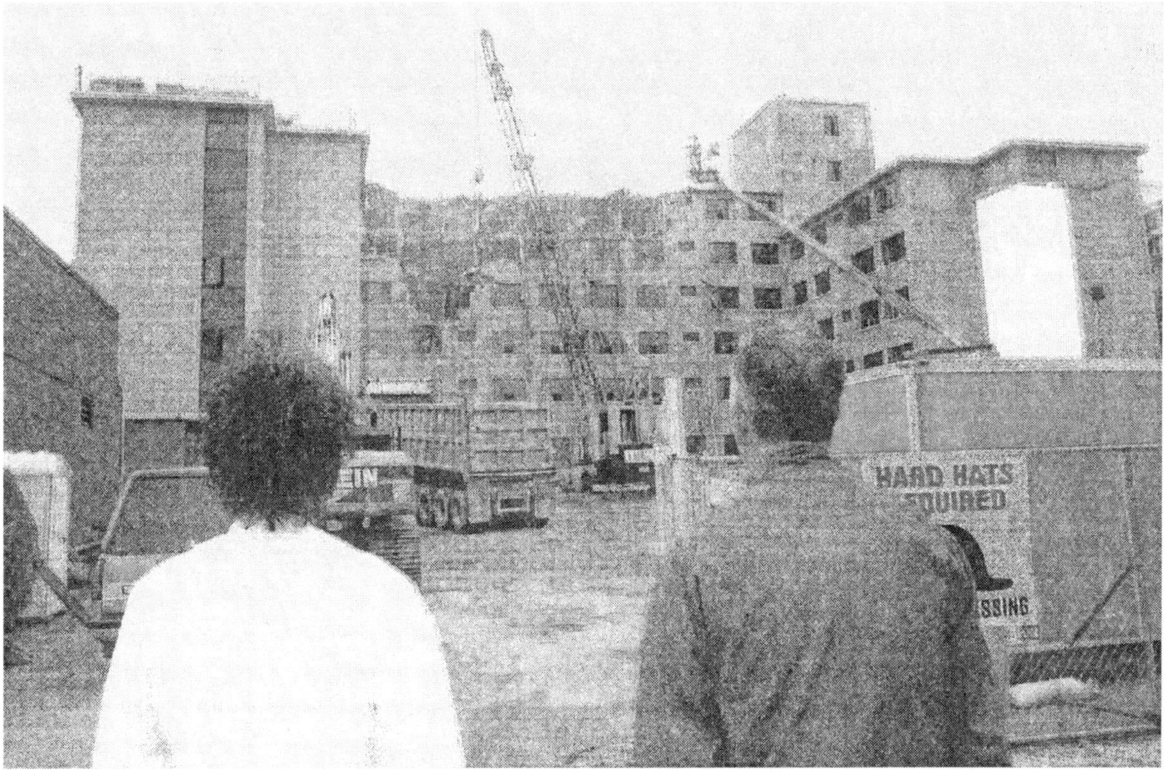

— Used with the permission of the KALAMAZOO GAZETTE.

223. (above) Martha Walker, a Bronson employee and Derwin Motyer, retired janitor of Bronson's Truesdale residence for over 34 years, watch as the wrecking ball begins to raze Truesdale Hall, May 1997.

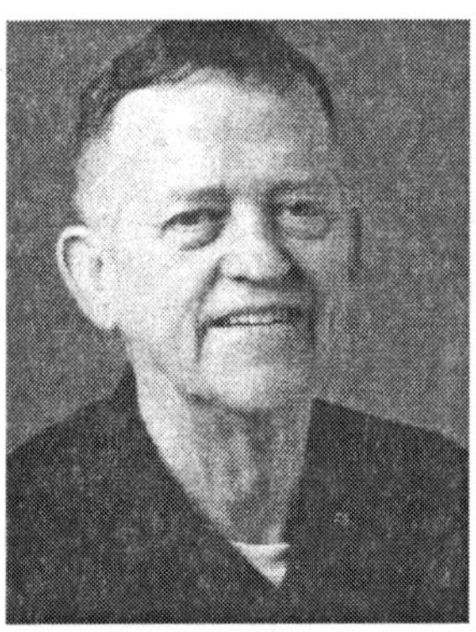

224. (left) Der Motyer cared for Truesdale during the 60s, 70s, and 80s.

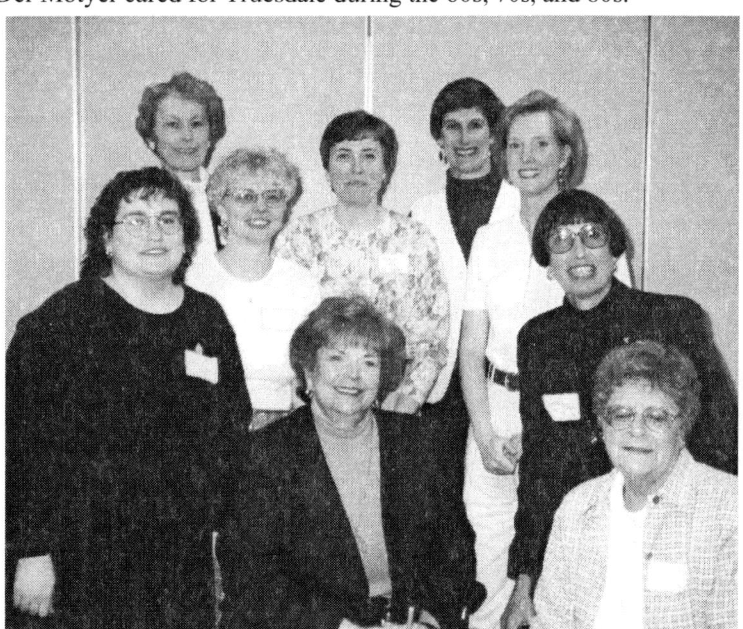

225. (right) Board of Directors, Alumni Association of Bronson Methodist Hospital School of Nursing: (foreground) Dawn Barnard; secretary Julie DeKorte; Ruth Matteson; (middle row) president Ruth Clemans, vice president Jackie Wylie; (back row) Anna Stryd, Sharyn Schlueter, Jan Walcott, Paula Ritsema, April 1997.

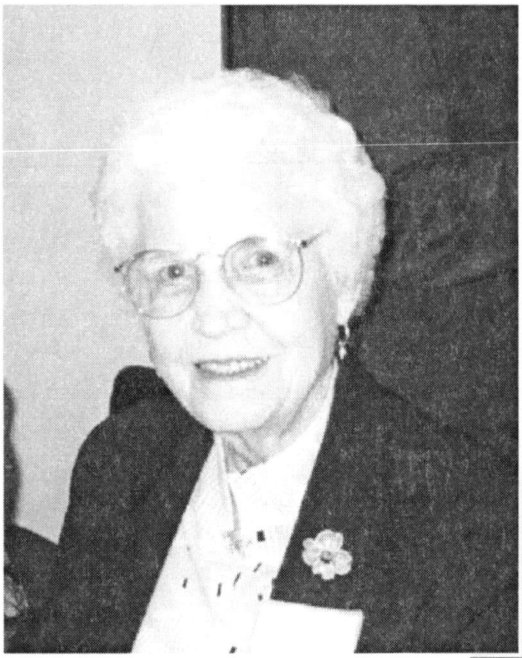

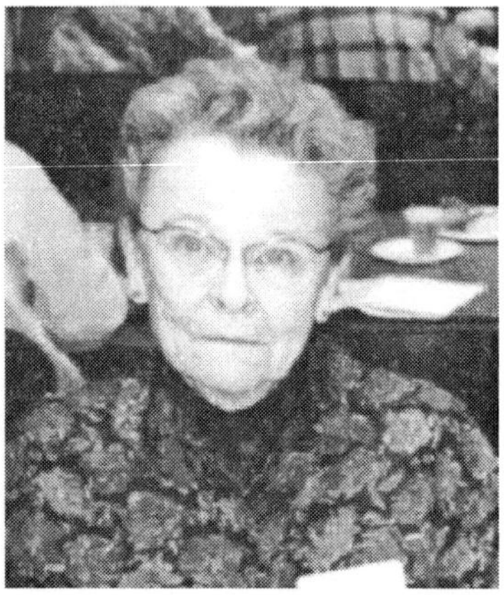

226. Alethea Utter, (above) Class of 1932, and 227. Winnie VanderMeer (above right) at the 1997 spring brunch. Alethea was the oldest alum present.

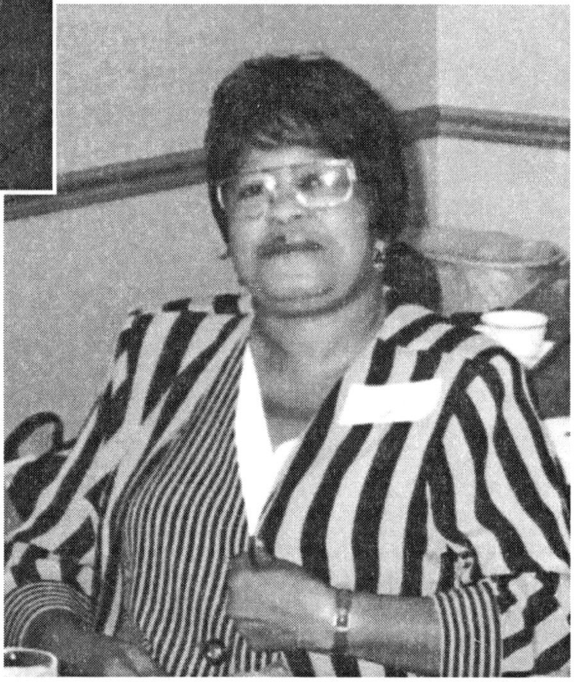

228. Gracie Harris enjoys a late 1990s brunch.

229. (below) Perkins Restaurant, Kalamazoo, was the site for reviving old memories, April 1996.

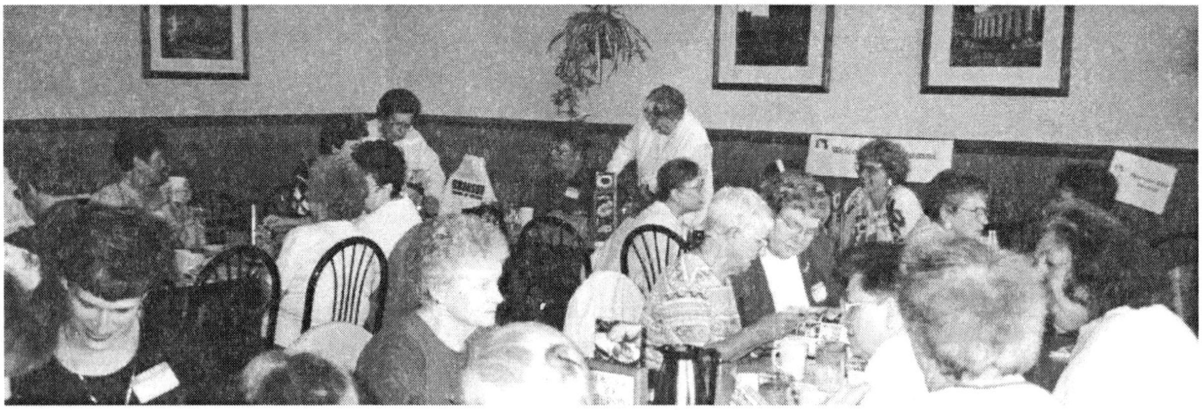

230. Diane Hamilton PhD, RN (right) was among the original and continuing faculty at the school.
231. Corrie Hitchcock (below center) member of the first WMU graduating class, April 1999.

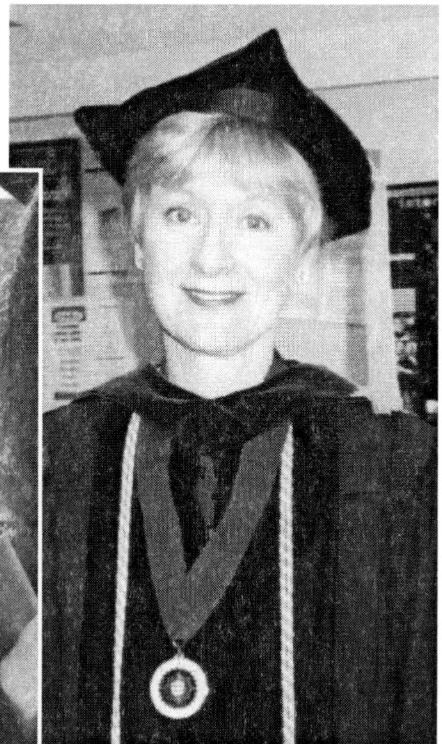

232. Bernardine Lacey EdD, RN, founding director, WMU Bronson School of Nursing.

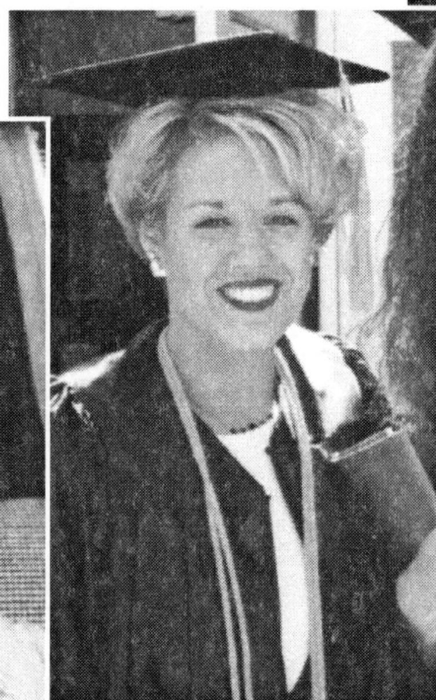

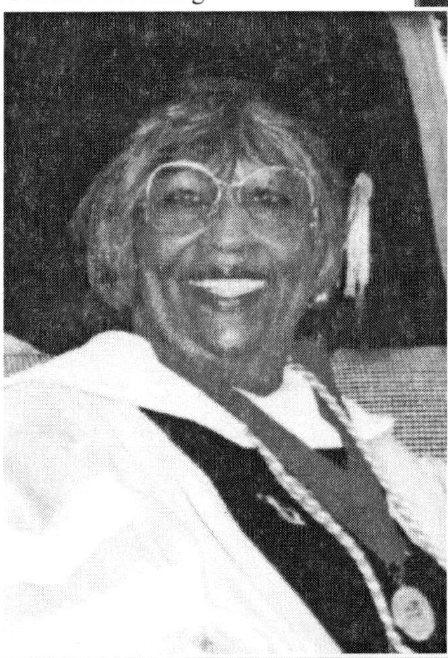

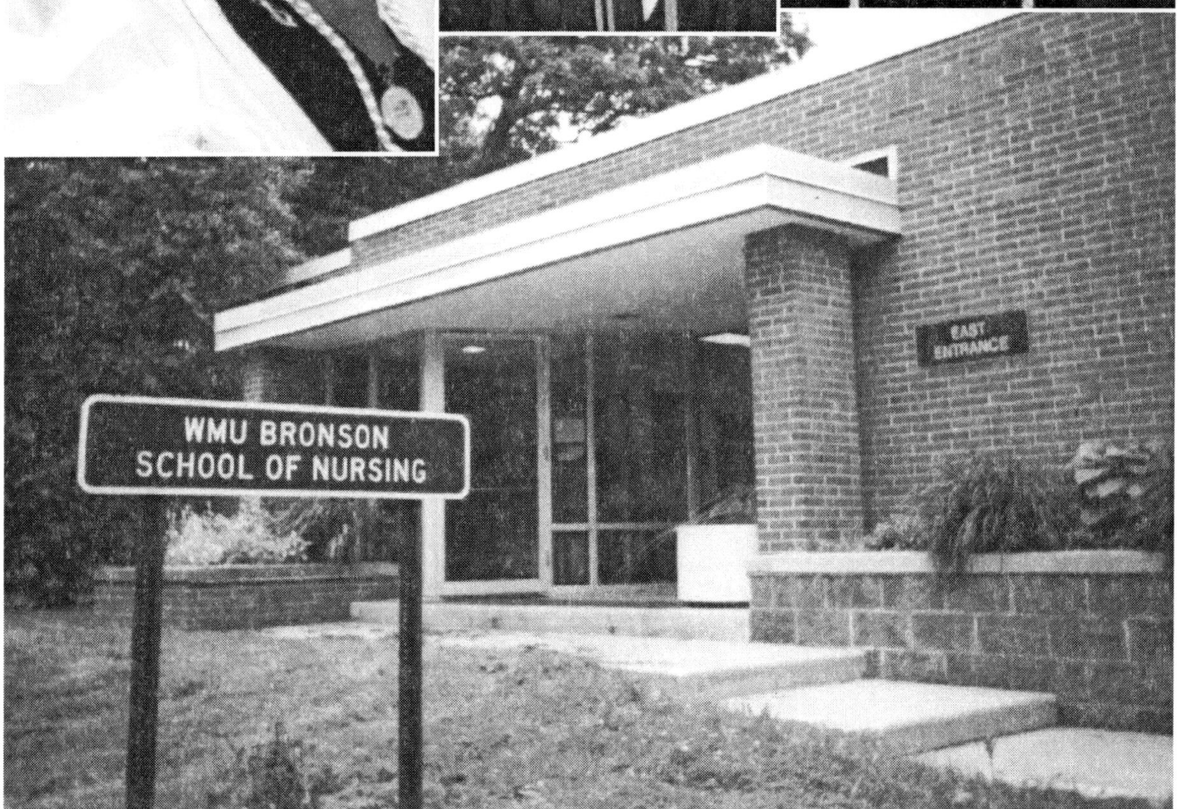

CHAPTER 11

TRANSFORMATION INTO THE NEW MILLENNIUM, 2000s

Four transforming events in the nineties changed the Kalamazoo nursing community, a series of losses and gains:

- ***First,*** Nazareth College closed in July 1992. It housed the sole local baccalaureate nursing program. That closure spurred WMU in adding a new School of Nursing. A WMU–Nazareth collaboration to create a graduate-undergraduate nursing program was discussed prior to closure, since healthcare challenges required more nurses to be prepared at the graduate level.
- ***Second,*** the Western Michigan University School of Nursing was established in 1994. Its first four RN graduates earned baccalaureate degrees with majors in nursing, in 1996. The reality of a public BS nursing program hit home when the 37 graduates in the first prelicensure class matriculated on April 23, 1999.[1] The new school of nursing was named the Bronson School of Nursing when a significant monetary gift added to the already existing legacy.

- ***Third,*** the Bronson Methodist Hospital School of Nursing made the decision to close in 1994, once WMU had established the new program. The hospital graduated its last class in May 1998, and a December 1998 closure date was submitted to the Michigan State Board of Nursing.
- ***Fourth,*** a new monument to women rose up just south of the existing Bronson campus—a new Bronson Methodist Hospital designed to be a healing house for the new millennium!

The new Bronson culture set the stage for a balanced design of high-touch, high-tech care that required conscious balance of feminine-masculine values. Patients were transferred December 3, 2000, from the old hospital in a well-orchestrated move into the new healing-house environment.

What to do with the oldest buildings was an issue. Expansion-year remodels and add-ons to increase beds left behind a maintenance nightmare that, if it could be fixed, would come at an exorbitant cost. The first building to be razed was the 1906 original hospital structure, followed in turn by Truesdale Hall, the Harding building, the 1940 hospital addition facing Lovell Street, and then the ten-story North Tower. East medical center and the newest section, the Center building, remained to be remodeled to accommodate future uses, including the first floor of the entire structure that connected the saved buildings and the Lovell–Jasper Street parking structure.

ESTABLISHMENT OF THE WESTERN MICHIGAN UNIVERSITY SCHOOL OF NURSING

Persistence and serendipity paid off! The work of the Council of Nursing Educators and Service Administrators (CNESA), as a collective and with the support of its individual members over the past ten years, kept the need for increasing educational requirements for nurses in front of the eyes of the public, nurses, nurse educators and nurse administrators.

Earlier during the 1980s, the groundwork had been laid for the WMU program when William Burian, Dean of the College of Health and Human Services (HHS), aligned the college with the CNESA. He managed the internal WMU political process for the development of a nursing program and supported CNESA in lobbying Lansing legislators for state funding for a WMU nursing program. After Burian's sudden, untimely, September 1988 death, the process slowed during the interim leadership of Dean Tyndall, who assumed the HHS helm from November 1988 to August 1989 when Janet Pisaneschi was appointed the permanent dean of the college. She resumed the challenging task of establishing a totally new nursing education program within HHS.

Both Borgess and Bronson hospitals supported the effort by originally donating $25,000 each. Local nurse educators and administrators volunteered their time with the external political process to convince the community and legislators that a public program was essential to the future of healthcare in southwest Michigan. Expert consultants in national and local nursing education gave time and attention to facilitate program development. Margaret Murphy, RN, PhD, a Wisconsin nurse educator, was one of the consultants who facilitated the new school establishment, along with members of the local CNESA.

Bernardine M. Lacey, RN, EdD, became the founding director when the WMU nursing program was established in 1994. She was the right person for the position in the first five years, establishing a community presence, and representing persons of color and cultural diversity. The enrichment of nursing was dependent on the transformation from white dominance in nursing practice to the inclusion of people who identified themselves as non-white.

Dr. Lacey's leadership was colorful in multiple and complex ways, not always appreciated nor understood by the School of Nursing faculty and staff. The faculty and staff challenge was to honor diversity in ways not done before, to be sensitive to people of color in white-dominated American institutions, and to build appreciation for a diverse community population. Lacey was a gift to the Kalamazoo community and, before returning to her home in the Washington D.C. area, she was honored by having a local philanthropic family give a $1 million for a WMU Community Nursing Endowed Chair in her name. This non-budgeted faculty position was program enrichment in itself! Dr. Lacey was a catalyst for a change long due in Kalamazoo nursing leadership. In a sense, she was "on loan" to the southwest Michigan community.

Community and State Gifts to Nursing Education

The John E. Fetzer Institute contributed to nursing program transformation both philosophically and monetarily by exalting nursing and the new university program in its 1998 annual report:

> Nursing is a profession that has often bridged the gap between conventional medicine and less conventional practices including relationship-centered care and mind-body-spirit health. With the support of the Fetzer Institute, a nursing program within Western Michigan University's College of Health and Human Services is piloting a unique curriculum that is community-based, relationship-centered, and holistic in its philosophy, design and content.
>
> The program's guiding philosophy is that a student's awareness of and progress toward balance in body-mind-spirit are prerequisites to assisting others. Students begin by assessing their own lifestyle and developing self-care skills for lifelong practice. Students then enlarge their focus from self-care to working with individuals, families, groups and communities. In addition to traditional biomedical skills, students are taught a variety of complementary approaches to healing including relaxation and therapeutic touch. In this way, the nursing program is graduating practitioners who can implement a complete and integrated approach to health care.[2]

In the larger community contributors to start-up costs were Bronson Methodist Hospital, Borgess Medical Center, the Irving S. Gilmore Foundation, and the W.K. Kellogg Foundation, along with the Fetzer Institute. The Fetzer Institute's enlightened philosophy for holistic health that embraced healthcare practices beyond the confines of an allopathic medical model was a major transforming factor in the local design of nursing education. The WMU College of Health and Human Services and the Fetzer Institute were long-time allies so that support for the School of Nursing was a logical consequence.

A New Bronson School of Nursing at WMU

Five years after its establishment, the WMU School of Nursing was publicly named the Bronson School of Nursing with an announcement at an awards ceremony the evening before the first pre-licensure class graduated on April 24, 1999. Bronson had pledged over $5 million, starting with a first pledge of $1.25 million, when the school opened in 1994. Said Frank Sardone, president and CEO of Bronson Healthcare Group:

> Transferring the Bronson School of Nursing name to WMU is the next step in a relationship between our institutions, which began more than 70 years ago when our School of Nursing students first enrolled in classes at WMU.[3] It is also a continuation of efforts which began in 1988 when Bronson and Western began working together to develop a BSN program with the idea that it would become the successor to the Bronson School of Nursing diploma program.[4]

Directly involved in the Bronson name negotiation and a $5 million endowment was Sardone; Robert Doud, vice president for public relations; Ken Taft, vice president of finance; and WMU's Carl "Bud" Bender, vice president for development. It was as if it had to be! The WMU–Bronson connection represented a legacy of conscious recognition of available resources and the need to move nursing into higher education in collaboration with local clinical services.

First Nursing Graduates from WMU

The Michigan Board of Nursing granted the School of Nursing initial approval in 1996 when four registered nurses graduated including two from BMH School of Nursing, Paul Kokales '87 and Lisa McMillan'93, plus Kim White and Danielle Kunza. A picture of this group, in graduation regalia gathered around Dr. Lacey, hangs in the School of Nursing lobby.[5]

The National League for Nursing (NLN) awarded five-year initial accreditation (1997–2002) to the WMU School when the submitted report met NLN standards for baccalaureate nursing education. In 2002, when that accreditation status ended, Director Marie Gates and the faculty chose to apply for accreditation with the Commission on Collegiate Nursing Education. The School exceeded the commission's standards and received recognition that will be effective to 2007.

INTEGRATION AND TRANSFORMATION OF NURSING EDUCATION

Jackie Wylie found it challenging to separate the first Bronson School of Nursing, initiated at the beginning of the 20th century, in the Kalamazoo Hospital from the new WMU nursing program established at the beginning of the new millennium:

> I knew how separate the two were, comparing roots and purposes of academia to those of a hospital-based educational program, and yet at an intuitive level they seemed so connected to me. The new WMU Bronson School of Nursing was my dream and that of Judy Stewart Hoelscher, Phyllis Nicolaou, Louette Lutjens, B.J. Shell, and other Kalamazoo staff nurses, educators and service administrators. It was a collective dream to better articulate professional nursing practice as the artful and caring science that it had always been.[6] The new WMU Bronson School of Nursing

> faculty, students and graduates have brought a new dimension of healthcare to southwest Michigan.

Several Bronson Methodist Hospital School of Nursing faculty joined the Western Michigan University School of Nursing faculty ranks during its first ten years, and included Mary Ann Stark, Helen Truss, Jackie Wylie '62, Sally Vliem '86, Elizabeth Phillips, Sally Sutkowi, Suzanne Nahan '75, Wendy Kerstner and Pam Moore. Stark earned a PhD from the University of Michigan with Phillips and Vliem working toward PhD's in the early 2000s.

"NEW BRONSON BLOOMS DOWNTOWN"

The new Bronson Methodist Hospital[7], with an address change to 601 John Street, covers the block surrounded by Walnut, Jasper, Vine, Burdick and John streets, just south of the original Lovell and John Street campus. With completion scheduled for November 6, 2000, the structure was designed to increase the amount of space devoted to outpatient services in keeping with changing healthcare practices, decreasing hospital lengths of stay and attendant new technology.

Hospital bed capacity was designed for 274 inpatients, down sized from the 343 state-licensed beds last approved for the old structure. Bronson, however, retained the right to all the licensed beds, given the numbers of frail aged, chronically ill, and younger populations with limited self-care skills and self-health management capacities in its service community. The cost of human suffering and monetary resources was an untenable burden on society. With additional beds added during the first four years of the new hospital's existence, 307 of the 343 licensed beds were staffed in the new building, including those in the north campus units.[8,9]

Beds reopened on the old campus when Semper Care, a nationally owned, long-term, acute-care service contracted for space in the newest part of the old campus. Remodeled space accommodated mostly elders who often needed more time to recover from their illnesses than the acute-care system allowed. Services for them complemented inpatient, short-term, acute and outpatient care for which the new hospital was designed.

One Bronson Nurse's Gift

The major nurse donor to the new hospital was Margaret Hannah Varney, a 1925 graduate and loyal supporter of Bronson throughout her lifetime, who funded the garden in the new hospital atrium. Varney dedicated a portion of the final bequest to her beloved Bronson Methodist Hospital as planned prior to her June 1997 death. Remembering Bronson, she " . . . bequeathed more than $4 million of her estate to the Bronson Health Foundation. . . . A portion of the bequest will go toward scholarships and the remaining amount will go into an endowment."[10] Throughout her lifetime she gave generous monetary gifts, mostly designated for hospital projects such as remodeling a family surgery waiting room. Varney, during the early nineties and long retired from nursing practice, often hosted the annual spring alumni event at the Parkview Hills Clubhouse, in the community where she lived. She was a reminder of Kalamazoo women who early in the 20th century gave their gifts of time, money and service to build the original 1906 dream—the first Bronson Hospital.

NURSING AND HEALTHCARE—
REVOLUTIONARY OR EVOLUTIONARY PROCESS?

Redesigning the Healthcare System

Cost containment pressures in the nineties failed to produce savings or enlightenment. Patients expected the most advanced medical technology to diagnose, treat, and cure their illnesses, seemingly without always owning responsibility for lifestyle, self-care and self-health management, or safe environment—major determinants of health. Cost shifts and cost reductions weren't the same entity: A paradigm shift was needed to move from expensive illness care to self-care responsibility. Nursing models of practice were a part of the solution, not alone, but within transformative, transdisciplinary team practice that included self-awareness, lifestyle changes, measuring and monitoring healthcare outcomes, cognitive reframing of healing and illness care, and family ability to provide extended care within their homes.

Colleges and schools of nursing with autonomy often managed nursing clinics for the uninsured and underinsured, working-class poor, and indigent, vulnerable populations that lacked access to expensive medical care. Often it seemed as if nursing was perceived as a second-class service for poor, second-class citizens who did not qualify for medical care due to lack of insurance. Nursing was about client advocacy, education and empowerment of the public toward more self-care and responsibility for outcomes. Nurses promoted health and disease prevention with lifestyle changes, not an easy sell. One such clinic was established at WMU.

Barbara Starke, a WMU School of Nursing faculty member, and Joan Ashley, WMU apartments manager, established a nursing-care site in 2000. It was called Community Connections and was housed in a campus apartment dedicated to support the self-care of WMU students. Meant as a healing place painted in rainbow colors, nursing students and other WMU students came to explore health promotion activities. Principles of holistic health were practiced. For example, presence and relationship building with diverse populations was practiced as intervention, along with non-invasive health awareness practices. Its benefits to the community went beyond roles for nursing in traditional services in hospitals, extended-care facilities, physicians' offices and public health departments.

National Nursing's Impact on Local System Redesign

At the national level, *Nursing's Agenda for Health Care Reform* complemented the Clinton administration's Health Security Act of 1993. The public had much to gain if access to affordable, primary care included patients and allied health professionals[11] as partners. With more shared responsibility for outcomes, physicians would be more partners than principals in decision making.[12] Nurses in primary care, however, were seen as a threat to the American Medical Association as shown in a report, "attacking nearly every aspect of nurses' ability to give adequate care, . . ." while the nurses gave, "an unexpected return volley from the extremely well-organized nurses' lobby."[13]

> A profession that had its origins in nuns' orders and had long been associated in the public mind with nothing more specific than furnishing generalized [medical] help, support and mercy—though, of course, the actual work always required far more than that in medical expertise—stands suddenly revealed as a highly specialized and regulated profession with a multitude of training programs and graduate degrees.[14]

Advance practice nurse (APN) privileges varied, with Michigan having more medical control than some states where nurses had sole prescription-writing authority, for example:

- ***Some 43 states authorized advanced-practice nurses and/or physician assistants*** to prescribe medications noted *USA Today* in 1993. If this approach was a bad idea, "Where is the flood of lawsuits? A number of studies show that qualified nurses provide competent, satisfying services. . . . Doctors don't hate nurses. But they do hate—or, at least, strenuously oppose—any erosion of their status as exclusive keepers of the health-care system."[15]
- ***Nurses lightened the workload***. They helped bolster profits. For routine visits, the doctor told the patient, in effect: "See the nurse, and have your insurance company send me a check."[16]

- ***"Nurse practitioners have been delivering primary care*** since 1965 . . ." and, reported in the *New York Times,* " . . . hundreds of studies have examined the quality of their work, including diagnostic ability and management effectiveness. There is not a single study that shows any lapses . . . and most of the studies have been done by physicians."[17]

People didn't mind seeing nurses for minor ailments and often felt more cared for because of the extra time nurses spent listening. The difference[18] between 1992 average salaries for physicians at $170,000 compared to nurses at $43,000 was $127,000, quite a cost saving that could relieve cost pressures if patients weren't charged the physician rate. Even in states where traditional medicine held control, APNs acted independently, were not directly supervised, and sought physician input when needed. Nurse managers supervised staff nurses, rather than the physicians who ordered medical interventions and expected competent nurses to carry out the medical treatment plan. Physicians wanted to retain exclusive privileges to provide primary care, although few were prepared to be generalists. Instead they chose more lucrative, specialty practices. If access to care were more equitable with more people served by use of more nurse practitioners, theoretically the costs of care per person would decrease. However, costs could rise due to increased numbers served. Would Americans then live healthier?

Relationship-centered Care

Significant nursing research brought its caring, evidenced-based practice into a new millennium. Outcomes of well-designed nurse studies demonstrated healthcare enrichment and began to receive the attention of hospital administrators' and the public.

Nurse shortages caused moments for pondering why the average staff nurse age was mid-forties and faculty mid-fifties. Making the nursing profession more attractive to young women and men required more than a simple reframing of healthcare relationships. When nurses with PhD's sat on interdisciplinary healthcare teams, doors were opened to new healthcare models.

Nurses' levels of achievement added new dimensions to healthcare, nursing education and practice opportunities. Relationships between novice nurse, doctoral and postdoctoral roles needed to be valued and honored. WMU nursing students learned and practiced relationship-centered care (RCC) as defined by the Pew-Fetzer Task Force in its report, *Health Professions Education and Relationship-Centered Care.*[19] Skill sets intended to enhance healing included competencies within the dimensions of self- awareness, patient–practitioner, practitioner–community and practitioner–practitioner relationships. Nursing was given credit for its " . . . long history of emphasizing caring relationships in its practice and ethos," although, "this focus has not become a defining force in healthcare."[20]

No conscious nurse or other healthcare provider would happily pursue his or her career without being in healthy relationship with self and other. Interdisciplinary teaming meant a team of experts with inclusion of all health professional classifications, not just nurses and physicians. Students of all healthcare disciplines needed more opportunity to practice together early in their clinical education to shape new transdisciplinary mindsets and together learn the competencies of RCC.

One dilemma was that most nurses were prepared at less than the baccalaureate level of knowledge. Differences in the years of nursing education posed a threat and intimidation within the profession itself. How could nurses honor their work and level of education in a way that promoted collaboration? It was difficult to see the richness in nursing education diversity and be able to maximize differences instead of feeling threatened by different educational levels and clinical expertise. Practitioner–practitioner affirmation could make the difference and relationship-centered care helped enlighten providers.

Nursing's educational ladder could be viewed as a hidden gift. Instead, it remained a problem among nursing and healthcare teams that rarely understood nursing education and levels of dependent to autonomous, interdependent practice. Registered nurse licensure appeared to be a leveling factor. Often heard in the work setting was that "a RN is a RN is a RN". The public and other healthcare professionals had to learn about differences in competencies for a positive shift and change in nursing practice that would lead toward a desired, respected, well-remunerated career choice. Honoring all levels of nursing education first needed nurse–leader champions.

Balancing Art with Science

Managed care and evidence-based practice became the buzzwords of the nineties. The focus was on achieving the best health outcomes for the least costly screenings, diagnoses and interventions. Twenty years of analysis described differences in preferred medical interventions and their costs for treating identical healthcare problems. Often there was no difference in outcomes to justify greater costs. Hospitalization for the same surgical procedure might result in a two-day hospital stay in the West and a five-day stay in the East, even when all patient variables were factored in. Practice, thought to be research-based, frequently happened more because of tradition—"it was always done that way." At the new WMU Bronson School of Nursing, baccalaureate nursing education focused on population-based care and epidemiological approaches as part of a holistic, relationship-centered care, critical decision-making, and community health curriculum. Students learned best practice.

MAGNET HOSPITAL STATUS INCREASES AWARENESS OF NURSING VALUE

The term "magnet hospital" came from a policy study commission in 1982, authorized by the American Academy of Nursing, which examined the organizational characteristics of U.S. hospitals that were successful in recruiting and retaining nurses during a national nursing shortage.[21, 22]

Roberta Utrecht's leadership in the 1990s focused on achieving professional nursing practice behaviors and new practice roles in healthy relationship with physicians and other providers. The nurses were often the glue for hospital clinical service collaboration within both administrative and clinical management roles. Shared governance models offered nurse's empowerment and authority to accompany their level of accountability and responsibility for clinical services. Patterns of practice were hard to break. Some nurses embraced the need for change and were willing to propose innovative programs, while others seemed to be intimidated by the dominant medical model or lacked consciousness about new practice possibilities. Katie Harrelson started the process for achieving Magnet Hospital designation once she was established in her role of chief nurse executive.

Preparation for Magnet Hospital status included meeting national nursing practice standards of excellence to promote more egalitarian hospital practices and the recognition of nurses as partners in practice with other healthcare professionals. Shared governance provided evidence that nursing morale was boosted along with the courage to learn new ways of being, thinking and doing. Practice recognition, authority and autonomy were essential to divert a growing nursing shortage by positively impacting recruitment and retention.

It took a unified management team of administrators and clinicians to deliver care that met high levels of patient and employee satisfaction and to develop a culture in which mutuality and mentoring was a daily occurrence. Physicians and patients were considered the hospital's major customers during the eighties, and sometimes nurses were forgotten, yet patients stayed in the hospital only as long as they needed 24-hour nursing care, no longer, and outpatient services often required professional nurse support. Nurses may have appeared only to do as physicians told them, but they accomplished much more. Application for Magnet Hospital status brought hidden roles to light.[23]

Nancee Himes Hofmeister '82 in Project Coordinator Role

Magnet status was a new concept described by McClure, Poulin, Sovie and Wandelt.[24] Nancee Hofmeister had graduated from Bronson just one year before the authors published their manuscript, and returned to Bronson in August 2002 to become part of the magnet development team. She was destined to become a leader in the transformation of nursing as nurse coordinator for the Magnet Hospital status application process. This transformation was supported by the efforts of all Bronson employees.

Years of research, including the findings of nurse researchers like McClure, that demonstrated the impact of professional nursing practice on patient outcomes, hospital recruitment and retention of nurses, was being published in the 1990s.

Nurses at Bronson did not have data to prove that the numbers of professional nursing staff and their educational levels made a difference to patient outcomes or the hospital's bottom line. So logically, nursing could be downsized for a more cost-effective, efficient organization. Fewer professional nurses to delegate less invasive, direct care to unlicensed personnel were believed able to save money while not impacting the quality of patient care, a team approach that worked in the fifties and sixties.

Hofmeister's career[25] began at Bronson after her 1982 graduation. Her first 13 years were devoted to Bronson's women and children's services, the Neonatal Intensive Care Unit (NICU) and serving as a nurse manager in Obstetrics. She left Obstetrics in September 1995 when an administrative reorganization eliminated jobs to streamline services and reduce hospital costs and she expected her job to be a target.

Actually, Hofmeister left Bronson for several reasons during the downsizing and reorganization when over 700 employees took advantage of "early-out" packages. Beside her belief that her job would be eliminated, it was next to impossible to meet her work responsibilities as a manager, care for her family, and complete a BSN at the University of Michigan. She needed a break and time to focus on home and school. The nineties were a challenging time in her life. She left Bronson with a sense of her worth as a nurse and confidence in finding a new position, plus her work evaluations had been positive.

The choice to complete her BSN and leave Bronson opened new career doors for Hofmeister. She found a less stressful, home care nursing position with the Visiting Nurses Association (VNA) in Kalamazoo, first assessing the health status of moms and babies and teaching the new mothers in their homes. She learned requirements of commercial payers, as well as rules for Medicare and Medicaid reimbursement for adults and children who were certified for Michigan case management, according to requirements of the Michigan Children's Special Health Care Services. Hofmeister was able to be part of a dramatic outcomes project, Immunize by Two, in Kalamazoo County, that increased documented children's immunizations from 68 percent compliance to greater than 90 percent. In the process she learned that many children had actually been over-immunized because of poor documentation.

Then, over a seven-year period, she transitioned from VNA to Borgess Medical Center (BMC) and was introduced to another side of patient services—adult medical-surgical nursing. This world was a new kind of case management in which she acquired more knowledge about Medicare; Medicaid; diverse private companies; utilization review; and documentation requirements for reimbursements; as well as meeting healthcare needs of adults living with chronic illness and acute episodes. One part of her practice was to analyze patient care records. In searching for co-morbidities and informing physicians about appropriate documentation not to miss diagnoses under insurance reimbursement, Hofmeister experienced ongoing care management with the ultimate goals to reduce the burden of patient suffering and cost to the system.

Hofmeister learned that advancing her education changed her thought processes in approaching nursing practice. She branched out and learned competencies for a new healthcare business world that ultimately prepared her for the position of her dreams at Bronson, when she was invited to reapply. In August 2002, she was hired as a general project coordinator for nursing. This appointment soon became known as the Magnet Project Coordinator when chief nurse executive Katie Harrelson received the administrative go-ahead to apply for Magnet Hospital status. Hofmeister was ready when the application was submitted in December 2002.[26]

Hofmeister and Stacey Brawer '92 participated in the 2003 Institute for Research, Education and Consultation, a workshop for achieving Magnet Hospital designation. Hosted by the American Nurses Credentialing Center (ANCC), it was held in Newark, New Jersey, at the Robert Wood Johnson (RWJ) University, part of the RWJ teaching hospital. Hofmeister also took advantage of workshop materials supplied by other Bronson Operations Improvement staff.

Achieving Magnet Hospital Status

Bronson contracted with Magnet Hospital expert and national consultant, Peggy Jones from the ANCC and the American Nurses Association (ANA), who came to Bronson to complete a gap analysis in 2003. She interfaced directly with Hofmeister to identify the magnet strengths in Bronson's professional nursing team and to describe which forces were missing to achieve the "best of the best" nursing services. Jones had been a chief nurse executive who had led her hospital team in attaining Magnet status and was the first chair of the ANCC committee that determined magnet criteria. She was also a reviewer of Magnet status applications, a position that kept her in touch with the ever-changing needs of patients and their nurses. A BMH steering committee was organized to include all nursing divisions with managers and staff nurses represented.

Fourteen "forces of magnetism," described by McClure and others in their 1983 Magnet Hospital study,[27] laid the foundation for building a hospital nursing service for excellence in patient care and the best culture and environment in which professional nurses could thrive:

- quality of nursing leadership with advocacy and a well-articulated philosophy
- a flat organizational structure
- participative management style
- personnel policies and programs with competitive salaries and flexible staffing models
- professional models of care
- quality of care based on national benchmark measurements
- quality improvement processes with an educational focus
- advance practice nurse consultation and resources
- autonomy within nursing practice standards
- a community and hospital presence
- nurses identified as teachers
- nursing image as part of the hospital whole
- interdisciplinary relationships of mutual respect
- professional development[28]

Magnet forces were integrated into a developing shared governance model, one that needed revamping at BMH in order to maximize nurses' daily input into patient care outcomes.

The Magnet Steering Committee included Beverly Anderson '67, Stacey Brawer '92, Barb Groh, Katie Harrelson, Nancee Hofmeister '82, Jane Janssen, Hilary Knight, Kelly Kulczyk, Michelle Link '81, Anne May, Betsy McGraw '78, Anika Meyers '96, Sally Ossewaarde '87, Nikki Romence, Julie Switek, Jan Tucker, Jackie Wahl, April Willard and Mary Woodhouse '76.[29] Within the complex hospital culture, the monumental task faced by its members required extensive analysis of nursing practice.

Analysis and development of all fourteen forces culminated in January 2004 when Hofmeister began leading Bronson's report writing team to provide evidence of Magnet status accomplishments. The report was compiled during the year, with November 2004 being the expected submission date for the report. An accreditation site date was to be scheduled by The *New* Bronson Methodist Hospital and the ANCC in 2005.

Other Hofmeister Roles

Continuous patient-care quality improvement was another Hofmeister role that provided Bronson the data that could be used to create positive changes and continued evidence for clinical practice excellence. She managed Bronson's contribution to the National Database for Nursing Quality, housed at the ANA. Some of the submitted benchmark data included staff mix, professional nurse hours per patient and total staff hours per patient day, patient falls with and without injury, pressure ulcers and other outcome indicators. Comparisons were made to other hospitals of similar size and patient demographics so that BMH would have accurate measurements of progress.

Hofmeister also tracked professional nurse educational credentials from the 2003 staff mix figures in the table on the following page. This step was necessary to track and keep growing a knowledgeable nursing staff and one commensurate with its accountability, responsibility and authority.

DEGREE	PERCENT
PhD	0.00
MSN	2.75
Other Graduate Degrees	1.17
BSN	23.32
BS	7.02
Diploma/ADN	65.75

Hofmeister's enthusiasm for nursing practice and patient-care contributions at Bronson in 2004 demonstrated a 360-degree turnaround from when she resigned in 1995. Hers was an exciting testimony to a future in which Bronson nurses, in collaboration with area nurse educators at local universities and colleges and other colleagues from diverse health professions, will do more than survive. The monument to women and their caring work was destined to thrive!

Nurse Staff Involvement in Movement Toward Magnet Status

Stacy Finley Brawer '92

Stacy Brawer[30] wasn't sure about the direction that she wanted to follow when she graduated from the BMH School of Nursing in 1992. Open to finding her niche, she accepted a position in the Medical-Surgical Nursing Float Pool.

Nursing cardiology patients became a love—a surprise, because in nursing school she was intimidated by the gravity of their illness and the nursing care demands needed to support their healing. It wasn't as much about the cardiology specialty as it was being a part of a dynamic team, one that respected the expertise each person brought to patients' bedsides. By 1993 she left the float pool to cross-train in the Coronary Care Unit (CCU) and Telemetry and at the same time learn the role of charge nurse. The next two years were glory days in Brawer's eyes! She had found the perfect work environment, never felt alone, and was always backed up by other professionals in clinical decision making. She felt rewarded!

The mass staff exodus in the 1995 early retirement and buyout turned her perfect world around. The loss of nursing expertise decreased the team support available for less mature nurses. By 1996, her role was that of CCU Charge Nurse and often included patient-care assignments, a type of double load.

She transferred to the Cardiac Catheterization Lab (CCL) in 1997, loving the impact of advanced technology on patient care. Working closely with expert cardiologists brought educational opportunities. Her learning curve was close to exponential. She couldn't believe how much more there was to learn about the medical care of cardiac patients.

Brawer was part of the nursing team managing the move to the new hospital in December 2000. She remembered the first case . . . how exciting it was to care for patients with new state-of-the-art equipment at your fingertips and knowing firsthand the use of state-of-the-art technology. Patient volume increased at least 40 percent, with two labs accommodating a patient load meant for three. Soon the third lab was added. She worked hard on 12-hour shifts that never seemed to end and took on additional "off" hours. No surprise that the load was too much and Brawer began to feel "fried." By the end of 2002, she felt like she wasn't a nurse anymore but just a glorified technician instead, going through daily rote motions.

Brawer recalled Barb Groh's words, "If you ever feel the need to leave nursing or Bronson please come see me first." She went to see Groh in 2003 to tell her, "I need to get out!" Groh encouraged her to talk with Katie Harrelson, new chief nurse executive, about her feelings. "I wanted to stay at Bronson, but I needed to stretch my wings," Brawer stated, "I called Harrelson's office. I suspected that Barb Groh had already told her my story."

Harrelson had an idea. The Magnet application process needed a staff nurse liaison and Nancee Hofmeister needed help writing the report. Harrelson asked

Brawer about her thoughts on Magnet Hospital designation and if she wanted to work part time in Operations Improvement.[31] Brawer said, "Yes." The opportunity appeared to be the needed change, a step away from the stressful bedside practice and another opportunity to learn and broaden her perspective about nursing contributions and how they fit into the whole hospital design. It was the right decision for her.

Brawer found that her passion for nursing was revitalized while working in the split position between Clinical Operations Improvement and the CCL. With her renewed enthusiasm she looked forward to continuing her formal education while practicing nursing in a variety of roles in the Bronson system.

Joyce "Jo" Ulrich '73

Jo Ulrich's story[32] is a positive example of nursing's integration into the greater hospital development picture and one of mutual mentoring (described earlier as a Magnet Hospital qualification). Ulrich was offered an opportunity to integrate her love of nursing with the creation of a new healing-hospital environment that included changes in its physical structure and organizational culture. She had a passion for blending the healing arts and science. She could see a futuristic hospital that would respond to patients and families by providing an inviting environment in which the family could be cared for and, in turn, care for its hospitalized loved ones.

Family involvement meant that comfortable furniture and overnight sleeping accommodations had to be available. Ulrich envisioned nurses listening to both families and patients and providing guidelines in which their unique needs could be accommodated, not simply enforcing a "one rule fits all" system. Caring for others was accompanied by listening and adapting to meet the needs of all people in the relationship, the public and employees interrelated according to holistic principles. She opposed rigid visiting hours, believing most families would respond to respect and caring relationships by owning personal responsibility for the best outcomes.

Families needed private, overnight space built into the environment. Ulrich's story unfolded:

> I reported to Art Littlefield [in 1992] as the nursing coordinator, overseeing the Nursing Quality Assurance and productivity programs. The organization had just begun work with two consultants to prepare for and to build a new building—Kurt Salmon Associates (KSA), and Deloitte and Touche in program development, building design, and organizational re-engineering. Reorganization included centralization of Quality Assurance (later called Performance Improvement) activities into one department, eliminating the nursing coordinator position that I held.
>
> At the same time, Al Balhorn (an architect with experience in planning hospital facility projects) was hired to begin the facility planning for the new building, and he needed someone who knew the organization to assist in the planning. Since my position was being eliminated, I was offered the opportunity to interview with Al who subsequently offered me the position. When a door closes, a window opens. To be in the midst of the exciting changes that Bronson was about to embark on was the opportunity of a lifetime.
>
> The position was created at a time when the "dream" was in the feasibility phase and not everyone believed the dream would come true. I initially felt like a fish out of water in a world that was foreign to me— construction, architects, engineers, design, and RFP's, but bit-by-bit Al taught me and believed in me. Frank [Sardone] and Jon [Dixon] took Pat Ludwig's dream and made it real. I witnessed exceptional leadership and innovation, and these colleagues stretched my abilities and involved me in this exceptional experience.
>
> The planning and move into the new building was a project that included all levels of the organization and all departments, especially nursing. Roberta [Utrecht], as the CNE, led the nursing managers' and directors' involvement. She had the ability to blend the individual nursing needs with the big picture goals and long-term vision of the healing environment as well as a view of the future.

Hundreds of meetings took place with staff and leaders to define their needs in designing The *New* Bronson. This project spanned at least six years from inception to reality, and nursing involvement impacted all of the process. A feeling that dreams can come true was realized, and the walls and barriers that often restrict innovation and true teamwork were eliminated.

Every day was not utopia—conflicts occurred, fear and discomfort presented challenges, but these were all part of risk and innovation. The *New* Bronson entailed a total change—a change in how the organization operated, the processes it used, and how it looked. This was an opportunity to start with a blank sheet of paper and discard some of the long-standing practices which led to growing pains for several departments, including nursing. Organizational leaders guided everyone to achieve the new vision, pain and all.

The staff was involved in layout, redesign of mock-up patient rooms, furniture styles, staffing levels, and even down to where light switches were placed. Nursing designed the head walls and chose the nurse call system. Staff was able to tour the facility as it was being built, redesign its processes, stock its own units, orient and participate in the plan to move patients into the facility.

Interdisciplinary teams and meetings brought departments together, not only within nursing but also in the organization as a whole. Our success was a result of each and every one of us doing our part and working together to bring to life a dream. The entire project brought great pride to the organization at all levels, and a part of each one of us animates the spirit and life of *The New* Bronson. Looking back, of course, there are decisions we may have made differently if we knew then what we know now, but perhaps, if we had made different decisions, the end result would not have resulted in the sensational *New* Bronson.

My role was broad, as were those of many others who were deeply involved in the project. I started by assisting Al [Balhorn] with minutes, analyses and research, as well as bringing myself up to speed on the project. Later my role extended to serving as a part of the team in planning and decision making.

> Under the direction of Al and Jon [Dixon], I coordinated and helped keep track of issues-related department meetings with the architects and the activation planning agencies. Activation planning included participating in all the teams to prepare for the occupancy of the building (Orientation, Marketing and Public Relations, Patient Care, Information Technology, Support Services and the Steering Teams). I worked with the designers to select finishes, furniture and signage, and to create the feel of a healing environment.

Jo Ulrich's supervision targeted a calming, healing presence. She emphasized the finding of inner strengths within an environment that offered opportunities for patient consciousness-raising balanced with soft external supports.

Visible Hospital Transformation Begins

Frank Sardone's leadership as the hospital CEO set the stage. He put together a team of people who came from different backgrounds and who worked together as colleagues, thus creating a single management team. Nursing was reorganized in October, 1996, to report to chief nurse executive, Roberta Utrecht. She believed the change was positive:

> I think nursing now has one voice, but I feel the pressure of just being one person trying to move healthcare in a new direction, and I find that pressure to be difficult. I'm without administrative peers who really understand nursing—they understand the medical-care industry—but to get them to understand nursing?

An example was the budget and the cost burden of vacation time for nurses. When nurses vacationed, if the patient census remained the same, replacement staff was needed. Often business administrators responsible for finance and budget said, "Don't replace the nurses." Education was needed for administrators to understand front-line patient care and imperative to maintain safe, effective nurse-to-patient ratios.

On the other hand, nursing consolidation under Utrecht's leadership provided strength and potential for greater nurse collaboration. At budget time, given a finite amount of money, the directors of nursing met to decide what equipment was needed on the clinical units and in surgery. Together the nurses prioritized according to the most critical unit needs, a process that eliminated competition for equipment that had existed before all of nursing reported to Utrecht.

The hospital hierarchy was changing with Sardone's leadership. As an administrative leader who supported a major cultural shift, he rethought and reframed administrator-clinical provider relationships that were essential to a more satisfying, healthy work environment.

Katie Harrelson, Chief Nurse Executive in 2002

A new nurse leader emerged when Katie Harrelson[33] accepted a staff nurse position on the Adult Oncology and Pulmonary Medical Unit, 3:00 to 11:00 P.M. shift, in March 1986. Her supervisor immediately recognized her leadership skills and positive, take-action attitude for creating a healthy, professional work environment. She was promoted to supervisor 11:00 P.M. to 7:00 A.M. in October of the same year, and in 1988 was once again promoted, this time to unit manager for all shifts. She was a natural-born leader who benefited from the polishing and experience provided by her nurse mentors.

Harrelson reported to Nancy Figel, who had a clear vision for professional nursing and an ability to mentor a young, energetic nurse who welcomed her guidance. Nancy was a gentle, positive presence in the organization—a quiet leader. Harrelson recognized the gift that she was given with Nancy as her supervisor and mentor.

Harrelson, however, was not a quiet leader—she visibly involved herself in any activity that looked like an opportunity to make healthy organizational changes for nursing practice. She attended employee hospital forums held by administration to improve relationships with employees. Many of the employees were reactive and feared potential changes in their jobs or layoffs. Some, including the nursing staff, saw themselves as victims without power. Not Harrelson. When information was shared and employee questions fielded, she was one of the employees who came to the forums with solutions and an interest in being part of positive change. She was developing a vision for nursing within Bronson that could build on groundwork laid by Utrecht's notions of hospital professional practice development.

Harrelson's story is about challenging the system during one of the early nineties' employee forums, when she asked the wrong question, one that embarrassed the administrative representative leading the discussion. She wasn't aware that there was a problem with the question until she was told that she had to report to Art Littlefield's office, then the chief nurse executive. Littlefield was another gentle guide and quiet advocate for young nursing staff. He helped Harrelson to understand that the question itself was not inappropriate, but he felt that she had put the administrator in an untenable position by the way she phrased the question. In other words, it was politically incorrect to embarrass an administrator but right to introduce new notions about nursing practice.

This encounter was a growth experience for Harrelson. She took a risk, challenged the system and, in the future, would have her voice heard in a politically correct way. By learning better ways to challenge the sacred cows, she was heard rather than demoted or fired and became the nurse champion for her peers by using self-directed internal energy as an organizational green light.

Harrelson's next assignment was that of Bronson nurse analyst. This position supported organizational transformation and championed nursing when consultants from Deloitte and Touche were hired. The consultants' presence disturbed fearful employees who referred to them as the Destroy and Torch Group in an attempt to salve their fears with humor. Why was she chosen to work closely with the consultants and become a conduit for change in Bronson nursing practice? She said, "I was told that I had a big vision, challenged the system and that I had thick skin."

Thick skin did not refer to a characteristic of insensitivity, but to her high self-esteem, confidence in her ideas, and ability to enrich the hospital nursing culture. She listened to others, heard their stories, and did not need to defend a professional nursing vision or the route the hospital was taking toward transforming patient-care practices. She could integrate experiences of other nurses whom she saw as practicing too often in mechanistic, robotic ways that did not fit with the professional nursing model needed to enrich the hospital culture and patient-care environment. Nurses' voices were heard with Harrelson's risk-taking ability to speak up as their champion and spokesperson.

In the mid-nineties she formed a mentee–mentor relationship with Frank Sardone, the new president and chief executive officer. Sardone's vision was inclusive. It balanced masculine and feminine values within an interdisciplinary team hospital model. Changing nursing staff dynamics from simply physician extender roles to be inclusive of a professional nursing practice model was essential. Harrelson's vision fit with Sardone's. She had the ability to lead toward shared responsibility for outcomes within the transformative, interdisciplinary Bronson team. Harrelson said that Sardone was a consistent, positive force moving the organization into the new millennium amid plans to build a totally new Bronson on property just south of the ten-story North Tower and Center Building, Truesdale Hall, and Gilmore Education Center. The new monument was a $175 million, massive new construction project that had been initiated by Bronson's CEO, Patric Ludwig. What a difference in cost from the original $50,000 inpatient structure built in 1906.

In the midst of the late nineties' changing environment Katie Harrelson worked on ways to bring the heart and soul of nursing back into daily professional practice. The completion of the new hospital in 2000 gave hope for the emergence of a new culture. In preparation for the new environment Harrelson watched the Human

Resources Department offer customer-service training, consciously re-teaching employees of their service and marketing roles. This approach helped in many ways to open the door for special caring behaviors in daily practice. Nurses were the experts in caring science—it was the root of their practice. Could the patient-care units be designed to support an environment of healing relationships for patients, families and all healthcare personnel (professional and support staff)?

With no more renovations and add-ons to the existing ten-story North Tower and Center Building, plans for a new hospital were in the making—a new monument to women who throughout the 20th century represented about 85 percent[34] of the total hospital staff.

Susan Ulshafer, Senior VP, Human Resources

Susan Ulshafer[35] left a position in Chicago when she was appointed head of the Bronson's Human Resources Department in August 1995 by Patric Ludwig. She soon became a part of Frank Sardone's management team after Ludwig's untimely 1996 death.[36]

Ulshafer was aware of Sardone's vision and leadership skills and was impressed with the quality of Bronson and the management team's desire to move the quality bar even higher. The vision for development of a service culture included external and internal customers, patients, families, businesses, physicians and Bronson employees. She was given the freedom to develop a service culture strategy that would complement the new Bronson's vision of excellence, not only a structurally healing environment but also one that demonstrated caring for all people entering its doors.

Ulshafer had known that Sardone was likely to become Ludwig's successor after his expected retirement, which was planned a couple of years from her hire date. She arrived one week before the mass exodus of seven hundred to eight hundred employees who had accepted the "early out" retirement or "buy out" options. Diverse community health positions awaited their exit.

From Wylie's perspective, Bronson inadvertently gave an ultimate gift to the community: well-educated experts who moved out into community healthcare positions, many with positive feelings and reports about their work at Bronson. The gift eventually was returned in numerous ways but left the hospital staff reeling with a sense of loss and Ulshafer with the amazing task of building a new expert staff and a new Bronson culture. Instant leadership education was required, with novices ready to fill vacated management positions and ready to learn how to fulfill their new job requirements.

BALANCING SERVICE AND TECHNOLOGY CULTURES— A NEW MONUMENT EMERGES IN THE 21ST CENTURY

Emergence of a superlative service-culture plan required leaders like Sardone, Ulshafer and numerous nurse administrators, managers, educators, other healthcare professionals and staff to bring the "Hi Touch–Hi Tech" balance that John Naisbitt described in his popular book, *Megatrends,*[37] back from a sense of "forced technology" only. High-touch behaviors were needed to complement high technology and, if not provided by the organization, people would find ways outside of the system for the touch component.

Bronson employees changed the way they looked outwardly and inwardly, with hiring practices focusing on the selection of people who knew what service orientation meant.

Organizational loyalty was built with the new building. Ulshafer mentioned employee comments about their good feelings toward their workplace as ownership of outcomes. Current employees, who were in turn rewarded with a small monetary compensation, referred 21 percent of newly hired employees in 2003.

National recognition was achieved based on employee surveys by *Working Mother* and *Fortune,* identifying the "100 Best Companies to Work For." Also, in 2004, Bronson received the Governor's Award of Excellence for Improving Care in the Hospital Setting from the Michigan Quality Improvement Organization.

Magnet Hospital status application-in-process after 2000 demonstrated the nurses' desire to step up to the plate with leader development, shared governance and participation in nursing research. No doubt, this status will be achieved given an organizational culture that values human capital. Ulshafer, a seasoned expert when coming to Bronson, listened, learned and responded as part of a team with a plan for a culture of empowered people, those served and serving. Caring had come full circle.

Mary Ann Eldred, 1998–2003

Mary Ann Eldred, senior VP operations/patient care services, in a telephone interview on June 3, 2004, told about the new hospital opening. The story was a labor of love and hope for a new healing culture, and it generated the same excitement as the first new hospital opening in 1906.

Eldred was hired by Frank Sardone in 1998. She arrived when the new hospital was a hole in the ground. Her work centered on the kind of caring environment that would rise up from the hole—a healing house, The *New* Bronson! It would be patient-centered and friendly, with privacy, and adorned in art and green gardens.

Eldred observed that the size of the project was massive and overwhelming—how to build it well, safely and without disruption in patient care would be a challenge. Nurse leaders most involved with Eldred were Roberta Utrecht, Jackie Wahl, Katie Harrelson, Lois Van Donselaar and Jo Ulrich '73, whose title at that time was facilities planning assistant.[38] The administrative team listened to nurse managers who had listened to nursing staff. All gave their input on important questions in hospital design:

- How to make the physical plant patient-centered and effective for all of the employees?
- How to furnish and supply?
- How to orient the staff, even for making the massive move of patients when that long-awaited day arrived?
- How would patient care change in the new building to be more focused on patient needs?

Managers often worked seven days a week to assure that the plan was realized—an exhausting but exhilarating schedule.

Eldred led the move to the outpatient facility, scheduled seven months ahead of the anticipated November 2000 inpatient move.[39] She recalled the special shirts and jean attire that staff wore as they pitched in on the weekend before the move to help the nurses unpack supplies and set up for their first outpatient customers. The air was filled with excitement when the outpatient facility opened April 3, 2000, after a well-orchestrated transfer. Equally exciting and more dramatic was the inpatient move on December 3, later that year. Spirits were high as staff rehearsed and practiced and planned for the transfer of patients. Eldred said,

> Utrecht was the "Grand Commander" for the transfer. It resembled the opening night of a play after so many rehearsals. It was a goose bump-producing event as the doors to The *New* Bronson opened. We were alive! It was the real triumph that felt so unreal for the first few hours. A mixture of excitement for entering the new and sadness for leaving the old was in the air.
>
> It was a momentous occasion when the first department, Trauma and Emergency, turned on the lights at 5:30 A.M. and opened the doors to receive patients. The old trauma area remained open to care for those patients who had been admitted in the hours prior to the new hospital opening. Slowly the old department wound down

> as patients were served and left the unit, winding down to one patient who was stable enough to transfer to the new unit.

Wonderful stories circulated about the first baby born in the new birthing center and of children on the old pediatric unit who transferred with their parents amid balloons and fanfare. The bricks and mortar were in place. The move had been made and staff adapted to a new environment that exceeded the expectations of the community.

Attention then shifted to exceeding standards in customer service. It took extensive in-service training to begin to build a healing-house culture—how to reframe interactions with patients and their families and within and between departments and how to be a healing house in the Kalamazoo and southwest Michigan community.

Questions came to Eldred's mind about the nursing staff mix and movement toward a professional practice model, which required an increase in nursing practice autonomy and a sense of ownership for patients' care experiences. Such a model would be more visible in its service to patients and RN self-respect. Eldred wanted nurses to recognize that they had a practice of their own that focused on total patient care, and that they could be accountable for the quality of patient care during the patient's hospital stay. Eldred felt that more graduate-prepared nurses would be needed to facilitate the development of a professional practice environment within *The New* Bronson. Hiring clinical nurse specialists, a role that Bronson accepted in the eighties but had lost within budget cuts of the nineties became a priority. The vision was facilitated by contemplating an application for Magnet Hospital status. Eldred's Bronson tenure was cut short when she and her husband decided to move to New York in late 2003.

Harrelson at the Helm

Accepting the chief nurse executive position in August 2001, to replace Roberta Utrecht who planned to retire in December 2001, Harrelson was excited about fulfilling her desire to lead the nursing management team into the new millennium. She would occupy one of the seats at the diverse administrative table, within a beginning era of transdisciplinary practice.

The timing was right. Frank Sardone shared her vision for transforming nursing into the professional model in which recognition and remuneration matched skills. Nurses were to be paid, not only for their work as skilled clinical technicians, but for their clinical judgment and ability to manage patient care and healthcare system complexities.

Harrelson approached the task with honesty and straightforwardness to encourage the nurses to hear themselves in situations of unwarranted submissiveness. Playing the victim only accelerated a downward spiral, not only for nurses themselves, but also for the community that they served. Some nurses, for example, were sharing frustrations in public, acting as if they had no power to change their professional direction and, in a sense, asking for help. Harrelson herself heard stories in the community that demonstrated the nurses' frustration and lack of insight as to changes needed in their own response. A shared governance structure provided one external support.

MOVING TOWARD SHARED GOVERNANCE

Stacy Brawer '92, became the first chair of the Divisional Council established in April, 2003; she was already the chair of the CCL Unit Council. Approximately 30 staff nurses, who were divisional unit chairs, met monthly to listen and collectively offer suggestions for clinical operations improvements. Staff nurses were expected to report back to their unit peers, nurse managers, unit clerks and patient-care assistants. The council encouraged the four groups to participate in meetings. A spin-off for unlicensed staff participation was potential nurse recruitment. The groups saw themselves as respected partners in a democratic process. It became clear that, with a nursing education, the unlicensed staff could offer more to patient care and also gain more for themselves and their families in the process.

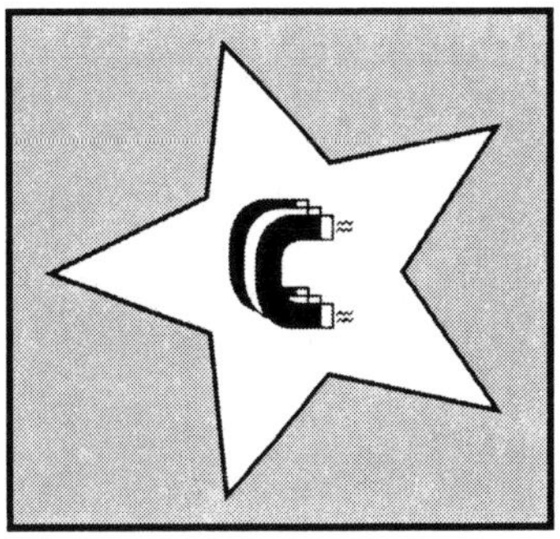

The Divisional Council created a symbol for the "magnet journey." It was a five-pointed star with three concentric, overlapping Cs and wavy lines extending from the two ends of the Cs to represent the magnetic forces. The three Cs represented Bronson's values of Clinical Excellence, Customer and Service Excellence, and Community Accountability and Long-Term Viability.

The council provided the same opportunity as it had in the past to take ownership of nursing practice, with awareness of the need for a legitimate interdisciplinary team. Harrelson persistently facilitated nurses' understanding that pleading would not get them to where they wanted to go. She used inclusive, non-threatening ways to increase nurse awareness—ways to regain the soul of nursing, inviting nurses to the table, not simply to listen to "poor pitiful me" stories, but to raise consciousness levels and to facilitate nurse empowerment toward becoming proactive members of the complex hospital team. Sometimes the dialogue was discomfiting to nurse managers who had difficulty recognizing that appropriate risk taking was useful in gaining new outcomes.

A deeper understanding of benefit versus risks, a part of managerial and clinical decision-making, was especially required in an era of accelerated change. Together, the nursing divisional unit chairs, created a mission with a caring philosophy that included several of the curriculum threads of the WMU Bronson School of Nursing: relationship-centered care; holistic practice; evidence-based outcome-oriented practice; critical thinking; shared decision making and more.

The second Divisional Council chair for the 2004-year was Eileen Negri, educational services instructor, whose expert area was trauma and emergency room nursing. Her "Magnet Moment" column was added to the in-house *Healthlines* publication in June 2004.

NEW BRONSON'S NURSING PHILOSOPHY

Bronson Methodist Hospital's Philosophy of Nursing Excellence[40] is founded on the principles of respect, compassion, expertise, impact and pride. We connect with patients, families, colleagues and community through relationship-centered caring, shared decision-making, evidence-based practice and accountability:

- ***Compassion*** – Patient and family focused, holistic, hopefulness, humor, kindness, relationship-centered caring, empathy and advocacy.
- ***Respect*** – Acceptance, forgiveness, celebration/recognition of talents and success, tolerance, patience, integrity, appreciation for diversity of mind, body and spirit, conflict management and professionalism.
- ***Expertise*** – Critical thinking, shared decision-making, evidenced-based practice, outcome-oriented, continuous improvement, confidence, technical skills and personal development.
- ***Pride*** – Coaching, education, modeling, mentoring, precepting, earning/ career pathways, attention to detail, promotion of a positive image, engagement, honesty and trust.
- ***Impact*** – Accountability, safety, cost effectiveness, peer review, empowerment, participation in Nursing Councils, responsibility, optimizing resources, communication, positive patient outcomes, influence on healing and leadership.

Standing with Harrelson, Bronson staff nurses regained an identity seemingly buried in previous decades of growing medical technology and physician-extender work. High-tech hospital treatments were balanced with visible high-touch nursing care. Nurses still were responsible for myriad medical orders, but there was a glimmer of what nursing presence meant in a culture that honored the nurse as a peer and professional.

The presence of a shared Bronson Methodist Hospital nursing mission and philosophy laid the groundwork for a new culture of professional caring in southwest Michigan. Nurses with their daily patient and family connections learned to listen with a third ear—patient expectations could be met with the outcome of measurable high patient-satisfaction reports. Nurse standards of care were recognized. Nurse articulation of healing through caring relationships was in the process of balancing medical technology. With opportunities to work directly with the WMU Bronson School of Nursing, faculty and researchers enhanced both education and practice outcome potentials. Physician practice was also changing, with an increased number of women graduating from medical school and attention given to relationship-centered care in some medical schools.[41]

Acute Care for the Elderly (ACE) Unit Exemplified Nursing Philosophy

Leading a new nurse team was Alison Dickinson. She helped plan and open the unique, first of its kind in Michigan, 20-bed unit for elders[42] on December 15, 2003, on the remodeled third floor of the old campus Center Building. Excellent nursing staff and PCAs had participated in the Geriatric Resource Nurse Program (GRN). RNs received 16 hours of training and the PCAs, eight hours, taught by Rita LaReau, geriatric clinical nurse specialist and nurse educators Jane Morrow and Bertha Stewart. Not only did the three teach Bronson nurses but they had also taught the GRN at other acute-care settings in Michigan. All nurses were expected to sit for geriatric certification to further demonstrate competencies in the nursing care of elders.

The model of nursing practice followed *Nurses Improving Care for Health System Elders* (NICHE) guidelines for promoting excellence in older adult nursing care from the John Hartford Foundation Institute for Geriatric Nursing. Nursing practice was visible and made a difference in patient outcomes and satisfaction! Length of stay in 2004 was four and one-half days, with patients discharged in improved conditions. Interventions included mobilization and integrated social support with walks to a community room. Families were welcomed as partners and each morning enjoyed complimentary continental breakfast in an environment that recognized their need for support as well as for learning more about the family care-giving role. Families sensed their value as much as the nurses sensed theirs.

The interdisciplinary unit, led by Dickinson, addressed challenges, such as poly-pharmacy—too many drugs—by reducing prescription numbers to a more manageable medication program whenever possible. Ferris State University pharmacy residents were part of the ongoing conferencing team.

Dickinson described a common elder problem of sleep deprivation which hospitalization often exacerbates. All patients were assessed for sleep habits and first offered interventions that did not require the use of medications but rather nurse presence and touch. Enthusiastic teams continued to build nursing excellence.

Dickinson was a spring 2004 recipient of the Nursing Excellence Leadership Award, a recognition initiated by Bronson nurses several years ago and retained to honor Hazel Latondress, beloved nurse administrator during the fifties, sixties, seventies and eighties.[43] At the same time Bronson Methodist Hospital was awarded the first John Hartford Foundation Award, given by the American Organization of Nurse Executives at their annual convention held in Phoenix, Arizona.

Jacqueline (Francisco) Wahl

Jackie Wahl[44] earned multiple promotions at Bronson after graduating from Nazareth College with her BSN in 1980 and an MS degree in perinatal nursing from the University of Michigan in 1986. Her career began as a staff nurse in 1980 in the Neonatal Intensive Care Unit (NICU), with the added responsibilities as a transport nurse.

Wahl became the nursing manager of NICU in 1986, then was appointed manager of applications, and advanced to an information technology position, project coordinator, director of operations improvement, and executive director of patient outcomes, April 2004. Her work in 2004 included management support for the Pharmacy Department, case managers, and medical social workers. Wahl led a unique recruitment strategy to introduce young people to the world of healthcare careers. Fourth, fifth and sixth graders were engaged in a four-week summer career camp to explore nine health-related careers including job shadowing hospital staff.

Wahl was involved in the early planning of the new hospital while she was project coordinator. Staff nurses were involved also in these stages of planning but were less involved as cost factors influenced building modifications that changed some of the original design plans. The outcome was not always based on the nurse's suggestions.

Originally, the plan was to have computerized, electronic documentation and record keeping. Time for developing a system with staff training fell short of the opening date operations so the new facility had to be adapted to accommodate paper records. In the last hours, new documentation equipment had to be purchased and homes found on every unit for charts and chart racks. Wahl was part of efficiently managing that process, with nurse managers stepping in to finalize the work on their units.

Research—Future Healing-Hospital Environmental Design

It was clear to Wahl that a perfect building was a dream to strive for, but the real world of building meant that moving toward environmental excellence would be an ongoing challenge. She continued to observe and discover what worked and what could be designed for future unit modifications to decrease nurse fatigue and other stressors. Researching the impact of hospital design on caregivers and care given has increased understanding of improvements that could enhance future Bronson clinical services. Wahl's work helped develop a rich database for improving the work environment.

She partnered with the WMU Industrial Engineering Department's Tycho Fredericks and Steven Butt to undertake a study of how nurses use their time during a shift. Susan Olsen, PhD, RN, and WMU educator, had introduced Wahl to the possibility of conducting this joint research with the Industrial Engineering Department.

Nurses were job shadowed on two units, Surgical Intensive Care and the General Medical Unit. They were monitored for impact of the environment on their work. Recorders outside of acutely ill patients' rooms monitored the minutes/hours they spent at the bedside. Indirect time was noted when not caring directly for patients. Also measured were nurses' heart rates throughout their shift and miles walked per shift with the use of pedometers.[45, 46]

What was learned? The building was designed for its patient customers, for all patients to have private rooms with space for family inclusion and personal space, plus every room had a window for connection with the world outside: sun, sky and an outdoor view known to be therapeutic. The expansive units meant that nurses, in the course of their work, averaged a daily hike of five miles with the range of three to ten miles—distances, one could assume, much greater than traveled by 19th century nurses in hospital wards that Florence Nightingale originally designed with the nurses' feet and physical abilities in mind. Unit and design differences such as the distance of patients' rooms from the nurses' workstation and supplies accounted for some of the differences in miles nurses walked each shift. The aging nurse work force, with the average Bronson staff nurse 43 years old, was a little lower than the national average of 45. Could the walking part of the staff nurse job be a healthy factor or another stressor? Stress is a part of one's perception, not only an external event.

Participation in Magnet Hospital Designation

Wahl applauded Nancee Hofmeister for her leadership toward gaining the Magnet Hospital designation for nursing excellence. She read every document and article she could find about magnet hospitals and had been one of the nurses who attended conferences to learn more about the process. Were Bronson nurses ready to move forward? Listening to presenters and conferees resulted in roller-coaster minds: First thought was, "Yes! We're ready to apply." Then, on the other hand, "No! We haven't accomplished that feat." It was up and down but finally, with Harrelson's enthusiastic, move ahead, and just-do-it leadership style, Bronson applied. It was the right approach to take.

Saying, "The final draft of our self-evaluation process is being fine-tuned! We will be ready to submit the report and plan for a site visit in 2005," Jackie Wahl brings this story to a point of closure. Her passion for professional nursing practice and upbeat, can-do attitude is built on a solid nursing education foundation with a participative management style—both necessary for third millennium healthcare. She brings positive energy to a futuristic transdisciplinary world.

As for the compiler of this Bronson history, Jackie Wylie is content to do the little tasks that individuals do to add small magnetic forces—an endless supply of energy that will continue to flow from the supportive Alumni Association of Bronson Methodist Hospital School of Nursing to its beloved alma mater and the new WMU Bronson School of Nursing.

> I am done with great things and big plans, great institutions and big success. And I am for those tiny invisible loving human forces that work from individual to individual, creeping through the crannies of the world like so many rootlets . . . yet which if given time, will rend the hardest monuments of human pride.
>
> —***William James***

CHAPTER 11 NOTES

---

[1] The Western Michigan University School of Nursing first enrolled registered nurses in 1994. Their objective was to obtain a baccalaureate degree with a major in nursing, a next step in the advancement of their education from matriculation in an associate degree or diploma program. Four RNs graduated in 1996, before the first 1999 graduating class of prelicensure students, paving the way for attainment of the National League for Nursing Accreditation, a voluntary recognition for meeting national nursing education standards which included the requirement that a class be officially graduated.

[2] Fetzer Institute, *Annual Report*. Kalamazoo, Michigan, 1998. p.22.

[3] BMH School of Nursing students received college credit from Western Michigan University's predecessors as early as 1926.

[4] *Healthlines*, 1999 April 27–May 10, "WMU's School of Nursing named, 'The Bronson School of Nursing'."

[5] Paul Kokales and Lisa McMillan Washington became the first double graduates of both Bronson Methodist Hospital and WMU schools of nursing.

[6] It became necessary to identify the closing school as BMH School of Nursing since the new WMU School of Nursing was named the Bronson School of Nursing in 1999.

[7] *Kalamazoo Gazette*, 1999 July 31, "New Bronson blooms downtown."

[8] The remodeled campus, including the old Center Building, north of the new John Street hospital was renamed North Campus.

[9] Oral interview with Jacqueline Wahl by Jackie Wylie, confirming current bed utilization and total licensed bed numbers, 2004 August 4.

[10] *Healthlines*, 1997 July 8–21, "Local resident leaves generous contribution to Bronson Health Foundation."

[11] Often health care disciplines other than medical doctors were called allied health professionals, a term that would imply alliance of all professionals to the dominant medical model of practice.

---

[12] *American Nurses Association,* 1993 December 15, "American Nurses Association declares strong support of Clinton's Health Security Act."

[13] *Washington Post*, 1993 December 21, "Docs and nurses: who prescribes?"

[14] *Ibid.*

[15] *USA Today*, 1993 December 10, "Nurses deserve a bigger role in patient care."

[16] *New York Times*, 1993 December 15, "Nurses on the advance."

[17] *Ibid.*

[18] *USA Today*, 1993 December 8, "Doctors and nurses dispute boundaries of medical 'domain'."

[19] Tresolini, Carol, and the Pew-Fetzer Task Force, *Health professions education and relationship-centered care.* San Francisco: Pew Health Professions Commission, 1994.

[20] *Ibid,* p. 21.

[21] Boyle, Suzanne, "Nursing unit characteristics and patient outcomes." *Nursing Economics* 2004, 22(3); 112–123. (The authors of the original 1982 work were McClure, Poulin, Solvie and Wandelt.)

[22] "Magnet" hospitals referred to hospitals in the 1980s, which had the capacity to recruit and retain nurses. It became formalized into an accreditation process for recognizing hospitals that had exemplar nursing practice.

[23] McClure, Margaret L. & Hinshaw, Ada Sue, eds., *Magnet hospitals revisited: attraction and retention of professional nurses.* Washington, D.C.: American Nurses Publishing, 2002.

[24] McClure, M.L., Poulin, M.A., Sovie, M.D. & Wandelt, M.A. *Magnet hospitals: attraction and retention of professional nurses.* Washington D.C.: American Nurses Association, 1983.

[25] Oral interview with Nancee Hofmeister by Jackie Wylie, 2004 June 1.

[26] *Bronson Nursing Notes*, 2004 Winter, "Magnetizing excellence: the journey towards magnet recognition at Bronson."

[27] McClure, M.L., Poulin, M.A., Sovie, M.D. & Wandelt, M.A., *op.cit.*

[28] McClure, M.L. & Hinshaw, A.S., Eds., *op.cit.,* pp. 106–107.

[29] *Healthlines*, 2004 June 15–28, p.2, "Meet the Magnet Steering Committee."

[30] Oral interview with Stacey Finley Brawer by Jackie Wylie, 2004 July 1.

[31] Operations Improvement was renamed Clinical Operations Improvement in 2004.

[32] Oral interview with Jo Ulrich by Jackie Wylie, 2004 June 21.

[33] Oral interview with Katie Harrelson by Jackie Wylie, 2004 February 4.

[34] Oral interview with Susan Ulshafer by Jackie Wylie, 2004 June 10.

[35] Oral interview with Susan Ulshafer by Jackie Wylie, 2004 June 10.

---

[36] Year provided by Kay Bennett, Bronson Methodist Hospital, 2004 August 4.

[37] Naisbitt, John. *Megatrends: ten new directions transforming our lives.* New York: Warner Books, 1984.

[38] Joyce "Jo" Ulrich's title in 2004 was planning manager. She is a 1973 Bronson graduate.

[39] The actual transfer of patients to the new Bronson Methodist Hospital occurred on December 3, 2000.

[40] Bronson Methodist Hospital, "Bronson's philosophy of nursing excellence."

[41] A relationship-centered care project at Indiana University School of Medicine, led by Tom Inui, MD, has been on going during the early 2000s.

[42] Oral interview with Alison Dickinson by Jackie Wylie, 2004 August 8.

[43] *Bronson Nursing Notes*, 2004 June, "Bronson celebrates nursing excellence."

[44] Oral interviews with Jacqueline Wahl by Jackie Wylie, 2004 July 29 and August 4.

[45] *International Occupational Ergonomics and Safety Conference,* 2004 May 19–22, Houston. Proceedings, XVII, edited by L.J.H. Schulze. "An evaluation of physiological work demands on registered nurses over a 12-hour shift."

[46] Butt, Steven E., Tycho K. Fredericks, Anil R. Kumar, Jacqueline Wahl, Katie Harrelson, Stephanie Means, Alana Dumasius, and Erin Brown, "An investigation of the relationship between patient acuity, time standards, and productivity," reported at the Pebble Meeting, 2004 March, Boston.

CHAPTER 12

BRONSON ALUMNI ASSOCIATION—PROFESSIONAL NURSING ORGANIZATIONS AND LASTING RELATIONSHIPS

The story of the Alumni Association of Bronson Methodist Hospital School of Nursing[1] offers a snapshot of member service and community activities that helped build the Bronson monument, 1904 to 2004. Bronson graduates, when not practicing nursing, served in diverse health-related capacities in the care of their neighborhoods and families and also within organizations such as their churches, American Red Cross, American Cancer Society and White Cross Guild.

Alumni minutes, available from 1923 until the present, document professional and volunteer services given and the lasting relationships that developed for those who participated. Generally, the minutes are boring to read, lacking the luster of detail. The minutes were for simple recordkeeping, not for telling the association's story eighty years later. Reflected is more a reactive rather than proactive stance toward changes in healthcare. Confrontation and the recognition of differences of opinion were not detailed, another reason the minutes lacked luster. Emotions such as joy, excitement, sadness or anger, when or if emotions were present, were well hidden and probably represent the quality of an objective minutes-taker. Although community service is recorded, humility was a living virtue. Acts of kindness and good deeds were not visible and rarely verbalized.

Alumni who worked behind the scenes did not share their good deeds in public or even in their own meeting minutes. Insight into the group member's minds, what pleased or displeased them, what long-term goals they envisioned or chose to accomplish for nursing practice, the school or hospital, is limited in annual reports or future planning documents. The Alumni as change agents for the betterment of nursing services and the profession is not expressed. What is evident? They found relationship and nourishment for their spirits in service and social activities. Very few were activists. They were not out to change the world but simply to care for others.

ESTABLISHMENT OF THE ALUMNI ASSOCIATION

There were 63 graduates, including the Class of 1917, when the association was founded.[2] While the earliest Constitution and Bylaws recovered by the authors was not dated, the original name was Bronson Hospital Alumnae Association of Kalamazoo District Association, Michigan State Nurses' Association. The 1917 date is based on a list of charter members, leading to the conclusion that the association was established sometime between 1917 and early 1918, before that class graduated. Official documents are missing from 1917 to the end of 1922, but the January 1923 minutes do refer to meetings held in 1922.

When the name of the association changed from the feminine case, alumnae, is not known. Minutes throughout the years are inconsistent, depending on the secretary who may have used either case. Several graduates were men, so *Bronson Women and the School of Nursing* uses "alumni" as gender inclusive of both men and women for all but its earliest years, even though a strong feminine presence was and is the reality of nursing.

On the back of a piece of letterhead stationery from Dr. R.E. Balch's office at 115 W. Lovell St., Kalamazoo, Michigan, someone wrote the names of 18 graduates and identified them as charter members of the Bronson Hospital Alumnae Association (*see* sidebar). This list is not dated. Since Mina Weber practiced nursing in the office of Dr. Balch, on whose letterhead the list appeared, it was likely that she was present at and part of the formal development of the organization. Perhaps she also was responsible for this casual record.

Bronson Hospital
Alumnae Association of
Kalamazoo District Association,
Michigan State Nurses' Association

CHARTER MEMBERS

Irene Lage '09	***Anna Heethuis '15***
Theresa Norberg '09	***Suzanne Bauer '16***
Josephine Cook '11	***Lena Bloem '16***
Nina Heath '11	***Cora Fetteroff '16***
Eva Knight '11	***Una Frisbie '16***
Mrs. Helen Makin '11	***Emma Schwartz '16***
Mina Weber '13	***Clara Olson '16***
Ruth Mumly '14	***Kate Bushhouse '17***
Ann Gemrich'15	***Edith Sweetland '17***

Another likelihood was that the association existed prior to its 1917 formalization. Eighteen members represented 28.6 percent of the 63 graduates in 1917, a surprisingly low percentage given their sense of sisterhood and their need to secure private duty positions, paid directly by families to care for ill members at home or in the hospital. Graduates who felt a sense of belonging shared their stories, giving a sense of a strong collective group, but alumni voice and power were not obvious, even though individual graduates were in positions of authority in hospital practice and community healthcare. Alumni seemed to look upon each other as a personal source of strength more than strength related to unity within their profession.

MEETINGS IN THE EARLY YEARS

Extant original minutes of the Alumni Association begin with the annual meeting and election of officers, dated January 2, 1923, with the presence of Misses Weber, Herrmann, Gemrich, Lemmer, Frisbie, Taylor and Hinds. They met at the

Osborne Nurses Home at 3:30 P.M. and at the same location for most of the additional eight meetings held in 1923. Most likely the nurses were on relief from 24-hour, private-duty assignments or were waiting for one.

Miss Mina Weber, the first Bronson graduate to become a superintendent of nurses at Bronson, was one of the few chiefs of nursing service and/or education whose name often appeared in minutes—testimony that she was instrumental in maintaining a functional alumni organization throughout the twenties and thirties.

Attention to membership in the first ten years is well documented in the minutes. For example, when Miss Weber, superintendent of nurses, was elected president at the first meeting in 1923, nine new members were approved: Misses Wilson, Veenhuis, Hooven, Baker, Garrison, Ilahbelle Finley, Gladys Finley, Healey and Frye. All but Miss Frye, who is listed as a nonresident member, became designated active members. Resident members were "in-district," whereas nonresident were out-of-district. Nonresident members most likely were expected to pay dues in their home district.

No record mentions rejection of a member application. These applications for membership, accounting for members and designating their status, comprise a large part of the minutes.

Functions described in 1923 included social events, especially for graduating seniors; the business of private-duty nursing; and managing the organization. A program by Miss Sarah E. Sly, secretary of the Michigan State Nurses Association, offered, "a very informal talk about the National Convention, Parliamentary Law, our Constitution and Alumni."[3] Details are absent for this account.

A social event that June was an outing to Oakwood Park, a popular amusement park on Oakwood Lake on the south side of Kalamazoo, which had rides, including a roller coaster, and a pavilion. It could be reached by trolley car or auto. Notes indicate that business was also conducted during this outing with the presence of six guests from the 1924 senior class. A banquet as well, at the Park American

Hotel in Kalamazoo, was sponsored for the graduating seniors that year. Banquets represented a formal way of welcoming new graduates into the "fold."

Throughout the 1920s, meetings took place at the Osborne Nurses' Home in the afternoon, except for occasional outings to local parks and for the annual banquet to honor graduating seniors. Two popular spots for a lunch or dinner meeting were the South Rose Street YWCA and the Gilmore Department Store's Tea Room on Burdick Street.

Most of the original local committees were an outgrowth of the prototype bylaws from the Michigan State Nurses Association: Membership and Credentials, Program, Publicity, Hospitality, and Nominations. The Publicity Committee was never activated, decreasing visibility of the group in the community. Sometimes Hospitality Committee was referred to as the Social Committee. A purely local committee, not set by national and state structures, was the Banquet Committee. An annual gala event honored graduating seniors provided a social outlet for all graduates. Time and attention were paid to planning and hosting the event with the few alumni resources available.

How could nurses ever attend meetings when most practiced private-duty nursing, 12 to 22 hours a day, well into the 1930s? Hospital shifts were 12 hours long, six days per week. Work schedules did not allow time to engage in many activities, although numerous written memories of fun within the daily work routine are interspersed with descriptions of occasional outings.

In 1927 came a decision to have more meetings of a social nature. This innovation seemed to be in response to poor attendance at meetings and less involvement by membership overall. Most likely the phenomenon represented a change in the numbers of graduates who married or had their own apartments or homes in which to entertain. Card games played after the meetings included bridge, fan-tan, and Five Hundred. This pattern continued into the 1930s, with single nurses gradually moving away from the nurses' home and hosting meetings in their own apartments or sponsoring a meeting at the home of another person. Occasionally the meeting was held at Osborne Nurses' Home, hosted by Mrs. Ann Gwinn Draher, director of nursing, and supervisors[4]. Refreshments were always praised as being, "delightful . . . delicate, dainty, delicious, *etc.*"

Rummage sales and bazaars were held periodically to help finance services and social events for graduating seniors. Opportunity to recycle trash and treasures was a time-honored tradition that supplemented dues income and met the needs of an organization requesting more of members' time than of their limited money. Rarely did members ask for hospital support, since most of the time their role was to give, not get. Contributions willingly came from alumni volunteers at any time and in any setting.

What is not said about finances tells the story. There were little to none. Even holidays were celebrated with white elephant gifts, often exchanged at Christmas gatherings. Money was collected to supply a family for the holiday.[5]

Decisions Concerning Uniforms and Pins

Minutes of April 29, 1924, document the adoption of, ". . . organdy caps. The caps to be . . . the same pattern and to be worn by all members of the alumni. Also a new style of uniform and introduction of capes—the capes to be decided on later as to color [and] style." Parliamentary procedure was followed with a motion made by Miss Weber and seconded by Mrs. Cessna. It carried. Seven members were present at the meeting.

The action regarding uniforms received more attention on May 27, 1924, when Miss Weber moved, " . . . that a committee be appointed to send letters to the alumni members and ask their opinion in regards to adoption of organdy caps, of adopting capes, their color and length, style. Also, what should be the pattern of the [student?] uniform?" Motion did not carry. That September's minutes referred to previous discussion regarding capes and noted that it was "impossible to adopt them."

This decision most likely related to the cost, although the reason for rejection was not given.

When and why was the blue enamel-faced pin changed to the raised Old English "B" for Bronson encircled with white enamel? In 1931, the March minutes cited the need to, "change hospital pin due to factory going out of business and inability of other factories to stabilize the blue dye." Other pin changes occurred over time (*see* Appendix E, Collectibles).

Regulation of Private Duty Fees

After graduation, nurses joined the "registry" to accept private-duty assignments. In the beginning nurses were on duty 22 of 24 hours until the patient recovered, died or the nurse was discharged and had time off—sometimes too much time off and too few calls for work. Only affluent families could afford to pay for nursing services, this work delegated to women who were most likely informally trained by their female family elders to give care.

American work patterns were changing and the nurses followed suit by planning for a shorter workday. Since the general pay rate of the day was not recorded at the alumni meetings, it is not evident what the change in pay rate meant when discussed at the February 24, 1925, meeting. Were Bronson nurses' fees higher or lower than Miss Kester's statement?

> Miss Kester brought the matter of ruling for regulation [of] fees for private-duty nurses before the meeting. She stated that all but Bronson nurses were charging $7.00 and $8.00. The president appointed Miss Kester as a committee of one to take the matter up with the district to determine what the custom has been regarding such regulation.[6]

The nurses controlled the rate, but the challenge was to find clients who could pay the set fee. Cornelia Veenhuis '21 did indicate she made $8.00 per day, and in one case made $10.00, which pleased her.[7]

In March, 1925, Miss Wagner wrote to the *American Journal of Nurses* regarding the regulation of fees for the private-duty nurses. Because "No definite information was received,"[8] the alumni decided to write to the Michigan State . . . [Nurses] Ass[ociation]."[9] Apparently members wanted to hear about more fee possibilities than were allowed by the ruling that must have come from the Kalamazoo District Nurses Association. The next month Miss Wagner motioned, with a second from Miss Kester, to set alumni fees. The motion carried and was followed by another from Mrs. Phelps, seconded by Miss Wagner. General discussion ensued and the motion carried,

> . . . that the private-duty nurse charge seven dollars per day for surgical and medical cases. Eight [dollars] for obstetrical, and eight [dollars] as a minimum for contagion and mental. Six dollars for 12-hour duty. In home or hospital an additional fee of one dollar for each added individual of the same family. Five dollars each for medical or surgical patients of different families.

A motion made by Miss Ward, " . . . that the twenty-hour duty be adopted for the 24-hour nurses: [was] seconded by Mrs. Phelps. Motion carried." [10]

The Bronson nurses needed more patient referrals and may have felt that they were in competition with the nurse registry. They went on record favoring an organized nurses directory under the direct supervision of the Kalamazoo District Nurses Ass[ociation]." [11] Private-duty price lists were printed and distributed. Once again, details were not recorded so specific prices remain unknown to us. [12]

Nurses Relief Fund

Minutes of December 1, 1925, indicate an involvement in the Nurses' Relief Fund. If a nurse had no family or chose to be independent of her family, how would she receive care if or when she became ill? Almost a year later, the minutes make "Mention of the subscriptions by the alumni to the Nurses' Relief Fund." A number of nurses subscribed individually to this fund.

THE ALUMNI MISSION

A mission defining nursing practice at Bronson is evident in the alumni Constitution and Bylaws, which set standards and quality in its opening statement, " . . . to establish and maintain ethical standards . . . to defend the law relative to the registration of nurses."[13] The School of Nursing and its graduates set a standard of care within the hospital. Caring for the sick and injured regardless of ethnicity, for example, clearly emanated in stories told throughout the years. No one was refused care according to graduate accounts. Most of the nurses were schooled in the Christian faith, so their beliefs and values about service and charity care fit well with the 1920 Methodist mission.

The alumni were student mentors, an unvoiced expectation of support and instruction. Students learned from graduates and peers. Few instructors were hired during the first 40 years, and the nursing superintendent had dual roles of directing service and education until the 1960s. When the first instructor was hired in 1920, the instructor could not possibly have been present 24 hours a day, seven days a week. Staff nurse tutoring was an expected role within this experiential learning model of on-the-job practice. The majority of Bronson nurses, during the first 25 years of the hospital's history, were those trained at Bronson and in other affiliated hospitals. Still, an amazing number of nurses, having received their education in other states, moved to the area and were hired, effectively diversifying the early nurse population.

One's duty to the healthcare of others seemed to be the strongest message—duty to patients by maintaining ethical and professional standards, to physicians and to the hospital, and to each other in a mentoring and censoring way. It depended on the individual's style as to whether his or her support leaned more toward that of an empowering mentor or of a controlling censor. Whatever, graduates had to fit in. Deviance was not viewed as a healthy difference and one's right; autonomy simply was not tolerated. Possibly this philosophy was the reason for limited evidence in the minutes of proactive change or dissenting voices. Service to the community and medical/hospital system was rewarded. Nurses were informed in ways of family health and the medical model in which they practiced. Occasionally, the graduates reacted to changes and shared their collective voice, but the phenomenon was rare. Mostly they accepted what was, fitting in consciously or unconsciously with minimal outward dissatisfaction. Loyalty to Bronson and medical care seemed to be incredibly strong as nursing care itself went unrecognized.

More visible and valued was the use of medical and surgical interventions, the preferred treatments of the allopathic physicians. Though often recognized individually for their healing contributions, nurses' wages were low. They did not publicly take credit for their part in the healing and recovery of patients or for a well-managed hospital. Pride in patient satisfaction was high. Low infection rates, an incredible nursing feat before the advent of antibiotics, attested to strict enforcement of medical aseptic practices and well-designed isolation of patients with communicable diseases. Nurses practiced behind the scenes and did not share glory in public. Acknowledgment of jobs well done was absent, except for individual messages from families grateful for the nurses' caring presence. It wasn't acceptable to share in any way what could have been construed as bragging.

ALUMNI CONNECTIONS—NEVER-ENDING RELATIONSHIPS

"Nursing . . . has long held as a central value the formation of caring relationships with patients [and with each other]. Relationships, however, have never become a defining force in healthcare."[14] A graduate collective was always actively involved in the work of the alumni. They kept the group together and functional; their ultimate goal was to engage all graduates in their pursuits. On the other hand, many graduates did not respond to the group's entreaties. Recruitment into the association was an ongoing labor of love, searching for those who did not belong or who failed to keep in touch by attending meetings and programs or providing forwarding addresses. Recruitment of inactive members and poor attendance at meetings were identified as an organizational problem in the early years, while lack of active member participation remained a concern throughout the group's recorded history.

Relationships and connections were so important to those who participated—any note or phone call from alumni was appreciated—whether graduates lived in the Kalamazoo area or in the far corners of the globe. Persistence and attention of the "joiners" kept the association together.

Meeting connections meant more than relationship. A community presence was also noted. Graduates in nursing programs across the nation who joined their respective alumni associations began a process of collective professionalism that benefited them and the public they served by raising nursing practice standards. They must have known that one nurse's voice most likely would not be heard. Few nurses were of the mind that speaking out was important. Most would not risk confrontation. Professional growth was possible only if there was a collective movement requiring inclusion, diversity and tolerance for practice variances. Maybe only those who thought in similar ways felt that there was a place for them in an association.

Stories were left untold by the numbers of graduates who did not choose to join the association. It's possible that some members perceived the association's style as a carry over from School of Nursing days—often judgmental and non-accepting of new ways in practicing. Possibly the cost of member dues was prohibitive when state and national dues were part of the total dues collected.[15] Some people were not joiners, no different than today. Another possibility is that graduates who married dropped out of their professional connections to manage family affairs. The number of married members continually increased over time as more nurses fit marriage and careers together. If a nurse had Mrs. in front of her name in the 1900–1920 era, quite likely she was a widow, like Mrs. Edna Wildermuth, the Superintendent of Nursing, 1917 to 1920. The alumni, however, kept the names of all graduates on their roster.

Given the powerful sense of sisterhood developed during school days, many alums wonder what set those non-participants apart who chose to maintain an inactive status—not at least to pay dues, to receive communications, and to be recognized for that level of involvement? Competition for work was one reason. Graduates who aligned directly with physicians were referred for private-duty practice to affluent members of the community who could afford personal nursing care. Since the medical model was dominant, some graduates may have felt that they could only be certain of income through their relationships with physicians. Nursing students were in demand in hospitals; graduates were not. Until the 1930s, nurses competed for paid work as private-duty nurses and for the few available hospital positions. They needed long-term family relationships or physician referrals to be considered for these opportunities.

Aligning with a power source is a common practice for people who believe they are powerless.[16] Nurses could be placed on a continuum from the least risk-taking (those who aligned closely with physicians) to more risk-taking (those who dared to align with their professional nursing organization). All of these women were also without the right to vote until 1920.

The alumni organization was never viewed as a prestigious or powerful group that one should join. There was pride in being a Bronson graduate that was accompanied by a sense of humility that fit with their education—nurses were taught humility as a virtue, but humility did not fit into the American entrepreneurial focus on economic success that brought recognition and status. Most nurses were left behind, in their level of formal education and professional advancement, by having graduated from hospital-based programs that offered diplomas rather than college degrees. They were experts in patient care and systems management. They learned experientially, heart wisdom interwoven with mind. Their vision, though enriching in spirit, did not swell their pocket books.

Building Professional Connections Beyond the Bronson Locale

Connections with the American Nurses Association (ANA) at local, state[17] and national levels are recorded in alumni Minutes from 1923 into the 1930s.

The Michigan State Nurses Association (MSNA) was founded in 1904. "Its first goal was to lobby the state of Michigan to establish licensure for nurses."[18] The right of educated nurses to define professional nursing standards was a major issue as were representing and advocating for nurses and nursing practice. Bronson Hospital acquired state approval to operate a School of Nursing in 1907.

The Detroit Graduate Nurses' Association led the state association movement. It called for all state graduates to " . . . meet in Detroit on May 10, 1904, for the purpose of forming a state association to secure state registration for nurses."[19] However, the first state meeting occurred the following year, March 1905, in Grand Rapids. Annual dues were one dollar. Legislative resistance blocked registration the first time it was introduced, but persistence paid off! House Bill 180, passed in 1907, provided for the registration of educated nurses and restricted the title only to those who had matriculated from an approved nursing program.[20]

The MSNA accomplished its next goal two years later when the first Nurse Practice Act in Michigan limited the use of the title to professional nurse graduates of schools approved by the Michigan Board of Nursing.[21] Mandatory licensure further controlled entry into the profession by requiring graduates to register and pass a state board licensing examination to call themselves professional nurses and use the title, Registered Nurse (RN). According to Amy Bailey Seward, Class of 1914, this period was difficult for nurses who had been practicing for years but now needed to pass a licensure examination to use the title professional registered nurse. Seward took the State Board examination in 1918 and passed![22] Standards had been raised by two mechanisms, (1) state control of school curricula and operations, and (2) an examination requirement before a graduate could use the title Registered Nurse.

MSNA and the BMH School of Nursing Alumni Association

The Bronson Methodist Hospital School of Nursing Alumni Association was part of the Kalamazoo District Association and Michigan State Nurses' Association (MSNA).[23] An undated Constitution and Bylaws proposed by the local organization were filed with the 1923–1948 minutes' notebook. The Constitution and Bylaws template had a fill-in-the-blank format from MSNA. The district included Kalamazoo and St. Joseph counties, plus the following townships in Van Buren County: Pine Grove, Almena, Antwerp, Porter, Decatur and Lawrence:

> **Article II. Object**
> The object of the Association shall be to establish and maintain ethical standards among nurses; to support and defend the law relative to registration of nurses; to promote the educational and social standing of the nursing profession; to cooperate with the Kalamazoo District Association, Michigan State Nurses' Association and the American Nurses' Association.
>
> **Article III. Membership**
> Membership in this Association shall be in accordance with the conditions laid down in the By-Laws of this Association. Members shall be in sympathy with the objects of the Association and express a willingness to work toward their accomplishment.

President Mina Weber, on January 27, 1925, read a letter from the MSNA during an alumni meeting. Discussion following the reading was not recorded. The action immediately following the discussion was that " . . . a committee of three be appointed to look over the opposed constitution." What the MSNA opposed about the constitution was also not recorded. Possible opposition related to two sections of the prototype that were lined out: Article I. Membership, Section 1(a) referenced to,

> Active members become automatically active members of the (underlined space to be filled in) District Association, the Michigan State Nurses' Association, the Mid-West Division of the American Nurses' Association, and the International Council of Nurses' through the American Nurses' Association.

The second lined out area was part of Article VII. Dues. Section 1, amounts of, " . . . $2.35 to the Michigan State Nurses' Association; of 50 cents to the American Nurses' Association; of 10 cents to the Mid-West Division; of 5 cents to the International Council of Nurses; of $1.00 to the National Nurses Relief Fund."[24]

Requirement to pay dues at all levels may have been opposed by the alumni. Similar to belonging to a union, paying multiple dues was not different from mandatory membership, a current practice by nurses who have organized into collective bargaining units. The argument was that it was unprofessional to organize for collective action. It was plausible that mandatory membership with the state association gave graduates a reason not to join, if the alumni bylaws could not allow for a non-paying, associate member status.

What did alumni get for the $7.00 dues paid to their alumni, the local Kalamazoo district, and state and national organizations? Four dollars was passed on to the district, state and national levels, leaving $3.00 dues to operate the District and alumni locally. An annual fee of $7.00 was a great deal of money in 1925! Alumni had to be committed to collective action and the potential positive outcomes to pay this price. It took commitment to fit the expensive dues into meager wages and budgets. Nurses with less family support may have believed that they could not afford to be without membership, while others saw no benefit, not unlike current-day beliefs and values. Associate membership was possible, however, if voting privileges were forfeited:

> **Article I. Section 1. Membership**
> (c) Associate members shall be those graduates from the Bronson Methodist Hospital School of Nursing, who for reasons satisfactory to the Board of Directors desire Alumni membership only. This membership does not permit voting on any question pertaining to the District, State, or National organizations, or of holding office. Associate membership confers social privileges only.

Associate status was awarded to members who married and were not actively practicing as RNs. Dues were needed from all members if their collective voice was to be heard, but dues continued to be an issue. Minutes on June 16, 1931, reflected that, "Miss Pike reviewed an article in the *American Journal of Nursing* in regards to back dues of alumni members. She stated we had never required back dues to be paid." Discussion followed but was not recorded. It appears the cost of belonging to MSNA and ANA was perceived as too great or the professional gain too small at a time when resources were scarce.

Dissociation from the MNA and ANA

The March 14, 1951, minutes record action to amend the local Constitution. Mabel Stell chaired the revision committee. It was February 14, 1952, before a report was given, asking for ideas, ". . . for revision of the constitution as it was written in 1925." At the next month's meeting a revised draft was presented to members by Mabel Stell and Shirley Evans suggesting that discussion occur in April after the amended constitution and bylaws were read to the assembly. The April reading and discussion occurred without changes or corrections. The document was approved on May 14, 1952, when Miss Mertie Dunavan so moved, seconded by Mabel Stell. The new constitution was accepted unanimously, and the alumni had moved to dissociate from the MNA and ANA. Their professional connection to the American Nurses Association seemed to have no benefit or interest. Dissenting voices, if there were any, were not part of the minutes and discussion.

In the fifties the thread connecting the Bronson alumni to the Michigan Nurses Association (MNA) and ANA further unraveled. Movement away from self-employed, private-duty status and toward hospital employment seemed to come with some loss of autonomy in nursing practice and a gain in certain, stable employment. The dues increase by the state and national associations appeared to be higher than many staff nurses were willing and/or able to pay. Not to be forgotten was the impact of the medical culture and a sense of powerlessness that consciously or unconsciously marginalized nursing practice. It created alignment with the medical model instead of with nursing practice and the risk of unemployment. Though licensed by the state, a payment mechanism for nurses, except for fee-for-service, did not exist. Most were dependent on two of the largest local nurse employers, hospitals and physicians.

Over the years, the object of the Bronson alumni Bylaws did not change except for severing nurses' relationship with the local district MNA and ANA. Recorded actions in minutes rarely connected the alumni with the MNA and ANA after the 1930s.

A note in the November 9, 1955, minutes about, "an error on amount of [MNA] district, local and state dues brought to our attention." Had the association failed to report the dissociation to MNA? No record of how many alumni belonged to MNA at that time was noted. Sue Murray VandeGiessen '51 was president of the Alumni Association in 1956 and had been an active member since graduation. She could not recall how the associations were interwoven but knew that the connection existed.[25] Graduate loyalty to their local alumni and Bronson was stronger than their connection with the state and national professional organizations. Excessive dues often became the reason, but there was more to the story than money alone. Where did most of the loyalty lie? With the Bronson family, even though the district and state nurses' viewpoints were in keeping with the alumni mission.

There never seemed to be outward animosity or antagonism toward the MNA and ANA. Goals and objectives of each organization were compatible, but state involvement seemed nonexistent and the connection ignored. Not until November 1995 were the Constitution and Bylaws actually changed to delete wording that led one to believe that a professional ANA connection existed. This revision was the most current document change and reflected an earlier attitude:

> **Article II. Objects**
> The objects of this Association shall be:
> to provide funds for nursing scholarships;
> to promote the professional standards of nursing;
> to secure and maintain good fellowship among graduates
> and the students of the school.

How many Bronson graduates belong to the ANA today is not known.

Professional Involvement

Names of alumni members and Mrs. Edna Wildermuth, then the superintendent of nurses, were submitted to the Kalamazoo District Nurses Association for positions of president, first and second vice presidents, corresponding and recording secretary, treasurer and directors. Later minutes do not indicate if they were elected.

Miss Ruth McLellan, superintendent of nurses from 1935 to 1937, demonstrated involvement in professional activism in reports to the alumni. Minutes were void of details: "Report by Miss McLellan on a District Meeting in Detroit that was very interesting to all present"[26] and "Interesting report by Miss McLellan on

State meeting of nurses."[27] What were the hot topics? What detailed news came back to Kalamazoo with Miss McLellan? Records do not provide evidence of directors' leadership in political activities, and rarely do alumni refer to politics. One exception was Marian Vanderweele's October reminder that everyone become acquainted with candidates and amendments and vote in the 1952 general election.[28]

Thirty years later, discussions about the establishment of a baccalaureate degree-granting program at WMU were intended to build alumni enthusiasm to support the transformation of their diploma-based program into a collegiate model. "Members [were] urged to contact board members at Western to encourage the establishment of the baccalaureate program."[29] For the most part, alumni seemed to remain loyal to their alma mater.

FINANCIAL DONATIONS AND GIFTS OF SERVICE

Main sources of revenue for years were member dues, rummage sales, bake sales, and bazaars. Even *Reader's Digest* subscriptions were sold in the 1950s for $1.00, with the alumni keeping half.[30] Occasionally members gave gifts directly to the hospital and School of Nursing.

Every time the Bronson board of directors and hospital administrators made plans for hospital expansion, the alumni supported the cause. Alumni record-keeping did not account for the actual dollar value of gifts given to several fund-raising campaigns over the years. Pledges were common, and though not representative of relatively large donations, they were consistent and meaningful over time.

Over 90 years, alumni services were given on a daily basis in a multitude of ways, but money was not the primary donated resource until late in the century. Most nurses and their families did not have extra money for gifting or building a nursing presence on dollars. Money contributed was often bestowed collectively in modest amounts as pledges to hospital building funds and individual student scholarships.

Monetary gifts were ongoing, never huge, but always delivered. Gifts of food were often presented to needy families at Thanksgiving and Christmas.

Pennies donated in 1933 bought amenities, such as drapes and curtains, for the alumni room in the hospital.[31] Post-depression days found many people without spare cash, and most nurses continued to come from the poorer class of hard-working laborers. The graduates were often the first in their families to advance their education beyond high school.

The use of the Guild Room at the hospital for meetings was dependent on providing hospital services such as making dressings (folding the material into the proper size and preparing it for sterilization) for surgical incisions and other wounds. It took a constant volunteer effort to keep the hospital supplied with dressings prior to the purchase of commercially-made dressing products. The formalized rule was that the room was not available for meetings unless service was provided during the meeting.[32]

Ongoing recruitment was one type of service provided during the 1940s and 1950s when Director of Nursing, Mary B. Anderson, asked for alumni help. The post-war shortage of nurses was a concern of Doris Dahlstrom, MD, who led an alumni discussion about the problem in the hospital, during which she encouraged recruitment.[33] Alumni were invited to join a School of Nursing committee in 1948 that selected entering students.[34]

A service effort in the late 1940s involved screening for early cancer detection. Mrs. Marian Vanderweele '31, reported that the Academy of Medicine had adopted the Hillsdale Plan for Cancer [Screening]. Forms were available in physician offices for anyone who desired this type of examination and who specifically asked to participate in the Hillsdale Plan. These patients' records were sent monthly to Dr. Prentice.[35] Vanderweele knew that, for cancer screening and detection to happen, more doctors had to be involved. At the November 9, 1949, meeting, she shared a plan with alumni for interesting doctors and others in the cancer detection program and Dr. Hazel Prentice backed the effort.

The Bronson School of Nursing Alumni Scholarship Loan Fund offered $100 annually as a recruitment tool:

> [It was] available to any worthy young woman who would be unable to pursue the course of professional nursing without financial aid. Scholarships are granted upon evidence of scholastic ability, strong character and financial need. The scholarship could be renewed for five years,[36] and, if the student withdrew, had to be repaid.[37]

A scholarship committee was appointed to manage the award process. The alumni news in the *Bronson Bulletin*, Spring 1949, mentions the establishment of this scholarship.

Free-will offerings in the 1950's supported graduates in financial distress, usually related to family illness, while ten years later donations to the Michigan Nurses Association building fund consisted of each alumna giving one completed book of Green Stamps to Eileen Roach '47, who was a MNA district member.

On February 14, 1952, ten members helped the Kalamazoo County Cancer Society survey men between the ages of 28 and 50. As many as 38 members participated in the committee structure, with a service entity coming into being in the early sixties. Cancer dressing assemblies became a routine event, making them especially for people who did not qualify for cancer society free dressings.

Beginning in the 1980s donations were solicited in addition to member dues for support of alumni services that were not part of the annual dues collection. This gave Life Members a special opportunity if they had the means and desired to contribute. These donations boosted the treasury when service volunteers were becoming scarce.

In 1985, Alumni Vice President Marilyn Luther invited members to support the School of Nursing's blood pressure clinics and other outreach activities when students were on vacation. Most members' commitments did not afford time for one more volunteer position. Alumni, as well as all nurses at Bronson and in local healthcare agencies, continued to be informal mentors where students practiced, but that role was never formalized within the Alumni Association.[38]

It became common in 1987 to support one-time donations at the request of participating members: Haitian healthcare, $200; Kenya healthcare, $200; Kalamazoo Hospitality House, $300 for use at Christmas and for office supplies; and Special Day Camp, $100. Long-term commitments to the one-time donations did not occur.

Since 1989, alumni have given a total of $42,915 specifically for scholarships.[39] A $10,000 endowment for scholarships was presented to the Bronson School of Nursing at Western Michigan University in 2001, with $13,000 bestowed to date. Recipients of the rest of the money were students at the hospital-based program. When that program closed in 1998, scholarships were awarded to students in the WMU Bronson School of Nursing, with first preference to Bronson Methodist Hospital graduates who were earning degrees with a nursing major at the new school. They became "double Bronson" graduates (matriculating from both the hospital and collegiate programs). As the WMU College of Health and Human Services constructed its first building to house all of the college's health-related disciplines, including the School of Nursing, in 2003 the alumni contributed $5,000 to the building fund with an additional $5,000 conferred in 2004.[40]

In return for decades of service, loyal alumni remained part of the Bronson family.

Hospital Gifts to the Alumni

Once in the late 1920s the alumni asked Dr. Puffer for the hospital administration's support to pay for the graduate banquet. He complied. In later years in-kind assistance was provided for publishing an alumni bulletin that was sent to members on a periodic basis. Funding was given for a gala commemorative celebration on May 1, 1998, when the final class graduated, and a last monetary gift was given to support publishing this Bronson School of Nursing story.

MAINTAINING RELATIONSHIPS

Meeting attendance was stable throughout the years and often drew 25 to 40 local graduates. The peak meeting attendance occurred in the 1950s. Hospitality and social committees always provided refreshments at meetings so that members lingered after meeting for social conversations and catching up with personal experience. From the beginning, at banquets as well as annual Christmas potluck parties, new graduates were welcomed into the fold and their active membership encouraged. The last Christmas party was held in 1994 at Truesdale Hall, when alumni attendance was low, around ten members, but it was supplemented with hungry students,[41] compared to 50 members who attended the annual Christmas dinner and gift exchange on December 12, 1950.

All active members periodically received *The Bulletin*, sent to inactive members once a year. Whereas the bulletin used a fair amount of the budget for postage and paper, the connection it maintained among graduates and to the hospital was worth the cost. From 1989 to 2004, that cost was $36,500, while member mailings took another $17,170. Other donations included $500 annually to the student yearbook and the annual scholarships. Since the hospital-based school closed, another $5,600 funded student and alumni requests for various activities.

Eight to nine business meetings a year, followed by refreshments and time to socialize, became the regular pattern until the 1990s. The group function that never changed was honoring lasting relationships and performing needed services in professional and personal ways. Alumni always took time for a social "hour" before or after business meetings, worked on service projects, and participated in educational programs. Conversation, tea, coffee and desserts, picnics and potlucks were interspersed with educational programs or local entertainment, whereas in the 1920s and 1930s members often played games.

In the 1950s the group tried to locate all graduates and map their locality, to encourage graduates to return to active status.[42] Active Life Memberships were awarded to alumni that had been graduated for over 40 years (to recognize those retirees on fixed incomes). The reward for perfect attendance for a given year was an exemption from paying dues the next year.[43]

Committee Structure in the Second Half of the Century

Personal relationships were the most wonderful part of belonging to the Association throughout time. The numbers involved in committee work attest to the caring and camaraderie needed to plan events, especially in the 1950s when member involvement in monthly meetings was high.

The Membership Committee accepted dues and donations and worked closely with the Bulletin Committee members to insure active member receipt of bulletins and meeting notices. Dues were increased from $5.00 to $10.00 at the September 11, 1985, meeting after thoughtful discussion on membership impact. Was it too much to ask? The main argument for the dues increase was the increasing cost of postage and paper for mailing bulletins.

Computers, since 1984, helped the board simplify the process of communication. Member recruitment that lagged was constant throughout the association's entire history. Nevertheless, communication between alumni still was quite phenomenal. Carol Van Antwerp '67, reported that 750 bulletins were mailed in October 1985.[44] The School of Nursing, which had been absorbing the costs of paper and printing as a service to its alumni, now requested that they consider paying their own costs for the bulletin to decrease expenses within its institutional budget. Alums agreed.

The dues were raised once more in September 1992 to $15.00 to offset inflation and the decrease in member participation. At the same time donations were solicited, providing the opportunity for graduates in the Life Member non-dues-paying category to contribute if they chose. Some gave directly to the scholarship fund; others added to the group's discretionary income. By the 1994–1995 year, dues paid totaled $4,675 and donations reached $4,370.[45]

In the 1990s, with fewer members available, Anna Stryd '61, managed both membership and bulletin responsibilities. Amal Mansour '85 took an active role in helping to manage membership activities, and she made arrangements for spring and fall semi-annual brunches that substituted for the numerous social events held in earlier decades.

The Bulletin connected hundreds of members with consistent publications—monthly became bimonthly, then quarterly, and finally semiannually by 2000. In the fall of 1991, 1927 bulletins were mailed,[46] but six years later the number had decreased by more than 1000, totaling 927[47], when bulletins were mailed only to active dues-paying members and Life Members who requested them.

The Ways and Means Committee, the service-arm, was led by Marie McLeieer '55 throughout the 1980s, 1990s, and into the 2000s, with a focus on the Annual Holiday Bazaar, often held in the hospital lobby and later in the Gilmore Education Center. Items collected for the December bazaars were wrapped and identified as an item for a man, woman or child, with the help of Winnie Vander Meer '42, for purchase at a variety of prices less than $1.00. They were fun, white elephant kinds of gifts, mostly purchased by hospital employees and alumni to add pleasure to holiday giving and receiving moments. Also, plants were often sold that had been nurtured over the year, and baked goods sold out early.

The Hospitality Committee provided refreshments and hosted most of the association's events. They planned for dinner meetings at modestly priced restaurants, such as Chicken Charlie's on the southwest corner of South Westnedge and Whites

Road, which didn't require a room fee or minimum number in attendance. Alumni volunteered to serve refreshments at graduation receptions held in Truesdale Hall from the 1960s until school closure.

A Christmas Party Committee planned that event to be held in a restaurant or hosted a potluck affair at the School of Nursing, while the Program Committee provided hours of both nursing and medical updates on the latest medical breakthroughs between 1950 and 2000.

The Remembrance Committee, dissolved in the 1990s, sent get-well wishes, while the Memorial Committee remembered graduates and family members who had died, acknowledging that remembrance of losses was a way to share sympathy and support healthy grieving. It purchased items for the school and donated to hospital campaigns with collected memorial contributions.

Each year the Senior Gift Committee purchased special gifts to surprise the graduates at a special dinner held in their honor. For some years in the 1980s, a silver charm replica of the school pin was presented. Gift giving became more of a challenge as student graduation dates became more individualized—a student could enter school and choose to take summer courses to accelerate program matriculation; others opted for the more traditional summer off. While it supported student diversity, this change did not build as close a tie with the Alumni Association, one of those unpredicted outcomes of change. The alumni gifts in the 1990s were baskets of fruit for consumption during final exam weeks.

PROGRAMS

By the 1950s, programs switched from games and entertainment to a more professional focus to learn about changing payment systems, nurse responsibilities in a civil defense climate, developing medical specialties, and the new specialty physicians establishing practices in Kalamazoo. Examples during this time included Dr. Edward Hall, who discussed the compulsory sickness tax;[48] Dr. DeLong, bone and skin grafts;[49] Miss Vanden Bosche, from the State Board of Nursing, professional nurses in civilian defense; and Miss Janet Ginter, former vice-president of the American Nurses Association, described "The New Partnership," in which nurses and doctors worked together toward great medical progress.

Dr. Curtis Hanson shared recent trends in orthopedic surgery;[50] Dr. Preston Weadon, aneurysms and arteriograms;[51] and Dr. John Neerken, lung disease and surgical corrections.[52] Not least was the popular Dr. Charles Peake who spoke on pelvic and breast cancer.[53] Mrs. Florence Friend of the Kalamazoo Civic Players, "very capably present[ed] several readings which were both thoughtful and entertaining,"[54] an event reminiscent of the 1920s and 1930s.

Laura Pleyte '31 presented member-led programs such as civilian defense and atomic nursing.[55] Lorraine Zimmerman '42 and Dorothy Beimer '42, who served as volunteers with the 1951 civilian defense effort, asked 15 graduates to become involved in atomic nursing training. The alumni held a May–June meeting that year and invited medical-civil defense co-chair physicians Hugo Aach and Harvey Bodmer to speak. Professional Nurses in Civil Defense classes were held that May.

Later program examples demonstrated the alumni's interest in medical changes:

- "Defenses against Impulses," by Dr. Berry, psychiatrist
- "External Cardiac Massage," a film
- the latest medical techniques
- the latest planned additions by a hospital administrator who also asked for pledges from alumni who willingly gave donations.

Programs took on a social problem pattern in the 1950s and 1960s: unwed mothers, domestic abuse, emotionally disturbed children, divorce, delinquency. They fit with that era's popular musicals, "Grease" and "West Side Story." Ministers from Christian denominations were occasional speakers. Members and nurses employed by Bronson and in the community in the 1970s, 1980s and 1990s often spoke about their specialty nursing practice or nurse involvement in medical specialties to lessen knowledge gaps.

Adventures were often topics shared by nurses and physicians. Programs by medical doctors commonly focused on their latest travels abroad. In 1962, Linda Weiandt '58, presented colored slides from a European vacation. A student adventure was highlighted on November 12, 1986, with a Hungarian dinner, when student nurse Shelley Buchler shared stories from her previous summer's attendance at the International Oncology Conference in Budapest. Based on her application and faculty references, she had been supported by the Helene Fuld Foundation Scholarship Fund.

Always of interest were activities at the School of Nursing. Mrs. Helen Weber, then its director, provided an update on nursing education and accreditation on February 9, 1966. It was the first time her participation was noted at an alumni meeting. Mrs. Weber, who lived in Gobles, did not drive, so her evening participation was limited. Prior to Mrs. Weber's tenure, Miss Anderson often attended to make requests or give updates and lead building/remodeling tours.

On September 14, 1977, one of the alumni's first advanced nurse practitioners, Marilyn Babcock Cardiff '49, described her role in a pediatric office and making patient rounds in the hospital. Programs of a social nature, such as flower arranging and interior decorating, provided relief from work-related programs.

SCHOOL OF NURSING CLOSES—ALUMNI ASSOCIATION CONTINUES

The last Bronson nursing students graduated in December 1998, with the last formal graduation held the preceding May. By then the School of Nursing program was flexible and asynchronous, allowing students to enter and exit to meet their learning goals and needs. In keeping with this philosophy, the last students were supported to earn the Bronson Methodist Hospital School of Nursing diploma along with a membership in the Alumni Association.

After 2000, it became a greater challenge to nominate new officers. The alumni were unable to find members willing to accept nominations, so many of them continued in their current positions. As part of an alumni board, they were open to new ideas and often published requests for members to step up and share the glory of giving and accompanying responsibilities.

Management of the alumni continued with Jackie Wylie '62, vice president, becoming acting president. In the meantime the board was searching for a graduate who would want to strengthen a résumé and was therefore willing to accept the leadership position. Sharyn Schlueter '78, became treasurer and has stayed in that role; Anna Stryd '61, maintained publication of *The Bulletin* and its distribution, and co-chaired the Membership Committee; Marie McLeieer '55, led the Ways and Means Committee that increased funding available for services; Amal Mansour '85, volunteered to co-chair the Membership Committee and continued her role on the Hospitality Committee, arranging for the two brunches held annually in the spring and fall; Kay Hanson '64, volunteered to serve as secretary in 2001. A scholarship committee composed of Dorothy Dunn '48, Sylvia Nicholas '74, and Jackie Wylie '62, supported awards to nursing students in the new Bronson School of Nursing at Western Michigan University. Co-historians were Wanda Boekhout '47, and Jackie Wylie '62, who agreed to care for memorabilia often sent to the Alumni Association by families of Bronson graduates who had died.

Alumni Association Board Members, 2004

Name	Position
Julie Betzler	Member-at-large
Wanda Boekhout	Historian
Dorothy Dunn	Scholarship Committee
Kay Hanson	Secretary
Amal Mansour	Membership and Hospitality

Marilyn McCarter-Davis	Member-at-large
Marie McLeieer	Ways and Means Committee
Rosemarie Nedeau-Cayo	Associate member, last Director of the School of Nursing and liaison to Bronson Methodist Hospital
Sylvia Nicholas	Scholarship Committee
Sharyn Schlueter	Treasurer
Anna Stryd	Bulletin and Membership
Lois Vermeulen	Member-at-large
Jan Walcott	Member-at-large
Jackie Wylie	Vice President

SUMMARY

Always low profile, almost never asserting their views, alumni quietly cared for each other and the community through their work and volunteerism. Alumni practiced in public schools, physicians' offices, health departments, industrial settings—the majority in Kalamazoo hospitals and offices. Those in global practice mixed nursing with their Christian mission. They were mostly women who listened, learned and responded to the needs of others, nurturing and caring not only for patients, but for all staff, including physicians. No job was too big or small.

Confrontation was rarely recognized. Avoidance of discomfiting issues was the chosen way to manage in both work settings and within the Alumni Association. Dissatisfaction and disappointment did occur when symbolic changes threatened alumni identity. When the Bronson logo was changed from the Old English "B" to a stylized modern logo in the 1980's, it was as if "the family" had changed its name. Most felt the new logo excluded past Bronson graduates and some of the older employees who identified strongly with the past. One concession survived: the School of Nursing pin retained the old English "B," as did the school's stationery and other school-related materials.

Many of the alumni worked for physicians in their offices and as their assistants, as private scrub nurses in the hospital operating rooms, as office managers, and in telephone triage and patient follow-up. This alignment prompted some alumni to join with the American Association of Medical Assistants (AAMA), newly established in 1956.[56] Pauline Peterman '41, a past alumni president, was a leader in the Kalamazoo chapter. As allegiance to the American Nurses Association had waned over the years, some nurses realigned with the AAMA. The definition applied to a medical assistant was, "Medical assisting is an allied health profession whose practitioners function as members of the healthcare delivery team and perform administrative and clinical procedures."[57] One- to two-year medical assistant training programs sprang up in community colleges in the 1960s.

Why Bronson nurses chose the alignment with the AAMA medical assistants seemed to be consistent with physician extender roles. Many nurses stayed faithful members of the Alumni Association at the same time they participated in Kalamazoo's AAMA chapter. There seemed to be no cognitive dissonance. The nurse's role in a physician's office involved clinical judgment within the practice of nursing, often offering counseling and care choices at visits and by telephone. No doubt the positions of RN and medical assistant in these instances became transdisciplinary. These professionals forged new relationships. Nurses, medical assistants and physicians worked together in mutual respect, a forerunner of the healthcare world to come in which all providers recognize how much they all cross over into each other's practice domain. Maybe this phenomenon occurred more frequently within small groups, like clinics and medical office teams. Future course similarities may blur practice boundaries and philosophical differences. In reality, all healthcare practitioners must be in healthy relationships in order to provide the best care.

The Alumni Association continued its work, similar to that of its past, but with aging members more often with monetary gifts for services and less direct care. Members were and are a dedicated group of professionals in diverse career paths. Accolades to all for their stellar performances and wholesome stories!

Alumni Association Presidents

From 1917–22, no records of officers or members have been located, except for the charter-member list that includes graduates through 1917

1923 Mina Weber
1924 Rose Taylor
1925 Mina Weber
1926 Sena Holke
1927 Hazel Kester
1928 Jennie Lemmer[58]
1929–30 Blanche Herrmann
1930–31 Frances Pike
1932–33 Ruth Siertsma
1934–35 Mrs. Jeanette Van Kersen Bordwell
1936 Mrs. Myrtle Burns Hatfield
1937–38 Eva Kingsley
1939 Reba Fitch
1940 Mrs. Marquita Land Vander Hoef
1941–43 Mrs. Mabel Wright Stell Meyle
1944 Mrs. Christine Gierman Jarchow
1945 Mrs Reitinga, presiding 1st VP
1946 Mrs. Marquita Land Vander Hoef
1947–48 Lois Neissink
1949 Pauline Peterman
1950 Katherine Blake
1951–52 Margaret Brown
1953 Ellen Emig
1954 Pauline Peterman
1955 Dorothy Dunn
1956 Sue Murray
1957 Madonna Blakely
1958 Beverly Francisco
1959 Louise Vanden Berg
1960 Beverly Francisco
1961 Minnie Tameling
1962 Eileen Roach
1963 Marge DeYoung
1964 Carol Rosin
1965 Lee Johnson
1966 Ellen Weston
1967 Barbara Hartman
1968–69 Nancy Weston
1970 Mary Ann Shaw
1971 Marilyn Boer
1972 Ellen Weston
1973 Marie Hicks
1974 Carolyn Lewis
1975 Marilyn Ely
1976 Marge DeYoung
1977 Linda Maag
1978 Beverly Anderson
1979 Ruth Schwoebell
1980–81 Betty Vander Molen
1982–83 Virginia Hill
1984–86 Nancy Weston
1986–88 Marilyn Luther
1988–90 Betty Vander Molen
1990–92 Carol Lawrence
1992–96 Sharyn Schlueter
1997–98 Ruth Clemans
1998–2000 Kelley Hempsall
2000–04 Jackie Wylie, presiding VP and liaison with WMU Bronson School of Nursing students, faculty and staff.[59]

CHAPTER 12 END NOTES

[1] This story of the Alumni Association of Bronson Methodist Hospital School of Nursing was drawn from its Minutes (handwritten in three legal-size ledgers), the first dated 1923 January 2–1948

September 8; second, 1948 October 28–1963 April 19; and third, 1963 May 9–1985 June 12, and also include perceptions of Jackie Clark Wylie.

[2] Bronson Hospital did not become Bronson Methodist Hospital until 1920.

[3] Alumni Association minutes, 1930 January 23.

[4] Alumni Association minutes, 1932 November 15.

[5] *Ibid.*

[6] Alumni Association minutes, 1925 February 24.

[7] Oral interview with Cornelia Veenhuis Cody by Jackie Wylie and Marge Kars, 1989 February 28.

[8] Alumni Association minutes, 1925 March 24.

[9] *Ibid.*

[10] Alumni Association minutes, 1925 April 28.

[11] Alumni Association minutes, 1926 March 30.

[12] Alumni Association minutes, 1927 October 25.

[13] A 1984 copy of the Bylaws reflects the same language as the first bylaws found, and the latest 1995 revision included language, ". . . to promote professional standards of nursing."

[14] Tresolini, C.P., & Pew-Fetzer Task Force. 1994. *Health professions education and relationship-centered care: report of the Pew-Fetzer task force on advancing psychosocial education*. San Francisco, CA: Pew Health Professions Commission.

[15] The date is not clear when the alumni quit paying state and national dues in favor of inexpensive local-only dues. Graduates of the 1950s have vague memories about when and whether they paid ANA dues or only at a local level to belong.

[16] Freire, P. *Pedagogy of the oppressed.* New York: Continuum Publishing, 1993.

[17] The state association was first called the Michigan State Nurses Association; later the word "state" was dropped to become the Michigan Nurses Association.

[18] Michigan Nurses Association, *Guide to the MNA House of Delegates Booklet,* 2002 March 22, "Historical highlights."

[19] Sincox, A, *Michigan Nurse*. 77(2): 2004 March. "The first MNA: turning RN into reality."

[20] *Ibid.*

[21] Michigan Nurses Association, *op.cit.*

[22] Oral interview with Amy Bailey Seward by Mary Lou Stewart, 1985 July 3.

[23] The undated copy of the constitution is after 1920 since Methodist appears in the alumni name. The American Nurses Association name is not included in the title.

---

[24] Constitution and By-Laws of the Bronson Methodist Hospital Alumni Association of the Kalamazoo District Association, Michigan State Nurses' Association.

[25] Conversation with Sue Murray VandeGiessen, 2004 March 14.

[26] Alumni Association minutes, 1935 March.

[27] Alumni Association minutes, 1935 May 20.

[28] Alumni Association minutes, 1952 October 8.

[29] Alumni Association minutes, 1987 November 11.

[30] Alumni Association minutes, 1950 November 1.

[31] Alumni Association minutes, 1933 February 21.

[32] Alumni Association minutes, 1949 November 12.

[33] Alumni Association minutes, 1946 September 11.

[34] Alumni Association minutes, 1948 May 12.

[35] Alumni Association minutes, 1949 September 14.

[36] Five years offered students the opportunity to receive financing while completing the baccalaureate portion through relationships with Western Michigan College and Albion College.

[37] Alumni Association minutes, 1948 November 29.

[38] Alumni Association minutes, 1985 September 11.

[39] Conversations with Sharyn Schlueter, 2004 March 28 and 2004 September 1.

[40] Expected completion and opening date for the new College of Health and Human Services building is planned for August 2005. It is located on Oakland Drive toward the north end of the property previously dedicated to the Kalamazoo Psychiatric Hospital.

[41] Numbers in attendance were not recorded. Jackie Wylie was present and remembered that students outnumbered alumni who stretched the food to feed the invited students.

[42] Alumni Association minutes, 1952 April 9.

[43] Alumni Association minutes, 1958 September 10.

[44] Alumni Association minutes, 1985 October 9.

[45] Alumni Association minutes, 1995.

[46] Alumni Association minutes, 1991 October 11.

[47] Alumni Association minutes, 1997 October 7.

[48] Alumni Association minutes, 1949 March.

[49] Alumni Association minutes, 1951September 12.

[50] Alumni Association minutes, 1953 October 14.

---

[51] Alumni Association minutes, 1958 January 8.

[52] Alumni Association minutes, 1958 April 9.

[53] Alumni Association minutes, 1958 October 8.

[54] Alumni Association minutes, 1958 September 10.

[55] Alumni Association minutes, 1951 March 14.

[56] American Association of Medical Assistants, "The history of the American Association of Medical Assistants," www.aama-ntl.org, 2003 September 13; 2.

[57] *Ibid.*

[58] Jennie Lemmer, during interview with Jackie Wylie, said that when she was admitted to nursing school, the Director of Nursing advised her to change her name to Jean. Her graduate records and diploma have that name.

[59] Wylie was employed at the WMU Bronson School of Nursing 1997–2004, served as the student advisor to WMU student nurses association and worked to build positive relationships.

Bronson Women and the School of Nursing

EPILOGUE

EPILOGUE

Being part of the faculty at WMU from August 1997 to April 2004 and participating in the commencement for the first WMU graduating class in April 1999 were peak experiences for Jackie Wylie '62. Hers was a dream come true of an academic connection the hospital needed for a new model of nursing excellence and for the evolution of nurses into third-millennium professionalism. The relationship between Bronson Methodist Hospital nursing staff as front-line student educators and novice nurses is evident in Corrie Hitchcock's and Jennifer Lemke's stories that spanned the years 1997–2004.

Corrie Hitchcock, WMU Bronson School of Nursing '99

I started my college education at WMU in the dietetics program.[1] The required courses and internship during my freshman year didn't appeal to me, so I went back to the drawing board, so to speak, to find what I wanted to do with my life. I thought about the reasons I wanted to be a dietician: to help people make healthy choices for their lives. Well, I thought, I can do that as a nurse on a grander scale. I looked into the new nursing program at WMU at the start of my sophomore year and liked what I saw. Accepted into the first class, I transferred into the WMU nursing program but, after the first two years, I felt the need for more clinical practice.

I applied and was hired at Bronson Methodist Hospital for a patient care assistant (PCA) position. That assignment meant working the Medical-Surgical Float Pool as a PCA for about six months before becoming a nurse extern at BMH in the same Float Pool. Diana Dahlquist '95 was my "buddy" for a year and a half. She had gone to Bronson Methodist Hospital School of Nursing and was a great resource and teacher. We made a great team, floating to all the units in Med/Surg areas where staff was needed, and we felt that we provided excellent patient care. We also had fun! Towards the end of my externship, other nurses often commented on our "team" and wanted us to work on their patient-care units.

After I graduated from WMU, I studied for "boards" while still serving as a nurse extern. I passed and went right into a RN position in the Med/Surg Float Pool where little formal orientation was needed because of my nurse extern experience. Then, seemingly very suddenly, there I was—the RN for my very own patients! When I had worked full time for about six months, Bronson decided to start an intern program for novice nurses to learn critical care. I was the first nurse accepted into this internship and started the program immediately. For six months I rotated orientation in each critical-care unit for about a month at a time and loved the experience. The preceptors were wonderful and I learned so much from all of them. After this critical-care internship, I took a position in the Post Anesthesia Care Unit (PACU) where I continue to work today (2004). Currently I am a relief charge nurse and preceptor for novice nurses and students, including those from the WMU Bronson School of Nursing.

I served on the Nursing Advisory Committee when it was functional, and have filled in for the PACU Division representative on occasion. I work with Julie Switek, who is a wonderful manager, and other great nurses! The teamwork is awesome, and we can depend on each other for support.

Bronson has been good to me during my education and employment because it offers flexible shifts and extends generous benefits; I would recommend Bronson to anyone seeking a position in hospital care.

Jennifer Lemke, WMU Bronson School of Nursing '01

My journey at WMU Bronson School of Nursing began in August of 1998.[2] After a few clinical experiences, I realized that I wanted to expand my clinical and patient-care skills. In the summer of 2000, I was hired as a patient care assistant (PCA) at Bronson Methodist Hospital. In order to make the most of the experience, I took a position in the VIP float pool. I "floated" between cardiology, general medical, general surgical, and ortho/neuro units working as a PCA. Skills that I developed included basic patient care such as bathing and transfers. Most importantly, I was able to increase my comfort when interacting with patients and family. As my experience grew in both school and work, I decided to move into an externship (a learning position for students to be precepted with RNs). My externship placement was on the Medical ICU floor. During the externship, I was able to take on more of the nursing role in a critical-care setting. It was a wonderful experience and fueled my passion for critical care nursing.

After graduating from WMU in December 2001, I applied for the critical care internship program and was invited to start the program when word was received that I had successfully passed the Michigan State Board of Nursing licensure exam. This program allowed me to begin my nursing career and gain valuable on-the-job training and experiences! I worked on the cardiology, general medical, general surgical, and ortho/neuro floors as a RN Throughout this program I was working with knowledgeable RN preceptors who patiently assisted me in the development of my own practice. After this rotation I was able to move into the critical care setting as a RN I rotated through the Medical and Surgical Intensive Care Units (ICU) as well as PACU and Cardiac Surgical Unit (CSU). Each of these rotations gave me the opportunity to expand my critical care nursing skills. After approximately seven months of the internship program, I bid on a full-time job in the Medical Intensive Care Unit (MICU). After two years every day is still filled with new clinical learning! I am participating in the Shared Governance committee and am a co-chair for the Keystone ICU project. Now most days are spent caring for patients while precepting new orientees through their own journey.

The Story Never Ends

Bronson School of Nursing and Bronson Methodist Hospital nurses will together teach, mentor and precept each other and their successors, in caring ways, within an ever changing healthcare system. Nurse stories will not be forgotten but will be ever enriched by caring relationships that extend hearts, hands and minds into the community.

And the Beat Goes On…

It's not easy,
this business of dinosaur-riding.
Hanging on,
while she gathers to
feed
herself and her young . . .

. . .and the beat goes on . . .
La di da di da . . .

Shoulder grinds and
massive movements
lumber, leaving
crater prints
for evolving
kin.
Path and praxis.

I cling, sharing
myopic view of future's
roads, redesigned for
revolutions'
swift
progressions.

. . .And the beat goes on . . .

She sees people lost
in populations'
management.
Feels rejection
of values left
behind.
Forgotten?

. . .And the beat goes on . . .
La di da di da . . .

She crys for
caring drown in customer
service standards.
For ethics evaded in
risk
management.

. . .la di da di da

Still, I hold on.
For old, singular styles and ways:
Touch and soul honored.
Caring respected.
OR
Is it fear

Keeping me
clutched to her heroic insistence?
Mammoth size mired,
bogged, stopped.
No
adaptation.

. . .and the beat goes on . . .

Then comes the tricky
business of dismount.
How? When? Rhythms
diminish, neck drops and
slides
me to safety.

. . .And the beat goes on . . .

Secured, I wait,
watch and weep for
lessons of death
with dignity. Her
life
ceases, leaving me

Alone. Now I
move, on foot, her fossil
fueling my
own, solitary
steps
into . . . ?

. . .And the beat goes on . . .
La di da di da. . . .

Barb Groh, May 1998

EPILOGUE NOTES

---

[1] Corrie Hitchcock's story as written in e-mail on 2004 July 6, was followed by a telephone interview July 17, 2004, with Jackie Wylie.

[2] Jennifer Lemke's story was written in e-mail on 2004 July 20.

BRONSON METHODIST HOSPITAL
B
SCHOOL OF NURSING

Section IV.
APPENDICES

APPENDIX A

CHRONOLOGY:

BRONSON METHODIST HOSPITAL HISTORY ENTWINED WITH EDUCATION AND MANAGEMENT

YEAR EVENT/ACTIVITY

1860 Forerunner to American hospital-based schools of nursing, the Nightingale School of Nursing was established at the St. Thomas Hospital, London, England with separate finances from the Nightingale Fund.

1900 Hundreds of hospital-based schools of nursing sprung up in America without funding resources. The students were necessary for inexpensive labor and were placed in a quasi, work-study model beginning the nursing journey towards professionalism. Diplomas granted verified the new graduate status as trained nurses.

Six physicians formed the Kalamazoo Hospital Association.

1901 Jessie Yancey, experienced nurse from Chicago appointed first superintendent[1] of newly established Kalamazoo Hospital in the Fish Home on Fish Lane.

1903 Four nursing students received certificates for completion of two-years of training and service.

1904 Irene VanPelt, from West Virginia, appointed Director of Nursing.

Hospital on Fish Lane closed June 1904 when construction started on a "real" 50-bed hospital. Its cornerstone was laid May 22, 1904.

Three-year School of Nursing officially established. It was first modeled after St. Thomas Hospital School of Nursing founded by Florence Nightingale with its two years of training; later increased to three years, as nursing standards increased education. Entrance requirements were changed from "just a doctor's statement of good health" to at least two years of high

620620———————————

[1]The director of nursing (earlier referred to as the superintendent of nurses) was responsible for both nursing services and the School of Nursing until the 1960s. Then Mrs. Helen E. Weber became Director of the School of Nursing with sole responsibility for the school, and Mary B. Anderson retained the position of Director of Nursing to supervise nursing services. The title of the chief nurse executive (CNE) changed when Mr. Littlefield was promoted to Administrative Assistant in charge of Nursing Services, as title changes occurred in the hospital and 1982 parent organization, Bronson HealthCare Group (BHG) changed form.

school. The program was to cover three full years, with a six-month affiliation with Women's Hospital and Infant's Infirmary in New York City. Irene VanPelt was Director of the School.

Jessie Yancey employed by the Women's Civic Improvement League to provide nursing care in homes. Students were trained in home care.

MATRON FOR NEW HOSPITAL HERE

MISS ELIZABETH LOUNSBURY, WHO WILL BE SUPERINTENDENT, ARRIVES IN CITY.

1905 Elizabeth Lounsbery appointed matron of Hospital. She was formerly Superintendent/ matron of the Presbyterian Hospital in Cincinnati, Ohio.

1906 Hospital name changed to "Bronson" in a public naming contest, for the founder of the city of Kalamazoo, Titus Bronson.

1907 First students officially graduated with the name of "Bronson Graduate."

1909 Minnie Goodnow, Superintendent of Hospital, achieved international recognition for writing a fundamentals of nursing textbook.

The New York affiliation (*see* 1904, item 3) was transferred to Michael Reese Hospital, Chicago, and training in the care of children was added.

1910 Bronson School of Nursing added to first list of accredited schools in Michigan by the State Board of Registration of Nurses. The first school pin, blue enamel and gold Maltese cross, was given at graduation.

Edith May Cowie Partridge appointed Superintendent of Nurses.

Requirements for student admission raised. "Applicant should be between the ages of 19 and 32; have a certificate of good moral character signed by three responsible persons, preferably from the local pastor, teacher or family physician; and be a high school graduate, if possible."

Florence Nightingale, at age ninety, died on August 13, and was buried at St. Margaret's of Antioch Church, East Wellow, Hampshire, England.

1917 Edna G. Wildermuth appointed Superintendent of Nurses.

The Alumni Association of Bronson Hospital School of Nursing organized, forming its constitution and by-laws in keeping with the Michigan State Nurses Association. The first meetings were held in the nurses/nursing student collective homes surrounding Bronson, with succeeding meetings held in the homes of members.

1920 Mrs. Blanche Earnest Prater appointed Superintendent of Nurses.

William Puffer, D.D., a Methodist minister, appointed Superintendent of Hospital. The Board of Trustees decided that a guarantee of financial security and progress could best be obtained by turning the hospital over to a church for its management. Approximately $45,000 was raised by subscription to eliminate all indebtedness, before the hospital was given outright and debt-free to the Methodist Episcopal Church. The name of the hospital changed to "Bronson Methodist Hospital (BMH)."

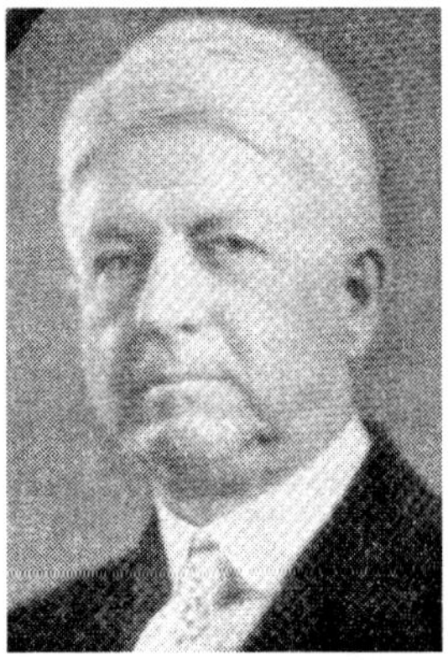

Dr. William Puffer

Decision made to continue with the School of Nursing, and a full-time nursing arts instructor hired. Hours of hospital duty shortened to twelve, with an additional two hours off—if and when work permitted. Students lived in the West Nurses Home, with its wide veranda, and under the watchful eye of one of the hospital supervisors. Classroom sessions met in the School Building (otherwise known as the Annex).

1921 Lillian Leason Daviell appointed Director of Nurses.

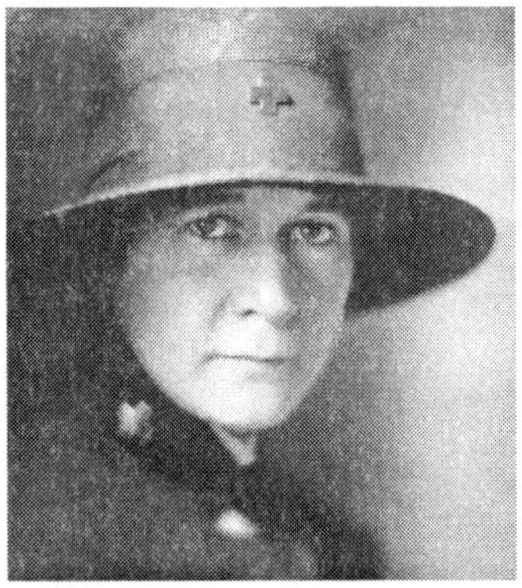

Mina Weber Macgrayne

The H.B. Osborne home and the Dewing property purchased for School of Nursing residence expansion. More applications received than could be accepted, and careful screening of applicants made and pre-entrance examination required. The school exceeded state requirements for classroom hours so new affiliations were secured: Children's Hospital in Detroit and Fairmont Hospital (for communicable diseases) added to the curriculum.

1922 Mina Weber Macgrayne, a 1913 graduate of Bronson School of Nursing, appointed Superintendent of Nurses.

1924 Herman Kiefer Hospital, Detroit, replaced Fairmont Hospital for Communicable Disease affiliation.

1925 Ann Gwinn Draher appointed Superintendent of Nurses and Principal. She had been Educational Director at Bethesda Hospital, Maryland.

Affiliation with Western Michigan College began with a course in Sociology.

1926 A new north wing was added to the hospital, increasing the total capacity to 110 beds.

1930 Two classes a year were admitted; this was discontinued in 1934, changing to once a year. Working hours shortened to allow students more time to study the expanded curriculum.

1931 The school pin, shaped like a Maltese cross, changed from a blue and gold background to one of glistening white and gold.

1934 S.W. Robinson, D.D., a Methodist minister, replaced Dr. Puffer as Superintendent of Hospital.

1935 Ruth McLellan appointed Superintendent of Nurses.

Student nurse uniforms changed from black shoes and stockings to white. In May the passing of black shoes and stockings was afforded full celebration by burning them at Gull Lake.

Women of Kalamazoo organized into the White Cross Guild.

1936 Blue and white striped dresses, stiff collars, cuffs, bibs and aprons were abandoned for the all-white uniform. Capes were added to the uniform. Black bands added status to caps for junior and senior years. The student purchased clothing and textbooks.

1937 Bernice Hammond, a graduate of Pacific Hospital in Los Angeles appointed Superintendent of Nurses, and Alfred Way, D.D., a Methodist minister, replaced Dr. Robinson as Superintendent of Hospital.

Bronson's staff numbered 150 and served 4,000 patients, 445 of whom were accident victims.

1940 Alberta Erhart Merritt, a 1935 BMH School of Nursing graduate, appointed Superintendent of Nurses, and Marguerite Sheckles became Assistant Superintendent of Nurses.

New five-story hospital building was dedicated, increasing hospital capacity to 175 beds.

Nursing school entrance requirements became more demanding; a year of chemistry was necessary, and a series of psychological examinations was given.

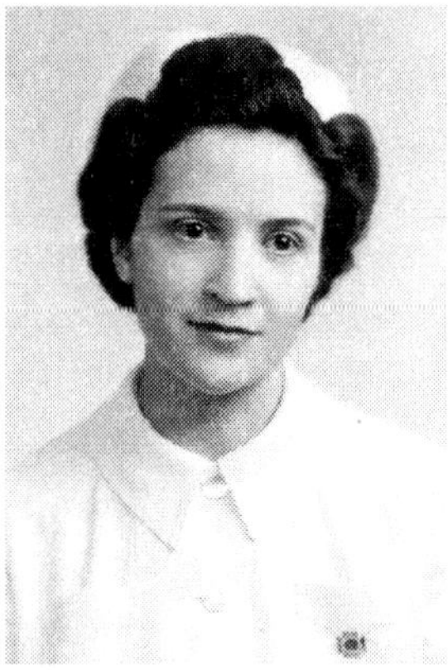

Alberta Erhart Merritt

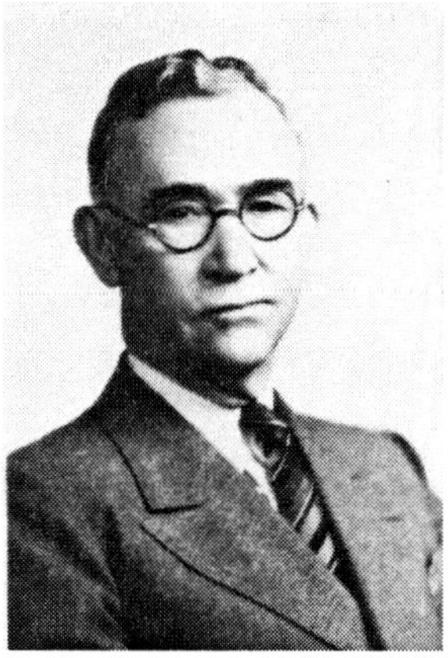

Dr. Alfred F. Way

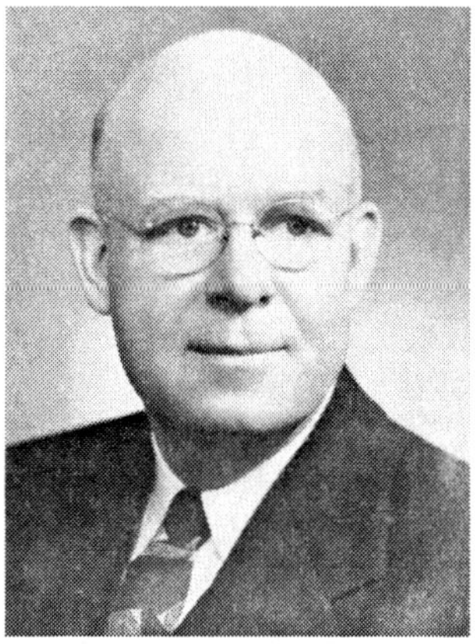

Dr. William C. Perdew

1942 Dr. Hazel Prentice established the Kalamazoo County Blood Bank at Bronson Hospital.

1943 Dr. Way semi-retired, and Dr. William C. Perdew, minister of the First Methodist Church of Kalamazoo replaced him as Superintendent of Hospital.

BMH became training center for the U.S. Cadet Nurse Corps.

To alleviate the nursing shortage, Amy Bailey Seward, Bronson School of Nursing graduate, appointed by Eleanor Roosevelt to head the nurse aide training center in Kalamazoo.

Affiliation with Children's Hospital in Detroit discontinued, and a two-month affiliation began with Mayberry Sanatorium, Northville, Michigan. A psychiatric affiliation with Kalamazoo State Hospital established.

BMH School of Nursing affiliated with Western Michigan University and Albion College to offer a baccalaureate degree with a major in nursing.

1944 Mary B. Anderson, graduate of Copley Hospital, Aurora, Illinois, appointed Director of Nurses, and Mrs. S.A. Lott became Assistant Director of Nurses.

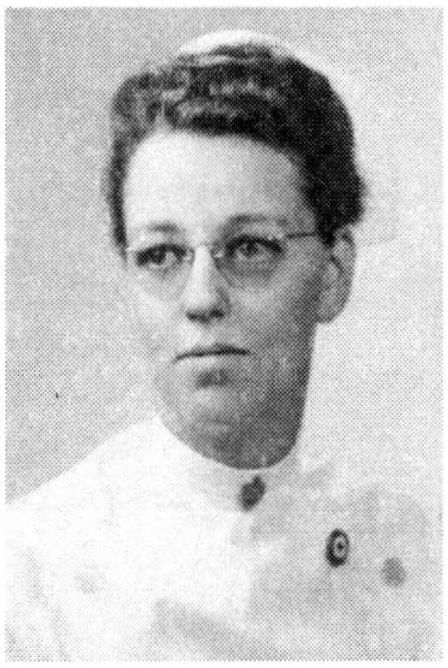

Mary B. Anderson

1945 Mayberry affiliation was dropped and replaced by a two month orthopedics rotation at Sigma Gamma Hospital, Detroit. The third floor of Harding School was acquired for classrooms, lecture and laboratory facilities. The Annex was assigned to residents and interns. Physicians maintained an active interest in the nursing program and gave freely of their time in both classrooms and wards.

1947 Dr. Harold Machin appointed first resident physician at Bronson Hospital Marguerite Sheckles appointed Assistant Director of Nursing in charge of nurse education.

1948 Mrs. S.A. Lott succeeded Marguerite Sheckles as assistant director of nurses in charge of nursing education. Mrs. Lott had a Bachelor of Science in nursing education from St. Louis University.

1949 BMH School of Nursing was among the top 25 per cent of the nation's basic nursing programs.

1950 Helen E. Weber hired as Assistant Director of Nursing Education, and promoted to Director in 1966.

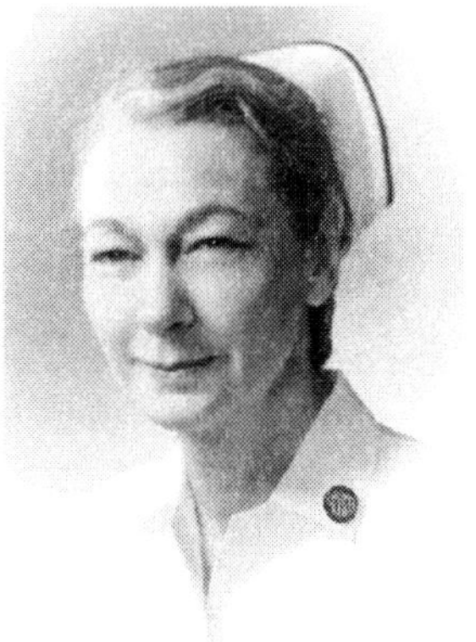

Helen Weber

New additions to the hospital included: medical center, beautiful lobby, pharmacy, snack bar; classrooms and extended teaching facilities for the school.

The option for the baccalaureate degree with a major in nursing from Western Michigan or Albion Colleges was eliminated.

1951 The main hospital addition dedicated.

A papermaking company, Kalamazoo Vegetable Parchment (KVP) gave $50,000 to the Chapel Fund in honor of Jacob Kindelberger. The Chapel was dedicated this year.

The White Cross Guild made many contributions to the Chapel and to the Student Nurses Fund.

1952 Emergency Room added a full-time charge nurse. The latest modern equipment acquired for surgery, obstetrics and medical floors. New complete units were: laboratory, x-ray, physical therapy, examining and consultation rooms for the many clinics and emergency. These additions benefited the students in new and wider experiences. Enrollment nearly doubled during the past 15 years, a much larger increase than experienced by most schools of nursing.

1953 A new nursing library opened separate from the medical library.

The Good Neighbor Fund established to pay for medical care for those in need of financial aid.

1954 The BMH School of Nursing celebrated its 50th Anniversary.

1957 Truesdale Hall dedicated. Classes of 1958, 1959, and 1960 were the first to live in its spacious quarters.

BMH School of Nursing received full NLN Accreditation.

1960 Dr. Perdew died suddenly after suffering a heart attack.

The Lovell Street Parking Lot opened—more cars and beds.

1961 John C. Pratt appointed Assistant Administrator for Professional Services, and Floyd E. Weddle appointed Assistant Administrator for General Services.

Daniel N. Finch appointed first Hospital Administrator since 1920 who was not a Methodist minister

1962 Virginia McPhail (1948 BMH School of Nursing graduate, 1951 BSN from Wayne State University, and 1960 MSN from University of Colorado) promoted to Director of Nurses.
Floors 4 and 5 were added to Bronson Medical Center West.

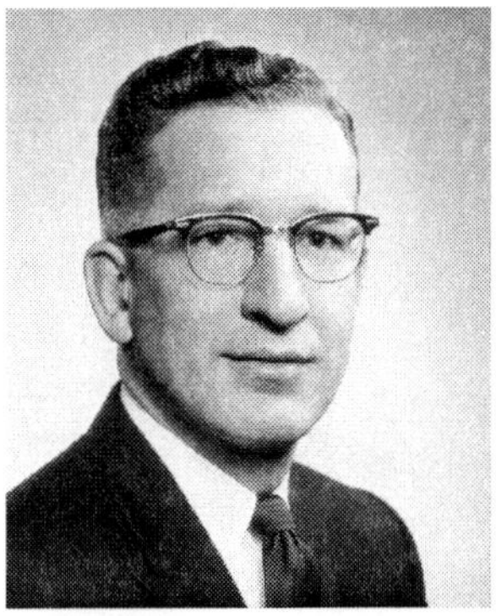
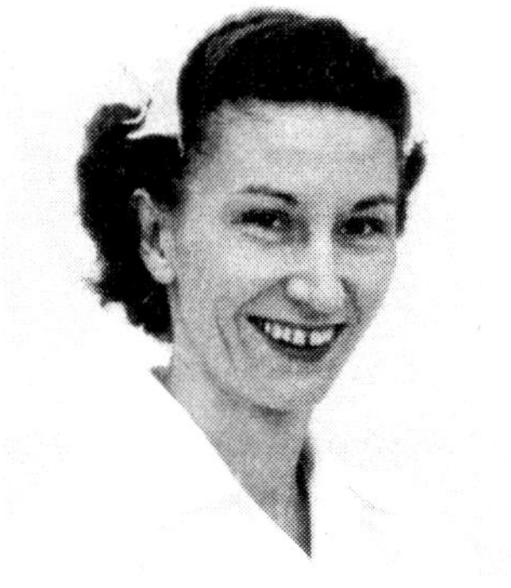

John Pratt

Hazel Latondress

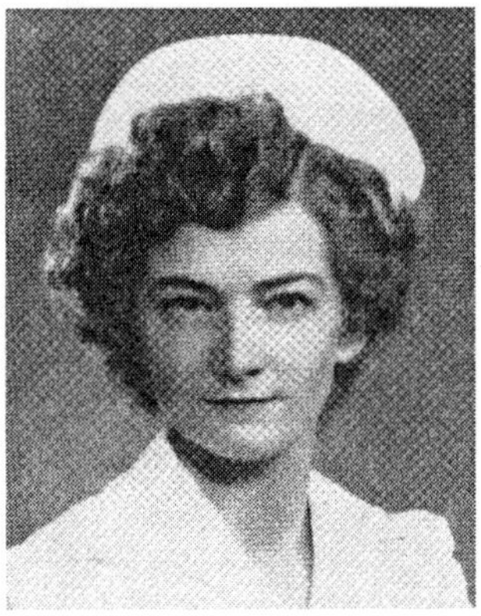
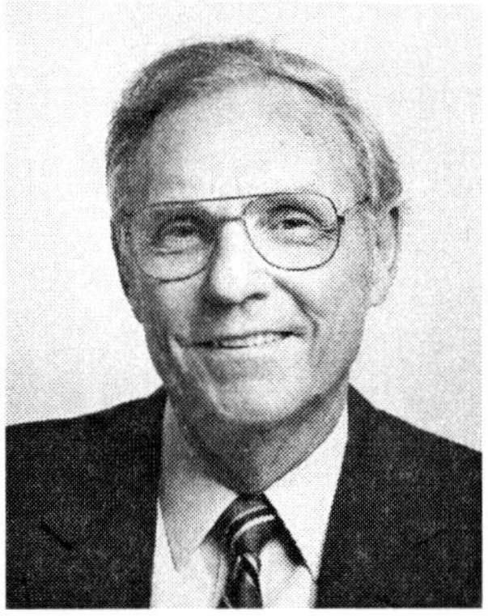

Virginia McPhail

Daniel Finch

The Harding Building, purchased from the Kalamazoo Public Schools, provided space for Outpatient Clinics to support indigent patients, residency programs, and a unique combined Nursing and Medical Library.

1963 Bronson and Borgess joined together in a spirit of cooperation to request $3.2 million from the Kalamazoo community for facilities expansion and with it sophisticated medical services. The campaign was successful.

1964 The first Dutch Market organized by the BMH Women's Auxiliary to raise money, was a successful annual event for years to come.

1966 Hazel Latondress, graduate of Kansas City General Hospital School of Nursing, promoted to Director of Nurses.

The Bronson/Borgess fund drive enabled the hospital to enlarge and complete a new laboratory addition and new power plant. Also, floors 7 and 8 were added to the 1951 main hospital addition, forever changing the skyline of Kalamazoo with a circular ICU. Floors 9 and 10 were roughed in.

On July 1, BMH received its first Medicare payment.

1967 A medical staff planning committee was organized to plan for medical/surgical advances in the next decade. An OB/GYN Residency Program was started.

1968 Intern apartments were built with a $300,000 gift from the Upjohn Company, and other medical services became a reality: hemodialysis (HDU), cardiac care (CCU), inhalation therapy, and nuclear isotope scanning.

1970 The Pediatric/Adolescent Center and the linear accelerator Radiation Therapy Unit opened.

1971 The BMH Women's Auxiliary opened the Gift Shop, raising money to finance service projects.

In cooperation with Mall City Ambulance, the first Bronson baby bus in southwest Michigan went into operation.

1972 A unique clinical research unit opened in cooperation with The Upjohn Company. It became the Bronson Clinical Investigational Unit in 1976.

The Trauma and Emergency Center and the North parking ramp opened.

The Neonatology Program was organized with a full-time neonatologist on staff.

1973 Bronson Medical Center East and Burn Unit opened.

Southwest Michigan Area Health Education Center (SMAHEC) developed by Bronson and Borgess for planning and operating their medical education programs.

1974 The School of Nursing graduated 74 students, its largest class to date.

1975 The high-risk newborn delivery service was established, and the Special Care Unit opened.

A new surgery unit opened.

1976 Bronson and Borgess cooperated for fund raising efforts.

The South Hospital Addition opened.

The BMH Auxiliary pledged $125,000 for a Coronary Care Unit (CCU).

1977 Opening of Pediatrics Intensive Care Unit, developed from the former Special Care Unit.

1978 Jacqueline L. Wylie, 1962 BMH School of Nursing graduate, promoted to Director of School of Nursing after a six-month appointment as Associate Director.

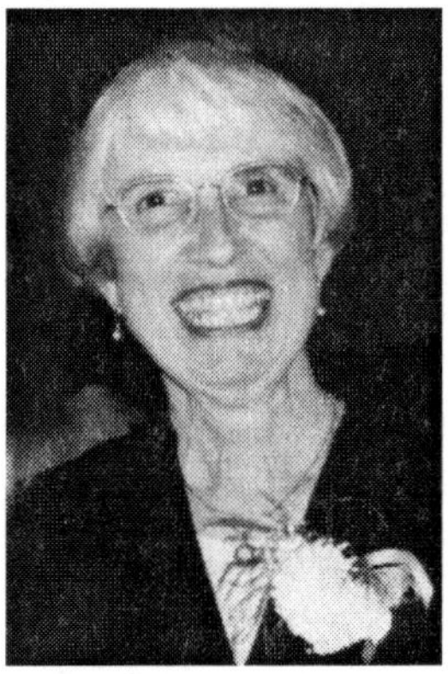

Jacqueline L. Wylie

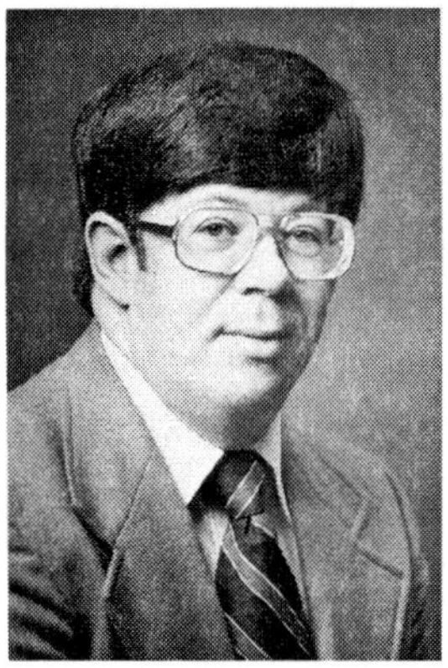

Arthur Littlefield

Arthur Littlefield appointed Administrative Assistant in charge of Nursing Services. Littlefield graduated from Kellogg Community College, Cook County School of Nursing, and served in the U.S. Army. He completed a Bachelor of Business Administration at WMU.

A CT Scanner was installed, and Floors 9 and 10 opened.

1979 The First Young People's Health Fair was held in Bronson Park.

Bronson School of Nursing celebrated its 75th Anniversary.

1980 The Oncology Unit opened with a more home-like environment for patients, families and friends, including a huge living room and kitchen for family use.

Bronson Hospital hired William Selinsky, a 1975 BMH graduate, as its first clinical nurse specialist (CNS).

1981 BMH was designated as a Regional Trauma Center by the State of Michigan.

"Portable" Self-Health Management Clinics, were transported to older adult residences, Senior Centers and Title VII congregate meal sites, providing community health educational opportunities for nursing students. The clinics were designed and managed by Barbara Groh, School of Nursing faculty member.

1982 Bronson Healthcare Group, Inc. (BHG) was formed—a movement toward comprehensive "seamless" care.

Bronson Health Foundation was formed.

Bronson Management Services Corporation was formed to diversify financial base.

BHG purchased the former Sears Building, located on the corner of South Burdick Street and Crosstown Parkway, and remodeled it as the Crosstown Outpatient Surgery Center.

The Short Stay Unit opened on Hall 9.

The new lobby on Lovell and John streets and the South parking ramp opened.

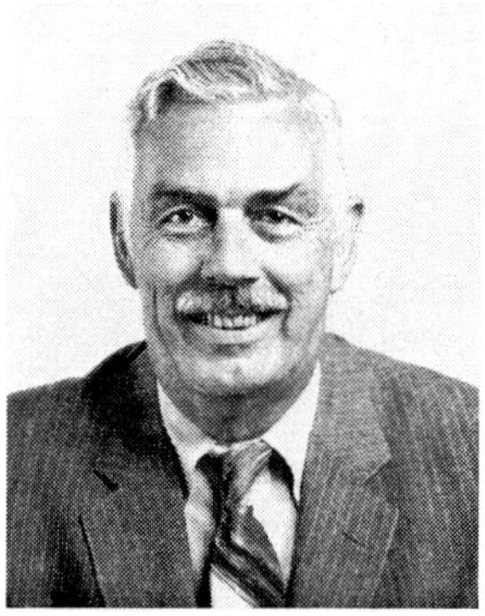

Russell P. Kneen

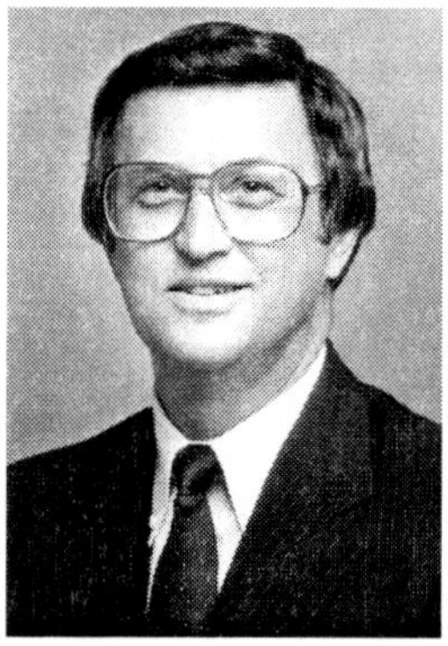

Peter W. Froyd

1983 Daniel Finch appointed Chairman of the Bronson Healthcare Group, Inc., and Russell P. Kneen, President. Peter W. Froyd appointed President of Bronson Methodist Hospital.

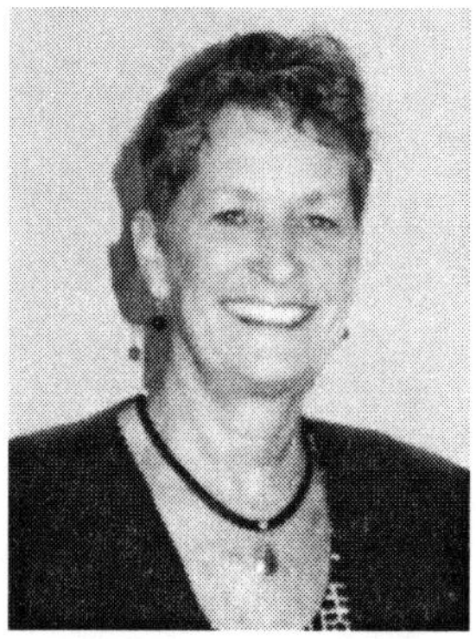

Judy Stewart Hoelscher

Judy Stewart (Hoelscher) Ed.D., R.N., appointed to Associate Director, School of Nursing. Previously Dr. Stewart had been at Nazareth College as a faculty member and director.

The Gilmore Center for Health Education construction completed.

Bronson Outpatient Surgery, (Crosstown Center) opened.

1984 The Nurse Extern Program was established, first accepting Bronson students and then extending invitations to students from ADN and BSN programs.

Federal government prospective payment system, and DRGs (Diagnosis-Related Groups) took effect as a method of controlling escalating costs of hospitalization and medical care.

CareFlite, Inc., helicopter flight ambulance service, established.

GoldenCare PLUS established and three specialized treatment services opened: Bronson Laser Center; Gastroenterology Laboratory; West Michigan Hyperbaric Unit.

The Rehabilitation Unit opened at Bronson Vicksburg Hospital (formerly Franklin Community.)

1985 Daniel Finch retired from Bronson Healthcare Group, Inc. Russell P. Kneen appointed Chairman and CEO and Patric E. Ludwig appointed President.

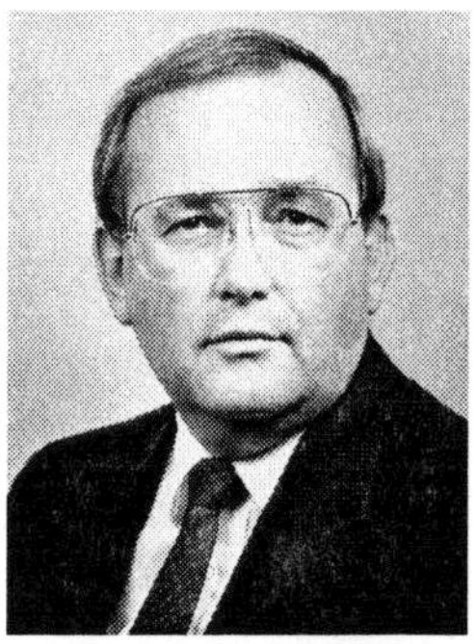

Patric Ludwig

Physicians Health Plan (PHP) joined the Bronson Healthcare Group.

The Trauma Care Unit, for inpatient intensive care, opened.

The first layoffs in the history of Bronson Hospital occurred for 260 employees, including 23 R.N.s and 37 LPNs.

Breast Screening Clinic opened and Women's Health became a specialty.

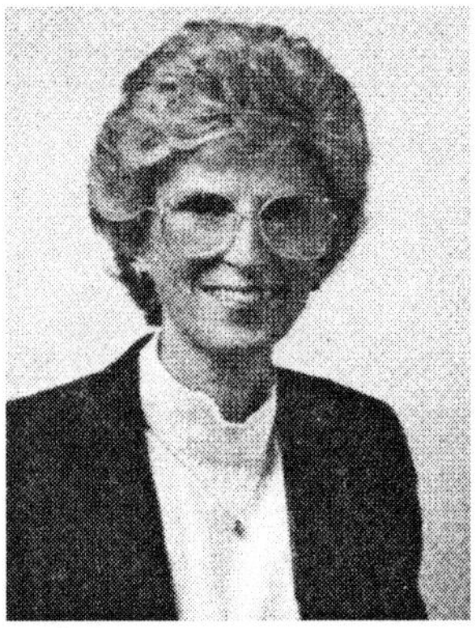

Anna Mae Spaniolo

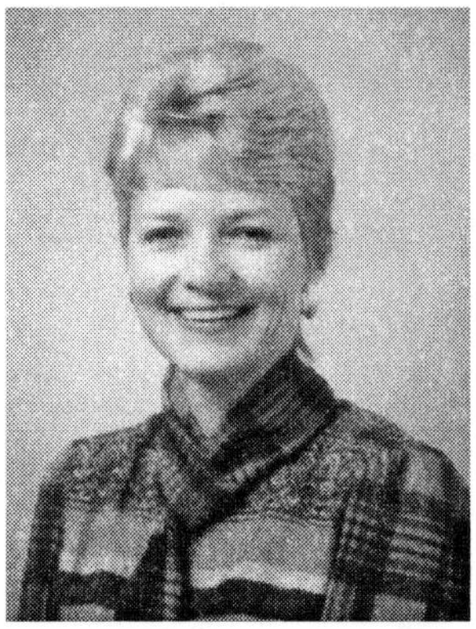

Carol Van Antwerp

Western Michigan University Family Nursing Center offered nursing students opportunities to meet the WMU international student population and to build skills in cultural competence, health assessment, nursing intervention, and evaluation. Carol VanAntwerp and Anna Mae Spaniolo, School of Nursing faculty, initiated this clinical practice.

Nursing student uniforms remained white with BMHSON sewn on breast pocket; caps and capes became obsolete. Community nursing students were equipped with navy blue canvas bags containing stethoscopes, sphygmomanometers, otoscopes, Bates' Physical Assessment texts, scales, and other tools needed for client assessment and diagnosis.

The School of Nursing became the first department of the hospital to have word processors; a small computer lab was built under direction of Linda Thede—with some of the funding from a Helene Fuld Foundation grant; and the nursing arts laboratory was extensively remodeled to include state-of-the-art equipment.

1986 Bronson purchased two area long-term care centers: Arboridge and Brookhaven..

The SIDS Apnea Center established.

The Bronson Breast Screening Center opened.

Bronson Methodist Hospital and IBA Health and Life Assurance Company joined forces to create the IBA HealthCare Plan.

1987 The Bronson Institute for Health Education (BIHE) formed.

Bronson Healthcare Group, Inc. reorganized into four divisions: Patient Services; Older Adult Services; Medical Affairs; and Business and Insurance Services.

Childcare PLUS, a daycare center, established adjacent to Crosstown Center.

Responsibility for Self Health Management Clinics transferred from School of Nursing to Bronson's Golden Care Plus and Older Adult Service Line.

The First Health Development Corporation created to promote cooperation between Bronson Hospital and Borgess Medical Center.

Bronson Hospital Gift Shop became a hospital function, costing the Bronson Auxiliary their major fund-raising source.

Rambling Road Pediatrics joined BHG.

The Gerontology and Outpatient Rehabilitation Centers opened at Crosstown Center.

The Great Lakes Institute of Hyperbaric and Diving Medicine established.

1988 Bronson approved to perform open-heart surgery.

A flexible curriculum structure and admission process initiated in response to nontraditional student needs.

Patric E. Ludwig replaced Russell Kneen as Chairman and CEO of BHG.

The Center for Women's Health at Bronson Crosstown Center opened.

Frank Sardone hired as Administrator of Inpatient Services.

Robert Doud, EdD appointed Vice President, BIHE.

1989 Bronson designated as the only Level I Trauma Center in the Southwest Region of Michigan.

1990 The new Trauma and Emergency Care Center opened.

1992 West Michigan Air Care Services contracted.

Jo Ulrich '73, Nursing Coordinator, worked with consultants to prepare for the building of a *New* Bronson Hospital.

1993 Bronson adopted a smoke-free environment.

1994 Bronson partnered with Western Michigan University to support the establishment of WMU School of Nursing.

1995 Jacqueline Wylie retired as Director of the School of Nursing.

Susan Ulshafer hired as Vice President of Human Resources with the transfer of the School of Nursing responsibilities from Robert Doud.

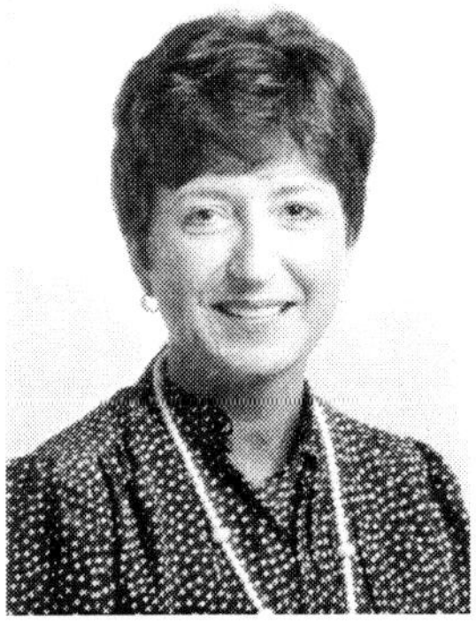

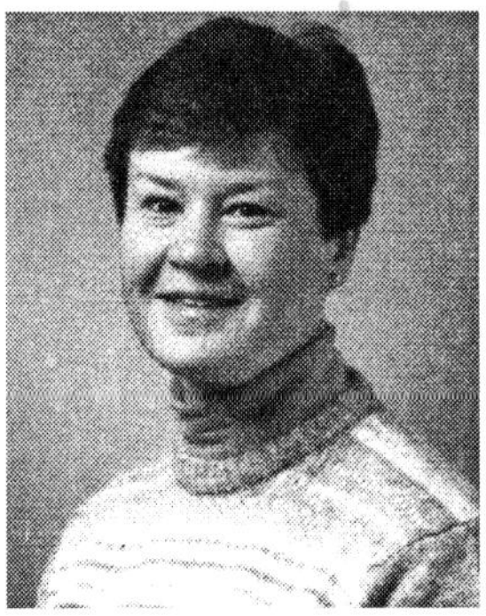

Roberta Hunt Utrecht, Rosemarie Nedeau-Cayo

Rosemarie Nedeau-Cayo promoted to Director of the School of Nursing. She was the last nurse to hold that position.

Roberta Hunt Utrecht promoted to Chief Nurse Executive (CNE).

1996 Patric Ludwig died following cerebral vascular accident (CVA) and related complications.

Groundbreaking celebrated the *New* Bronson Hospital, immediately south of the old campus, beginning with a new parking structure on the corner of Burdick and Vine streets.

Frank Sardone promoted to Bronson Methodist Hospital CEO.

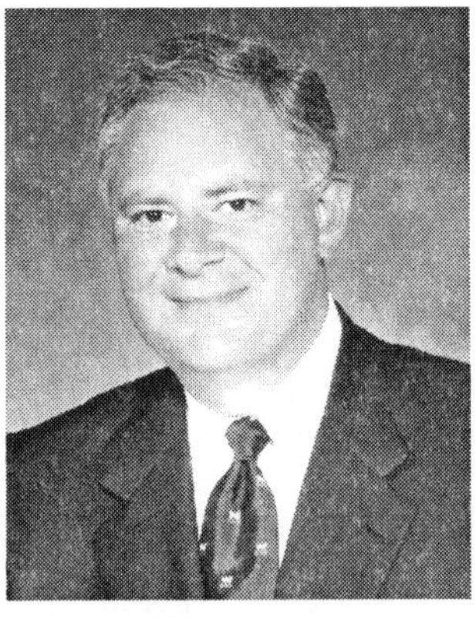

Frank Sardone

1997 Truesdale Hall razed. The School of Nursing moved into the Center Building adjacent to Educational Services.

1998 A May three-day commemorative event hosted 800+ graduates, Bronson Staff, family and friends, including a gala and dinner at the Radisson Hotel.

December marked the closure of BMH School of Nursing.

The nurse extern program transitioned from the School of Nursing to the Educational Services department.

Mary Ann Eldred, appointed Senior Vice President Operation/Patient Care Services, joining Roberta Hunt who continued as CNE.

1999 WMU's School of Nursing named "The Bronson School of Nursing," in conjunction with its first graduation ceremony.

Thirty-seven graduate from WMU Bronson School of Nursing in April, its first graduation.

2000 Dedication of the *New* Bronson; Outpatient facilities opened in April and Inpatient units opened on December 3.

2001 The original hospital (later called Wesley Hall) razed.

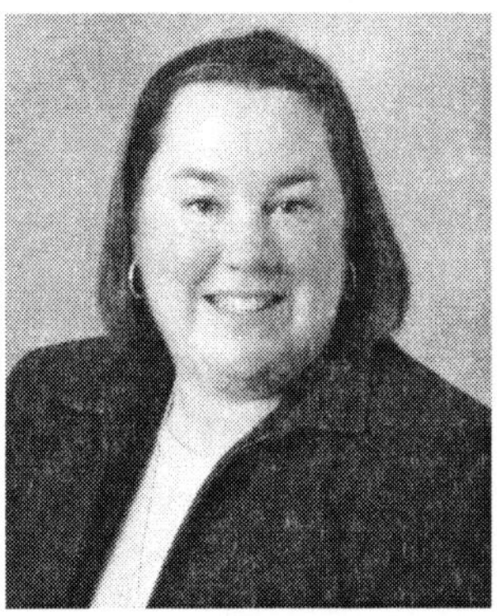
Katie Harrelson

Bronson celebrated its Centennial year.

Bronson Hospital won the State of Michigan Quality leadership award.

Katie Harrelson appointed Chief Nurse Executive.

2002 Nancee Hofmeister '82, returned to Bronson Hospital as a general project coordinator, to further develop professional nursing practice toward the achievement of Magnet Hospital status.

2003 Bronson Healthcare Group named among "100 Best Companies for Working Mothers," by *Working Mother* magazine.

The ten-story and 1940 hospital buildings razed.

2004 Nursing administrators lead the process to achieve Magnet Hospital Status designation.

2005 The Alumni Association of Bronson Methodist Hospital School of Nursing continued to support professional nursing practice with gifts of scholarships and other donations to the WMU Bronson School of Nursing.

APPENDIX B

FACULTY:

BRONSON METHODIST HOSPITAL SCHOOL OF NURSING

Names are listed in the decade in which they first appear as nursing faculty, and an asterisk (*) denotes a Bronson Methodist Hospital School of Nursing graduate.

Prior to 1920

Wildermuth, Edna

1920s

Atwood, Hazel
*Evans, Lucy
*Holke, Sena
*Mohney, Mary
Showerman, Myrtle
Walker, Ellis
Wood, Mrs. Lavender

1930s

Draher, Ann Gwinn
Kunkle, Miss

1940s

Browne, Geraldine
*Crofoot, Helen
Danielson, Alfreda
*Erhart, Alberta
*Evans, Shirley
Godley, Leo F.
*Groat, Thelma
Haines Day, Allene
Heinzelman, Roberta
Hunger, Pauline
*Kiewiet, Joanne
Lott, Beatrice
*Mc Phail, Virginia
Melson, Maude
Miller, Ethylene
Newell, Betty
Parmalee, Maxine
Sheckles, Marguerite
Sweet, Leone
Wantz, Marie
Wolters, Dena

1950s

*Bailey Ambrose, Ione
Boomgaarden, Tebina
Brown, Mae
*Brown, Margaret
Campbell, Dorothy
Cripe, Irene
*Curtis, Phyllis
Damvelt, Barb
Dasler, Louise
*Dunn, Dorothy
*Emig, Ellen
File, Mary
Flower, Ethel
Forsythe, Eleanore
*Gould, Margaret
Gutermuth, Shirley
Hammond, E. Bernice
Heneveld, Elizabeth
Huffman, Louise
Klute, Helen
Kohrman, Joan
Kromminga, Johanna
Lewis, Marian
Maatman, Eunice
Mabee, Ruth
Mac Vean, Eleanor
Mason, Mary Lou
McCarthy, Sarah
McVean, Margaret

*Meninga, Dorothy
*Murray VandeGiessen, Sue
Nelson, Helen
Olech, Ruth
Parren, Margaret
Reibel, Mary
Tiedeman, Mae
*Van Boven, Adriana
Van Vranken Lord, Edna
Weber, Helen
*Wilkinson, Lois

1960s

*Barney, Kathleen
Barron, Shirley
Barta, Patricia
Beisel, Janet
Bellfy, Marylynn
Burton, Rose
Camburn, Lulabelle
Dennany, Lillian
Dobson, Joann
Gamber, Ruth
*Greene, Sandra
Grubb, Sarah
Hoffman, Alice
Holman, Judi
Hoogerhyde, Marie
*Horst McCarty, Carol
*Huston, Isabelle
Kaiser, Mary
Kavalhuna, Dorothy
*Kimber, Erlene
Kingsley, Ruth
Knee, Lynn Jo
Koteskey, Everilda
*Howard Leonard , Linda
Lutz, Carroll
*Mac Donald, Patricia
Mayville, April
Mc Cord, Carmen
Mc Cracken, Betty
McCann, Suzanne
Miller, Kathleen
Monticello, Margaret
Morrey, Joyce
Moulton, Maxine
Mukasa, Idella
Reinsma, Shila
Rhinehart, Jacqueline
Schoolfield, Roberta
*Sheperd, Helen
Shepherd, Anne
Sloat, Eleanor
Spaniolo, Anna Mae
Sullivan, Judith
*Sweet, Diane
*Tameling, Minnie
Tate, Virginia
*Van Bruggen, Kaye
Van Dyke, Mary Lou
Wirtz, Joan
Wybrecht, Barbara
*Wylie, Jackie
Zuidema, Marie

1970s

*Bahlke, Sarah
Broyer, Marjorie
Bush, Harriet
Carr, Carol
Crouch, Lorraine
Crow, Sondra
Dunstone, Deborah
Fuller, Janet
*Gren-Bailey, Elizabeth
Groh, Barbara
*Harper, Kathleen
Holland, Isabelle

Jernstadt, Mary
Heinrich, Gail
Koster, Judy
Leppke, Edith
*Luther, Marilyn
Mange, Virginia
Mouser, Judith
Meholic, Irene
Nedeau-Cayo, Rosemarie
Olsta, Nancy
Orr, Anne
*Schiltz, Sandra
Schneidenbach, Lorraine
*Selinsky, William
Shaw, Karen
Stansky, Roberta
*Tanner, Beth
Truss, Helen
Vogel, Margaret
*Witteveen, Diane
*Zolp, Felicia

1980s

Cervone-Brown, LuAngela
Christian, Arlene
Corbin, Brad
Creager, Susan
*Hargis, Dianna
Haveland, Alicia
Ingersoll, Gail
Mc Evers, Julie
*Mc Graw, Betsy
Moore, Pamela
Passero, Virginia
Potts, Barbara
Proos, Rosalind
Remick, Dolores
Stewart Hoelscher, Judy
*Taylor, Kay
Thede, Linda
*Van Antwerp, Carol
Vedrody, Joan
Wheaton, René

1990s

Albery, Linda
*Blades, Rebecca
Carpenter, Cyndi
Clark, Susan Kay
Creameans, Joan
Davis, Teri
Deitzen, Denise
*DeLeeuw, Joan
DeWeerd, Jerald
Grimm, Rhonda
Hall, John
Ingraham, Ray
Kershner, Wendy
Leadley, Jeanne
Lennan, Gail
Manifold, Susan
*Ossewaarde, Sally
Parker, Shelley
Phillips, Elizabeth
Richman, Crystal
*Sander Jones, Mary Beth
Stark, Mary Ann
Stevens, Marsha
Sutkowi, Sally
*Themins Nahan, Suzanne
Veltman, Rebecca
*Vliem, Sally
Vrobel, Susan

NOTABLE STAFF:
SPANIOLO AND VAN ANTWERP

This message was written for the Michigan Nursing Diagnosis Association, *Newsletter*, 7 (1), by its President Cindy Coviak:

> With this newsletter, it is time for me, as for most of us, to look back on the old year, while looking forward to the new. For members of MINDA, it has also been a sorrowful one, as we learned of the death from cancer of a valued colleague and active supporter of nursing diagnosis.
>
> Anna Mae Spaniolo, MSN, RN, was a faculty member at Bronson Hospital School of Nursing in Kalamazoo for many years. As an educator in this program, she not only served as a role model in clinical practice for her students and colleagues, but also was innovative in her work to serve children and their families. With her colleague and co-worker, Carol VanAntwerp, a clinic was begun to serve students' families at Western Michigan University. As well as serving as a clinical site for the Bronson students, this clinic offered services to an "invisible" group of underserved healthcare clients. For its innovation, the project won the esteemed M. Jeanette Juntti Award from the Michigan Nurses Association.
>
> Across the state, Anna Mae and Carol were active in the Michigan Chapter of the Association for the Care of Children's Health. More than once, the two presented at the national conferences of this multidisciplinary group, while keeping the Michigan chapter viable. As this occurred, Anna Mae and Carol both became active in MINDA. More than once, MINDA members were fortunate to learn of the contributions of these nurses to nursing diagnosis research and to the

> education of new practitioners in the diagnostic process. As presenters at MINDA Research Symposiums, their contributions were timely.
>
> As practitioners in the nursing of chldren, they were in the forefront of those who recognized the value of nursing diagnosis for the care of children and their families. As scholars, they searched for ways that nursing diagnosis could be used to improve care for children. They were able to impact nursing students across the country, as well as practitioners and other educators, as contributors to Lynda Carpenito's books on *Nursing Diagnosis.*
>
> MINDA joins with Carol VanAntwerp, the family of Anna Mae Spaniolo and her other colleagues in mourning her death. We look to the new year inspired by her professionalism, courage, and determination, to continue our own professional lives in her manner."

Lippincott editor Lynda Carpenito noted in her 1992 test, "Anna Mae died in March 1991 after a long illness. Her contributions to this book are evidence of her expertise in pediatric nursing. Her compassion and spirit for others will continue to live in each of us. We all grieve her loss but celebrate her life."

AWARDS

1985 and 1987, M. Jeanette Juntti Education Award, Category 111, Division of Maternal Child Health, Michigan Nurses Association, Anna Mae Spaniolo and Carol Van Antwerp.

1987 October 21, 11th Annual Writing Contest, Instructional Category, Assembly of Hospital Schools of Nursing, American Hospital Association, to Anna Mae Spaniolo and Carol Van Antwerp.

1988 April 30, Outstanding Nursing Alumni Award, Michigan State University, to Anna Mae Spaniolo.

ORIGINAL PROJECTS

- Development of the Pediatric Assessment Tool, based on Marjory Gordon's "Functional Health Patterns."
- Development of the Lifestyle Questionnaire for School-aged Children

PUBLICATIONS

Spaniolo, A.M. & Van Antwerp, C., 1986. "Case study of a child with meningococcemia," *Journal of Pediatric Nursing*, 1(6), 1986 December; 396–403.

Spaniolo, A.M & Van Antwerp, C., 1987. "Potential for injury related to maturational age," in Carpenito, Lynda Juall *Nursing Diagnosis Applications to Clinical Practice*. 2nd ed. Philadelphia:J.B. Lippincott Co.

Spaniolo, A.M. & Van Antwerp, C., 1989. "Potential for injury related to maturational age" in Carpenito, L.J., *Nursing Diagnosis Applications to Clinical Practice*, 3rd ed. Philadelphia:J.B. Lippincott Co.

Spaniolo, A.M. & Van Antwerp, C., 1992. "High risk for injury related to maturational age and pediatric considerations" in Carpenito, L.J., *Nursing Diagnosis Applications to Clinical Practice*. 4th ed. Philadelphia:J.B. Lippincott Co.

Van Antwerp, C., 1993. "High risk for injury related to maturational age, pediatric considerations, altered growth and development" in Carpenito, L.J. *Nursing Diagnosis Applications to Clinical Practice*, 5th ed. Philadelphia:J.B. Lippincott Co.

Van Antwerp, C., 1995. "Risk for injury related to maturational age, pediatric considerations, altered growth and development" in Carpenito, L.J., *Nursing Diagnosis Applications to Clinical Practice*. 6th ed. Philadelphia:J.B. Lippincott Co.

Van Antwerp, C., 1995. The Lifestyle Questionnaire for School-aged Children: A Tool for Primary Care. *Journal of Pediatric Health Care*, 1995:Nov/Dec; 9(6), 251–255.

Van Antwerp, C. & Spaniolo, A.M., 1988 "Nursing services to families with children in a nursing clinic." *American Hospital Association Nursing Educational Communique*, 1988 Spring; 3–9.

Van Antwerp, C. & Spaniolo, A.M., 1991. Checking out children's lifestyles. *Maternal Child Nursing,* 1991:May/June; 16(3), 144-147.

Van Antwerp, C. & Spaniolo, A.M., 1992 Nursing services for children of families living in university housing. *Journal of Pediatric Nursing*, 1992, June; 7(3):211–215.

Date

Child's first name

Child's age Grade

Lifestyle Questionnaire for School-age Children*

Activities that promote health	Yes	No	Sometimes
1. I sleep at least 8 hours every night.			
2. I brush my teeth twice a day.			
3. I visit the dentist every year.			
4. I watch less than 2 hours of TV every day.			
5. I exercise (running, biking, swimming, active sports) one hour every day.			
6. I eat fruits.			
7. I eat vegetables.			
8. I limit my intake of salty snacks and high-sugar snacks.			
9. I have a physical examination every 2 or 3 years.			
10. I stay away from cigarettes.			
11. I stay away from alcohol.			
Injury prevention	**Yes**	**No**	**Sometimes**
12. I wear a seat belt in an automobile			
13. I look both ways when crossing streets.			
14. I follow bike safety rules.			
15. I stay away from lighters or matches.			
16. I never ride ATVs (all-terrain vehicles).**			
17. I wear a helmet when I go on bike trips.			
18. I swim with a buddy.			
19. I wear a life jacket when I ride in a boat.			
20. I take medicine only with my parent's permission.			
21. I stay away from real guns.			
22. I tell my parents where I am going.			
23. I say "no" to drugs.			
24. Our home has a smoke detector that works.			
25. Our home has a fire extinguisher.			
26. If there is a fire, I know a safe way out of my house.			
Feelings	**Yes**	**No**	**Sometimes**
27. I think it is okay to cry.			
28. I enjoy my family.			
29. It is easy for me to fall asleep at night.			
30. My appetite is good.			
31. I like myself just the way I am.			

**The American Academy of Pediatrics recommends that children do not ride on these vehicles.

146 May/June 1991 Vol. 16 **MCN**

APPENDIX C

BRONSON METHODIST HOSPITAL SCHOOL OF NURSING
CATALOG RETROSPECTIVE, 1900–1998

GROWTH AND DEVELOPMENT, ADMISSIONS, CURRICULUM AND TUITION

HOSPITAL VS. ACADEMIC MODELS

For years the question was argued, were hospital-based schools of nursing more houses of labor than learning? How many repetitions were needed to perfect technical skills, clinical judgment and caring practices? What competency development was the responsibility of the nursing program and what did employers need to provide for the orientation of novice RNs into their expected roles?

Another question often argued was whether the professional practice model taught in colleges and universities was distinctly different from hospital-based diploma education in which the model focused more on nursing as an art, learned in an experiential vocational way than the science side—researched knowledge expected to be part of university curricula. According to many nurse educators, nursing could not become a true profession until entry level for practice became no less than the baccalaureate degree and others argued that graduate education was the level of entry as evidenced by most professions in 2000. These questions are not addressed in Appendix C. Content is from verbal reports of graduates, faculty and the school bulletin and represent the growth and development of one hospital-based school of nursing curriculum.

The shift from experiential learning within the labors of daily nursing practice to increased classroom activities and selected clinical experiences occurred in an evolutionary way at Bronson, spurred on by changing expectations of the public, the Michigan State Board of Nursing school approval process and the National League for Nursing's (NLN) voluntary accreditation process. NLN accreditation provided criteria for educational standards and controls that qualified programs for participating in federally directed Basic Educational Opportunity Grants (BEOG) and entry into some baccalaureate programs.

Evolutionary changes to meet academic and practice standards in Bronson's diploma program design began with integration of nursing students into college and university courses and gradually built consistent course lengths, hours and credits that were awarded. Three years of education and practice with little vacation was changed to reflect similarities to college academic years, with breaks given between semesters. For example, second and third year nursing courses until the 1970s often were completed on a Friday, with the next course beginning on the following Monday without a break for students or for faculty preparation.

Curriculum changes in the 1970s and 1980s courses reflected similarities in collegiate lower-division nursing courses and raised the potential for the awarding of transfer credit from hospital-based and associate degree programs to colleges and universities. Students sometimes transferred to Bronson from associate degree programs with transfer credit granted based on course similarity.

Medical concepts (physician-extender practices) were never lost from nursing courses. A movement toward using standardized nursing language from the North American Nursing Diagnosis Association (NANDA) attempted to articulate interdisciplinary work and the interdependence of the professions in the provision of caring services. The curriculum included the expectation of nursing practice competency achievement while not ignoring expectations and necessary competencies to provide for medical care as extensions of physicians hands. Knowledge of the medical school culture was essential.

Curriculum changes in the 1990s drastically cut courses and hours of content and practice, lessening the time at Bronson and hopefully encouraging students to continue their education to advanced levels of practice. Learning strategies in the 1990s engaged students in life-long learning and self-directed, individualized contracts based on sound educational principles while facilitating program downsizing.

Principles, Theories and Common Practices

Bronson's School of Nursing was built on this foundation:

- Caring for others was a constant curricular theme. The first 70 years of the School of Nursing program of study focused more on self-sacrifice and caring for others, often at the expense of the nurses physical, mental and spiritual health. Inclusion of self care filtered into the curriculum during the last 28 years, 1970 through 1998. Sometimes it was recognizable in course titles.
- Discipline, order, frugality and efficiency were expected behavior with residential life, an extension of the total learning experience. Students lived in nurses' residences close to the hospital until the 1960s when nurse staff expectations changed.
- Clinical judgment: graduates were prepared to monitor patient changes in condition and to call attending physicians when progress toward recovery or complications dictated changes in medical interventions. Physicians assessed patient progress when making their rounds once or twice a day. A nurse accompanied the physician who was updated on condition changes and patient concerns. The nurse listened to physician's

judgments about patient progress and newly ordered interventions. Often, technical assistance was offered with new dressings and treatments that could be managed in the patient care area.

- Ethical judgments and behaviors were always an expectation.
- Suspension of value and cultural judgments was expected in the care of patients, though student behavior was judged with rigid, unbending rules, meant to enforce traditional nursing principles practiced that were not culturally sensitive. In the last 20 years, cultural competency for patients and students as human beings was a skill learned and practiced by faculty. Attention was paid to learning styles and teaching students assessment skills for the education of future patients as well as themselves.
- Doing technical competencies—how to—was taught years before the logic of why. The shift to logic connected with practice occurred in the middle decades, and theory before practice as a way to design policy and direct practice during the last 25–30 years.
- Teaching and learning strategies were sequential, a progressive process of acquiring complex skills that built on simpler, basic health and illness concepts. Though rotation of second and third year courses prevented a "perfect" progression, it was expected that students' critical thinking skills and judgment would increase with each clinical practice opportunity. The bar was raised daily.

1900–1904 The Kalamazoo Hospital, A 12-Bed Facility

First established was a two-year training program similar to Florence Nightingale's first nursing school in England, which was focused on laws of God and nature as they related to health and illness care in the hospital and home for individuals and families. A probation period of three months sorted students who were judged both capable and able to manage crises, or incapable, without the aptitude for nursing. No vacation time was planned. Student assignments varied with hospital census and patient need and on-call 24 hours/day was required. Student practice hours were similar to a full-time job so that two years of practice, averaging 12 hours per day, six days a week equaled 7488 hours of practice plus sporadic classroom learning. Curriculum was less of a concern than the students' abilities to learn experientially and respond to the cultural needs in context.

Training included all housekeeping duties, such as laundry, mopping floors, and assisting the cook, plus activities oriented to direct patient care and making supplies such as bandages. A strong body was considered as much of an asset as an intelligent mind and unwavering spirit.

Classes, chiefly lectures by doctors, were held when convenient, with the students often having to dash from the classrooms to answer patient calls and physicians responding to patients' crises.

—*Bronson Bulletin* (1954 Summer)

1900–1916

Records of admission requirements prior to 1916 are reported in unofficial documents and include: a 1913 letter of reference from applicants' pastors, and in 1914, a letter of recommendation and an 8th grade diploma. Students had a 2–3 month probationary period after which they were accepted as official students.

1906

A three-year general training program was adopted, with entrance requirements changed to include at least two years of high school, a sign of the growing need to understand theory and logic behind practice. An affiliation with a New York City hospital provided enrichment and diversity. Curriculum details were not found.

Common student practice was 12 hours per day, six days a week with time off for attending Sunday church services. Classes still came second after patient care demands were met. Practice hours of on-the-job training could easily have exceeded 10,000 hours.

1909

Nursing care of children was added to the curriculum when the New York affiliation was ended and one initiated with Michael Reese Hospital in Chicago.

1916–1918

The 1916 Application Requirements for Training School (see form on following page) specified requirements for applicants who wished to become trained nurses. Applicants were required to be between 18–35 years of age, have at least one year of high school with women of superior education preferred. She received "tuition compensation" of $6.00 after the probationary period. This sum was used for uniforms, textbooks, etc. and was not considered a wage. Their payment was considered to be part of the education they received and services they provided (the work-study model). After completion of the program, graduates would then have a means of livelihood. In 1918 admission requirements were the same; however, applicants were required to provide three references.

1916 APPLICATION REQUIREMENTS FOR TRAINING SCHOOL

The Trustees of the Bronson Hospital are prepared to give a three-year course of instruction in Medical, Surgical and Maternity Nursing to women desirous of becoming trained nurses. Those wishing to enter must apply personally or by letter to the Superintendent of the Bronson Hospital, Kalamazoo, Michigan, who will furnish application blanks. The application should be filled out and returned at once, even though the applicant is not prepared to enter immediately. In returning the application blank, a letter from a clergyman, testifying to the good moral character of the applicant, and from a physician, stating that she is in sound health, must be enclosed.

Applicants are received at any time of the year when there is a vacancy. Pupils are boarded and have their laundry work done at the Hospital; they reside in the Nurses' Home. Nurses receive six dollars a month after acceptance, during their training, this sum being allowed for uniforms, text-books, etc., and is not intended as wages, it being considered that the education given is a full equivalent for services rendered.

Applicants must be between the ages of eighteen and thirty-five years, and at least of average height and physique.

They must have at least one-year high school education, but women of superior education being preferred.

Candidates will be received on probation for two months. They are not permitted to join the School formally until the end of the second month, when, if approved, they must make an agreement to complete the prescribed course and conform to all rules.

They are required, after the two months probation, to wear, when on duty, the hospital uniform.

The day nurses are on duty from 7 A.M. to 7 P.M. with two hours off each day.

They are given an afternoon each week, and four hours off duty on Sunday.

Nurses are allowed two weeks vacation each year. All time lost by sickness, or for any reason, must be made up. Pupils are cared for gratuitously when ill.

When the full term of three years is completed, the nurse will, if she has passed satisfactorily all examinations, receive a diploma certifying to her knowledge of nursing and to her ability to perform the duties of a trained nurse.

The instruction includes:

1. The managing of helpless patients in bed, changing the bed and body linen with patient in bed, giving baths, prevention and treatment of bedsores.
2. The administration of enemata and use of the catheter; observation of pulse, respiration and temperature.
3. Bandaging, making of bandages and rollers and preparation of splints; names and uses of surgical instruments.
4. Dressing of blisters, bruises, sores and wounds; application of fomentation, poultices and minor dressings; cupping administration of anaesthetics, and subsequent treatment of surgical patients.
5. Massage.
6. The cooking, preparing and serving of food and delicacies for the sick.

7. They are also given instruction in the best practical methods of ventilating sick-rooms, and are taught to take proper care of rooms and wards in the Hospital; in keeping all utensils perfectly clean, disinfected, etc.; to observe accurately the sick in regard to the state of the secretions, excretions, temperature, pulse, breathing, skin, eruptions, sleep, mental state, condition of wounds, administration and effect of medicine, obstetrical nursing.

1920

The first nurse instructor was hired. Prior to this time the Nursing Superintendent of the hospital was also responsible for the program of study and the students' learning experiences. She taught nursing arts and supervised students in developing the prescribed skill set. Physicians lectured on diseases, illnesses and treatments.

Students were required to practice a set number of days to graduate. If illness meant absence time had to be made up to successfully complete program requirements.

During the 1920s as practice and educational requirements were enhanced, admission requirements were also raised. Applicants were required to have at least two years of high school and a reference from their high school superintendent. They were also required to have a physical exam after their admission. They continued to receive $6.00 per month, which was used to purchase their books, etc.

1926

Sociology was the first college course in which Bronson students enrolled at Western State Normal School.

1929

By 1929 applicants were required to have a vaccination. The type of vaccine was not recorded.

1930

Physicians continued to teach classroom content within an allopathic medical theoretical framework in formal classroom lectures and then taught informally during patient care rounds. Students were well schooled in current nursing and medical practice.

Course work was structured and defined. Practice hours required regular shifts following work hours for practicing nurses. Twelve-hour-a-day shifts dropped to three 8-hour shifts. A specific number of prescribed practice days continued to be a requirement for graduation.

1931

The probationary period was increased to four months in 1931 and a registration fee of $55 was charged for uniforms. The school purchased uniforms for students, but the aprons were still made by students, using a pattern sent to them prior to admission. They also were charged a $3.25 diploma fee.

—Handwritten graph, BMH Alumni Archives

1933

The registration fee increased to $95 to cover books and uniforms, except aprons. They were also required to provide a small photo, a duplicate high school transcript, and evidence of having received a typhoid vaccination as well as Shick and Dick tests for diphtheria.

—Handwritten graph, BMH Alumni Archives

1934–1935

Year 1, Preliminary and Beginning Students	
Ethics (Preliminary students)	15 hr.
History of Nursing	8 hr.
Anatomy	26 hr.
Chemistry	15 hr.
Principles and Practices of Nursing	64 hr.
Bandaging	18 hr.
Personal Hygiene	15 hr.
Drugs and Solutions	20 hr.
Hospital Housekeeping	14 hr.
Year 2, Intermediate Students	
Obstetrics	8 hr.
Medical Lectures	9 hr.
Medical Nursing	8 hr.
Case Study	4 hr.
Surgical Technique	9 hr.
Year 3, Senior Students	
Case Study	4 hr.
Total number class hours	**237 hrs.**

— Report of Director of Nursing (1934 October), Miss Ruth McLellan, Bronson Alumni Archives; Bronson–Western State Training College (later WMU), 1935.

Affiliations

Herman Kiefer Hospital in Detroit, Contagious diseases
Fairmount Hospital in Kalamazoo, Contagious diseases

—Oral interview, Christine Jarchow

1936

Applicants were required to finish in the upper third of their high school class.

—Handwritten graph, BMH Alumni Archives

1940

Multiple classes were added with expanding nursing and medical science. Nurses continued to teach nursing arts, ethics, history, etc., and physicians provided guest lectures on diseases, illnesses and treatments. Patient care had to be prioritized above student learning so if the nurses on duty called a physician instructor, classes were cancelled or rescheduled. Experiential, on-the-job training continued to be the teaching method of choice.

Admission requirements were expanded to include one year of high school or college chemistry and applicants had to meet college entrance requirements.

1941

Psychological testing of applicants was initiated.

1943

Affiliations

- Western Michigan College science courses moved to the first year instead of being taught during two years. To speed the training of nurses, approximately 95% of the theoretical learning occurred during the first two years of training. The third year was reserved for special affiliations and the small amount of class work necessary.
- Children's Hospital of Michigan, pediatric nursing, three months in length.
- Kalamazoo State Hospital, psychiatric nursing, three months in length.
- Freshmen students, who entered training at Bronson in June, took their first basic science classes at the University of Michigan for three months.

A birth certificate was required as part of the application process.

—*Bronson Bulletin* (1943 June)

1944

Subjects and class hours (60-minute periods) for the three-year course leading to the Graduate in Nursing diploma met or exceeded minimum hour requirements mandated by the Michigan State Board of Nursing for all schools of nursing. The subjects marked (*) were Western Michigan College courses for 19 semester hours of college credit. The six college science courses were the basis on which nursing practice was built. Chapel attendance at 6:30 A.M., though not a curricular activity, was required for all beginning students and those scheduled for duty at 7:00 A.M. Designated evening study hours reinforced the need for study or remediation for upper classmen who had not maintained a "B" average in the preceding semester.

Michigan State Board of Nursing

First year	**Minimum Hours Required**
Nursing Science and Arts, including Massage and Personal Hygiene	150
*Anatomy 211A and Physiology 211B	90
*Chemistry for Nurses 106	45
*Bacteriology 212A and Hygiene 112	45
*Principles of Sociology 244	15
*Nutrition 211	30
*General Psychology 200B	30
History of Nursing	15
Professional Adjustments I	15
Materia Medica	15
Medical Nursing	20
Pharmacology	45
Operating Room Technique	20
Surgical Nursing	20
Diet Therapy	15
Second year	
Social Problems	15
Surgical Specialties, including Urology, Orthopedics, Eye, Ear, Nose and Throat, Gynecology and Medical Staff lectures	45
Medical Specialties, including Communicable Diseases, Dermatology, Neurology, and Medical Staff lectures	45
Obstetrics	45
Pathology	15
Advanced Nursing and Electives, including First Aid	30
Public Health	30

Third year

Pediatrics and Specialties (Affiliation)	45
Psychiatry and Specialties (Affiliation)	30
Professional Adjustments II	30
Total Minimum State Board Requirements	**900**

—BMH Alumni Archives

1945

A BSN was granted between 1945–1949 for students choosing a five-year course of study that met graduation criteria for Western Michigan College or Albion College and Bronson Hospital School of Nursing. Bronson affiliated with Western Michigan College of Education and Albion College. Students attending for one year prior to entering nursing school and one year after completion of nursing courses and graduation, received a BS degree with a major in nursing from that college. Affiliation at Sigma Gamma Children's Hospital in Mt. Clemens exposed students to rehabilitation from many ailments (polio, congenital hip, cerebral palsy, etc.).

Class hours increased dramatically from the 1930s from 237 to 900 hours. The hour increase appears to have been in response to the minimum hour requirement in schools of nursing, as mandated by the Michigan State Board of Nursing.

As hours of study increased and the number of service hours decreased, the cost for education grew. The tuition fee increased to $340, which included tuition at Western Michigan College, affiliation fees (Albion College and Sigma Gamma Children's Hospital), textbooks, uniforms, laundry, board, room and health fees.

—Bronson School of Nursing Bulletins (1945–1949)

1947

In addition to being in the upper third of her high school class, applicants were required to have a "B" average for the four years of high school, and include 16 units of credit from her accredited high school. After approval of her application, additional requirements for students included the following:

- An aptitude test at the Psycho-Education Clinic of Western Michigan College, with a $10 charge
- Vaccination for small pox within three months previous to admission
- Shick test; if positive for diphtheria, the applicant must have immunizing sera
- Wasserman or Kahn test for syphilis

- Tuberculin test
- Typhoid inoculation
- Thorough physical exam by applicant's physician, including chest X-ray
- Thorough dental exam by applicant's dentist, and necessary work completed

Tuition costs continued to rise with the decrease in work-service hours. The three-year cost was $400 which included tuition and fees at both Western Michigan College and Bronson School of Nursing; room and board, health and medical services; textbooks; nurse's cape, uniforms and laundry; and affiliation expenses and student activity fees.

> It costs the hospital approximately $2,500 to provide three years of education for a student nurse including board and room, textbooks, uniforms, health services and many other items. Of this amount the student pays $400 in cash, the balance representing the value of her nursing practice in the hospital.
>
> —*Bronson School of Nursing Bulletin* (1947)

1950

The option with graduation from Western Michigan or Albion Colleges was eliminated. One reason given for the program's demise was the small market for the degree. More reasonable causes may have been the growth in academic sophistication and the need to justify and control courses for which college credit was granted. Hospital-based nursing apprenticeship models were not part of most colleges unless work-study or service learning was an integral part of programming.

Tuition increased a minimal amount and reached $650 in 1959. The age limits for admission continued to be 17–35 years of age, these high school units of credit were recommended:

English	4 units
Science	3 units with Chemistry required
Social Studies	2 units
Mathematics	2 units
Electives	5 units

1955

Classroom and laboratory courses totaled 24, with nursing practice on three shifts, 7 A.M. to 3:30 P.M., 3 to 11:30 P.M. and 11 P.M. to 7:30 A.M. Split shifts on days were common for freshman practice. Shifts were split into two parts, with time out for classroom work between floor duty stints. Required autopsy attendance was intended to reinforce anatomy, physiology and pathophysiology.

First year
Western Michigan College
Bronson Methodist Hospital

Second year, Bronson Methodist Hospital
Operating Room, 13 weeks
Obstetric Nursing, 13 weeks
Diet Kitchen, 6 weeks

Third year, Bronson and Clinical Practice Affiliations

- Kalamazoo State Hospital, 13 weeks nursing practice with psychiatric patients
- Oaklawn Hospital, Marshall, Michigan, 8 weeks rural nursing and 2 weeks with handicapped children
- Bronson Methodist Hospital, 8 weeks nursing management acting as an assistant to the head nurse on a selected patient care unit

—*Bronson School of Nursing Bulletin* (1955 Spring)

1958–1959

Although religion was not recognized as a part of the curriculum before the 1950s, morning chapel attendance was mandatory before beginning clinical practice. Bible was added, then deleted in the fall of 1959.

Freshman Year (Seventeen freshmen courses were the main reason for unacceptably high attrition rate. Several of the Bronson courses were two credit offerings with homework that felt equal to three or four credits.)

Semester 1

Anatomy and Physiology	Nursing Arts I
Chemistry	Pharmacology I
Nutrition	Professional Adjustments I
Psychology	Bible

Semester 2 (20 weeks, including 2 weeks of vacation)

Microbiology	History of Nursing
Sociology	Communicable Disease I
Diet Therapy	Medical Surgical Nursing I
Public Health	Nursing Arts II
	Pharmacology II

First summer term (12 weeks including 1 week of vacation)
Operating Room Technique and Post Anesthesia Recovery
Religion and Health

Junior Year
Semester 3 (20 weeks)
Operating Room Technique, including
Emergency Room and Central Supply
Nutrition and Diet therapy
Obstetric Nursing
Medical-Surgical Nursing II
Semester 4 (18 weeks, including 4 weeks vacation)
Medical-Surgical Nursing III
Communicable Disease II
Professional Adjustments II
Second summer term (14 weeks)
Medical Surgical Nursing IV

Senior Year
Semester 5 (17 weeks)
Pediatric Nursing
Tuberculosis Nursing
Semester 6 (22 weeks)
Psychiatric Nursing
Professional Adjustments III, including Ward Management
Community Aspects of Nursing
Third Summer Term (13 weeks, including 3 weeks of vacation)
Surgical Nursing IV

—*Bronson School of Nursing Bulletin* (1958–1959)

1959–1960

Courses continued to be described in numbers of weeks enrolled and hours of attendance, not credit hours. Bible was eliminated from the first year curriculum in 1959–1960.

—*Bronson School of Nursing Bulletin* (1959–1960)

1960

The 1960s saw an increase in vacation time for students and additional recommendations for applicants.

1963

This was the first year that course descriptions were published in the School Bulletin, moving toward an academic model. The three-year curriculum included 12 weeks of vacation. Two weeks at the Christmas or New Year holiday and two weeks in the summer. Four 12-week clinical rotations gave all students similar practice opportunities during the second and third year of the program.

> The profession of nursing requires women of integrity and intelligence who are motivated by a spirit of service. Personal as well as education qualifications are therefore considered in the selection of students . . . [students were interviewed as a means to determine character.]
>
> Applicants must be between 17 and 25 years of age, a change from 17 to 35 years of age. Character references must show that the applicant is emotionally stable, has a sense of responsibility and is of sound moral character . . . .
>
> Graduation from high school should be in the upper third of the class. A transcript of credit will be sent directly from the high school showing that the applicant has at least 12 units of credit from grade 10–12.

English	3 units
Science	2 units (Chemistry)
Social Studies	2 units
Mathematics	1 unit
Electives	4 units

Tuition fees continued to rise with curriculum changes:

1961–1964	$1,000
1965–1967	$1,300
1968–1969	$1,760

—*Bronson School of Nursing Bulletin* (1963–1964)

1965

Freshman Year

First Term (15 weeks)

Anatomy	105 hours
Chemistry	45 hours
Psychology	45 hours
Sociology	45 hours
Fundamentals of Nursing I	45 hours
History and Trends of Nursing	15 hours

Second Term (15 weeks)

Physiology	90 hours
Bacteriology	60 hours
Fundamentals of Nursing II	45 hours
Pharmacology	15 hours
Nutrition	30 hours
Introduction to Nursing	45 hours
Nursing Laboratory Experience	30 hours

Third Term (6 weeks)

Fundamentals of Nursing II, continued	45 hours
Introduction to Nursing, continued	45 hours
Public Health	15 hours
Nursing Laboratory Experience	60 hours

Junior Year, student schedules rotated with the class divided into four courses and companion clinical practice groups. Conference and practice groups were further divided by patient care units and work shifts.

First Term, Medical-Surgical Nursing I (12 weeks)

Class	60 hours
Medical Nursing Conference	30 hours
Nursing Laboratory Experience	300 hours

Second Term, Medical-Surgical Nursing II (12 weeks)

Class	60 hours
Surgical Nursing Conference	30 hours
Nursing Laboratory Experience	300 hours

Third Term, Medical-Surgical Nursing III (12 weeks)

Class	60 hours
Operating Room & Recovery Nursing Conference	30 hours
Nursing Laboratory Experience	300 hours

Fourth Term, Obstetric Nursing (12 weeks)

Class	60 hours
Obstetric Nursing Conference	30 hours
Nursing Laboratory Experience	300 hours

Senior Year, student schedules rotated with the class divided into four courses and companion clinical practice groups. Conference and practice groups were further divided by patient care units and work shifts.

First Term, Pediatric Nursing (12 weeks)	
Class	60 hours
Nursing Conference	30 hours
Nursing Laboratory Experience	360 hours
Second Term, Leadership in Nursing (12 weeks)	
Class	45 hours
Nursing Laboratory Experience	435 hours
Third Term, Psychiatric Nursing (12 weeks)	
Class	108 hours
Psychiatric Nursing Conference	65 hours
Nursing Laboratory Experience	300 hours
Fourth Term, Out-Patient Nursing (6 weeks)	
Class	20 hours
Nursing Laboratory Experience	200 hours
Fifth Term, Medical-Surgical Nursing IV (6 weeks)	
Class	10 hours
Nursing Laboratory Experience	230 hours
Sixth Term Orientation to Staff Nursing (6 weeks)	
Class	15 hours
Nursing Laboratory Experience	225 hours

—*Bronson School of Nursing Bulletin* (1965–1967)

1968

Numbers of courses taught during the freshman year were reduced to eight, creating a course load that would meet educational standards and decrease attrition. However, freshmen nursing students were expected to meet 200–level Western Michigan University sophomore course requirements in all courses except Chemistry, without the benefit of freshman biology courses. Student achievement was similar to the Western Michigan University students who had taken freshmen level biology courses.

1969

Married students were allowed to live away from the dormitory at their own expense.

1970

Freshman Year

First Term (15 weeks with semester credits)

Biology 210, Mammalian Anatomy	105 hrs.	4 credits
Chemistry 106, Chemistry for Nurses	45 hrs.	3 credits
Psychology 200, Psychology I	75 hrs.	3 credits
Sociology 200, Principles of Sociology	45 hrs.	3 credits
Nursing I, Fundamentals	45 hrs.	3 credits

Second Term (15 weeks with semester credits)

Biology 215, Bacteriology	75 hrs.	3 credits
Biology 219, Systemic Physiology	90 hrs.	4 credits
Nursing II, Fundamentals	150 hrs.	9 credits

Junior Year, student schedules rotated with the class divided into four courses and companion clinical practice groups. Conference and practice groups were further divided by patient care units and work shifts. Quarter credit system was used to accommodate 12-week course length versus the 15-week course length at WMU.

First Term, Obstetric Nursing, 16 credits (12 weeks)

Class and Conference	96 hours
Nursing Laboratory	288 hours

Second Term, Medical Nursing, 16 credits (12 weeks)

Class and Conference	96 hours
Nursing Laboratory	288 hours

Third Term, OR/PAR Nursing, 16 credits (12 weeks)

Class and Conference	96 hours
Nursing Laboratory	288 hours

Fourth Term, Surgical Nursing, 16 credits (12 weeks)

Class and Conference	96 hours
Nursing Laboratory	288 hours

Senior Year, student schedules rotated with the class divided into four courses and companion clinical practice groups. Conference and practice groups were further divided by patient care units and work shifts. Quarter credit system was used to accommodate 12-week course length versus the 15-week course length at WMU.

First Term, Pediatric Nursing, 16 credits (12 weeks)

Class and Conference	96 hours
Nursing Laboratory	288 hours

Second Term, Psychiatric Nursing, 16 credits (12 weeks)

Class and Conference	96 hours
Nursing Laboratory	288 hours

Third Term, Leadership Activities in Nursing, 16 credits (12 weeks)
Class and Conference 66 hours
Nursing Laboratory 366 hours
Fourth Term (12 weeks split into 2–6 week courses)
Introduction to Intensive Care Nursing, 8 credits
Class and Conference 32 hours
Nursing Laboratory 176 hours
Out-Patient Nursing, 8 credits
Conference 24 hours
Nursing Laboratory 192 hours

—*Bronson School of Nursing Bulletin* (1970)

Western Michigan University courses were listed with actual course numbers and semester-hour credits. Chemistry was dropped from the first semester. Intensive care nursing was added to the senior year, a more accurate description for the previous Medical-Surgical Nursing IV course. Fundamentals of nursing care was expanded in focus during the first year to include both wellness and illness components, how to promote health and prevent illness/disease.

The curriculum was changed to enhance student learning and decrease repetitious experiences. The school eliminated the purchase and laundering of uniforms in 1970 and towel and washcloth laundering was stopped in 1973. A cap charge was added, and transportation costs became the student's responsibility; bed linen supply and laundering was eliminated and students purchased meal tickets in 1974; and in 1976 housing was no longer furnished. Change occurred in the tuition and fee payment schedule. Students paid their tuition for Western Michigan University courses directly to the university. As tuition rates increased and work-study time decreased, total expenses increased:

Academic Year	Fees Paid to Bronson	Fees Paid to Western Michigan University	Total
1970–1972	$1600	$510	$2110
1973–1974	$2000	$590	$2590
1974–1975	$2000	$610	$2610
1975–1976	$2000	$656	$2656
1976–1977	$2025	$758	$2773
1977–1978	$2050	$822	$2872
1978–1979	$2050	$939	$2989

Any student could live off campus at his or her own expense. "Beginning August 1, 1976, a dormitory fee of $75 per 15-week term and $50 per 10-week term will be charged; students applying to live in Truesdale Hall will be assigned rooms according to available space."

Fees for living in the dormitory also increased during the late 1970s. For the 1977–78 school year the fee was increased to $150 per 15-week term and $100 per 10-week term; the 1978–79 fee was $187.50 per 15-week term and $125 for 10-week term.

1971

The upper age limit for admission to the school was removed.

1975

Nursing courses were given numbers, using a progressive numbering system, similar to college courses. Psychiatric Nursing was moved to the Junior year and became Nursing 204 with the three Medical-Surgical Nursing courses numbered Nursing 201, 202, and 203 respectively. Obstetric Nursing was moved to a senior-year experience as N302. The other senior nursing courses were Nursing 301, Pediatric Nursing; Nursing 303, Nursing Management and Leadership; Nursing 304 Intensive Care Nursing; and Nursing 305, Community Health Nursing.

When courses were changed, new numbers were assigned for the purpose of accuracy in student transcripts and course descriptions should the student chose to continue their education at a college or university.

1976

Attempting to differentiate hospital-based diploma from baccalaureate education, Nursing 305, Community Health Nursing, was eliminated from the curriculum based on the argument that it was an upper-division baccalaureate nursing course to be taken if students continued to pursue nursing education at that level.

The program of study was reduced in length, shortening the actual time in school and increasing vacations and term breaks. Decreasing program length was intended to make the diploma school of nursing compatible with the length of associate degree programs and a type of "2+2" model—two years of lower division courses, then two years of upper division courses, for students choosing to continue to BSN. In reality, programs were most often 5–6 academic years when combined.

The program, including 22 weeks of vacation, extends over 132 weeks. Students are admitted in September; graduation occurs in March of the third year. Vacations include two weeks each Christmas season, breaks between levels and six weeks each summer.

—*Bronson School of Nursing Bulletin*, (1975–1976)

1980

Preparation for the eventual transformation of the Bronson School of Nursing into a baccalaureate program depended on political and financial resources. The curriculum transitioned to a college-look in the 1980s. Changes were designed to support hospital-based school credit transfers to colleges and universities. Content integrated into nursing courses, such as growth and development, pharmacology and leadership needed "stand alone" course recognition with their own credit allocations. Over the decade, credit hours were reduced to remove repetitious content. It was a time of frequent modifications, discovering new ways to combine nursing content, practice and learning. Students were resilient and succeeded, given an open, supportive learning environment! Informatics, the use of computers and word processing was integrated into all practice courses with a Helene Fuld Fund Grant that provided computer hardware and software.

Nursing courses were adapted to move content, previously taught by nurses, to discipline-specific college departments in keeping with standards of academia, for example, concepts of growth and development were removed from the pediatric nursing course with the content taught at Western Michigan University. Nursing instructors taught nursing science; first, in concepts basic to all nursing practice, and then to the care of specific populations of well and ill persons.

Subsequently, WMU courses Occupational Therapy 225, Growth, Development and Aging, (3 credits) and Social Work 572, Community Agency Resources, (2 credits) were added to the second year. Sociology 200 was moved to the second year when English 105, another transferable college credit was added. Nursing 205, Pharmacology, later was revised and accepted as a three-credit variable field course numbered HHS 530, and taught through the Distance Learning Department. Pharmacology was designed as a separate course; previously being integrated into clinical nursing courses during the 1970s.

English 105, a WMU course, was added to enhance communications skills of scientific writing, technical writing, and general informative writing.

Interpersonal communication skills and medical record documentation had a long history of integration into nursing courses.

Communications Arts and Sciences 355, Leadership, was added to give college credit to the leadership component previously integrated into the nursing leadership and management courses, titled in various ways. Reduction in nursing course credits is notable and progressive with practice hours decreasing. For students desiring a work-study option, the Bronson Nurse Extern Program was established.

Individual, personal health and self-awareness was added to the first year. The assumption was that people with poor self-care skills, low self-esteem and little or no self-awareness would be less able to provide care to others. They would be unable to reenergize themselves to the detriment of self-health and patient care.

Changes in entrance requirements during the 1980s were:

- Entrance testing waived on college graduates at Director's discretion
- Acceptable ACT or SAT scores (40th percentile or above) accepted in lieu of Ohio State Psychological Inventory Test given at WMU
- High school graduate or GED
- LPNs granted credit for Nursing 101–102 on committee approval, current LPN licensure, and graduation from a state approved practical nursing program.
- ACT or SAT scores required for admission in 1983, and WMU testing eliminated
- 10 year limit on transferable college credit
- All age requirements were removed.

1981

Written descriptions accompanied course numbers in the School Bulletin. The first level introduced Nursing within a humanistic and holistic health continuum framework. In Nursing 101, Concepts of self-care were integrated. Nursing process, in Nursing 102, provided a critical thinking approach to practice (scientific method applied to nursing), including health assessment and history-taking skills, diagnosing in nursing language, goal development, choosing interventions with patient partners, and evaluation care outcomes. Nursing 103 focused on care of patients with psychological and physiological distress.

The second level courses N201, N202 and N203 focused on the nursing care of acutely ill, chronically ill or terminally ill adults with physical or mental health problems. Nursing 204's central theme was care of the family in the home and community, an overview of the health-care delivery system and measures for improving health care.

The third level courses N301, N302, N303 and N304 continued to provide content in family centered maternity nursing, care of well and sick children, critical care nursing, management, leadership, group process, professional trends and issues.

—*Bronson School of Nursing Bulletin* (1981–1982)

1982

First Level

Fall Semester (15 weeks)

WMU, Biomedical Sciences 210, Mammalian Anatomy	4 credits
WMU, Psychology 194	3 credits
WMU, English 105	4 credits
Nursing 101	6 credits

Winter Semester (15 weeks)

WMU, Biomedical Sciences 232, Microbiology and InfectiousDiseases	3 credits
WMU, Biomedical Sciences 240, Human Physiology	4 credits
Nursing 102	6 credits

Spring Session (8 weeks)

Nursing 103	8 credits

Second Level

Fall Semester (15 weeks)

Nursing 201 or Nursing 202	12 credits
WMU, Sociology 200	3 credits
Occupational Therapy 225	3 credits

Winter Semester (15 weeks)

Nursing 201 or Nursing 202	12 credits
WMU Social Work 572, Community Agency Resources	

Spring Session (8 weeks)

Nursing 204	4 credits
Nursing 205	4 credits

Third Level courses were not sequential; students were expected to demonstrate increased clinical judgment skills with successful completion of each course.

Spring Session (10 weeks), Fall and Winter Semesters (15 weeks)

Nursing 301, Parent-Child Nursing	12 credits
Nursing 304, Advance Nursing (Critical Care Nursing)	12 credits

Nursing 305, Family and Community Health 1	2 credits
Nursing 306, Perspectives on Nursing (professionalism, legal and ethical issues)	3 credits
WMU, Communications Arts and Sciences 355, Leadership	

—*Bronson School of Nursing Bulletin* (1982–1983)

1983

Nursing courses were modified to clearly articulate the use of nursing process and nursing diagnoses. Nursing 103, Self Health; Nursing 104, Nursing Process; and Nursing 105, Nursing Skills, honed the most critical skills that needed to be mastered for successful progression. WMU course offerings stayed the same.

—*Bronson School of Nursing Bulletin* (1983–1984)

1984

A transitional plan for the class graduating in 1987 looked like this:

First Level

Fall Semester (15 weeks)	
BMed 210 Mammalian Anatomy	4 credits
Psych 194 Psychology	3 credits
Eng. 105 Writing	4 credits
Nsg 103 Health Promotion	5 credits
Winter Semester (15 weeks)	
BMed 240 Human Physiology	4 credits
Bmed 232 Microbiology & Infectious Diseases	4 credits
Nsg 104 Nursing Process	5 credits
Spring Term(8–10 weeks)	
OT 225 Growth, Development and Aging	3 credits
Nsg 106 Nursing, Self-Care Deficits	5 credits

Second Level

Fall Semester (15 weeks)	
Soc 200 Sociology	3 credits
Nsg 220 Nursing Concepts I	6 credits
Nsg 221 Nursing Concepts II	6 credits
Winter Semester (15 weeks)	
Nsg 205 or WMU HHS 530 Pharmacology	3 credits
Nsg 222 Nursing Concepts III	6 credits
Nsg 223 Nursing Concepts IV	6 credits

Third Level

Spring Term (8–10 weeks)	
WMU Family theory	3 credits
Nsg 320 Behavior & Relationships	6 credits
Fall Semester	
Nsg 321 Expanding Family	6 credits
Nsg 322 Nursing Management of Families with Children	6 credits
WMU Elective	3 credits
Winter Semester	
Nsg 323 Nursing Practice with Families in Community	6 credits
Nsg 324 Nursing Management of Client/Family in Situational Crisis	6 credits
Nsg 306 Perspectives in Nursing	3 credits
Total Program	**106 credits**

WMU = 34 credits
BMH = 72 credits

Program Length = 106 weeks including vacations
Total Practicum = 1450 hours

In the academic year 1983–1984, the School of Nursing moved from a "flat fee" tuition to a "per credit hour" tuition charge.

Tuition charges published combined WMU and BMH School of Nursing fees. Charges increased when Western Michigan University classes were added. Students often had attended college and were prepared to transfer credit so that Bronson courses needed to reflect a credit hour charge as opposed to the past flat fee charge. Students were learners not workers. They were no longer considered primary caregivers who boosted hospital staff, and the increase in tuition reflects the philosophical and functional change.

A summary of tuition changes in the 1980's follows:

1980–1981	$3687.50	
1981–1982	$3880.00	
1982–1983	$5237.10	
1983–1984	$5237.10	
1984–1985	$6046.25	106 credit hours
1985–1986	N.A.	
1986–1987	$6211.25	105 credit hours
1987–1988	$6644.50	103 credit hours
1988–1989	$7937.50	102 credit hours
1989–1990	$7937.50	102 credit hours

Housing charges were optional since students were no longer required to live in the dormitory. Charges ranged from $2100–2330 for the three-year program, still a value at $58 to $65 per month.

1990

Program modifications evolved further to reduce practice and credit hours to 76 from 106 as a way to align the program with baccalaureate nursing education, which required approximately 120 to 130 credits to receive a Bachelor of Science degree with a major in nursing. Credit hours for the WMU Bronson School of Nursing, revised for initiation in the Fall 2004, was 127 to successfully complete the program to earn a baccalaureate degree.

The Bronson Methodist Hospital School of Nursing program transitioned to align with baccalaureate nursing education, in a sense, following the two plus two model: two years of under division, then two years of upper division nursing courses. More non-traditional students were entering the nursing program and required university courses became pre-requisites for admission to the school of nursing.

Applicants were required to have college credits in the following areas: anatomy, physiology, microbiology, general psychology, and growth and development. They also were required to have completed a chemistry and algebra course either at the high school or college level. Basic requirements also included experience in the healthcare field or a transfer-nursing student who had completed clinical nursing courses in another nursing program. This model was less labor-intensive for faculty since students who came to Bronson had successfully completed science courses and were less likely to fail nursing courses, and required less support.

Science course credits were transferred to Bronson from colleges or universities. Bronson faculty taught nursing courses.

The cost of tuition for the 1990–1991 year was $6515, less than the previous year with basic courses already taken and the program reduced to 48 weeks. Total cost for the program declined, as fewer credits were needed for graduation. In May of 1995 admission for students without completion of all science courses was discontinued. A summary of tuition changes in the 1900s follows:

1990–1991	$6515.00	78 credit hours
1991–1993	$6856.00	76 credit hours
1993–1995	$7058.00	75 credit hours
1995–1998	$4908.75	57 credit hours

1991

Literature provided for students encouraged them to continue their education to earn a Bachelor of Science in Nursing following completion of Bronson's program. Most universities with nursing programs offered specific programs for RNs who had received their initial pre-licensure education in two to three year programs.

Validation tests for proficiency in nursing practice, such as standardized examinations prepared by American College Testing or National League for Nursing or instructor-prepared examinations were required by some colleges for awarding transfer credit when students chose to apply for the RN–BS completion option.

1993

First year

WMU	
BioS 211, Human Anatomy	4 credits
OT 225, Human Growth and Development	3 credits
Psy 100, Introduction to Human Behavior	3 credits
BioS 232, Microbiology and Infectious Diseases	4 credits
BioS 240, Human Physiology	4 credits
BMH	
Nsg 100, Introduction to Nursing Practice	3 credits
Nsg 107, Nursing Process	4 credits
Nsg 108, Nursing Fundamentals	3 credits
Nsg 109, Nursing Technologies	3 credits

Second year, nursing courses could be taken in any sequence over five 8-week academic periods.

WMU	
HHS 530, Pharmacology,	3 credits
BMH	
Nsg 230, Essentials of Psychiatric Nursing	7 credits
Nsg 231, Essentials of Obstetric Nursing	7 credits
Nsg 232, Essentials of Pediatric Nursing	7 credits
Nsg 233, Nursing of Adults with Acute Illness	7 credits
Nsg 234, Nursing of Adults with Chronic Illness	7 credits
Capstone course, all courses had to be successfully completed prior to enrolling in the final course.	
Essentials of Managed Care	7 credits
Total Program	**76 credits**

Nursing Course Contact Hour Equivalency

Instruction	= 15 hours/1 credit
Clinical Laboratory	= 30 hours/1 credit
Clinical Experience	= 45 hours/1 credit

—*Bronson School of Nursing Catalog* (1993–1995)

1995–1998 Closure

Curriculum objectives of the School of Nursing (shown below) became the same as those of the National League for Nursing's *Roles and Competencies of Graduates of Diploma Programs in Nursing*, 2nd edition, revised 1989:

A. Provides nursing care for individuals, families and groups by utilizing the nursing process
B. Provides for the promotion, maintenance, and restoration of health and support and comfort to the suffering and dying
C. Utilizes management skills including collaboration, coordination and communication with individuals, families, groups and with other members of the health care team
D. Assumes a leadership role within the health care system
E. Teaches individuals, families and groups based on identified health needs
F. Functions as an advocate for the consumer and the health care system to improve the quality and delivery of care
G. Practices nursing based on a theoretical body of knowledge, ethical principles and legal standards
H. Evaluates nursing practice for improvement of nursing
I. Accepts responsibility and accountability for professional practice
J. Utilizes opportunities for continuing personal and professional development
K. Participates in health related community services
L. Utilizes critical thinking in professional practice

CONCEPTUAL FRAMEWORK/RATIONALE

Our philosophy provides beliefs and values that guide our caring relationships and learning within seven conceptual areas: CARING, NURSING, INDIVIDUAL, HEALTH, ENVIRONMENT, LEARNING and COMMUNITY. The areas are not mutually exclusive.

The focus is CARING. All school personnel and students model CARING relationships. Caring is demonstrated in the attainment of all school competencies within a holistic, total person approach. No one nursing theory is favored. An eclectic approach encourages diversity to meet individual needs.

Program Competencies

- Uses caring behaviors of respect, nurturance, confirmation and responsiveness for self and others
- Meets regulations for professional practice using critical thinking, interpersonal and technical skills
- Facilitates choices and growth for self and others in learning and care management
- Promotes health based on beliefs and values of community, client and self
- Manages own responses within a given system(s) toward health promotion.
- Manages self-directed learning
- Changes behavior to fulfill program competencies using and evaluating resources available in the environment
- Meets requirements of the community in which nursing is practiced
- Students demonstrate program competencies at planned evaluation points as they matriculate. All courses contribute to the program competencies (*see* Curriculum Plan, see page 675).

Crystal B. Richman, assistant director, edited the school's final handbook that included the progam of study on the following page. This curriculum plan remained in place until the Bronson Methodist Hospital School of Nursing closed in December 1998.

A-4

PROGRAM OF STUDY

PRE-REQUISITE COURSES

The following pre-requisite requirements are completed prior to nursing course enrollment:

- ♦Anatomy
- ♦Human Physiology
- ♦Microbiology
- ♦General Psychology
- ♦Human Growth, Development and Aging

REQUIRED SUPPORT COURSE

COURSES	HOURS	HOURS	HOURS	CREDITS
PHARMACOLOGY	45	0	0	3

REQUIRED NURSING COURSES

COURSES	INSTRUCTION HOURS	LAB. HOURS	CLINICAL HOURS	CREDITS
NGS 120 ESSENTIALS OF SELF MGMT.	15	0	0	1
NSG 121 INTRO TO NSG PRACTICE I	45	30	90	6
NSG 122 INTRO TO NSG PRACTICE II	45	30	90	6
NSG 230 ESSENTIALS OF PSYCH. NSG.	45	30	135	7
NSG 231 ESSENTIALS OF OBSTET.NSG.	45	30	135	7
NSG 232 ESSENTIALS OF PED. NSG.	45	30	135	7
NSG 233 NSG. OF ADULTS WITH ACUTE ILLNESS	45	30	135	7
NSG 234 NSG. OF ADULTS WITH CHRONIC HEALTH PROBLEMS	45	30	135	7
NSG 310 ESSENTIALS OF PATIENT CARE MANAGEMENT	45	30	135	7
TOTAL NURSING COURSE HOURS	**375**	**240**	**990**	**55**
TOTAL PROGRAM HOURS	**420**	**240**	**990**	**58**

—Bronson Methodist Hospital School of Nursing, *Handbook 1995-1998,* revised August 1995, page A-4

BRONSON METHODIST HOSPITAL SCHOOL OF NURSING
SAMPLE CURRICULUM PLAN – FALL ENTRY

Effective Fall 1995

Completed Prior to Nursing Enrollment	**Fall (16 weeks)**	**Winter (16 weeks)**
Anatomy Physiology Microbiology General Psychology Growth, Development, & Aging **Optional:** Pharmacology	NSG 120 Essentials of Self Mngmt. . . . . 1 credit NSG 121 Intro to Nursing Practice I . . . . 6 credits NSG 122 Intro to Nursing Practice II . . . . 6 credits HHS 530 Pharmacology/16wk . . . . 3 credits	NSG 230 Essentials of Psychiatric Nursing . . . . 7 credits NSG 231 Essentials of Obstetric Nursing . . . . 7 credits
Spring (8 weeks)	**Fall (16 weeks)**	**Winter (8 weeks)**
NSG 232 Essentials of Pediatric Nursing. . . . . 7 credits	NSG 233 Nursing of Adults with Acute Illness . . . . 7 credits NSG 234 Nursing of Adults with Chronic Health Problems . . . 7 credits	NSG 310 Essentials of Patient Care Management . . . . 7 credits

Course Descriptions are located in the Student Handbook

PROGRESSION NOTES:

- Anatomy, Physiology, Microbiology, General Psychology, and Growth, and Development, & Aging must be completed with a grade of C or better, prior to enrollment in first nursing course. Pharmacology may be completed prior to nursing enrollment or while enrolled in 100- or 200-series nursing courses.
- All nursing courses are taught in sessions 8 weeks in length.
- 100-series nursing courses must be taken in sequence. The five 200-series nursing courses may be taken in any order.
- All 100-series and 200-series nursing courses and Pharmacology are pre-requisite to NSG 310.

Updated: 6/6/95 CB/CURRPLNP.CAT State Board Approval: 3/21/90; Board Approval of Modified plan: 8/9/91, 6/21/93

BRONSON METHODIST HOSPITAL

B

SCHOOL OF NURSING

APPENDIX D

BRONSON METHODIST HOSPITAL SCHOOL OF NURSING GRADUATES[1]

[1] Under each class year, names at time of graduation are followed by subsequent last name/s. These names are current in Alumni Association files as of July 2004. We apologize for any inadvertent errors. The symbol (*) designates graduates who contributed oral or written memories as sources for the text of this book.

1903

Johnston, Minnie
Koster Bosker, Rena
Legge, Mary
Pyle Dayton, Bessie

1907

Campbell Sprague, Harriet
Collier Spitler, Josephine
VanHartesveld Jacobs, Sophia

1908

Cowlbeck, Earl
Ruckoft, Mary

1909

Brody, Nellie
Carr York, Evarilla
Fye, Mae
Lage, Irene
Norberg, Theresa

1910

Cumbers, Eva
Meengs Russell, Grace

1911

Brown Barker, Bertha
Cook Clark, Josephine
Eaton Haskett, Amy
Farthing, Anna
Flower Kennedy, Frances
Heath Patterson, Nina
Houghton Thompson, Hilda
Knight, Eva
Maul Makins, Helen
Ramsey Schemerhorn, Isabell
Warfield Richardson, Buelah

1912

Briggs Miller, Hazel
Crosby, Harriet
Gitchell Holmes, Minnie
Houghtout Hodge, Willetha
Simons Gitchell, Bernice

1913

Huber, William
Teller Johnson, Mina
Ward Streeter, Grace
Weber Macgrayne, Mina

1914

Baarman Buell, Anna
*Bailey Seward, Amy
Cady Evans, Madge
Garrison, Charlotte
Miller, Stella
Mumby Bien, Ruth
Whitcomb, Belle

1915

Gemrich Richmire, Anna
Heethuis Bosker, Anna
Lemmer, Nellie
Zerwis Hicks, Lois

1916

Arnold, Emma
Bauer Bauchman, Suzane
Bloem White, Lena
Campbell Laneko, Edith
Elmer White, Emile
Fetterhoef Beers, Cora
Frisbie, Una
Olson Carbinier, Clara
Schwartz Bryant, Emma
Sullivan, Nellie

1917

Bushouse Wade, Katherine
Frisbie Bouwens, Ida
Heckleman Bullock, Arvilla
Rowe Fuller, Bessie
Sweetland Dankert, Edith
Ward Thompson, Ruth

1918

Beck Newton, Ella
Demoor Doos, Mary
Luyendyke Tenninga, Lydia
Nash Mopps, Gladys
Nielson, Sophie
Notely, Jane
Plumb, Elsie
Smith Hurni, Fern
Wygent, Elsie

1919

Fisher Haight, Naomi
Hermann Winslow, Blanche

1920

Carr Simmons, Jennie
Difendefer Beuker, Jean
Jenkins, Leona
Kester, Hazel
Laroy Cessna, Nancy
Taylor Peck, Rose
Thorn, Florence
Verhage Popiwich, Dorothy
Wightman Wheaton, Lillian

1921

Baker Nunan, Mildred
Beadle Poe, Gladys
Finley Davis, Gladys
Finley Whalen, Ilahbelle
*Hinds Phelps, Ruth
Hooven, Myrtle
*Veenhuis Cody, Cornelia
Wilson Bengfeld, Honora

1922

Garnaat Gibbs, Cena
Healey Hamilton, Susan
Lemmer Vander Molen, Jean
Matthews Danielson, Marvel
Olephant Reeder, Mildred
Rutherford Meyer, Belle
Tribolet Moody, Louise

1923

Anderson, Kerstin
Evans, Lucy
Holke Hayes, Sena
Kingsley Rose, Eva
Ory Stone, Bertha
Pike Wood, Frances
Sootsman Wagner, Irene
Wagner Kinney, Clara
Warner Loetz, Ferne

1924

Badder, Grace
Boughner, Belva
Hill Peck, Sarah
Lee Young, Mildred
Mohney Wallenstein, Mary
Pallister Brown, Frances
Stillwell Groat, Thelma
Winters Kievit, Ellen

1925

Boers Decker, Marian
Bond Trent, Alfrieda
Bush Lancaster, Fannie
Carrol Knoblock, Hilda
Hanna Varney, Margaret
Harding Meyers, Laura
Hicks Rogers, Clara
Hollenbeck Cook, Donna
Holmes McRobbie, Oril
Kelley, Grace
Moody Cairns, Nina
Reynolds Cleary, Olive
Wilcox Skamfer, Susan

1926

Brown Reid, Latona
Edgar, Hattie
Langworthy Bell, Ruth
Matthews Ernst, Marquerite
Nottle Goodwin, Eliza
Olson Simpson, Anna
Wright Meyle, Mabel

1927

Agan Triestram, Marian
Brickell Winans, Elvra
Burns Hatfield, Myrtie
Cook, Eleanor
Hutchens Fry, Dorothy
*Kitzmiller LaMar, Margaret
Moore Kitzmiller, Georgia
Page Smith, Cora
Rice Palmer, Ruth
Roper Wilson, Dorothy
Royal Fritz, Lettie
Troxell Stetter, Harriet
Whiteman Kitzmiller, Rena
Wren, Evaray

1928

Abbott, Beula
*Bast Bell, Jennie
Beebe Reitenga, Elda
Berry Hycoop, Doria
Bittrich, Gertrude
Heaton Dutmers, Neva
Homer Lambert, Ruth
Lamphere Wharram, Fern
Littlefield Noel, Frances
Meng Cookingham, L.O.E

Ostrom Tefft, Anna
Robertson Schneider, Bertha
Ten Houten Jennings, Edith
VanWagner Perron, Ercyl
Williams Cole, Hettie
Zimmerman Rogers, Minnie

1929

Beck Fry, Ida
Finney, June
Fischer Ford, Mable
Harmon, Gertrude
Lee Wixon, Esther
*Reiff Raisch, Anne
Siertsema Brown, Ruth
VanKersen Bordwell, Jeanette
VanWingerden, Verna

1930

Allen Brown, Lucy
Allen Johnson, Bernice
Bixler, Kathryn
Bowen Henderson, Jessie
Bozer Douglas, Doris
Brooker Curtis, Annette
Cross, Ruth
Edson, Beulah
Hitzeman Lowe, Dorotha
Jorgensen, Gladys
Kennedy, Irene
MacRitchie Littlefield, Kathryn
Mater Powers, Mabel
Purdy Harrison, Susie
Shoemaker Fisher, Edna
Stephens, Mary
Voyce Sturgis, Edith
Wallis Harding, Grace

1931

Archer Sabo, Arlyne
Bush Neal, Wilhelmina
Clark Crocker, Grace
Doster Lamb, Ruth
Edwards Fuller, Lucille
Forman Lippert, Isabel
France Pleyte, Laura
*Garlock Crockett, Doris
Graves Theis, Estella
Hager Bertram, Bertha
Hallan Burgwald, Ivah
Hanna Blake, Catherine
Holmes, Marylois
Lawrence Grimes, Anna
May Collier, Mary
McKnight Splithoff, Gladys
Moshier Harris, Evelyn
Pellows MacRitchie, Iris
Pohl Terry, Eva
Pooler Freemier, Annabel
Robertson Brown, Bertha
Rowlson Bacon, Olive
Shepard Kain, Ila
Shipway McEndarffer, Iris
Sinclair Holdstock, Hilda
Titus Pallet, Dorothy
Vandenberg Vanderweele, Marian
Warren Lake, Gertrude
Watson Miles, Cheridel
Wells Miller, Belva

1932

*Armstrong Chase, Dorothy
Baker, Edna
Britton Ford, M. Frances
*Crawford Utter, Alethea

Dainer Carey, Iva
Harding Thill, Marian
Holmes Tucker, Ruby
Hudgins Arthur, Ruth
Johnson Davenport, Margaret
*Kraft Jackson, Ena
Leach Downey, Wanda
McCormick, Mary
McKinley Nelson, Mary
Minogue, Virginia
Moser Witters, Annis
Nelson Bertolissi, Elizabeth
Pascoe Klok, Hazel
Pearson Bossard, Leta
Putney Smeltzer, Ruth
Rowe Smith, Wilma
Sharpe White, Mae
Wallis Lampe, Charlotte
Wilcox, Beatrice

1933

Beal Meyer, Gertrude
Charlebois Richcreek, Margaret
Coom Tracy, Margaret
Dell, Dorothy
Ditlow Niewoonder, Lois
*Gierman Jarchow, Christine
Hansbarger Burrows, Gaylia
House Hopps, Gertrude
Jorgenson Comstock, Violet
Klotzback Leedy, Grace
Lowe, Dorothea
Lynn, Maxine
Mead Neidlinger, Neva
Monroe, Ardath
Moore Sherman, Arlene
Niegarth Mott, Jean
Sumner Hoffman, Leora
Tegrootenhuis, Fern
*Thomas Brandeberry, Nora
Tobias Meyer, Thelma
Wieble Hannan, Bessie

1934

Becker, Lucille
Brainard Crawford, Adelaide
Brown, Ruby
Burns Beesing, Margaret
Carley Binns, Irene
Ellinger Simmons, Jessie
Farley Merritt, Roxia
Grieder Fiedorek, Florence
Hoshal Metcalf, Martha
Ireland Schroen, Mary
Knoblack, Mary
Ringel Allen, Alberta
*Schanzlin Lietzke, Mary
Talbot, Dorthea
Thorley Proudfit, Margaret
Tornga Burleigh, Grace
VanBoven, Adriana
Ward Stillwell, Myrtle
Wood Beedle, Ida

1935

Carey Lower, Frances
Carr Bauchan, Irene
Dykstra Brink, Jennie
Erhart Merritt, Alberta
Fishel Draper, Helen
Forsman Spann, Lillian
Harding Mather, Joyce
Hartman, Louise
Hilles Wilson, Imogene
Howard Conklin, Myrtle
Jaeger DeHaan, Zelma
Johnson Lutz, Lillie
Kmuth Bentley, Maebelle
Land Dunnington, H. Eleanor

*Land Vanderhoef, Marquita
Lindsley Funk, Virginia
Martin Burns, Helen
Nash Stiglich, Irene
Oates Collins, Shirley
Parker Hoppe, Mildred
*Peck Ollila, Marjorie
Robins, Marjorie
Thomas Vivian, Alice
Vandenberg Isenharts, Hattie
Wheaton Churchill, Lillian

1936

Carrow Cole, Helen
Crawford Fredericks, Edith
Dunavin, Myrtie
Eckstrom Haack, Sarah
Filarski Farrin, Deanne
*Green Ramsay, Doris
Hansen Wilson, Kathryn
Harger Sabin, Helen
Houghtaling Collver, Mary
Housel Shaw, Irma
*Kemp Kanaar, Ruby
Kobelt Hopkins, Mildred
Kumler Brown, Charlotte
McCoy Niessink, Katherine
McDaniels Cox, Jean
Montgomery Nash, Doris
Nicholls, Hilda
Olli, Aino
Richards Mitchell, Miriam
Tregonning Spitler, Bernice
Walker, Roma
Wivell Leavens, May

1937

Betz, Evelyn
Brown Lievense, Carlie
Carncross Weaver, June
Conklin Cowgill, Alta
Fitch Robinson, Reba
Frohriep Gazella, Viola
*Hjortholm Molyneux, Helen
Ingle Labar, Germay
Luttenbacher, Ruth
Maloy Delaney, Charlotte
Nelson Joslin, Dorothy
Raymont Cook, Lorraine
Ringle Ray, Marjorie
Rose Bryant, Lucretia
Schaller, Hazel
Sherrod, Estina
Simmons, Mary
Steketee Jappinga, Grace
Stover Leibrock, Elaine
VandenBerg Hardy, Nola
Walton Johnson, Doris

1938

Brill Hively, Grace
Frutig, Elizabeth
*Gall Zook, Ruth
*Martin Correll, Margaret
Martin Schascheck, Theodora
May Moore, Anna
Smithz Alloway, Velma
*Thornburg Richards, Gladys
Walker Luginbill, Mildred
Watts Sebright, Marian
Wyers Hess, Frances

1939

Abbe Holland, June
Althaus Klerk, Elizabeth
Crane Wooton, Geraldine
Cunningham Cope, Mary

Denaway Robinson, Arlene
Geschwendt Dunlap, Marian
Ingle, Jennie
Kinney Clement, Thelma
Latimer Gorman, Helen
Luttenbacker French, Ruth Anna
McNeal Cain, Margaret
Newell Kitzenger, Jena
Paull Weiser, Dollie
Pohly Harrison, Kathryn
Schulke Newton, Hazel
Seymoure Schrier, Elizabeth
Smith Meninga, Dorothy
Vanderweele Chase, Mary

1940

Bedford Maurer, Charlotte
Bouwhuis Boyd, Gerda
Bradley Bray, Elizabeth
Davis Crapo, Enid
Heavener Nye, Grace
Jason Harris, Dorothy
King Dykehouse, Lucille
Klager VanBruggen, Kathryn
Moon Jacobsen, Grace
*Munger Neiderlander, Paulene
Plass Odle, Margaret
Porter Mattson, Elsie
Streeter Gravlin, Madeline
Tyler Ramsey, Audrey

1941

Bedient Tetzlaff, Irene
Boekhout Workman, Ann
Boers Bell, Stella
Bosworth Bockstanz, Carol
Clancy Whiteley, Paula
Currey Kowalski, Eleanor
*Curry Pikkaart, Jewel
Davis Cook, Helen
Evans Cornish, Peggy
Feasel Klapp, Rowena
Halbert Howe, Mary
Hopping Butler, Mildred
Housel, Virginia
Johnson Vanmelle, Betty
Jones Allen, Alene
Large Lockwood, Edythe
Lee Frase, Maruerite
Mahieu Gabel, Margaret
Muir Harmer, Jean
Pioch Turner, Lorraine
Pryor Peterman, Pauline
Shellington Kidder, Ruth
Stockton Shell, Elinore
Vanek Roberts, Anna
Watts Kruba, Annette
Winterle Ellis, Elzada

1942

Abbott Richter, Margaret
Archer Craner, Shirley
Budd Naffziger, Gwendolyn
Carr Swinehart, Florence
Chase Mejeur, Mary
Davis Barton, Ruth
Dell Reinertson, Marian
*Gerard Vandermeer, Winifred
Hastings Caplan, Janice
Houseworth Hughes, Betty
Middlebush Jennings, Dorothy
Moffett Pippenger, Helen
Morrison Broxton, Frances
Peterman Zimmerman, Lorraine
*Ramsay Sheppard, Gwen
Rogers McMonagle, Elizabeth

Smith Uschuk, Ella
Steinen Beckius, Elizabeth
Van Eck Smarr, Janet
VandeStreek Smith, Joanne
Wheeler Shaffrey, Alice
Wilson Krupp, Pauline

1943

Colby Somers, Orvilla
DeBoer Dingman, Frances
Dyer McWee, Harriet
*Fox Glittenberg, Elaine
Francis Fair, Elizabeth
Hawkins, June
Housel, Janet
Matthews Beard, Winifred
Nidy Simmons, Greta
Noel Boers, Doris
Norton Appelquist, Lois
*Pettyjohn Ockerman, Phyllis
Pio Allsup, Mary
Raymont Scott, Dorothy
Robinson Bunge, Helen
Rohl Berndt, Margaret
Simpson McClain, Juanita
Underwood Pascoe, Gladys
Westfall Langhoff, June
Young, Mary

1944

Baird, Jeannette
Bryan Cherry, Eunice
Davidson Hoxsie, Wilma
Doster Shaffer, Jean
Evans Robbins, Shirley
Fletcher Trumbull, Marjorie
Howard Fowler, Barbara
Hubbell McCabe, Jean
Kline Giddings, Joyce
MacDonald Swanson, Elaine
Mack Farrell, Mona
*Mein Terpstra, Winifred
Newcomb Clement, Betty
Pioch Benacker, Maxine
Schneider Graham, Jean
*Sherwood Burrell, Martha
Smith Yeske, Barbara
Tousain Mooney, Louise
Van Patten Taggert, Dorothy
Walker Hughes, Arlene
West Grossbart, D. June
Wilson Stuut, Eleanor
Wright Hathaway, Dora

1945

Case Fieberkorn, Mary
Crone Taber, Miriam
De Bruyn Petersen, Marian
Dunning Johnson, Velva
*Edgerton Brown, Margaret
Fennell Large, Beverly
Fowle Champion, Alta
Garrett Champion, Marie
Hanson Christopher, Frances
Hard Thomas, Wilma
Hecht Renner, Elaine
Hunt Wagers, Joyce
Kamps Edgerton, Gladys
Kenyon Blakely, Madonna
Lawrence Netzley, Elizabeth
Lulofs, Evelyn
*Newton, Marilyn
Price Norquist, Helen
Rimkus Wager, Veronica
Shaw May, Floy
Sherman Allen, Vivian
Terwilliger Johnson, Phidora
Turner Johnson, Eleanor
Van Eyk, Cecile

Wardwell VanNimar, Ruth
Washburn VanWelden, Constance
Welsh Heath, Donna
Whitney Winchell, Janice
Williams Larsen, Mable

1946

Albrecht Edwards, Margaret
Bailey Herbert, Jean
Brown Crawford, Elizabeth
Crofoot Hazen, Helen
Curtiss Burnham, Mero
Drolen Brown, Margaret
*Ellinger Jirikovic, Beth
Follett Kaeppeli, Ardys
Haugen Evans, Arlene
Houghtaling Shirah, Amber
Huss Purdy, Olive
Johnson Mandrick, Freda
Lounsberry Lynn, Barbara
McClung Wich, Sarah
Melin Schrader, Marie
Miles Finley, Marion
Oranje Gibson, Gertrude
Orr Depaola, Darlene
Porter Schwantes, Helen
Swigart, Grace
Whitehead Sinclair, Veva

1947

Albright Bader, Madelaine
Andrews Carr, Marian
Barber Crawford, Vera
Baxter Park, Cleora
Beachum Windon, Bernice
Beard Dickes, Nancy
Blake Kobe, Jean
Bode Bayless, Betty
Borton Sawyer, Marilynn
Broxholm Bale, Marilyn
Calkins Nahikian, Jane
Comfort Langley, Carol
Culverwell, Jean
Garrod Sparks, Gertrude
*Gould Carter, Margaret
Grauman Boekhout, Wanda
Kanable Hatfield, Irene
Kiewiet Miller, Joan
Kimball Higgins, Ellen
Latter Benefiel, Joyce
Madden Fitzpatrick, Bette
Mayfield Bird, Jane
Owen Carlson, Jo Ann
Quick Sutton, Barbara
Roach, Eileen
*Savage, Joyce
Schultz Meyer, Phyllis
Shoemaker Vermeulen, Lois

1948

Afman Gren-Bailey, Elizabeth
Banker Rennie, Reva
Beagle Teusink, Etta
Benson Gassen, Dorothy
Carpenter, Norma
Claflin Wright, Constance
*Emig Gunter, Ellen
Freer D'water, Ethelyn
Greenman, Jacqueline
Guenther Spink, Evelyn
Hafer Scott, Leila
*Macgrayne Camery, Janet
McPhail, Virginia
Miersma Schipper, Betty
Miller, Madeline
Moler Dowdy, Emma
Morgan Thompson, Helen
Oranje, Jeanette

Patow Dunn, Dorothy
*Spitters Olin, Bertha
Sweeney Goodrich, Patricia
Van Vorst Brown, Phyllis
*VanderLinde Phillips, Joan
Ward Nakken, Marcia
Wardell Swift, Lois
White Maurer, Wilma
*Willis Shepard, Nancy
Wilson Page, Lois

1949

Babcock Cardiff, Marilyn
*Bailey Ambrose, Ione
*Bouws Cole, Marjorie
*Cardiff Matteson, Ruth
*Clementz Manning, Florence
Cooley Gillam, Mary
Drenth Cunningham, Theresa
*Goodenough, Mildred
Graves Bacon, Mildred
Griner Michael, Ellen
Hamamura Holt, Tomo
Harder Mansberger, Joyce
Kraft Hart, Lucille
Kruizenga Winn, Grace
Luedders Moler, Mary
Motyer Perry, Gwendolyn
Peek Dunn, Betty
Scheffers Jepkema, P. Ruth
Snow Crossley, Laura
*Tageson Schumacher, Betty

1950

Buckholz Koning, Mary
Chute Palmiter, Kathleen
Cook Murdock, Evelyn
Cowling Hopkins, Harriet
Douglas Vincent, Elizabeth
Evans Price, Bonnie
Fox Naumann, Mary
Freyermuth Berry, Janet
Ganley Graves, Evelyn
*Gardner Henry, Barbara
Haight Barrie, Betty
Hillman Herbst, Florence
Johnson Eldred, Janet
King Forrester, Patricia
Lewis Jones, Eleanor
Lietzke Garrod, Rachel
Marr Zimmer, Maxine
Martin Krogel, Marvel
McKee Wyse, Marilyn
McLeod Van Nus, Margaret
Motyer Ehman, Shirley
Rapp Ward, Mary
Reis Tiernan, Marilyn
Ring Rogers, Andrece
*Robertson Bigelow, Patricia
Sheldon Boyce, Mary
Shutes Fox, Ethel
VanderVen Longyear, Christine
*Watkins Herndon, Carolyn
*Weenink Ossewaarde, Phyllis
Williams Marr, Helen
Yerke Swearingen, Marian

1951

Allen Armitage, Doris
Baulch Stevens, Joane
Baum Gutermuth, Barbara
Bennett Fenwick, Bertha
*Berkey Esenwein, Suzanne
Burgess Burbank, Nancy
Burk Kyne, Nancy
Butler Lewis, Beverly

Carns Ely, Marilyn
Casler Covey, Caroline
Dent Baker, Marie
Fox Kozar, Ruth
Fuller Kelley, Dororthy
*Gosling Vander Molen, Betty
Hanshew Galvin, Marjorie
Jones, Lois
Kriser Noss, Donna
Krueger, Patricia
Lapham Richards, Darlene
Martin Bowers, Marilyn
Murray VandeGiessen, Sue
Phares Harner, Joyce
Rogers Wire, Betty
Roney Milham, Joan
Rosemurgy Dye, Ruth
Ryefield Wheeley, Esther
Schultz Sowerby, Jacqueline
Shaffer Bond, Sara
Soule Benzenberg, Beverly
Spriggs DeWitte, Ruth
Stephenson Hagenbarth, Laura
Sutcliffe Haines, Margaret
Woker Tache, Maxin

1952

Aldridge Schneider, Nancy
Allen, Virginia
Belyea Ridley, Dawn
Churchill Dudgeon, Dorothy
Cook White, Donna
Cutler Osterling, Gloria
Dipert Monk, Mildred
Edinger, Eleanor
Engel Kozak, Ruth
Fridwall Forbush, Gloryann
Hall Petersen, Margaret
Hargan, Geraldine
Harrison Johnson, Aleitha
Hayes Kane, Della
Hendra Mainville, Jeanne
Hill Carroll, Shirley
*Hoogstraten Kaub, Betty
Keeler, Mary
Kinkead, Christine
Laroy Doorlag, Luella
LeCronier Curtis, Phyllis
Meske Niec, Joyce
Newland Freid, Shirley
Post, Beverlee
Prause Swartz, Joanne
Rasmussen Koopsen, Jennie
Robinson Rantz, Mary Jane
Schaus Childress, Mildred
Shafer Noto, Ona
Shine Page, Betty
Strunk, Eleanor
Swigart Rizzo, Betty
Wilkinson Gonder, Mary
Woodruff, Marilyn

1953

Anderson, Roxanne
Bailey Garson, Alice
Boomgard, Ardra
Bradley Wilkinson, Lois
Brown Bierman, Marilyn
*Bush-Logan Berry, Katie
Bushhouse, Mary
Cribbs Huffman, Janet
Delger, Marjorie
Gould Arends, Barbara
Hazle Milford, Winifred
Hewson Drenth, Alta
Hicks Duffey, Mary
Howard Leonard, Linda
Huffman Depagter, Gladys
Keizer Battjes, Marilyn

Long, Inez
McConkie, Mary Lou
*McClellan Duryea, Janice
Moffatt Gunning, Joan
Moyer Korita, Mary
Olds Johnson, Barbara
Proxmire, Betty
*Rosser Calkins, Gwendolyn
Thibedeau Korcal, Eunice
VandenBerg Smith, Louise
*VanDyken, Suzanne
VanStelle Gentzler, Ruth
Wall, Mary
Warren, Mary
*Weston, Ellen
Wilson, Lorraine

1954

Benson, Nola
*Bos Heath, Dolores
Bouwman Ward, Joan
Burns Singrey, Alline
Crane Hungerford, Dixianna
Davis Marciano, Nancy
Fleming, Lauretta
Funk Hawkins, Barbara
Gale, Barbara
*Gifford, Katherine
Haight Norcross, Peggy
Hiler Buel, Beverly
Hill, Virginia
Jackson Denning, Gwendolyn
Kalhorn Adkin, Ruth
Kesselring McAvoy, Margery
King Rosin, Carol
Kuhn VanDyk, Phyllis
Lapham Morrill, Donna
Lundstrum Cooke, Marilyn
Martens, Shirley
McNally McMurray, Joan
Mendicki Bloom, Gloria
Mendicki Heeringa, Eleanor
Munson Hodgkinson, Carole
Nelson Hasenick, Clara
*Newcombe Bryant, Marilyn
Pearson Smith, Beverly
Richards Echols, Lael
Stiner Cohen, Judy
Terry Siddall, Suzanne
Tuck Cramp, Mary
Tucker, Lora
VanHartesvelt Vandenberg, Jane
Waite Waller, Marlene
*Webb Schwoebell, Ruth
Wheeler Hess, Lois
Wolfle Glotfelty, Marlene

1955

Amann Lancaster, Helen
Beals Bertrand, Sarah
Brown James, Barbara
Currie Buttery, Mary
Fox Harrett, Florence
*Hauke Dahlman, Patricia
Jeske McLeieer, Marie
Johnson Richter, Meredith
*Juday Kracko, Marlene
Kniebes Kosher, Theda
Loker, Dolores
Lord Niedringhaus, Cynthia
*Martin Moffatt, Shirley
McCrea Huff, Ann
Osborn Kile, Joan
Parkin Powell, Myrna
Pelton Daly, Pauline
Puschel Opperman, Leonora
Rogers Newell, Patricia
Sanborn, Lorraine

Speers Pifer, Marjorie
Temple Sutherland, Jean
Truax Shier, Rosalee
Weller, Judith
Wise Baker, Marilyn
Wright Stacer, Delores
Yonkers, Louise

1956

Abramson Fritts, Bonnie
Adams Serbenski, Lorraine
Asbury Chapman, Marilyn
*Culver Brouse, Virginia
Damson Mattmueller, Sally
Dietz Saddler, Helen
Dockter Rorick, Doris
*Engle Smith, Virginia
Fenwick Harrington, Jane
Fredenburg, Mary Ellen
Fritts Kohler, Melva
Garrett, Joan
Graeber Sugden, Suzanne
Geschwindt Hilligus, Joanne
*Harper McKenzie, Clarice
*Hoyt Brown Richmond, Lois
Johnson, Nancy
Johnson Kidd, Ada
*Jolley Cook, Joan
Krieger Griffin, Joyce
Labadie Gebauer, Ruth
Lichty Carew, Phyllis
Marks Beane, Shirley
Marr, Betty
Mattson Grammel, Shirley
McClure, Ethelyn
Meaker Bowser, Helen
Nelson Macomber, Annette
Noteware Tyler, Betty
Paul Anderson, Eleanor
Penning Tameling, Hermina
Richter DeVries, Beverly
Rogers Davy, Dorothy
Rolfe Warner, Connie
Schott McDermott, Nancy
Shier Riddle, Nancy
Shoemaker, Katharine
Stokes Reshman, Beverly
Welburn, Sally
Wellfare Starkey, Barbara
Weston, Nancy
Youker Miller, Sandra

1957

Bradley Judge, Beverly
Bradstreet, Lucile
Brady Johnson, Shirley
Christie, Avis
Courtright Gearhart, Mary
Crandall Michael, Rhea
Demeester Beale, Betsy
DeYoung Wilson, Barbara
Drilling Enos, Ann
Fetters, Shirley
Gardner Ball, Thelma
Garn Haring, Melissa
Getty Yeager, Evangeline
Hinkel Banhidy, Alice
Howe, Alice
Keirnan Churchill, Carol
Kenyon Spychala, Bonnie
Lovett, Mary
Lubavs Smith, Karmena
Mayer, Janet
McGregor Booth, Carol
Morrill Finch, Sharon
Peacock Davidson, Barbara
Resh Thomas, Jane

Robinson Hawkins, Shirley
Russeau, Audrey
Seegraves, Barbara
Shepard Smith, Margaret
Siebelink Maursey, Joan
*Smith Deland, Linda
Vallieu Wikle, Jeannine
VanNess Rossin, Sandra
Ventres Tynes, Patricia
*Williams Kimber, Erlene
Woodhams Ritter, Mary
*Wyman, Esther

1958

Allen Niskala, Suzanne
Aukerman, Marguerite
Bjorklund, Gloria
Bowman, Marie
Brown, Lois
Campbell Hartman-Arnold, Barbara
Chaney Larke, Georgia
Curry Baur, Rosemary
Drake Duggan, Janet
*Gabriel, Marlene
Golinske Lakin, Barbara
Gribble, Kathleen
Griffin, Mary
Hierholzer Bey, Lois
Huepenbecker Powell, Janet
Klock Bonfoey, Joyce
Lane Babbitt, Virginia
Laurin Sweers, Loretta
Malek, Ruth
Ossenheimer Lowell, Rita
Pirnie, Saundra
Rupp Patzer, Darlene
Schleder, Phyllis
Smith, Kathryn
Spann Spain, Sandra
VanNaarden, Joanne
Weiandt Mayer, Linda
Weller Tolson, Ruth
Williams Wardell, Marcia
Wolf Forestal, Jeannine

1959

Albrecht Sundholm, Stephanie
Andrews, Kay
Bowman Jager, Barbara
Brott Beach, Peggy
Cooke McLeland, Sandra
Crookes Campsmith, Carol
DePond Dull, Mary
Fought Dibaba, Nona
Ginther Davis, Nancy
Gipson, Gaydene
Hack Tellonan, Eva
Harman, Juliene
Hunt Gagnier, Mavis
Hunt Norton, Kathleen
Hurd Massey, Patricia
Johnson Lucas, Doris
Joslin Hawkins, Jane
Karrar, Marian
Klenk Holmes, Barbara
Klimp Bloomquist, Beverly
Kubizna, Julia
Lewis, Carrie
Litzer, Barbara
Martin, Ann
*Martin Daniels, Sharon
Miller, Joyce
Mindrum Welch, Susan
Perrott, Hellen
Poll York, Joyce
Post Boucher, Jeanette
Roberts Kellogg, Mary
Robinson Ware, Sheila

Sabel Wilson, Laurel
*Simpson Fletcher, Elizabeth
Smith Overley, Carol
*Van Voorhees Bower, Elizabeth
Woodland Ryan, Barbara

1960

Bailey Nelson, Cynthia
Behnke Smith, Marilyn
Bohner Hartman, Judith
Briggs, Ruth
Bryant Metz, Polly
Burdick Harmon, Elaine
Collins DeKoster, Mildred
Dahnke, Esther
Geerligs DeWolf, Lois
Grote Coleman, Judith
Hazle Rawlings, Elaine
Horst McCarty, Carol
Landon Johnson, Shirley
Lewis, Carolyn
McDonald, Karen
Mercer Kruger, Margaret
Moored Ziegler, Marilyn
Osborn Lambright, Janet
Peterson Dees, Nancy
Pontz Brown, Ann
Resh Gallo, Judith
Trombley Pore, Kathryn
Trommater, Kay
VanderVeen, Ruth
Walker, Leola
Williams Forman, Kay

1961

Aebli Betten, Judith
Bartels Brown, Elaine
Baum Harris, Janice
Bumstead Bruining, Nancy
Burch, Jacqueline
Carruth, Jane
Daniel Derks, Beulah
Dann Hickman, Jeanne
DeGoffau Farmer, Joan
DeHaan Hansen, Sharon
DeYoung Kaak, Kay
Euans Schultz, Janet
Frank, M. Sharon
Galloway McClelland, Judy
Gambill Burnett, Sandra
Gilbert Adams, Geraldine
Goodshaw Woell, Tamara
Gunthorp Kackmeister, Jo Ann
Hansen, Mary Jo
Henry Hovingh, Barbara
Hiatt Branch, Joyce
Hill, Mary
Holben Bricker, Sue
Hollister Quimby, Phyllis
Howard Hashmen, Susan
Ingram Bourke, Eileen
Krickhahn Dunn, Janet
Krisov Casper, Althea
Ladd, Dixie
Lamphere Mackey, Janet
Lugten Veldhoff, Patricia
McDonald Paton, Patricia
McLeod Tripp, Kathryn
Milligan, Patricia
Naghtin, Marilyn
Nash Gowens, Kay
Nutt Gould, Judy
Prescott, Carolyn
Radabaugh, Nancy
Rayner Fisher, Sharon
Samborn Finch, Gail
Schaller Wilson, Sharon

Schippers Frederick, Mary
Sherman Lalone, Vernice
Starkey Gomes, Rosemary
Stone Stout, Janet
Turner Lemaire, Sharon
*Van Dyke, Linda
*van't Zelfde Stryd, Anna
Ward Bryant, Charlotte
Wright, Lucille

1962

Baker Pursel, Elaine
Baker, Wanda
Bear Erskine, Janice
Boysen Bellingham, Janice
Bradley Konstantine, Bonney Anne
Campbell Cloutier, Carol
Chapin McCuaig, Patricia
Charron, Sue
*Clark Wylie, Jacqueline
Cole Garvey, Donna
Esch Traer, Maribeth
Essenberg Shaw, Kathleen
Georgeau, Betty
Haschle Boer, Marilyn
Hastings Newhouse, Margaret
Hoke Cook, Karen
Hovey, Judith
King Dew, Frances
LeValley McKitrick, Jean
Lonsberry Smith, Betty
McRae Braun, Bonnie
Merrill Riske, Kathleen
Neher Boswell, Beth
Peters Rundio, Joan
Ranson Fornnarino, E.Catherine
Rawlinson Hansen, Barbara
Reed Amador, Sally
Rolland Walter, Kathleen
Schanzlin Woods, Elise
Shultz Ruelle, Judith
Smit, Joanne
Smothers Beadle, Patricia
Stahlbaum, Wanda
Stanger Perry, Sharon
VanOosterhout Wakefield, Dian
Williams Althaus, Nancy
Wiseman Goszczycki, Joanne

1963

Ames Decker, Carol
Atkari, Marilyn
Baker Stephens, Diane
Batten Tharp, Sally
Bauman Taylor, Mary
Bowman Kramarz, Rebecca
Bullington Oliver, Judith
Burpee, Karin
Cutright McLennon, Linda
Dalman Dorgan, Marcia
Daugherty, Brenda
*DeBruin DeKorte, Julianne
Ellinger Fassett, Joanne
Emmert, Marcia
Esman Peter, Janet
Essenberg, Judith
Graves, Carol
*Gunneman, Carol
Hamilton Gallagher, Mary
Hattendorf, Kay
Higgins Burk, Rosemary
Hover, Julie
Humenick Lind, Elaine
Johnson Watson, Louise
Johnson Whitt, Janice
Kinnisten, Penny
Kleyenberg Stockton, Donna
Korendyk Blackard, Clara

Lam Terbeck, Ruth
Lutz Robinson, Harriette
Lutzka Noble, Linda
*Marshall Fanson, Elaine
Metzler Greene, Jean
Meyer, Carol
Nap Rose, Evelyn
Newhouse, Ruth
Pangman Wood, Lois
Pratt Smith, Susan
Purlee, Jo
Rierson Jackson, Gwendolyn
Rothoff Hulit, Linda
Schants Darman, Kathleen
Schmierer Weaver, Sybil
Seat, Kathleen
Struckman Cox, Sharon
Stulp Spangler, Karen
Sweet McLeod, Diane
Ullrey Hawks, Dana
Voorhorst Hartgerink, Barbara
Wardeberg, Deanna
*Wigent Burr, Linda
Williams Morrow, Sharon
Witmer, Sharon

1964

Aalderink, Cloverlynn
*Abel, Faith
Adams Rinker, Janet
Alverson Odin, Barbara
Baldwin Hood, Judith
Bayha Tew, Bertha
Becker, Linda
Bristol Philip, Terrie
Broekhuizen Compaan, Rena
Broker Reetz, Jane
Brown Lutchka, Joan
Bunting, Carol
Casteel Fauss, Judy
Cavitt, Marilynn
*Cook Hanson, Kay
DeWitt Droppers, Joyce
deWyk, Cinda
Dickens, Barbara
Dykstra, Mary
Emig McCarter-Davis, Marilyn
Gay Hilboldt, Carol
Hartson Smith, Patricia
Hess Leshner, Sharon
Hutson Kiefer, Patricia
Johnston Klauda, Corene
Kroll, Florence
Lang, Jenny
Lutz Anderson, Gaille
McKane Speck, Barbara
Miller Parker, Marilyn
Munger Fassett, Barbara
Nagy, Delsie
Nordman Stob, Nancy
Owen Littlejohn, Cheryl
Rennhack Walters, Karen
Roundy Hayward, Bonnie
Schott Bristol, Jean
Smit Hopkins, Myra
Smith McNally, Katherine
Stamann Amrose, Judith
*Stapert Triezenberg, Phyllis
Stromsta Clark, Karen
*Taylor Wilson, Gail
Teusink Seabold, Jeanne
Unfried, Nancy
Van Valkenburg Johnson, Marjorie
Wagoner Guy, Shirley
Warner, Kathy
Wiessner Haug, Beverly
Willis Kerlikowske, Mary

1965

Anderson Beck, Susan
Anderson Misner, Linda
Barney Harper, Kathleen
Bos Stamm, Carol
Bosch Arendsen, Delores
Buelke Borgeson, Karen
Burke Elyea, Jill
Bushouse Hall, Karen
Castle Foust, Sharon
Coffman Bagby, Jane
Cramer VanderNoot, Jacquelyn
Crum Doubblestein, Karen
Curtiss Webb, Susan
DeFields Randall, Pamela
Edlund Liverance, Diane
Elson, Mary
Fisher Achterberg, Juanita
*Goldstein Collison, Sara
Grazier, Mary
Greene Schiltz, Sandra
Harmon Roehm, Carol
Heward Anderson, Mary
Homkes VanderSluis, Karen
Hood Vermeulen, E. Ruth
Irvine Newman, Sandra
Johnson Bair, Sandra
Keasey Sears, Martha
King Burge, Judith
Knickerbocker Wagner, Mary
Kreighbaum Baxter, Joyce
Matson Husted, Barbara
McKale Rockwell, Ruth
Mol Kamer, Constance
Nixon Meisner, Kay
Ott Alten, Joann
Overweg, Dianne
Reed Myers, Janet
Rose Telgenhof, Ruth
Schafer Peterson, Susan
Schroeder Moser, Arlene
Shaffer Montgomery, Sharon
Sheridan Stroud, Susan
Sholly Shaw, Jennie
Strachen Magney, Judith
Taber Austin, Marcia
Wales VanDosen, Kay
Wheeler Wheeler-Stroud, Jacqueline
*Whitbeck Bartell, Doris
Woodward Ritterbusch, Joyce

1966

Achterhof Hendriksen, Lois
Akin Van Dyken, Janice
Allen, Ruth
Anderson Anderson-Hadden, Karen
Barram Munson, Lois
Barratt Bloomquist, Catherine
Baurs Lightbody, Mary
Bohnsack Roberts, Bonita
Breen Downing, Barbara
Breneman Wilcox, Janice
Brower Brandsma, Lynne
Brower Rutherford, Ruth
*Burke Kakabeeke, Frances
Cochran Beck, Dorothy
Cody Irish, Linda
Corwin Fabiano, Judith
Crockett Bowman, Susan
Dannenberg Beckman, Carla
*Delobel Conner, Cheryl
Dunn Zabell, Sue
*Easton Meninga, Donna
Ely, Gwendolyn
Emerson, Laurel
*Emery Luther, Marilyn
*Fink Rebert, Mary
*Gamble Raseman, Lynne

Garrison Kuipers, Sally
Hammond Smuk, Kathy
Hoffman, Barbara
Houtman Brigham, Sandra
Howe Levy, Marguerite
Husek Rutlin, Evelyn
Huston Trenholm, Isabelle
Jackson King, Joan
Jepson Kleynenberg, Judith
Judy Gruizenga-Sahr, Phyllis
Kamer Sims, Patricia
Kirvan Ball, Nancy
Kleinheksel, Nancy
Kowalski Aardema, Adele
Lamberts, Linda
Lewis Priester, Faith
*Lingle Kleynenberg, Patricia
Matthews Jackson, Joy
Meier Dennis, Mary
Miller Daleiden, Marilyn
Pollard Boutell, Jean
Raak Knooihuizen, Arloa
Reynolds Rothfuss, Cheri
*Rivers, Edythe
Sanders Ferguson, June
*Santinga, Nellie
Schiedel, Carol
*Sheperd, Helen
Sinke, Brenda
Sipe, Barbara
Solley, Susan
Stone Childs, Joan
Vanderbeck Gast, Elaine
Watts Brown, Rebecca
Werner Martinez, Sharon
White, Marion
Whitmor Guilfoil, Mary
Wight Thurow, Evelyn
Wilt Yerkes, Carole

1967

Anderson, Beverly
Ayres, Jill
Balgoyen Waigan, Susan
Benner McKechnie, Susan
Birch Wadell, Patricia
Blackwell Mack, Karen
Buckman Modlin, Judith
*DeFeyter Chavez, Marian
*Dwan Poole, Diana
Everts Resh, Ethel
Fisk Harper, Arlene
Guise Lehman, Laveta
Hafer Kimmer, Lavay
Hart, Patty
Hicks, Betty
Holland Driver-Brown, Annette
Hovarter McCausland, Sharon
Howard Pufpaff, Donnya
Ide Sturgill, Sharon
Jenks Krampe, Patricia
Johnson, Janet
Johnson Krill, Cynthia
Krill Carter, Janet
Leeson Hunn, Janet
Lincoln, Diane
Lowrance, Gloria
Lutke, Marlene
Mac Dowell, Carolyn
Moore Martin, Mary
Pellow Bergum, Carol
Prince Adams, Beverly
Ries Carpenter, Janice
Schermer Vanderklay, Ruth
Shaver Axe, Jacqueline
Sherman Shutt, Carol
Sievers Wilt, Sandra
Sincock Ensign, Carol
*Sny Hartman, Jane

Spillers, Carol
Story Stratton, Kathleen
Stratton Frey, Maureen
Thompson Hinman, Nancy
Upson Stager, Sharon
Veltman Roehl, Carol
Vugteveen Pikkart, Barbara
Watson VanAntwerp, Carol
Wieling, Sally
Wirsing Scidmore, Bonnie
Wise Harthorn, Janice
Yagerlener, Sharon

1968

Acker Turner, Sharon
Badger Meoak, Betty
Balyeat Wells, Kathleen
Baszler Yoder, Pamela
Benz, Mary
Bliss Crawford, Mary
Borst Wierman, Denise
Bour Crawford, Deborah
Bryers Anderson, Sharon
Colwell, Vicki
Cooper Roberts, Sally
Durbon Lyles, Carol
Dykehouse Drayton, Gail
Frazier, Evelyn
Frye Miller, Deborah
Griffen Stearns, Linda
Griffendorf Leidy, Sandra
Hannon Strank, Carol
Harrison Middleton, Sharon
Henderson Dommert, Carol
Hofmeister Lewis, Carolyn
Horton Smith, Barbara
Houseman Welfare, Kay
Karsten Dokter, Laurel
Keith Ames, Lois
Keltner Chambers, Patsy
Kidd Lashbrook, Anna
Kiger Mitts, Mary
Lawrence Anusewicz, Linda
Lokers Moore, Linnay
Lutterloh Root, Linda
Marshall Bardin, Linda
Mast Hansen, Mary
May Palmer, Jewell
McCraner, Kim
McNichol Bickel, Constance
Mead Gaishin, Sally
Miller Bellware, Diana
Morgan Buyzelak, Nancy
Nelson Powers, Susan
Piper Borton, Beverly
Powers Mazique, Susan
Pratt Roosa, Lynn
Rohrback, Vicky
Schipper, Carol
Schipper Heystek, Linda
Schlinkert Decator, Gail
Shaver McDermott, Linda
Shaw Tobis, Barbara
Sheppard Ashton, Linda
Smith Brey, Mary
Smith Maag, Linda
*Taylor, Kay
Thaler Alberding, Linda
Thomas Brewer, Darlene
Todd Oosterhouse, Margaret
Vandenbelt Lungaro, Roberta
VanderBeek Olson, Nancy
Vorce DePree, Kay
Warren, Marilyn
Willson Glittenberg, Diane
Wiseley Oelberger, Dianne
*Wycoff Prouty, Sandra
York, Susanne

1969

Alberti Lindholm, Ruth
*Backus Patterson, Marilyn
Basner, Carla
Blowers Rick, Sharon
Brink Tanis, Pamela
Brown Zemitans, Jacquelyn
Carlson Olson, Christine
Conger Bader, Linda
Corey Porras, Lois
Davis Westfall, Rolleen
Diedrich Golna, Pricilla
Dilley Armstrong, Diane
Eiler Moore, Christine
Epley Donohue, Mary
Fox McBrien, Suanne
Francis Hooker, Lola
Gleason Duff, Donna
Grebel Carver, Janie
Grin Nemrava, Mina
Hawker Groom, Marian
Hoffman, Shirley
Hulst Robey, Doris
Hurd Lindsey, Susan
Jones Black, Merlene
Kamradt Johnson, Mary
Klynstra Mol, Lynda
Koetje Salsich, Janice
Kreitner Scholar, Carol
Large Bonebrake, Gail
Lewis, Linda
Lindsay Woods, Janice
McCourt Spreeman, Carlene
Meints French, Linda
Mielens Kuehnemund, Walda
Myers Pardee, Connie
Niebling Weurding, Carol
Nienhuis Ramos, Mary
Olson Curtis, Kathleen
Osborn Boxer, Jean
Polasky Taylor, Dawn
Pries Kuipers, Andrea
Prins, Karen
Randall, Penny
Randolph Green, Brenda
Rynd, Jill
Schaap Call, Karen
Schneider Dodge, M. Joanne
Shields Wegner, Theresa
Slager Fonger, Linda
*Starks Winzenz, Sandra
Stickel, Ann
Swart Terbeck, Nancy
*Tennant Farthing, Carolyn
Townsend, Linda
Travis Rankin, Ruth
Traxler Couzens, Suzan
Tucker Miller, Kathryn
Tuinstra Hickman, Sharon
VanHam Waldron, Phyllis
VanHellen Topp, Barbara
Walsweer Green, Nancy
Welch Bloor, Susan
Wood Miroballi, Barbara
Zook Phillips, Karen

1970

Anders Caroselli, Irene
Arens Kamper, Myrna
Barber Daam, Penny
Brautigam Hall, Mary
Brown Hargis, Dianna
Carlson Doctor, Linda
Chamberlain Miller, Dawn
*Conte Swander, Mary
Crimmins, Martha
Davis Ridinger, Sara
Delaney Feldmeier, Janice
Dell Kaplan, Elisabeth

DeMott Pashby, Glenna
Driy Callicoat, Marcia
Durbin, Diane
Ellis Campbell, Eileen
Haley Gafney, Sue
Heisler French, Charlene
Jipping, Delores
Kaeding Dolphin, Marcia
Kauffman, Lois
Kerby Konrad, Cynthia
King, Delores
Koeman, Nancy
Koops Moerland, Wanda
Kraynak Bremmer, Maryann
Kressley Daves, Marilyn
Levsay Bucha, Janis
Martinson Carman, Nancy
McElmurry Jackson, Paulette
Meyers Long, Christine
Monaghan Coles, M Kathleen
Mutschler Vincent, Ruth
Neville Buscher, Nancy
Orth Dechert, Marcia
Prince Budzinski, Dawn
Raak Bonner, Nancy
Ricketson Venn, Kathleen
Roe Schrock, Sandra
Rose Knapp, Virginia
Sink, Bonnie
Southwell Jex, Kay
Squiers Melson, Carol
Stehouwer Burden, Linda
Stelter Gelesko, April
Stemm, Joanne
Stevens Shaneberger, Kathy
Stewart Showers, Sharon
VanderHam Witteveen, Diane
VanDyke, Carolyn
Warsen, Leone
Wiesenhofer Price, Janice
Zuverrink Green, Sharon

1971

Annen Lintner, Judith
Appleton, Martha
Baird Wescott, Linda
Bosch Koning, Constance
Boucha Rohn, Susan
Brenner, Julie
Broadworth Rakoski, Gayla
Clark Higley, Marilyn
Cogswell Hohenberger, Linda
Delobel Luce, Carol
Dempsey Zipf, Marilyn
Eishen Creech, Nancy
Evans Anderson, Lea
Fink Schrock, Mary
Fleming Evans, Bonnie
Fox McMillan, Susan
Frazee Nelson, Geri
Ganton Demar, Connie
Geribo Witmer, Deborah
Glenn Doherty, Karen
Halstead Palmer, Bernadette
Harris Warren, Sharon
Haskin Nickel, Lois
Hayes Thurber, Elaine
Hoffman Johnston, Linda
Holmes Proctor, Cassandra
Hunt Henson, Susan
*Jorgenson Kneebone, Ruth
Keith Walker, Kay
Kelley Nelson, Martha
Kelly VanderVeen, Linda
Kibby, Brenda
Kole Stephenson, Jacqueline
Luckett Korytowsky, Mary
McPhall Comried, Lynn
Messenger Pierce, Joann

Miller Hunt, Deborah
Nakken, Sherilyn
Neal Posly, Kathleen
Nieboer Schuiteboer, Constance
Northridge Elberg, Nancy
Nunn Griggs, Elizabeth
Peterson Rathburn, Kathleen
Pippenger Magerlein, Joyce
Plank Wykstra, Linda
*Quick Richards, Sandra
Retberg Anderson, Phyllis
Roddy Teffner, Jean
Rouwhorst Nienhuis, Bette
Schipper Scholten, Donna
Sharp Stauffer, Barbara
Sheldon Chupp, Carolan
Smallegan Adema, Laura
Spencer Cairns, Marcia
Sprague Quinn, Sonja
Trepky Humphrey, Kathleen
Warren Takimoto, Cynthia
Wentzel Cox, Kathleen
West Watson, Barbara
Whitman, Diane
Winter, Rebecca
Woodman Mackinder, Mary
Yunker Holtz, Lois
Zolp, Felicia

1972

Anderson Hoover, Debra
*Arens Kleinheksel, Nancy
Bauer Hall, Jeanie
Bell Harrell, Ronnee
Berry, Linda
Bittner Hawk, Diane
Brenner Johnson, Janice
Brown Ford, Mary
Burk Hinderliter, Ella
Burns Bonga, Kathy
Church Dane, Carleen
Cushman Deming, Kathleen
Cuyler, Sharyn
Darbee Kobylinski, Margery
DeHaan McCormick, Pamela
Demilio Lamoureux, Suzanne
Diekema, Marcia
Doster Roth, Jade
Erskine Austin, Mary Lou
Fast Noble, Kathleen
Faust Chellis, Joyce
Fillmore Trudgen, Carolyn
Fischmeister Long, Janet
Fredrickson Beutter, Mary
Frizzle Albrecht, Connie
Fullriede Scheid, Patrice
Greer Tolis, Carol
Hand Dnochowski, Sue
Hess Loftness, Deborah
Hoogstraten Anderson, Marsha
Huizenga Strick, Carol
Isbell Abshagen, Linda
Jendrzejewski Cosgrove, Patricia
Johnson Ellis, Lee
Kapenga Scheerhorn, Mary
Laird Helm, Susan
Lucas Trevethan, Elizabeth
Lucking Hoekstra, Joan
MacGregor, Virginia
Mahaney Karr, Janet
McKeown, Lois
Meeusen Abshagen, Diane
Melnik Meyer, Cheryl
Miller Graber, Marsha
Morgan Curtiss, Ellen
Nystrom Shively, Darlene
Oonk Pollard, Nancy
Page Mielke, Jacquelyn
Peterson Hadley, Linda
Preston Perry, Patricia

Robinson Dedee, Lynda
Schrantz McLellan, Claudia
Schreuder, Grace
Shippy, Maureen
Spitters DeVries, Debbie
Stratton Bauman, Kathleen
Streur Kopp, Valarie
Switzer Shahan, Gail
Thompson Degrush, Carol
Thompson Weaver, Ellen
Treadwell Robertson, Judith
VanderRoest Smith, Nancy
Veldkamp Flikkema, Mary
VerBeek Hoffman, Sally
Walker Brown, Pamela
Williams Pfeifer, Kathleen
Winters Walicki, Susan
Wolters Smith, Marcia
Zandstra Gaiser, Elizabeth
Zandstra Howe, Deborah

1973

Alphenaar English, Peggy
Anderson Kern, Linda
Austin Schneider, Wendy
Bahlke Jacobs, Sarah
Bos Shelley, Lila
Bosch, Linda
Brouwer Klunder, Joy
Burnes McNeely, Barbara
Carter Gingrich, Carol
Conley Delancey, Denise
Cooper Devowe, Deanna
Creason Frey, Kristen
Davis Rineveld, Valerie
Far Umberger, Mary
Faust Jansen, Judith
Fitzgerald Barndt, Christine
Ford Clark, Janet
Franc Swierbut, Linda
Goudzwaard Williams, Joan
Goulooze Ryan, Hendrika
Haglandr Bolen, Janice
Hall Susens, Sandy
Heller Guthars, Paula
Hidenfelter Luce, Sheri
Hogle Hogle-Heyn, Christine
Hostetter VanOeveren, Mary
Hurley, Kathleen
Ippel Ausema, Nancy
Kampf Lin-Tuttle, Abey
Kiel Piechowiak, Carol
Kinsley, Melodie
Kline Savage, Barbara
Knope Berry, Diane
Kuipers Potterff, Jan
LaForge, Gayle
Leibrandt Yoder, Virginia
Lesman Cesler, Judith
Lowry Timpe, Rebecca
MacKenzie, Susan
Mattox Anderson, Marjorie
Meerdo Janus, Janice
Mull Goodacre, Debra
O'Dell Bloom, Deborah
Redder Vanhill, Sally
Roberts, Rhonda
Romanowski Kalinowski, Nancy
Schabbel Shinabarger, Jean
Schipper Foreman, Gwen
Shanahan Lewis, Norma
Simmonds Cvetnich, Barbara
Sopjes Van Emon, Marianne
Tamminga Geskus, Mary
Tindall Szwejda, Debra
Traxler, Marsha
Trumbull Chamberlin, Pamela
*Ulrich, Joyce
Van Noord DeHaan, Phyllis
VanDellen Castleberg, Geneva

VanDragt Bloomensaat, Laura
Veenstra Schloesser, Cynthia
Walters Lang, Deborah
Weaver Baker, Wendy
Wortz Carpenter, Loui

1974

Adle, Barbara
Anderson Olsen, Kristen
Anderson Dittmer, Peggy
Armstrong Pearson, Eileen
Ashworth, Lesley
Ausbon Hines, Janet
Ballard Ramseyer, Mary
Bartels, Shelly
Beerthuis VandenBerg, Barbara
Bogema Brost, Deborah
Bottecelli, Paula
Cobb Burtch, Carol
Coney Powell, Barbara
Cullitan, Jill
DeJonge Wolbers, Connie
England Heckman, Michele
Fargo, Carol
Fortin Wiegenstein, Debra
Gipson, Pamela
Harris, Amy
Hendon Bloomer, Diana
Holland, Sarah
Holzaepfel, Barbara
Houghtby Nicholas, Sylvia
Houghton Krafft, Pamela
Imanse Franck, Cindy
Kandt Dale, Shelley
King, Lisa
Klaker Dean, Carol
Kuhlman Bradley, Kandis
Kuhnmuench Ashley, Monica
Lancaster, Elizabeth
*LaRoy Triemstra, Lesley
Levitt Hnatiuk, Martha
Lewis, Marsha
Lindsay Socia, Beth Ann
Loedeman, Marcia
Long, Jeri
Lynn Mordy, Kathy
Mapes, Judy
Mashke Iannelli, Nancy
Mathieu Gaylor, Sharon
Matteson Parker, Deborah
Maynard Irvine, Nancy
McArthur, Sandra
McClain Allan, Melanie
Menke Leavens, Sharon
Metcalf Nuyen, Martha
Moormann Morganroth, Susan
Nelson Pishko, Carol
Newton Deno, Joyce
Orskey Debell, Shirley
Pastorick Spencer, Deborah
Penny, Peggy
Petee Mayberry, Jane
Picklesimer Hicks, Kathleen
Reed Diebel, Janine
Roberts Fest, Mary Beth
Rodewald Balsis, Marilou
Rogers Gunn, Karen
Rosteck Morgan, Suzanne
Sackett Harlow, Diane
Sanborn, Karen
Schipper, Patricia
Shinn, Martha
Shull Spafford, Andrea
Slagh, Carol
Snyder, Jacquelyn
Stimson Stimson-Eastman, Lynett
Strick, Faye
Strom, Christine
Taylor Keen, Carol

Twining Mao, Kristine
VanBuhler Cleary, Gwen
Weber Maxey, Katherine
Welborn Rowe, Deborah
Winnell, Diane
Yeiter Simmons, Crista
Young White, Susan

1975

Barnes Koss, Sandra
Bevins, Sharon
Black, Pamela
Blair Richardson, Linda
Blose, Barbara
Bowden Marland, Amy
Brown Moore, Cathryn
Cauley, Theresa
Coder Holeman, Christine
Dalman Toepper, Kathryn
Diorka Stafford, Kathryn
Doornbas, Margie
England, Pamela
Ewing Barger, Catherine
Fannin West, Kathleen
Gay Girard, Kathy
Gritter Zandstra, Beth
Hamlin Perjesi, Wendy
Hayes Cygan, Belinda
Henshaw, Nancy
Heyboer Van Nuil, Marcia
Hogan Mero, Deborah
Irving Ditto, Leslie
James, Barbara
Jensen Meeker, Judith
Johnson, Paul
Kauffman Jautakis, Pamela
Kelly, Katherine
Kimble Williams, Rebecca
Kline Cheeseman, Jane
Kotesky, Dawn
Larson Ivan, Karen
Locklin Atlas, Patrica
Maniaciz Stetler, Mary
Martin Kakoczki, June
McKay Alexander, Mary
Mericle, Susan
Merryman Mast, Donna
Moulton, Susan
Norburg Grossman, Nancy
Ott, Judith
Pechumer, Ila
Pontius McAllister, Denise
Prentice Keim, Jean
Price, Dianne
Pulaski Kopitzke, Joni
Rezin Nuyen, Kimberly
Robinson, Karen
Robinson Rutland, Myrtle
Ryan Misiasz, Rhonda
Saur, Catherine
Schwarz Rau, Nancy
Selinsky, William
Selner Dick, Sheila
Seyfred Genson, Cynthia
Shadley Buis, Pamela
Smith Wise, Suzanne
Steggerda deVries, Kathy
Steketee Thiebault, Debra
Stoops Baumann, Goldie
Szekely Nahan, Suzanne
Terry, Elizabeth
*Thompson Guyer, Lynette
VanHall Glenn, Kimber
VanHill Austhof, Debra
Vonehr Trippy, Cheryl
Westendorp Venhuizen, Barbara
Weston Muzic, Janice
Wilhelmsen Wheeler, Joyce
Wolcott Hamilton, Christine

Woodman Forker, Sally
Wright Wright-Riley, Tracy
Zeller Scully, Corinne
Zwiers Whited, Mary

1976

*Anderson Kusebuski, Pamela
Artz Artz-Howard, Theresa
Baehre Loneraan, Nadine
Ball, Suzanne
Bekes Marcoux, Stephanie
Bell Wolfe, Roberta
Blachowiak, Thomas
Brouwer Klunder, Debra
Brown, Dona
Bullen Downs, Linda
*Busick Crum, Ruth
Case, Deborah
Clover Winger, Debra
Cochran Waugh, Patricia
Coleman, Jo
Dave Slobogin, Cynthia
DeForrest Hefner, Susan
DeYoung Francisco, Cynthia
Diroff Kelly, Sharon
Doerr Penshorn, Brenda
Draper, Susan
Engels, Jill
Ericks Bosch, Cheryl
Ferris, Kimberlee
Finsterwald Finsterwald-Watts, Wendy
Garrod West, Kathryn
Grant Brennan, Janet
Guay Martin, Catherine
Hammond, Janelle
Helms, Dana
Heyboer Blystra, Lisa
Kaiser Pickard, Elke
Keeler Clements, Lee Ann
Kieft Smith, Yvonne
Kovacevich, Debra
Kroske Markovitz, Susan
Larson Glines, Nancy
Lightner Hamlin, Wendy
Link Woodhouse, Mary
Lobsinger Coppiellie, Holly
Lockwitz, Diane
Madole Faust, Jacqueline
McAllister, Margaret
McKeage Heyboer, Patricia
McMullen Sharp, Colleen
Nykamp Meringa, Ruth
Ott, Penny
Patranc Kelley, Wendy
Payne Kammers, Susan
Rabb Douglass, Karen
Reutter Blaney, Brenda
Seelhoff Haley, Sue
Senek Correia, Phyllis
Stemple Saylor, Diane
Strumpfer, Rivka
Swanchara, Nancy
Tuls Rozema, Judith
Turner, Mary
VanKeuren Shugar, Kelsey
Vredeveld Stob, Sandra
Weagley, Rebecca
Wheeler Mays, Mary
White Lilly, Susan
Wilbur Jambeau, Suzanne
Willbur Lockhart, Patricia
Zimmerman, Vicky

1977

Adkin Wohlfert, Holly
Alphenaar Schwabauer, Susan

Balkema Naugle, Nancy
Batterbee Wood, Verna
Buffenbarger Wood, Sue
Burns, Connie
DeKock Nyhuis, Cheryl
Diekema Kraai, Patricia
Doyle Lowe, Carol
Elzer Sequin, Paula
Ensing Jongekrijg, Pat
*Foglesong Gosling, Leslie
Frye, Lu Ann
Genzink Reimink, Sharon
Graveling Sheen, Cheryl
Hall Taplin, Leslie
Hartman Babij, Jill
Heimerl Holden, Debra
Hilton, Melinda
Hoogstraten Bremer, Susan
Kartheu Alday, Debra
LaForge, Edward
Landon, Linda
Leugs Bobroff, Patricia
Ludwa Rebant, Mary
Lupina Webster, Rosemary
Marutz Doublestein, Pamela
Masselink VanNette, Sandra
Mazlewski Copeland, Susan
Merriam Cole, Rebecca
Naugle, Carol
Nedervelt Batts, Linda
Nelson, Ruby
Palmer Hanover, Cristy
Pegram, Susan
Pell, Carole
Pfau, Patricia
Pillsbury Bonzelaar, Carol
Prince Lewis, Patricia
Rhind Toepper, Beth
Richardson, Alice
*Ringler Sponseller, Debra
Scheffers Mulder, Jill
Schiefer Gilbert, Beverly
Schlack, Theresa
Schultz Schuen, Elfie
Schurtz Leach, Susan
Smith Anderson, Barbara
Sowles Whalen, Kimberly
Swenson Magnante, Diane
Trinite, Miriam
Tucker, Shirley
VandeStreek, Janet
Van Dyken Winfield, Connie
*Verhoog, Petronella
Walley Tucker, Diane
Winfield Kerrins, Rosemary
Wolf Wilkening, Carol
Wonnacott Jacobs, Ilene

1978

Adgate, Cynthia
Albertson Vitarelli, Ruth
Bails Vemich, Mary
Beeke Timmer, Joanne
Behnke, Karen
Berghorst Mascorro, Sheryl
Bond Rubey, Susan
Bos Weatherwax, Patricia
Bouck Martzke, Laura
Calkins Pavilanis, Charlotte
Carey, Ellen
Cunningham, Rosie
Curry Fouch, Pamela
Curtis, Mary
Curtis, Susan
Deboe VanBaal, Barbara
Delger, Cherie
DeVries, Jane
Diaczenko Conolly, Mary
Dobson DeYoung, Dorothy

*Doctor, Linda
Dykstra Sportel, Cathye
England Arp, Deborah
Fort Brown, Eileen
Geyer Davio, Julia
Good, Mary
Gormely Neveux, Colleen
Greer Tinney, Carol
*Grimes Laeder, Cynthia
Hacker Maynard, Lynn
Henderson Collins, Brenda
Hoeksema Noordyke, Elayne
Hoogewind McGraw, Betsy
Huftile Fischer, Pamela
*Hughes, Anne
Huizinga, Beth
Hutchinson Boyne, Margaret
Iveson Kroll, Cathie
Jenkins Perkins, Linda
Johnson Taylor, Yvonne
Jolliffe VanderWeele, Barbara
Klein, Diane
Kleinheksel Hall, Kathleen
Kramer Nichols, Karen
Louis Schwabauer, Jane
Maat Bouwens, Beverly
Maynard, John
Mejeur Jepkema, Susan
Merriken Johnson, Beth
Moerdyk Ekema, Alice
Moerman, Marcia
Morrell Huber, Paula
Nie Schlueter, Sharyn
Phelps Kelly, Martha
Pratt Karn, Joan
Render Johnson, Kay
Ritsema Jacobsen, Paula
Roberts Angvick, Debra
Rochefort Crouse, Rhonda
Sandelin Breisach, Tobi
Street, Shirley
Sweet Brockway, Laura
Taeckens Nicolette, Nancy
Toaz Peck, Kathryn
Tuck Wahl, Bonny
VanHaitsma Shane, Sherril
Visser Root, Patricia
Vollmar Strand, Laura
Wagner Groggle, Catherine
Whitmore, Marilyn
Wilhelm Shorter, Diane
Wisner Cronkright, Robin
Wolthuis Wells, Cheryl
Zaleski Straubel, Janice

1979

Baudoux Piwowarski, Laura
Bennett, Kaye
Beyerlein Bowes, Joanne
Blakely, Jayne
Bosman, Kathy
Boss Busman, Denise
Boyes, Annice
Brunner, Sharon
Buckley Christ, Kathryn
Burns, Karen
Bush, Mary Ellen
Cogan, Cindy
Colton Cummings, Sheila
Cosgray Reed, Yvonne
Culham Recker, Cynthia
Curtis Smith, Joan
*Dimitroff, Ann
Dow Hepner, Monica
Ecker Veldt, Tamara
Eitelbuss, Karen
English Hercules, Ramona
Faust, Pamela
Fitzpatrick Lawrence, Carol
Gehlmann Bernard, Marjorie

Gelder Van Singel, Wanda
Genther, Jill
Groters Warren, Diane
Guy Trinks, Diane
Haley, Linda
*Hempsall, Kelley
Jones Thompson, Sara
Kleis Richey, Nancy
Kobiska Blevins, Pamie
Kovats Kovats-Bell, Sue
Kristofik Harder, Donna
Lown Hart, Julie
Mead Anasis, Connie
Meulenbelt Hoeksema, Mary
Mikula Hicks, Jacqueline
Miller VandenBerg, Judy
Miller Waldron, Sheri
Miyamoto, Sharon
Mohr, Carol
Nieman Myhand, Debora
Paull Kopec, Melinda
Paulsen, Jeffery
Payne, Brenda
Peekstok Shadley, Jill
Pilatowicz, Linda
Poll Johnson, Lynda,
Powers, Vicky
Radant Altoft, Karen
Richey VanEck, Janice
Rosier Maharey, Carol
*Sass Jones, Joni
Schneider, Pamela
Schoenheit Burnell, Lisa
Sherbert Kimbrell, Debora
Souden, Karla
Stam Padding, Kathryn
Thick Krajewski, Patricia
Thomas Gray, Debora
Tomecek Dam, Teri
VanderSchaaf Hulst, Cheryl
VanderSluis, Nancy
Wehrmeyer Solis, Nancy
Willis Fliearman, Leigh
Wilson Retberg, Carol

1980

Anstey Sweet, Kathleen
Babcock Carpenter, Cynthia
Bacon, Kimberly
Beers Gillespie, Lori
Binkley Fowler, Kathryn
Blades, Rebecca
Bushhouse, Joye
Capezza Holmes, Julie
Chadderdon Lejoncour, Jean
Cochran Sponsler, Mary
Compton Turner, Cynthia
Conklin Lebiecki, Cynthia
Coutts Riordan, Diane
*DeVries Walcott, Janice
Dragoo Slager, Katrina
Drake Kemp, Karyn
Dreyer Israels, Debra
Feikema, Brenda
Francisco Boyle, Gwendolyn
Froeschke, Monica
Fuller Parker, Cindy
Gunderson, Patricia
Harris Aldini, Theresa
Hoard Tackwell, Karie
Horrocks Knape, Judy
Hudson, Leonzo, Jr.
Hufford, Teri
Hughes Hutson, Peggy
Hysell, Kimberly
Irion Hogan, Valerie
Jeske DeGram, Debra
Koning Voss, Jan
Kremer Kieft, Elizabeth
Lang, Deborah

Lusso Beaty, Rebecca
MacIntosh, Cathleen
Mazzara, John
Milbrandt Godke, Heidi
Morison, Elizabeth
Moroz Barlow, Janet
O'Dell Tenbusch, Gretchen
Pastunink Steinbeck, Mary
Peekstok, Kimberly
Petee Zinderman, Martha
Phelan Skuta, Anne
Powell Williams, Sandra
Reidenbach, Gwen
Robinson Gunderson, Karen
Rudgers, Dawn
Ruggles Tomczak, Beth
Schuur Schweighoefer, Heidi
Seedorff Myers, Judy
Shockley, Mary
Skinner Budzinski, Lisa
Stroud Benzing, Kim
Syrjamaki, Anne
Tallman Johnson, Ann
Trasky, Robert
Turner Wardius, Laura
Tyler Grewe, Rebecca
Vandenburg Kotecki, Carrie
VanKuiken Bradford, Mary
VanSlooten Weststrate, Jane
Vermeersch Hasper, Kristy
Waffle Burkhardt, Cynthia
Wagner Mian, Patricia
Wahl Kish, Julie
Weaver Howard, Jackie
Worden, Kathleen
Young Phelan, Kimberly
Ziebart, Jill

1981

*Ammon Robinson, Susan
Babcock Sherry, Bernadine
Barlage, Denise
Bedford Dunfield, Nancy
Bills Tokarski, Laurie
Birge, Nancy
Borgman Heyboer, Jayne
Breneman Reed, Lisa
Brink Mulder, Sally
Bullinger Ballow, Julie
Butler, Janice
Butts, Leisa
Condo Bommarito, Annette
Conner, Margaret
Dennehy, Sandra
DeVries, Jacob
Dormady, Thomas
Douglas Jamieson, Barbara
Dunn Kalleward, Carrie
Easterday Learner, Luann
*Eberly Mercer, Gail
Froelich, Diana
Gildersleeve Waldner, Marybeth
Gooch, Susan
Grit Tharpe, Debra
Grotenhuis Quinn, Patti
Guth Goff, Karla
Haeger, Jennifer
Haverkamp Tiller, Shelly
Hawker Wdowicki, Kristin
Helmer Van Dyk, Catherine
Hochstetler, Rhonda
Houtman, Marian
Howard, Nathalie
Hull, Amy
Israels, Michelle
Jackson Cheesebro, Kathleen
Johnson Hunt, Trudy
Kamp Walters, Laurie
Kelsey McCrea, Jeanne

Kiser, Kent
Knapp, Cheryl
Kniebes Homister, Cynthia
Kremers Howey, Cynthia
Krueger, Mark
Kuenzel, Cheryl
Makowski, Barbara
Martin Robertson, Cathy
Mills Bronson, Tammy
Naylor Vlietstra, Robin
O'Connor Van Leuven, Angelynn
Omlie, Stephanie
Popowski Lehman, Janine
Riggin Colvin, Karen
*Retsema Laughlin, Deborah
Scheffers, Terri
Sedlarik Millard, Shelly
Slater Feret, Eileen
Stennett Missias, Julie
*Tokarz, Cindy
Turner Link, Michelle
Vlietstra Tuinier, Marsha
Wagner, Susan
*Wank Passow, Alecia
Winter Commissaris, Cindy
Winters, Kathleen
Zuverink McCleery, Nancy

1982

Adrian, Joan
Ahlers Kirklin, Leone
Baker Carr, Sarah
Baker Sornig, Joy
Benford Nason, Tracee
Bienz, Janice
Brockway Hassan, Sharon
Brown, Lillian
Brown Ekblad, Michelle
Bruner Minor, Brenda
Caplis Jonas, Maureen
Clark Van Tongeren, Anne
Clarke, Rhonda
Cobb, Barbara
Decker Thornton, Debra
*Dell Tibble, Patti
Dennery Dennery-Francis, Rosemarie
Doroshko Sager, Anna
Edder Turtle, Shelly
Elston Nash, Pamela
Ferris Poole, Natalie
Fooy, Chrysanthe
*Himes Hofmeister, Nancee
Hosner Smola, Joan
Irvine Tiner, Linda
Jacob Schacht, Kay
Johnson Lentz, Kathy
Kelly MacEachern, Patricia
Lindhout Gortsema, Jamie
Love, Carolyn
Maginity Chahbazi, Nora
McCulley, Miranda
McFarland, Nancy
McGaffick Campbell, Brenda
McKenzie, Lori
Meyers Petty, Michelle
Myers Breza, Kellie
*Parker Sanchez, Michele
Pritko Sergi, Deborah
Ranson Zimmerman, Mary
Raschke, Susan
Ratliff DeLeeuw, Joan
Reed Thomas, Kimberely
Rice, Steven
Rohwetter Turnquist, Sandra
Salisbury, Lonna
Schock, Robin
Schock Marineau, Vicki
Schrotenboer Dekker, Michele

Scott Remynse, Marshe
Shannon, Lisa
Slentz Ignelzi, Marcia
Smith, Russel
Stevenson Karns, Sharon
Stockham Labbe, Stephanie
Swanson, Janet
Tinklenberg Spek, Rachel
Triezenberg Dockweiler, Beth
Van Valkenburg Garrison, Kiya
VanDenBosch, Mary
VanOss, Linda
Varner Wells, Laura
*Vestal, Carolyn
Wade Ezelle, Cynthia
Walsemann, Wendy
Zoodsma Powell, Ellen

1983

Bachman, Cheryl
Baron, Lori
Barton, Kelly
Bauer VanderKolk, Shelley
Berg Makela, Tracy
Bicanich Laprade, Sandra
Brazill, Evelyn
Brown, Rebecca
Bush Darling, Julie
Cameron Funk, Mary
Carlson Champion, Carol
Chambers, Jill
Cholometes Newcomb, Lisa
Conrad Morgan, Diane
Cowels Studemann, Camille
Cummings, Jennifer
Deming, Linda
Derr, Janine
Diekema Evans, Katherine
Dorrier Ressler, Sara
Doubek VanTuyl, Marianne
Drenth Bertolissi, Robin
Eddy Storteboom, Carol
Eshuis, Brenda
Fischer, Thomas
*Flanders, Patricia
Foote Foote-Jury, Judith
Forbes, Julie
Geary, Teresa
Gill Castro, Rebecca
Godwin Alman, Debra
Green Payne, Jodi
*Harner, Patricia
Harris, Judith
*Hilla, Cheryl
Hope, Ruth
Horsfall Nadelin, Patricia
Hufford Brant, Linda
Johnson Wilson, Laurel
Karsonovich Goethe, Laura
Kidston, Cynthia
Kleis Harper, Sally
Lee Longe, Barbara
Maniaci Gibbs, Michele
McNichol Madson, Patricia
Michalik, Doreen
Miller Gemmill, Sheryll
Mixon, Johnnie
Moore Williams, Margo
Norton, Annelore
Nystrom, Jeffery
Phelan Firsich, Nancy
Rohloff Sullivan-Botma, Robin
Rowekamp, Kelly
Sanborn VanZoeren, Lori
Schlack Warman, Lori
Shinn, Kathy
Skelley Adams, Elizabeth
Snider Shinners, Kathleen
Teisan Schnur, Carolyn

Timmer, Sharon
Trudell Retter, Karen
Van Heukelum, Rebecca
VanDenBerg Buursma, Debra
Vigansky Ciuzio, Beth
Vroegop VanderPloeg, Kimberly
Warren Gallagher, Patricia
Williamson Hendricks, Elizabeth
Wilton Harrington, Christine
Young, Katrena
Zimmer Hibbard, Vivian
Zingery Cary, Laurie

1984

Abraham Keller, Marlaine
Albert Howell, Julie
Aldridge Gifford, Elizabeth
Baker Ulrich, Patti
Beattie, Cheryl
Bornhardt McCoy, Jennifer
Boschma Ide, Connie
Bosma, Darlene
Burza Schlieter, Deborah
Carrigan Moeggenborg, Maureen
Catherwood, Nancy
Cattell, Debra
Chobey, Theresa
*Crampton Crabill, Paula
Dice, Karen
Dillenbeck, James
Dotson, Angela
Fronius Bruinsma, Lynne
Fruin Pilibosian, Leslie
Herlein Boekeloo, Karen
Herman, Kae
Hosack Sheckler, Pamela
Huckendubler Wetzler, Julie
Jones Peterson, Cristy
Kellogg Reyes, Loretta
Kretchman Wagner, Laura
Labadie Mangold, Elizabeth
Langeland Landon, Margaret
Laupp Theaker, Deborah
Legris Willbrandt, Kathleen
Linabury, Olivia
Marsh Rademacher, Linda
Mollitor, Jan
Moyer Walter, Deanna
Nelson Wiedmayer, Rebecca
Neubauer, Kimberly
Olson, Robert
Parish Parish-Bowers, Donna
Phelan Westrick, Susan
Probst Wedgwood, Janeen
Pruss, Susan
Puma, Ivy
Raczniak, Dianna
Riedel, Monika
Rogers Hofstra, Christine
Roman Bundy, Marianne
Rossi, David
Ruggles, Kimberly
Sredzinski Ford, Sharon
Stevenson Pyrek, Mary Beth
Sticken Brief, Caroline
Stilwell Solomon, Sharon
Stiver, Julie
Stocker, Julia
*Stoline, Marie
Taylor Fleet, Susan
Topel Young, Sharon
Ufkes, Timothy
Villars Ponder, Sharon
Vining, Lori
Walsh Woofter, Kimberly
Warner, Karen
Wixson Eggleston, Rebecca
Yancey, Elizabeth

1985

Allen, Ladonna
Ash Braganini, Susan
Austin Nicholas, Sandra
Bankes Kirkemo, Dana
Baum Marshall, Marsha
*Beals Cox, Sharon
Bellardo Laszczak, Amy
Benthin, Marcia
Birman Kent, Karen
Bischoff, Kathryn
Blaney, Donna
Borger Weir, Lisa
Brewer, Gwendolen
Brown Rothering, Susan
Burlington Sterling, Jean
Chase, Patricia
Chumas Killman, Ann
Craig Chilla, Jeanne
Creswell Thompson, Kimberly
Crim, Patricia
Dealba McPartlin, Carla
Dice, Judith
Dillenbeck, Joseph
Duncan, Patricia
Emerson Burgess, Barbara
Erb, Susan
Essar Roessler, Cathy
Fladseth Spicer, Bonnie
Flatt, Beverly
Fredenburg Haskin, Kimberly
Fuller Malavasic, Cecilia
Gipson Graham, Marcia
*Hamblin Mitchell, Margaret
Hansen Abrams, Julia
Haywood, Deborah
Higgins Wright, Kimberly
High Beimfohr, Suzanne
Hildebrand Hirsch, Constance
Janousek Sherrill, Karin
Jennings, Linda
Johnson Johnston, Shawni
Kennedy Holmes, Wendy
Kilty, Daniel
LaForge, James
LaLonde, Linda
Lennon-Lukas, Shelly
Long Phelps, Janna
Lum, Tryna
Mansfield Smith, Maureen
Mansour, Amal
Marineau, Kimberly
Mastenbrook, Julie
May Fuller, Melissa
McIlvenny, Jina
Michelson Shimokochi, Susan
Miller, Rebecca
Miller Eavy, Susan
Moyer Hartley, Kelly
Nielsen Goodman, Susan
Olsen Klan, Teresa
Ostrander Reich, Polly
Parker Grantham, Lori
Pickard, Leslie
Pitt Eaton, Nancy
Powers, Cheryl
Rogge, Patricia
Rumsey Bradley, Diane
Salvati, Kathryn
Scott, Crystal
Sherrard Carpp, Frances
Stein White, Kristine
Strasser, Heidi
Taylor Martin, Renee
Ullrey, Jane
VanderLugt, Karen
Wahl, Mark
Walters, Barbara
Wooley, Linda
Wright Fulton, Elizabeth
Wrubel, Karen

1986

Archambault, Cindy
Bagley, Debra
Benson, Bonnie
Bishop, Marlene
Black Varney, Tina
Boonstra, Todd
Bryer, Kathleen
Buchler, Shelley
Burg Bessler, Marie
Campbell, Dawn
Coon, Monica
Daniels, Jennifer
Davis, Lola
DeForrest, Michael
Devereaux Flynn, Margaret
Dormer Gochanour, Elizabeth
Douglas Wahl, Rebecca
Fowler, Virginia
Garcia, Vicki
Germain Ludwig, Kelli
Gippert McLaren, Colleen
Harriman Matelic, Karen
Hauke, Allison
Hayden, Brenda
Heath Morgan, Karla
Hunn, Julie
Iacoboni, Mary Jo
Jancasz Mora, Nancy
Jones Bittle, Laurie
Josten, John, Jr.
Jutzi, Nancy
Karnemaat, Julie
Kaufmann Michele
Kozan, Cynthia
Laske, Michelle
Linington Brown, Denise
Long May, Deborah
McCarthy Chapman, Yvonne
McEwen Callan, Lisa
McKeever Sanislow, Laura
McLauchlin, Ann
Mendles, Ellen
Merlo Gustafson, Lisa
Miller Crotser, Laura
Minger, Jean
Moore Patterson, Kelli
Murray, Teeshia
Myers Shake, Pamela
Nicholas, Janet
Nolan Nolan-Solis, Kimberly
Norman Morrison, Kristy
Northrup Noel, Jane
Poel, Kathleen
Pratt, Joyce
Reardon, Brian
Rexford Griffioen, Janice
Richardson, Myrna
Ringle, Lori
Ruth Douglas, Wendy
Scofield, Kathy
Sellen Mitchell, Laura
Shaffer Leader, Lisa
Sheehan, Ann
Shegina Tomlinson, Rhonda
Siebert Haring, Agnes
Simonds, Sara
Stantz Vels, Laura
Stautz Morris, Carol
Steinke Carson, Karrie
Stewart, Susan
Stringham, Wendy
Sullivan, Rhonda
Sutton Grimes, Julie
Thompson, Sharon
Thompson, Wendy
Thorlund Wolthuis, Denise
*Vander Molen, Richard, honorary
VanEvery Moshier, Sarah

Vliem, Sally
Vohlken Kokales, Teresa
Wells Schmidt, Debra
Wichman Wichman-Culbertson, Julie
Williams Bergman, Karen
Williams, Lori
Wiltse, Mary
Yarger, Marlena
Young, Ruby
Zientarski, Nancy

1987

Bauman VanderSloot, Teresa
Baumeister, Katherine
Berg Hartwig, Jennifer
Blackman, Heidi
Bolender, Jennifer
Braunz Rice, Collette
Coppernoll, Theresa
Cory, Christine
Davidson, Cindy
DeWald, Rebecca
Diebel Wright, Kimberly
Dishmon, Valarie
Dorgan Ruark, Kelly
Draffen, Kristin
Dzubak Dzubak-MacFarland, Lynn
Evans Harvey, Christine
Fleet Ostman, Angela
Gale, Lori
Galow, Frances
Golding, Jill
Gorby Olsen, Tammy
Grossman, Kimberly
*Harris, Gracie
Howland Feagin, Susan
Jacobs, Betty Jo
Kemp Nagel, Paula
Kim Woolfolk, Myunghee
Knickerbocker Bosanic, Karrie
Kokales, Paul
Kozaczewski, Mary
Kunselman, Connie
Lovett Hazard, Lisa
Marshall, Kathleen
Menser, Lori
Mersino Engelke, Deberra
Miller Martin, Cindy
Morris Nuelken, Amy
Nguyen Hamann, Lien
Olsen, Peter
Ossewaarde, Sally
Parrott, Deborah
Perry, Eleanore
Phillips Kadwell, Susan
Potter Northrop, Laurel
Robinson, Shelly
Rollins, Sarah
Schaaf Dillenbeck, Karen
Scott, Amy
Shellman, Shirley
Snyder Camp, Heidi
Sprick, Lorraine
Stamm Weessies, Stacey
Terrell, Lessie
VanBrugge Vergunst, Melanie
Wagner McDowell, Lana
Williamson Huitt, Carma

1988

Bensley, Katherine
Bodman Baker, Maribeth
Boyer Boyer-Lahring, Nancy
Brady Ray, Kristin
Bun Gendron, Tina
Day, Tracey

Downing Cole, Linda
Esper Martin, Lori
Gallup, Cheryl
Giesbrecht, Michelle
Gustine, Jane
Hammill Rogers, Tonya
Hassan, Daniel
Hinkle, Kimberly
Jolman Welborn, Patti
Key, Dorothy
Kretzschmer Casasanta, Kendra
Krzyzaniak, Louise
Mack Reasoner, Maureen
McCloud, Amy
McCool, Brian
Monroe, Stephen
Morris Otero, Pamela
Mullins, Sharon
Ramsdell Shubnell, Sandra
Rapczynski Dayton, Denise
Reasoner O'Neill, Cheryl
Rentfrow, Sandra
Rice, Susan
Rogers, Angela
Rolph Schultz, Lori
Schuring, Synthia
Scothorn Strong, Elizabeth
Sielken Hodson, Renee
Sikkenga Proksch, Kyle
Sisson Carpenter, Kelley
Slack, Susan
Springer, Teresa
Strozewski Matejovsky, Joan
Thatcher Jaworowski, Liia
Tincknell, Marie
Todd Sherman, Jolene
Williams Hempstead, Cambi
Zimmer, Sharon
Zomer Martin, Wendy

1989

AcMoody DeBault, Kristen
Anderson, Linda
Arias Roehr, Nydia
Brown, Kimberly
Cato, Kimberly
Darscheid Rickhoff, Sonia
Disselkoen Boeve, Jolene
Fanke, Janice
Fillingham, Debra
Flager, Michelle
Fox, Dawn
*George, Nancy
Gray Aigner, Lisa
Gruizenga, Shirley
Haring, Lori
Hoopingarner, Victoria
Howard Eichenauer, Cheryl
Hulewicz, Tanya
Janssen McCormick, Kelly
Korhorn Segalini, Marcia
Kotecki, Christopher
Lindgren, Debbie
Logan Braunz, Monica
Mercer Heering, Kathleen
Monday, Gina
Noel, Ernest
Phillips, Michael
Raines, Ruth
Smith Aldendifer, Susan
Smith Keenan, Stephanie
Splear, Mary
Troccko Miller, Katherine
VanDenBerg, Cynthia
VanKalker Mather, Ruth
Vigansky, Ruth
Visscher Taylor, Teri
Wearne, Marlene

1990

Ballentine, Christine
Black, Mitchell
Bos Kennedy, Lori
Burgess, Kathryn
Carter, Michael
Curtiss, Susan
Daily DeHaan, Grace
Drago Daman, Mary
Esmail, Reem
Foster, Deborah
Hackman, Amy
Hastings, Cheri
Hathaway Tarner, Holly
Hawkins, Rosemarie
*Heath, Denise
Hoke Vogel, Tracy
Kaup, Lori
Koehler, Michael
Leduc, Barbara
Leske, Terry
Mattern, Janese
McIntyre, Lynn
Miles, Gloria
Munro-Rice, Lori
Nickrent Flynn, Laura
Notten, Martha
Odden, Jeretta
Shaw, Marian
*Smotherman, Sharon
Stephens Richardson, Laurie
Thirtle Peterson, Elizabeth
Vite, Susan
Webster, Duana

1991

Andridge-Mendel Sommerfeldt, Susan
Ballard Betzler, Julie
Beatty, Mary
Bennett Powell, Christine
Blackerby, Jessica
Bollen, Carie
Bowers, Katherine
Chisholm, Kathleen
Copprue, Gloria
Cox, Patricia
Crider, Jana
Csom Neel, Lorri
Czubachowski, Kevin
Dobbins, Sailor
Edgel, Gloria
Ellinger VandeLinder, Alissa
Faski, Christine
Fauson, Jamie
Feutz, Karen
Gardner, Brian
Garretson Harter, Beth
Gibala Fulton, Maryann
Gourdie, Chanda
Graber, Janalee
Hainen, Christina
Hall, Kimberly
Hiemstra, Sharon
Kauserud Teiber, Dagny
Lamer Bruner, Camilla
Lawson, Stacey
Leavitt, Peggy
LeCronier, Luann
Lincoln Cooper, Terry
Livingston Pohl, Dawn
Luntz, Cynthia
Madden, Kathleen
McEllis, Jamie
Meier, Lauret
Mercier, Laura
Miller, Camilla
Nagelkerk Quick, Jill

Nicholas, Karen
Nicholas Capps, Lisa
Peterson Knobloch, Shannon
Pierce, Shirley
Purpura, Victoria
Quayle, Debra
*Robinson, Jerri
Roggelien, Jill
Ruden, Christina
Seat Boyd, Sara
Segerdahl, Carol
Seifert Hannafius, Susan
Smith, Kathy
Stewart, Wendy
Terbrueggen Rank, Dawn
Terry, Michelle
Travis, Michael
VanGiessen Vroegindewey, Joan
*Voikin Berkenpas, Deborah
Weaver Warren, Kalee
Williams Schanz, Kimberly
Zomer Martin, Tamera

1992

Ackerson, Kelly
Amador, Tressa
Barlond, Jaqué
Barnum, Jill
Campbell Campbell-Quispe, Jacqueline
Clark, Melissa
Curtis Osmus, Caryn
Cuyler, Deborah
DeJonge, Tracy
Diljak, Michael
Dobson, Stacey
Dow, Rebecca
Dusek, Michael
Eis, Lorna
*Finley Brawer, Stacey
Garcia, Jodi
Griffioen Matherly, Cally
Guarniere Bruno, Daniela
Harestad, Beth
Hastings Eubank, Kimberly
Hyatt Macke, Angela
Jenkins, Victoria
Johnson, Jennifer
Kase Hodshire, Amy
Kingscott Robbins, Jill
Lachman, Char
Lavery, Pamela
Lind, Lien
Loew, Tonya
Lotter Bolyard, Julie
Martin, Lori
Mayes, Bobbi
McEachern, Ronda
*Meeder, Andrea
O'Day, Shannon
Oreskovich, Julie
Pushie, Ruth
Sanfilippo, Christi
Schapman, Amy
Scothorn, Robert
Siewert, Marjory
Simmons, Margaret
Smith, David
Stermer, Kelly
Street, Jana
*Towne, Jonathan
Vance Sellin, Julie
Vriend, Carolyn
Westhoff, Laura
Wikel Wikel-Brown, Dawn
Withers, Jon
Withers, Jori
Wogerman, Tracy
Zimmer, Jennifer

1993

Aquino, Miosotis
Barrie-Feaster Barrie, Nichole
Begeman, Christine
Blackwell, Natalie
Blades, Robyn
Bolenbaugh, Carol
Brown, Jessica
Bunse, Heather
Burgess Burgess-Wright, Joanne
Butler, Cheryl
Clark Beatty, Stefanie
Dimock, Teresa
Donewald, Kristin
Dykstra, Michael
Engelke, Eric
Fern, Susan
Forster, Julie
Frazier, Denise
Godush Richardson, Jami
Green, Sandra
Green, Virginia
Guizzetti, Jamie
Hamman Fenchak, Laurie
Hays, Katrina
Heineman, Nancy
Hesse, Lisa
Hughes, Tina
Johnson, Jennifer
Keen, Glenda
Killarney, Tracey
Kindle Kooi, Janessa
Koch, Julie
Krueger, Cindy
Lantis Ford, Susan
Lewis, Diane
Little, Rodney
LoDico LoDico-Morea, Nicole
McCarthy, Michael
McMillan Washington, Lisa
Merillat, Toni
Mersdorf Tarnow, Angela
Morea Carpenter, Julie
Mott, Susan
Munch Bronkema, Roxanne
Nord Hubbard, Susan
Norman, Lynne
Otteman, Amy
Pandya, Terry
Peterson, Pamela
Pio, Deborah
Richardson Coney, Joni
Ring, Jane
Roder, Debra
Rosselot, Susan
Schoen, Dayna
Sculley, Danielle
Seelig Gilbert, Kimberly
Seiwell Keefe, Michelle
Sharpe, Sarah
*Speedy, Amanda
Stevens, Marla
Stockinger, Scott
Sweat, James
Switzer, James
Taylor, Shaunna
VanderRoest Bailey, Shannon
Waite, Heather
Wolfe, Jennifer
Worsham, Shirl
Wright Ianello, Julie

1994

Aaron, Cecelia
Adams Oakleaf, Robin
Amos Meintz, Aimee
Barnard, Dawn
Battle Renfrew, Michelle
Beebe, Amy

Bell, Douglas
Bestervelt, Janet
Blissick, Lisa
Bray, Derek
Brovont Conner, Lynnae
Burkhard Ebbert, Kristine
Burleson, Lynette
Chandler, Stephanie
Compton, Jennifer
Cooley, Leslie
Dolan, Julie
Dorey, Christina
Fisher, Kelly
Fort, Dana
Gamel Marrell, Liza
Gillette, Janet
Gomez, Trina
Good, Mary
Goodman, Karla
Gray, Shirley
Green, Charles
Hakes Grant, Melissa
Keefe, Aaron
Klinger Weststrate, Wendy
Kruithoff, Joyce
Laughlin, Barbara
Lewis-Broussard, Kathryn
Marvin, Patricia
McFarland, Amy
Michaels, Jennifer
Mikowski, Monica
Monroe, Joely
Moored Rhodes, Jennifer
Most Van Sweden, Jennette
Opicka, Tricia
Pavlak, Sarah
Pelong, Polly
Pennington, Jennifer
Piell Hansen, Kari
Polum, Stephanie
Ransbottom, Lori
Ray, Robin
Rice Clement, Noelle
Rodgers, Michael
Seals, Christine
Sirlin, Katharine
*Smith Miller, Kelli
Swafford Rehr, Rebecca
Turner, Linda
Van Buskirk, Julie
Vazana, Mark
Wagoner, Gail
Walls, Monica
Westra, Colleen
Wierenga, Wendy
Wiles, Esther

1995

Ballinger, Lorie
Bartholomew, Anne
Bates Asselin, Katrina
Bayma, Stephanie
Bickley, Kimberly
Bierenga, Jennifer
Blades, Benjamin
Bodway Burhans, Jennifer
Born Westers, Judy
Brenn, Bruce
Cavanaugh, Karen
Clapp Beison, Jill
Clough Wells, Kimberly
Combs, Tina
Connor, Kathy
Conrad, Jody
Crill, Michaela
Daenzer, Denise
Dahlquist, Diana
Damstra, Renee
DeMaagd, Kristin
Eby, Roland

Eisenberg, Dinah
Flower, Susan
Frederickson Berryman, Kristie
Goebel, Carrie
Hall, Marilynn
Harmon, Hope
Hartman, Lydia
Hatfield, Dorothy
Hemingway, Christine
Hoeksema Rusinek, Julie
Janette, Ellen
Johnson Barber, Amy
Kendzior Oetman, Kacey
Kloosterman, Christine
Kneller, James
Komrska, Melissa
Koster Deary, Tanya
La Vigne, Rachelle
Locker, Jackie
Martin, Carol
Mezo, Kelly
Mickey, Debra
Mihelich, Gloria
Miller, Beth
Mizikar, Carolyn
Myers, Janice
Newton McLogan, Heather
Niezink, Jodi
Otten, Dorothy
Retberg Miller, Sheila
Runyan, Krista
Russell, Jennifer
Severance Layne, Ruth
Slayton Basso, Jan
Stuck Posey, Laura
Terpstra, Deb
Thompson, Kristan
Tomsic, Diana
Tonus, Anthony
Trumps Shean, Karyn
VanStreain, Andrea
Vestal, Joyce
Walenga, Kassie
Warmuskerken, Martin
Webb Forbes, Laura
Williams, Nicole
Witt Bronkema, Jodie
Wyman, Carol

1996

Amundson, Jan
Anderson, Kimberly
Arnsman, Johanna
Augustus, Sue
Bacon, Pamela
Barrett, Mary
Blodgett, Deborah
Blowers Beach, Melissa
Brain, Jennifer
Brigman, Karen
Brock Smith, Amy
Buck Cole, Teresa
Burk, Eric
Chamberlin, Kimberly
Cummings, Nicole
Dean Zamarron, Tara
Dennany, Larry
Dennany, Teresa
Diaczenko, Anna
Downey Kavanaugh, Anne
Earls, Andrea
Eldridge, Rebecca
Ensley, Teresa
Fisher, Maria
Freeman, Pamela
French, Tracy
Garcia, Blanca
Hall, Melodie
Heinzman Beck, Marci
Hoover, Dina

Hybels, Jon
Johncock, Cindy
Johnson, Marie
Kieft Howland, Jean
Knight, Shawn
Koeman, Michelle
Koetje Lehoczky, Kristen
Kreslins, Jennifer
Lee, Theresa
Lincoln, Mary
Madison Hughson, Kristin
McCallum, Nicole
McCaskey Freeland, Jennifer
Mellinger, Randy
Minger, Jennifer
Moeller, Julie
Mony Meyers, Anika
Mostrom, Linda
Peckham, Justin
Rankens, Heather
Reinbolt, Melisa
Ritchie, Michelle
Roedel, Marisa
*Sanders-Jones, Mary Beth
Schroeder, Diana
Schwab, Erica
Shoemaker, Margaret
Smith, Laurie
Smith-Engle Engle, Amy
Souers, Amy Jo
Spiegelberg, Kristine
Squires, Amy
Stone, Abbey
Sween Brzezinski, Karen
Thayer, Molly
Tomey, Vickie
Truax, Amy
VanDerMolen, Angela
VanHorn, Jenny
Walker-Talsma, Brandi
Whitten, Tonya
Wygant, Avalyn
Yax Kamp, Erica
Yonkers, Judith

1997

Allen, Sylvia
Baker, Julie
Barone, Michelle
Benson, Kathryn
Bingaman, Gregory
Bogema, Rebecca
Bolton-Knowles, Jennifer
Bosch, Melissa
Brown, Kimberly
Carnell Turbett, Rebecca
Compagner, Sheryl
DeMeester, Betty
Diebold, Mary
Dreyer, Janet
Duma, Jennifer
Dunfee, Mary Ann
Durren, Mark
Golba, Beth
Goulding, Kathleen
Hayes, Audrey
Herman Hahn, Denise
Hester Hester-Overton, Kimberly
Kafritsas, James
Kancauski Warden, Karen
Kesteris, Denise
Krause, Wendy
Lockwood, Darren
Mack, Uchechi
Martens, Nathan
Mast, Danielle
Mc Kenzie, Wendy
Meiste Griffioen, Debra
Meyer, Nathan
Mohlman, Sherry

Moravek, Ann
Murray, Wendy
Pamment, Susan
Parker, Shannon
Powers, Judy
Przygocki, Cathleen
Purgiel, Nacole
Rhoda-Crissman, Jennifer
Riemer Angersbach, Shannon
Sanchez, Sharon
Sharp Bingaman, Lyndsay
Simmons, Andrea
Simpson, Sarah
Smith, Tonisty
Sonnie, Musu
Stearns, Gaylene
Stockwell, Andrew
Striker, Jennifer
Van Zantwick O'Neal, Tricia
Watson, Michael
Whalen, Brian
Wilson, Phyllis
Wise, Michelle
Wise, Robert
*Witteveen, Mark
Worden, Lorraine

1998

Bailey, Heather
Bates, James
Bell, Juanita
Carson, Charles
Collins, Chris
Damon, Todd
Eklund, Heidi
Erickson, Joyce
Ertman, Heidi
Frick Milanowski, Michelle
Fritz, Denise
Garland Zanke, Meghan
Hill, Stephanie
Johnston, Angela
Kolff, Cari
Kurtz Stenger, Gwendolyn
McCann, Emily
Middlemas, Amy
Mitchell Wurtzel, Angie
Moravek, Ann
Murillo, Charles
Myers, Christine
Nequist, Julie
Oorbeck, Michael
Ozomaro, Paulette
Paeglis, Debra
Pankey Duncan, Sherry
Peckens, Natasha
Quertermus, Christopher
Simpson, Duane
Skupien, Linda
Tooman, Leigh
Tyler, Dana
VanDyke, Ronald
Zagarell, Laura
Zanke, Matthew
Zen Al Abidin, Nurah

APPENDIX E

ALUMNI ASSOCIATION OF BRONSON METHODIST HOSPITAL SCHOOL OF NURSING

Kalamazoo, Michigan

CONSTITUTION

ARTICLE I
Name

The name of this organization shall be the Alumni Association of Bronson Methodist Hospital School of Nursing.

ARTICLE II
Objects

The objects of this Association shall be

A. to provide funds for nursing scholarships
B. to promote the professional standards of nursing
C. to secure and maintain good fellowship among the graduates and the students of this school.

ARTICLE III
Membership

Graduates of the Bronson Methodist Hospital School of Nursing and all registered nurses in good standing are eligible for membership in this Association. Membership shall consist of active, inactive, life, associate, and honorary members.

A. active members shall be graduates of Bronson Methodist Hospital School of Nursing who have paid the dues for the current year.
B. inactive members shall be graduates of the Bronson Methodist Hospital School of Nursing who have not paid the dues for the current year.
C. life membership is automatically conferred forty years after graduation from Bronson Methodist Hospital School of Nursing. Life members are not required to pay dues.
D. associate members shall be graduates of other schools of nursing who have paid the dues for the current year and will have voting privileges.
E. honorary membership may be conferred by the Association, upon recommendation, on persons who have rendered service to this Alumni Association and whom its members wish to honor. Honorary membership confers social privileges only.

ARTICLE IV
Officers

Section l. The officers of this Association shall be graduates of the Bronson Methodist Hospital School of Nursing. The officers shall be: President, Vice President, Secretary, Treasurer, and two Directors. The six officers shall constitute the Board of Directors.

Section 2. All officers shall be elected at the Annual Meeting and shall continue in office two years or until successors are elected.

Section 3. The term of office of all officers shall commence at the adjournment of the Annual Meeting at which the election is held.

Section 4. All officers shall be Active or Life members of the Association.

Section 5. The President and Secretary of the Association shall be the President and Secretary of the Board of Directors.

ARTICLE V
Meetings

Section 1. The Annual Meeting of the Association shall be held in the spring of each year.

Section 2. Regular meetings shall be held as prescribed in the By-Laws or as determined by the Board of Directors.

Section 3. Special meetings may be called at any time by the President, by a majority vote of the Board of Directors, or on written request of five members of the Association. Active members shall be notified of special meetings in advance.

ARTICLE VI
Quorum

Section 1. Two officers and three additional Active or Life members shall constitute a quorum at any Annual or regular meeting.

Section 2. Two officers and three additional Active or Life members shall constitute a quorum for a special meeting.

Section 3. Three members of the Board of Directors shall constitute a quorum at any meeting of the Board or Directors.

ARTICLE VII
Revision

The Constitution and Bylaws of the Alumni Association of Bronson Methodist Hospital School of Nursing may be amended, adopted, or repealed by the following procedures:

A. reviewed by at least two Active or Life members appointed by the President.
B. submitted to the Board of Directors.
C. read and discussed at a Board meeting.
D. ratified at the next regular meeting by a two-thirds vote of all Active members present and voting.

BY-LAWS
ARTICLE I
Dues

Section 1. The annual membership dues shall be $15.00.

Section 2. All dues shall be paid to the membership chairman.

Section 3. Members failing to pay annual dues by December 31 shall be considered Inactive.

Section 4. Notification of payment of dues will be mailed to all Alumni in August of each year.

ARTICLE II
Election of Officers

Section 1. Elections shall be by secret ballot, except when the number of nominees does not exceed the number to be elected, in which case elections may be by voice vote.

Section 2. A simple majority of all votes cast shall be necessary to constitute an election.

Section 3. Vacancies in office shall be filled at any regular meeting of the Association or the Board of Directors by a simple majority vote.

ARTICLE III

Duties of Officers

Section l. The President shall:

A. preside at all Association meetings.
B. preside at all meetings of the Board of Directors.
C. appoint all standing committees and shall be an ex-officio member of the same.

Section 2. The Vice President shall:

A. assume all presidential duties in the absence of the President.
B. assist the President in the performance of duties.

Section 3. The Secretary shall:

A. record the minutes of each Association and Board of Directors meeting.
B. be responsible for the correspondence of the Association.
C. provide a written report of all Constitution and By-Laws changes to the Bulletin Committee for publication.
D. present a copy of the current Constitution and By-Laws to any member upon request. All officers shall have a current copy.

Section 4. The Treasurer shall:

A. collect all monies due the Association and shall deposit the same in a designated bank.
B. pay all approved bills.
C. keep a record of all money received and disbursed and shall submit a report of each at meetings of the Association.
D. collect, record, and acknowledge all memorial contributions.
E. transfer $10.00 from the Treasury to the Memorial Fund in remembrance of Alumni.

Section 5. The Directors shall participate in the action of the Board of Directors.

ARTICLE IV
Board of Directors

Section 1. The Board of Directors shall:

A. approve a place of deposit for the funds of the Association.
B. provide for auditing the accounts of the Treasurer.
C. keep constant supervision of the affairs of the Association.
D. transact the business of the Association between meetings.
E. devise and develop measures for the growth and prosperity of the Association.
F. prepare and present the Annual Budget to the Association.

ARTICLE V
Committees

Section 1. There shall be the following committees: Bulletin, Hospitality & Program, Membership, Nominations, Student & Alumni services, and Ways and Means.

Section 2. The Bulletin Committee shall collect and have printed current news of interest to Alumni Association members.

A. the *The Bulletin* shall be published and distributed four times yearly to all Active, Life, and Honorary members.
B. notices announcing the meetings shall be mailed to all local Active, Life, and Honorary members if not included in a regularly published *The Bulletin.*

Section 3 The Hospitality & Program Committee shall:

A. arrange for all meetings of the Association.

Section 4. The Membership Committee shall:

A. keep current data on all members to include (but not limited to) name, address, social security number, year of graduation, type of membership.
B. collect and record membership dues and give money to the Treasurer.
C. provide a current membership list to the Bulletin Committee and others as requested.

Section 5. The Nominations Committee shall prepare a ballot consisting of more than one consenting candidate, if possible, for each office to be filled.

Section 6. The Students & Alumni Services Committee shall make recommendations for services to the students and Alumni, and arrange for those services chosen by the Alumni.

Section 7. The Ways and Means Committee shall promote projects to reimburse the Treasury.

ARTICLE VI
Meetings

Section 1. Meetings of the Association shall be determined annually by the Board of Directors.

Section 2. The Order of Business at regular meetings shall be:

A. Call to Order
B. Reading of the minutes of the previous meeting
C. Communications
D. Report of the Treasurer
E. Report of the Standing Committees
F. Report of the Special Committees
G. Old Business
H. Announcements
I. Adjournment

Section 3. The Annual Meeting shall include year-end committee reports and the election of officers.

ARTICLE VII
Fiscal Year

The fiscal year of the Association shall be from June 1 to May 31.

ARTICLE VIII
Parliamentary Authority

The rules of parliamentary practice comprised in Roberts Rules of Order, Newly Revised, shall govern the proceedings of the Association and the Board of Directors.

Revised 10/16/80 Dorothy Beimer, Marilyn Ely
Revised 9/1/83 Marilyn Ely, Virginia Hill
Revised 11/1/86 Jo Carlson, Virginia Hill, Nancy Weston
Revised 10/16/92 Mary Ellen Fredenburg, Carol Lawrence, Sharyn Schlueter
Revised 10/15/94 Sharyn Schlueter, Dawn Barnard
Revised 11/95 Board of Directors

TRANSCRIPTS

ACADEMIC TRANSCRIPTS:

If you are requesting an academic transcript, please send the following information:

- Your name and complete mailing address.
- A daytime phone number where you can be reached in the event there are questions about your request.
- Your student ID number (social security number)
- Your name at the time of attendance
- The dates of attendance <u>or</u> date of graduation or date you withdrew from the program. Please specify you attended **Bronson Methodist Hospital School of Nursing** (not to be confused with WMU Bronson School of Nursing).
- The address where you would like your transcript sent.

The cost of each transcript is **now $5.00.** A check can be made payable to: Western Michigan University. Payment can also be made by credit card. Please provide card number and date of expiration.

A request form can be obtained from WMU online at:

www.wmich.edu/registrar/transcripts.html

Again indicate the request is for a **Bronson Methodist Hospital School of Nursing** transcript. Your signature is required to release information. Requests can be faxed to 269-387-4170.

Or, send your request to:

Office of the Registrar, Attention: Transcripts
Western Michigan University
1903 W. Michigan Ave.
Kalamazoo, MI 49008

FINANCIAL AID TRANSCRIPTS

Financial aid transcripts are no longer being processed. A letter, verifying Bronson School of Nursing is closed, meets the requirements for a financial aid transcript. You may obtain a verification of closings letter by writing to the following address:

Federal Student Aid Information Center
P.O. Box 4129
Iowa City, IA 52244

Be sure to indicate in your letter that you are requesting written verification that Bronson Methodist Hospital School of Nursing is closed. Include your name, social security number and the address you want the verification letter sent to.

For FURTHER INFORMATION contact:
Office of the Registrar, Western Michigan University
269-387-4300 follow the phone prompts.

COLLECTIBLES

DIPLOMAS

Diplomas are still available; however, we are no longer able to obtain covers. The cost of a diploma is $35.00. Make your check payable to Western Michigan University. Credit card payment will be accepted. See information above under transcripts. Send your request to:

Office of the Registrar, Attention: Transcripts
Western Michigan University
1903 W. Michigan Ave.
Kalamazoo, MI 49008

Include in your letter:

Your name and complete mailing address.
Your full name at the time of attendance (as it should appear on the diploma)
The year you graduated.

—Data above accurate, as of July 2004

PINS

Pins can be replaced. Please send your request to Eric Underwood or Steve Carlson or Recognition Sales, a Herff Jones Company representative by phone 517-641-6954. They will need your name at the time of graduation and the year of graduation. They will have all the information related to cost and shipment and arrangements for payment. The cost will depend on your choice of 10K or 14K gold, or 10K or 14K gold -filled.

History of the School Pin

The Bronson school pin received minor changes over it is lifetime of eighty-six years, 1906-1998, in color and wording but not in the base metal, gold, or maltese cross design. There was no pin or record found of a graduate pin from 1900 to 1906 when Bronson's predecessor, the Kalamazoo People's Hospital existed.

Design for the pin was a modified Maltese cross, similar to many school pins because of our hospital connections.

The mid-Mediterranean fortress island of rock-bastioned Malta has given its name to one of the most distinctive and best-known forms of cross—the Maltese. This symbol is of the square variety, having fishtail, indented ends. Its arms taper toward the intersection. The eight points gave rise to the 'Knights of the eight-Pointed Cross'—brave warriors of the military order of St. John, called the 'Knight Hospitaler' because of their founding hospitals for sick pilgrims to Palestine and elsewhere on the pilgrim route from Europe to the Near East. From *A Treasury of the Cross*, by Madeleine S. Miller. New York:Harper & Brothers, 1956.

The first pin was a flat gold cross with a blue enamel circle. Its center held the graduation date, and Bronson Hospital was printed on the blue enamel circle.

Later, the center was modified to an old English "B" which was the logo of Bronson Methodist Hospital.

Design changes were minimal over the years. In 1929 the words, "School of Nursing" were added, and white enamel replaced the blue. Other additions in the metal work occurred with the "B" raised within an indented circle, and detail was added to the edges of the cross.

In 1944 the words, Kalamazoo, Michigan, were added in a concentric fashion around the old English "B".

When Bronson Methodist Hospital changed its logo in the 80s, the Alumni Association of the School lobbied Bronson administrators to retain the pin design with the old English "B". The pin was not redesigned and continued to be awarded at commencement until the school closure in 1998.

CAPS

The Alumni Association of Bronson Methodist Hospital School of Nursing is no longer responding to requests for caps for those who may need or want one. The company has all but gone out of business, and contacting and ordering caps has become a difficult task.

Cap Folding Guidelines

One picture is worth a thousand words! Find a yearbook in which several caps are pictured on heads of students, displaying several angles. Sets of all available Bronson Methodist Hospital School of Nursing yearbooks are housed at the Kalamazoo Public Library. Students often modified the size of the pleated area on the gathered back of the cap so that the wingspan of the starched brim varied from 8 to 12 inches. Cap folding was learned by watching others. Uniformity was the outcome. Requisites for folding include the Bronson cap, 2 safety pins, and 1 white button with loop on underside of button.

Introduction: Prior to folding, notice the shape of the cap. It looks like an old-fashioned sunbonnet without ties. Before folding, a small safety pin is secured at the center, underside gathered material where it connects to the brim. The starched brim will cover the safety pin once it is folded over the gathered, soft material. Why the safety pin? It is used as the anchor for a bobbie pin that will secure the cap to the nurse's head.

Folding Procedure:

- The permanently starched brim is folded at the seam connecting the brim to the soft-gathered material, so that the gathered seam is no longer exposed but is covered by this wide brim. Do not crease the starched brim. (Notice that you can only see about ¼ to ½ inch of the safety pin, i.e., not the entire pin that should be covered by the brim.) A bobbie pin is placed on this tiny exposed area of of the safety pin in order to secure the brim of the cap to hair.

- Identify the center point on the soft material by making a crease or a tiny pencil mark at this center. (The exposed, gathered material will be pleated together, as directed below.) Finding the center ensures that the wings of the brim will have a balanced, even appearance.

- Measure in from where the tips of the starched brim meet the soft material, ½ to 2 inches on the soft material. (Make a crease at the measured points or make tiny pencil marks to identify the points at which the ½ to 2 inch-pleats will be brought to the center point.

- The ½ to 2 inch-pleated materials (both at once) are brought to the center mark/crease on the cap to be secured, side by side, with a safety pin (on the non-exposed side) and the white, round, button exposed on the outside. The safety pin passes through and secures the pleats together and to the center material under the button.

- You will notice small soft "wings" exposed on each side, under the "poofy" gathered soft material. They are used to anchor the back of the cap to hair with bobbie pins.

UNIFORMS

The crisp and starched white uniform and cap impressed many young women and reinforced their desire to become a nurse. Uniforms evolved through the past century from the stiff, heavily starched white dress uniform to a very informal trouser, scrub suit style.

Stories of early 1900 uniforms tell about gray and white striped uniforms with high starched stand-up collars, wide white cuffs, and stiffly starched white aprons and bibs. The skirts were precisely six inches off the floor. The aprons were gored to protect the uniform from soil in daily work and to give the uniform a finished appearance. After a three months probationary period, first year students were allowed to wear caps, with a narrow black band attached during the second year and a wide black band in the third year. The cap was white organdy poof shaped which was worn on the crown of the head. Black cotton stockings and black oxfords completed the uniforms. After graduation white uniforms were worn.

By around 1910 the white cuffs were narrowed to three inches and one that was V-shaped replaced the white stand-up collar. A full gathered apron replaced the gored style around 1916. The organdy cap was changed a cotton cap.

By the late 1920's the uniform was described as blue and white striped trimmed with a detachable stiffly starched white collar and cuffs plus a gathered white apron which matched the hem length of the dress. Students were required to make their own aprons, which covered their uniforms, using a pattern, which was sent to them upon acceptance into nursing school. The front band on the cap was folded wider and the back folded to fit the back of the head where it was worn.

In 1935 white shoes and hose replaced the black styles and sleeves on the uniform were shortened.

Navy blue capes with gold lining were introduced in 1936. A new all-white belted cotton one piece dress uniform with a Bronson emblem attached to the left breast pocket modernized the student dress; aprons were no longer required.

In the early 1940s there is mention of a white headband that was worn by probies before they earned their caps, which were awarded at the end of the first six months of training. The 1945 guideline for the length of the uniform dress was 13 inches from the floor. Students were clearly identified as Miss . . . on the pocket. No first names were used.

By the mid-1950s capes were no longer being issued to students and blue dress uniforms were issued for duty in outpatient services. Capes were still worn by 1960s students who purchased them from earlier graduates.

The uniform style remained the same until the 1970s when society became less formal and permanent press material became available. The pantsuit was adopted in 1976 as an option, and dress uniforms were noticeably shorter and not of a prescribed length.

The 1985 class protested the requirement to wear caps citing unhealthiness and difficulty of working on some units, such as orthopedics, while wearing a cap. Though for students it was a dysfunctional object, the real message of the cap was one of servitude and not connected with professional practice but with housemaids who wore dust caps. In the fall of 1985 caps were no longer being required uniform dress, but were worn for the graduation picture and ceremony. Fall of 1986 saw the introduction of the name pin, displaying the first and last name of the student. The school insignia was worn on either the breast pocket or on the sleeve. Navy blue uniforms were no longer issued for outpatient service duty and names on the uniforms were changed to first names with last initial. 1989 graduates remember no required student uniforms.[i]

Students purchased their own white uniforms, which stayed the standard for the school. At the same time, often they were encouraged to wear uniforms congruent with the agency or Bronson unit dress codes. For example, professional casual street dress was often worn in community agencies and the pediatric unit wore brightly colored or printed smocks or scrub suit tops.

---

[i] Uniform memories, as related by Sonia Darscheid, Shawni Johnston, Karen Bergman, Sally Vliem and Amal Mansour, late 1980 graduates of Bronson Hospital School of Nursing, to Rosemarie Nedeau-Cayo.

Bronson Women and the School of Nursing

PICTURE CREDITS

BMH = Bronson Methodist Hospital

1. Kalamazoo Valley Museum
2. BMH Archives
3. Bronson Bulletin Summer '54
4. BMH Archives
5. Kalamazoo Valley Museum
6. Florence Nightingale Museum
7. Alumni Archives
8. Alumni Archives
9. Kalamazoo Valley Museum
10. Kalamazoo Valley Museum
11. Kalamazoo Valley Museum
12. Alumni Archives
13. Kalamazoo Valley Museum
14. BMH Archives
15. Private Collection, Dick Vander Molen
16. Kalamazoo Valley Museum
17. Alumni Archives
18. Alumni Archives
19. Alumni Archives
20. BMH Archives
21. Alumni Archives
22. Private Collection, Dick Vander Molen
23. BMH Archives
24. Kalamazoo Valley Museum
25. Kalamazoo Valley Museum
26. Kalamazoo Valley Museum
27. Private Collection (Dick)
28. Alumni Archives
29. BMH Archives
30. BMH Archives
31. BMH Archives
32. BMH Archives
33. Alumni Archives
34. Alumni Archives
35. BMH Archives
36. Alumni Archives
37. BMH Archives
38. Bronson Archives
39. Bronson Archives
40. Alumni Archives
41. BMH Archives
42. Alumni Archives
43. BMH Archives
44. Bronson Bulletin April 1944
45. Kalamazoo Valley Museum
46. WMU Archives
47. Kalamazoo Valley Museum
48. Alumni Archives Bronson Bulletin April 1945
49. Private Collection, Jackie Wylie
50. Kalamazoo Valley Museum
51. Kalamazoo Valley Museum
52. Kalamazoo Valley Museum
53. Bronson Bulletin April 1944
54. Kalamazoo Valley Museum
55. Kalamazoo Valley Museum
56. Bronson White Caps 1952 p3
57. Private Collection, Dick Vander Molen
58. Bronson White Caps 1952
59. BMH Archives
60. Kalamazoo Gazette
61. Kalamazoo Valley Museum
62. Kalamazoo Valley Museum
63. Alumni Archives
64. Kalamazoo Valley Museum
65. Bronson Bulletin April 1947
66. Kalamazoo Valley Museum
67. Kalamazoo Valley Museum

68. Kalamazoo Valley Museum
69. Private Collection, Dick Vander Molen
70. Private Collection, Dick Vander Molen
71. Bronson Bulletin Spring 1949
72. Private Collection, Dick Vander Molen
73. Private Collection, Dick Vander Molen
74. Private Collection, Dick Vander Molen
75. BMH Archives
76. Private Collection, Betty Hoogstraten Kaub
77. Alumni Archives
78. Private Collection, Ruth Schwoebell
79. Private Collection, Ruth Schwoebell
80. Private Collection, Ruth Schwoebell
81. Private Collection, Ruth Schwoebell
82. Kalamazoo Valley Museum
83. Bronson Bulletin Spring 1952 p3
84. Bronson White Caps 1952 p43
85. Bronson White Caps 1954 p92 and Bronson Bulletin Fall 1952
86. Bronson White Caps 1952 p32 and Kalamazoo Valley Museum
87. Kalamazoo Gazette
88. Private Collection, Jackie Wylie
89. Bronson White Caps 1952 p 35
90. Bronson White Caps 1954 p 75
91. Bronson White Caps 1953 p 59
92. Bronson White Caps 1953 p 83
93. Bronson White Caps 1954 p 84
94. Private Collection, Jackie Wylie
95. Alumni Archives
96. Kalamazoo Gazette
97. Alumni Archives
98. BMH Archives
99. Private Collection, Dick Vander Molen
100. Bronson Bulletin Spring 1955
101. Kalamazoo Valley Museum
102. Alumni Archives
103. Alumni Archives
104. Bronson White Caps 1956 p 80
105. BMH Archives
106. Bronson White Caps 1957 p 76
107. BMH Archives
108. Private Collection, Dick Vander Molen
109. Bronson White Caps 1957 p 78
110. Alumni Archives
111. Kalamazoo Valley Museum
112. Kalamazoo Valley Museum
113. BMH Archives
114. BMH Archives
115. BMH Archives
116. Private Collection, Dick Vander Molen
117. BMH Archives
118. Private Collection, Beth Simpson Fletcher
119. Kalamazoo Valley Museum
120. Private Collection, Dick Vander Molen
121. Alumni Archives
122. Kalamazoo Valley Museum
123. Kalamazoo Valley Museum
124. BMH Archives
125. Kalamazoo Valley Museum
126. Kalamazoo Valley Museum
127. Kalamazoo Valley Museum
128. BMH Archives
129. Private Collection, Dick Vander Molen
130. BMH Archives
131. Private Collection, Ruth Schermer VanderKlay
132. Private Collection , Jackie Burch
133. Private Collection, Dick Vander Molen
134. Private Collection, Anna van't Zelfde Stryd
135. BMH Archives
136. Bronson White Caps 1960 p 32
137. Florence Nightingale Museum
138. Private Collection, Anna van't Zelfde Stryd
139. Alumni Archives
140. Private Collection, Anna van't Zelfde Stryd
141. Kalamazoo Valley Museum
142. Bronson White Caps 1961 p 44
143. Kalamazoo Valley Museum
144. Kalamazoo Valley Museum
145. Kalamazoo Valley Museum
146. Kalamazoo Valley Museum
147. Bronson Catalyst June 1968 p3
148. Private Collection, Diane Dwan Poole
149. Private Collection, Diane Dwan Poole
150. Alumni Archives
151. Alumni Archives
152. Kalamazoo Valley Museum
153. BMH Archives
154. Kalamazoo Valley Museum
155. BMH Archives
156. Private Collection, Deb Retsema Laughlin
157. Private Collection, Sue Rosteck Morgan
158. Kalamazoo Valley Museum

159. Alumni Archives
160. Private Collection, Deb Retsema Laughlin
161. Private Collection, Deb Retsema Laughlin
162. Private Collection, Deb Retsema Laughlin
163. Alumni Archives
164. Alumni Archives
165. Alumni Archives
166. Alumni Archives
167. Private Collection, Deb Retsema Laughlin
168. BMH Archives
169. Private Collection, Deb Retsema Laughlin
170. Alumni Archives
171. BMH Archives
172. Private Collection, Deb Retsema Laughlin
173. BMH Archives
174. Alumni Archives
175. BMH Archives
176. Alumni Archives
177. BMH Archives
178. Kalamazoo Valley Museum
179. BMH Archives
180. BMH Archives
181. BMH Archives
182. BMH Archives
183. Private Collection, Jackie Wylie
184. BMH Archives
185. BMH Archives
186. Alumni Archives
187. Private Collection, Dick Vander Molen
188. Bronson School of Nursing Yearbook 1991 p 34
189. Private Collection, Carol Watson Van Antwerp
190. Private Collection, Carol Watson Van Antwerp
191. Private Collection, Carol Watson Van Antwerp
192. Bronson Catalyst March 1983 cover
193. Bronson Catalyst May 1981 p 5
194. BMH Archives
195. Private Collection, Dick Vander Molen
196. Alumni Archives
197. Alumni Archives
198. BMH Archives
199. BMH Archives
200. BMH Archives
201. Catalyst September 1978 cover
202. Alumni Archives
203. Alumni Archives
204. Alumni Archives
205. Alumni Archives
206. Alumni Archives
207. Alumni Archives
208. Alumni Archives
209. Alumni Archives
210. Alumni Archives
211. Alumni Archives
212. Alumni Archives
213. Alumni Archives
214. Alumni Archives
215. Alumni Archives
216. Florence Nightingale Museum
217. Private Collection, Jackie Wylie
218. Private Collection, Jackie Wylie
219. Private Collection, Jackie Wylie
220. Private Collection, Jackie Wylie
221. Alumni Archives
222. BMH Archives
223. Kalamazoo Gazette
224. BMH Archives
225. Alumni Archives
226. Alumni Archives
227. Alumni Archives
228. Alumni Archives
229. Alumni Archives
230. Alumni Archives

INDEX

Notes: **Boldface** indicates photographs, and the italic letter *n* refers to chapter notes. Indexed surnames of BMH School of Nursing graduates are most recent. Birth names of graduates or their names at time of entry into the School are arranged by class year in Appendix D.

C

H

O

P

Q

R

T

Bronson Women and the School of Nursing

To order more copies of

Bronson Women and the School of Nursing:

Journeys Through One Hundred Years

by Jacqueline Wylie and Anna Stryd

Soft cover ISBN 0-9763413-0-1

Each copy is $25.00 with 40% discount for 10 or more copies

\# copies ______ x ______ = $ _________

Hard cover ISBN 0-9763413-1-X

Each copy is $40.00 with 40% discount for 10 or more copies

\# copies ______ x ______ = $ _________

Shipping and Handling (soft and hard cover)
USA $4.00 for first book,
$1.50 for each additional book. $ _________

Tax: Michigan residents, add 6% sales tax $ _________

Total $ _________

Checks payable to:
Alumni Association of BMH School of Nursing

Mail order form and payment to:
Alumni Association of BMH School of Nursing
1417 Lakeview Drive
Portage, MI 49002

Send book/s to (please print):

Name____

Street ____

City____

State/Province______________________________Zip ______________

Phone (______)_____________________E-mail ____________________

Please allow three weeks for delivery.